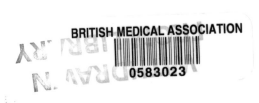

Informed knowledge of the outcome of disease and its treatment are of critical importance to patients and clinicians throughout the medical world. As treatment technology
becomes increasingly sophisticated and costly, health care planners and providers are
also looking to this information to make decisions on cost-effective services.

In many specialties, such as neurology and neurosurgery, the absence of extensive
outcome studies and agreed measures of outcome in different conditions can make this
information difficult to obtain. This book seeks to help in providing a succinct and
practical review of the clinical course, treatment options and rehabilitation possibilities
for the majority of conditions encountered in clinical practice. Particular attention has
been given to the evaluation of severity and outcome of each disorder and to advice on
comparing risks and benefits of treatment. Some treatments are of course well supported by data, others are empirical and yet others disappointingly poorly documented.
This resource will therefore prove invaluable to all involved in informing patients of
treatment options and making important cost-efficient decisions on care. It should also
be welcomed in the planning of clinical trials for potential new therapies and as a
reference in medico-legal work.

Outcomes in neurological and neurosurgical disorders

Outcomes in neurological and neurosurgical disorders

Edited by

MICHAEL SWASH

Professor of Neurology

St Bartholomew's and Royal London School of Medicine and Dentistry, London, UK
Royal London Hospital, London, UK

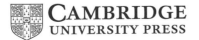

CAMBRIDGE
UNIVERSITY PRESS

PUBLISHED BY THE PRESS SYNDICATE OF THE UNIVERSITY OF CAMBRIDGE
The Pitt Building, Trumpington Street, Cambridge CB2 1RP, United Kingdom

CAMBRIDGE UNIVERSITY PRESS
The Edinburgh Building, Cambridge CB2 2RU, United Kingdom
40 West 20th Street, New York, NY 10011-4211, USA
10 Stamford Road, Oakleigh, Melbourne 3166, Australia

First published 1998

Printed in the United Kingdom at the University Press, Cambridge

Typeset in Utopia 9.25/13.75, in Poltype™ [vN]

A catalogue record for this book is available from the British Library

Library of Congress Cataloguing in Publication data
Outcome in neurological and neurosurgical disorders/edited by Michael Swash.
    p. cm.
1. Nervous system – Diseases – Treatment – Evaluation.   2. Nervous system – Surgery –
Evaluation.   3. Outcome assessment (medical care) I. Swash, Michael.
[DNLM: 1. Central Nervous System Diseases – therapy.   2. Central Nervous System Diseases –
surgery.   3. Outcome and Process Assessment (Health Care).   4. Informed Consent. WL 300
094 1997]
RC349.8.094 1997
616.8 – dc21
DNLM/DLC
for Library of Congress   96-40340 CIP

ISBN 0 521 44327 x hardback

CONTENTS

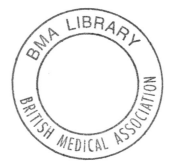

CONTRIBUTORS

C. BASSETTI
Department of Neurology, Inselspital, University of Bern,
CH-3010 Bern, Switzerland

J. BOGOUSSLAVSKY
Department of Neurology, CHUV, CH-1010 Lausanne,
Switzerland

A. BOWLING
Centre for Health Informatics and Multiprofessional Education,
University College London Medical School, 4th Floor, Archway Wing,
Whittington Hospital Campus, Highgate Hill, London N19 5NF, UK

J. BROTCHI
Department of Neurosurgery, ULB-Hôpital Erasmé,
808 Route de Lennick, B-1070 Bruxelles, Belgium

K. J. BURCHIEL
Department of Neurosurgery, Oregon Health Sciences University,
3181 SW Sam Jackson Park Road, Portland, Oregon 97201-3098, USA

D. B. CALNE
Neurodegenerative Disorder Section, University Hospital, UBC Site,
2211 Wesbrook Mall, Vancouver, BC v6t 2b5, Canada

N. E. F. CARTLIDGE
Department of Neurology, Royal Victoria Infirmary,
Queen Victoria Road, Newcastle upon Tyne, NE1 4LP, UK

P. R. COOPER
NYU Medical Center, Department of Neurosurgery,
550 First Avenue, New York, NY 10016, USA

W. J. K. CUMMING
Neuroscience Unit, Alexandra Hospital, Mill Lane, Cheadle,
SK8 2PX, UK

R. A. FELDMAN

Department of Epidemiology & Medical Statistics,
CELC at Queen Mary and Westfield College, Mile End Road,
London E1 4NS, UK

H. L. FRANKEL

Stoke Mandeville Hospital, Aylesbury HP21 8AL, UK

M. G. HAMILTON

Alberta Children's Hospital, Division of Neurosurgery,
1820 Richmond Road SW, Calgary, Alberta T2T 5C7, Canada

M. HOMMEL

Centre Hospitalier Universitaire Vaudois, CH-1011 Lausanne,
Switzerland

A. HOPKINS

Research Unit, Royal College of Physicians, 11 St Andrews Place,
London NW1 4LE, UK

J. HSIANG

Section of Neurosurgery, Virginia Mason Medical Center, 1100 Ninth Avenue,
PO Box 900X7-NS, Seattle, WA 98111-0900, USA

F. G. I. JENNEKENS

c/o Division of Neuromuscular Diseases, University Hospital Utrecht,
PO Box 85500, 3508 GA Utrecht, Netherlands

W. KOLLER

Department of Neurology, University of Kansas Medical Center,
39th and Rainbow, Kansas City, KS 66103, USA

E. R. LAWS

Department of Neurological Surgery, Health Sciences Centre Box 212,
Charlottesville, Virginia 22908, USA

L. F. MARSHALL

Division of Neurological Surgery, University of California Medical Center,
225 Dickinson Street, San Diego, CA 92103-8893, USA

F. B. MEYER

Department of Neurosurgery, Mayo Clinic, 200 First Street SW,
Rochester, MN 55905, USA

K. R. MOORE

Department of Neurosurgery, Oregon Health Sciences University,
3181 SW Sam Jackson Park Road, Portland, Oregon 97201-3098, USA

A. MORITA

Department of Neurosurgery, Mayo Clinic, 200 First Street SW,
Rochester, MN 55905, USA

C. NORMAND
Department of Health Policy, London School of Hygiene and Tropical Medicine,
Keppel Street, London WC1 7HT, UK

E. H. OLDFIELD
Surgical Neurology Branch, National Institute for Neurological Disorders and
Stroke, Building 10, Room 5D-37, Bethesda, Maryland, MD 20892, USA

A. PARRENT
Department of Neurosurgery, University Hospital, 339 Windemere Road,
PO Box 5339, London, Ontario N6A 5A5, Canada

J. M. S. PEARCE
304 Beverley Road, Anlaby, Hull, HU10 7BG, UK

M. R. PUUMALA
Department of Neurosurgery, Mayo Clinic, 200 First Street SW,
Rochester, MN 55905, USA

I. H. ROBERTSON
MRC Applied Psychology Unit, 15 Chaucer Road,
Cambridge CB2 2EF, UK

H. I. SABIN
Department of Neurosurgery, Royal London Hospital, Whitechapel,
London E1 1BB, UK

B. SCHUKNECHT
Universitatsspital Zurich, Departement Medizinische Radiologie,
Frauenklinikstrasse 10, 8091 Zurich, Switzerland

M. K. SHARIEF
Department of Neurology, The Royal London Hospital, Whitechapel,
London E1 1BB, UK

D. D. SPENCER
Section of Neurological Surgery, Yale University Medical School,
333 Cedar Street, New Haven, Connecticut 06510, USA

S. S. SPENCER
Department of Neurology, Yale University Medical School,
333 Cedar Street, New Haven, Connecticut 06510, USA

R. F. SPETZLER
Barrow Neurological Institute, 350 West Thomas Road,
Phoenix, Arizona 85013, USA

M. SWASH
Department of Neurology, St Bartholomew's and Royal London School of
Medicine and Dentistry,
Royal London Hospital, London E1 1BB, UK

R. R. TASKER

Toronto Hospital, Division of Neurosurgery, Suite 2-431, McLaughlin Pavilion, 399 Bathurst Street, Toronto, Ontario M5T 2S8, Canada

A. J. THOMPSON

University Department of Neurology, National Hospital for Neurology and Neurosurgery, Queen Square, London WC1N 3BG, UK

T. A. TRAN

Department of Neurology, Northwestern University, 645 North Michigan Avenue, Suite 1058, Chicago, IL 60611, USA

G. URWIN

Department of Medical Microbiology, The London Hospital Medical College, Turner Street, London E1 2AD, UK

A. VALAVANIS

Department of Neuroradiology, University Hospital of Zurich, Frauenklinikstrasse, 10, 8091 Zurich, Switzerland

L. H. VAN DEN BERG

Division of Neuromuscular Diseases, University Hospital Utrecht, PO Box 85500, 3508 GA Utrecht, Netherlands

D. T. WADE

Rivermead Rehabilitation Centre, Abingdon Road, Oxford OX1 4XD, UK

H. L. WEINER

New York University Medical Center, Department of Neurosurgery, 550 First Avenue, New York, NY 10016, USA

B. WILLIAMS

(deceased)

J. H. J. WOKKE

Division of Neuromuscular Diseases, University Hospital Utrecht, PO Box 85500, 3508 GA Utrecht, Netherlands

As neurology and neurosurgery become more and more concerned with therapy there is a need to consider the results of the different treatment options in a strictly comparative mode. As new strategies for treatment of these disorders are devised the question has to be asked whether any new treatment supersedes, becomes part of the management of a condition, or is used only in certain circumstances. Since much treatment in neurology and neurosurgery has been developed empirically, evidence for efficacy is, in many instances, surprisingly sparse. Other treatments, for example, the treatment of cerebral aneurysms, or the use of aspirin in stroke prevention have been subjected to rigorous evaluation in multi-centre and, in some instances, in international clinical trials. In this book most conditions treated by neurologists or neurosurgeons are discussed in relation to the outcome of treatment. Only when the outcome of a given therapy is known can its value in relation to other treatments be considered, and full, informed advice be given to a patient. In a sense, this process is an extension of knowledge about prognosis. The reader will notice in this book the different approaches to the problem of outcome taken by the authors of the different chapters, and reflect that these relate to the differing levels of effectiveness of treatment, or of understanding of the disease under discussion. In some areas it is apparent that there is much data but, in others, the data are more descriptive than analytical. Clearly, there is a long way to go in the search for conquest of neurological disease.

Information about the outcomes of different treatments is important not only to the physician or surgeon and the patient and family but also, in an era of cost constraints, to the health provider and the health purchaser. Indeed, decisions about the availability of treatments are increasingly made, not by individual physicians and patients, but by the health providers and purchasers with whom they are associated. The media throughout the world are full of stories concerning health care denied by such organisations, and it is clearly important for all concerned to have access to a source of information that can be used in approaching such decisions, both when they have to be made and when they have to be argued. In addition, there is a need for a source of data suitable for those physicians and surgeons, and lawyers, engaged in medico-legal practice in describing the expected outcome of certain procedures. This book may provide a source for such searches. In our individual clinical practices we all must aspire to achieve results comparable to the best. Only by knowing what is best practice can we begin to realise this aim.

This book consists of the contributions of many authors. As editor, I am grateful to them for their contributions, for their work in agreeing to the task set them in considering the outcomes of treatments in neurological and neurosurgical disease, and for their forbearance in modifying their contributions when unforeseen delays occurred in completing the project. I have been delighted to have been able to assemble such a distinguished group of authors. I am especially pleased to acknowledge the support of the staff of Cambridge University Press, particularly Richard Barling and Jocelyn Foster. I would also like to thank Mr John Wilden, who helped to formulate the plan of the book but who, unfortunately, was unable to continue to work on the project through to its completion. No book, of course, is ever completely up to date, and there is always something missing, however hard authors and editors strive to ensure that it is not. I hope, nonetheless, that readers will recognise the value of the reviews contained in this volume.

I record, with deep sadness, the untimely deaths of two contributors, Dr Anthony Hopkins and Mr Bernard Williams, during the preparation of this book. Bernard Williams' death occurred before his contribution was complete.

MICHAEL SWASH
Department of Neurology, The Royal London Hospital, London

1 The measurement of outcomes of health care

ANTHONY HOPKINS*

There are a number of reasons for the increasing interest in outcomes of health care interventions over the last few years. Foremost is the realization that in all health care systems, resources are limited, and should be directed towards those interventions that are of proven effectiveness, and producing outcomes that are valued by patients. As will be discussed below, deciding upon the outcome to be achieved is a necessary prerequisite for determining whether any treatment is effective.

The next stimulus to outcomes research is the realization that there are large variations in practice, not only throughout the world, but within the same health care system, and indeed in neighbouring cities. For example, Wennberg's comparison between Boston and New Haven, two university cities on the East coast of the United States, showed that in Boston people had twice the chance of having a carotid endarterectomy compared to New Haven, but only half the chance of having coronary bypass surgery (Wennberg et al. 1987). These differences were apparent even when corrections were made for the age and sex distribution and other variables between the two local communities. Another striking example is that rates of hysterectomy correlate more closely with the number of gynaecologists per head of population than they do with the number of women within a population. Such variations indicate that much of what doctors do is a matter of practice style, is imprecise, and is not related to procedures of proven effectiveness. Belatedly, the precision that has been brought to bear in biomedical research is now being brought to health services research. However, as in many other areas of research measurement of the variable concerned is not straightforward, and careful attention to methods is necessary if gross errors of measurement and interpretation are not to be made. The third pressure to develop outcome measurement is the increasing strength of consumer movements. Consumer pressures now affect more strongly not only the medical profession, but teaching, the law, and public service. The public now demands that all professions are more accountable for their work. The public is far more likely to leave self-regulation to health professionals if they can be assured that reliable systems of outcome measurement are in place, monitored by clinical audit.

* Dr Hopkins died suddenly on 6 March 1997, after this book went to press.

1

Definition

An outcome is a change in state that is attributable to a process; in terms of health, a change in health status (however defined) that is attributable to a health care intervention. Sometimes the intervention prevents a change in state. For example, pertussis immunization changes the recipient's immune state, and prevents whooping cough.

The population

Much of this book will be devoted to measurement of health status but first, we must consider the target population whose health states we are measuring. This may range from an individual to a nation.

For a nation, perinatal mortality has traditionally been taken as an overall measure of its health, because it reflects important components of the system, namely antenatal care, including nutritional support to pregnant women, good obstetric care, and good neonatal care. Furthermore, there is no doubt about the outcome measure – the baby is either alive or dead. An improvement of perinatal mortality has therefore been taken as a proxy for a measure of the health of the nation as a whole. It may indeed be a better proxy than expectancy of life at birth, which in developed societies may depend more upon the genetic pool than on health care interventions. For example, the expectancy of life for Japanese men is longer than for caucasians in the UK. This difference may be, but is not necessarily, due in large part to the lower incidence of coronary artery disease in the Japanese.

Years of life free from disability

There is increasing concern that extending the expectancy of life into older age will add years to life, but provide a poor quality of life in very old age, with the last years being spent in increasing infirmity. Put another way, have the gains in longevity increased the number and percentage of very ill, frail people who require protracted and expensive medical care and whose wellbeing is severely compromised? As a portmanteau measure for the outcome of the health care system of a nation, therefore, years of life free from disability is gaining increasing prominence. To measure this, of course, requires an operational definition of freedom from disability, but several are available (Grimley Evans 1993). Disability-free life years as a measure is particularly relevant to neurological practice, insofar as non-lethal impairments, such as persisting disability after stroke, significantly impact upon this measure. Research efforts should concentrate on delaying the onset of such diseases if we are not to have longer life but worsening health.

Inter-agency working

Although perinatal mortality and expectancy of life at birth and at different ages might be taken as good proxies for the outcome of health care systems, it must be remembered that both these indices are dependent upon other structural qualities in society, such as the provision of adequate nutrition, good sanitation, safe roads, government policies related to smoking, and so on. The United Kingdom is prominent amongst all developed nations in recognizing the need for inter-agency collaboration between the different Departments of State in order to improve health. However, it is to be much regretted that such collaboration does not extend to more rigorous financial disincentives to smoking and excessive consumption of alcohol.

Regional and local services

Descending from the national level, outcomes are also of importance in regional planning. For example, there are significant regional variations in mortality from stroke in the UK (Department of Health 1992). Although knowledge of these outcomes cannot benefit those who have already suffered a stroke, or who are dead, such measurements of health outcome should alert public health physicians working in localities with high rates to redouble their work to ensure adequate efforts in primary care to detect and treat hypertension, and to develop local incentives to encourage people to stop smoking, such as the establishment of smoking clinics, as two examples. There is now in the UK a national effort to develop a number of health care indicators, the so-called phase 3 indicator project of the Department of Health. The potential use of these and other indicators when considering comparability between outcomes of different service units must also be considered, but neurologists and neurosurgeons alike must be aware that there is now a developed public interest in the aggregated outcomes of the work of their service. All of us in clinical practice therefore need to understand something of the field, both so that we can influence policy when irrational 'league tables' are published, but, more particularly, so that we can use them as indicators for exploration within our own service for improvement of the quality of the care that we are delivering.

Outcomes for the individual patient

For many practising neurologists, however, the principal focus of outcome measurement is centred upon the consultations taking place between individual patients and their doctors and the supporting team of nurses, therapists and so on. For neurosurgeons, perhaps, the focus is more upon the outcomes of technical procedures, but the principle is the same. In this context an outcome of a consultation, a therapy or a procedure can be rephrased as follows: 'What is it that I, as a neurologist or neurosurgeon, am hoping to achieve with my management of this particular patient?' Rephrasing the term 'outcome' in this way has at least three benefits. It underlines the duality of the interaction between doctor and patient, so that patient values are pre-eminent; it provides a focus for action; and it should encourage before and after measurement, however informal in the first instance.

Attributability, efficacy and effectiveness

All neurologists have had occasional initially satisfactory consultations with patients who say that their epileptic seizures have stopped, the neurologist attributing this to his carefully chosen therapy, only to be disabused by the patient sheepishly confessing that he or she has not taken the tablets anyway! This raises an important point about outcome measurement; its *attributability*. In order to be sure that a health care intervention is effective, one has to have a sound epidemiological basis of the natural history of disease. It is impossible, except on probabilistic terms, to generalize from epidemiological studies to the course of an individual patient's illness, but, without a crystal ball, that is the best that we can do. Clearly, health care systems should only be interested in funding interventions to which an effect can be attributed. Research funding has in the last 40 years often supported randomized controlled trials in order to determine the *efficacy* of different therapies. In most trials, however, the outcome measure defined at the beginning of the trial is usually comparatively straightforward – in the case of tuberculosis, survival, or eradication of the bacillus from the sputum; in the case of hypertension, reduction in blood pressure to a previously defined range. Such trials can determine reliably the *efficacy* of interventions, but there is increasing realization that what may be efficacious in a randomized controlled trial, with the research team chasing up and supervising the therapy of individual patients, may not be *effective* when translated into routine health care delivery. For example, some antituberculosis regimes may be ineffective in developing countries unless systems are introduced, in parallel with the provision of the drug, to ensure supervised taking of the drug. With regard to the example of therapy for hypertension, there is no doubt from randomized controlled trials that beta-adrenergic blocking drugs reduce blood pressure. However, in practice many patients are non-compliant with medication because of the adverse effects of impotence, cold extremities and so on. In theory, one of two drugs might be more efficacious in randomized controlled trials, but less effective in practice because of lesser compliance.

Clinical importance of an intervention

The example of therapy for hypertension can be used to illustrate another point: that is, *clinical importance*. For example, very large-scale trials of drugs used in the management of hypertension may show that the reduction in diastolic blood pressure by drug A is, on average, 2 mm greater than drug B, and that the difference is highly statistically significant. The fact that the difference is statistically significant is not necessarily important if, for example, drug A is ten times the price of drug B, or accompanied by

Table 1.1. *Effect of combination of clinical features upon rate of recurrence at 1 year after a first seizure in 304 adults (late entry group excluded)*

Age < 50 Seizure between midnight and 8.59 am Family history of epilepsy/febrile convulsions	% recurred	Estimated probability of recurrence (95% confidence interval)
28 had none of these features, 5 recurred	18	0.18 (0.075–0.28)
177 had one of the features, 54 recurred	31	0.30 (0.25–0.36)
84 had two of the features, 35 recurred	42	0.43 (0.35–0.51)
15 had all three features, 9 recurred	60	0.56 (0.42–0.70)

more unwanted effects. Furthermore, although true in population terms that drug A is more efficacious than drug B, it becomes difficult to conceptualize, in relation to the prognosis of an individual patient rather than of large-scale trial populations, as to what a difference in 2 mm of mercury actually means. To bring this example back into the context of neurology, Hampton calculated on the basis of the MRC trial of therapy for mild hypertension that more than 800 person years would have to be treated in order to prevent one stroke (Wilcox *et al.* 1996). Other similar examples are given by Laupacis *et al.* (1988). It is increasingly clear therefore that randomized controlled trials can provide highly important evidence about efficacy, but can only be a rough guide as to what is fruitful to put into everyday practice, when health care expenditures and patient preferences become pre-eminent.

Case severity and co-morbidity

Many clinicians feel that those who are interested in aggregating outcome measures into indicators of performance fail to recognize the impact of case severity and coexisting illnesses upon outcome. To take an obvious example, no neurosurgeon would be interested in a study about the outcome of surgery, radiotherapy and chemotherapy for cerebral glioma unless the study took into account markers known to predict poor outcome, such as disability at presentation and histological grade (Davies 1996). Table 1.1 illustrates another example from my own work with Garman and Clarke on the risk of recurrence after a first epileptic seizure.

First seizure patients with different attributes have different risks of relapse. Almost certainly there are other risks yet to be discovered. Unless such factors or 'case-severity' measures are taken into account, it is meaningless to compare outcomes of care, so there is a tremendous research effort in all branches of medicine to determine factors that predict good and poor outcomes in the natural history of any disease.

Unless case severity is taken into account, aggregated outcomes from tertiary or university hospitals may appear to be worse than the outcomes from what may be termed 'ordinary' secondary care, until it is realized that the most complex and difficult cases tend to end up in the most academically and technically advanced centres.

Many older patients suffer from diseases that coexist with the primary diagnosis for which the outcome is being measured. For example, the outcome of a patient with a stroke who has extensive vascular disease, manifest by coronary artery disease and peripheral vascular disease, and who also has diabetes is likely to be significantly worse than someone of the same age who has stroke without any of these co-morbidities.

There are two dangers here: first, as already mentioned, the complexity of case severity and co-morbidity, and the difficulties in measuring the impact of these, will be inadequately recognized by those who construct aggregate outcome measures; the second is that units knowing that their outcomes are likely to be looked at, will turn down cases for therapy or for operation, simply because taking on these cases will make their results 'look bad', even though individual patients within the aggregate may be strikingly helped by an intervention. In the United States, case severity is often estimated by commercial software systems that require the clinical record to be reviewed to collect data. Examples include MEDIS groups and Systemmetrics. However, retrospective record review is expensive. Nonetheless, striking examples of the effectiveness of an academic analysis of case severity are the APACHE system in intensive care, which measures case severity by a number of physiological variables in the first 24 hours (Rowan *et al.* 1993), and the CRIB system in neonatal intensive care, which does much the same (The International Neonatal Network 1993). There is now good evidence that the outcomes of survival in both these intensive care situations can be predicted with a high degree of accuracy by such measures of case severity. Furthermore, it is proposed that, having corrected for case severity, survival can be used as an audit measure for the success of a unit. For example, no district general hospital achieved a survival rate corrected for case severity using the CRIB scale for neonatal intensive care that was as good as any teaching hospital. This is circumstantial evidence that care in the latter is better.

Retrospective record review is expensive, and there is now good epidemiological evidence of factors that do predict a poor outcome in many disorders. For example, in neurological practice in relation to stroke, there are a number of prognostic scores (e.g. Allen 1984). It might be feasible to audit the effectiveness of rehabilitation units by considering the functional status of those with stroke, modified by the prognostic score. That is to say, a patient who failed to walk again after a stroke, having been predicted to walk again on the basis of a measure of case severity, might be assumed, other things being equal, to have had inadequate rehabilitation.

Although the case severity and comorbidity, if adequately measured, can sometimes be considered as satisfactory 'explanations' for less than satisfactory outcomes, age and, in particular, ethnicity should not be accepted as 'excuses' without scrupulous self-appraisal. For example, old people with coronary artery disease may have poor outcomes simply because they are not offered effective interventions such as angioplasty or coronary bypass surgery as often as they ought to be (Krumholz *et al.* 1993); in the field of neurology, old people may not be considered to be 'worth' spending the money on effective rehabilitation. With regard to ethnicity, poor outcomes may be too readily attributable to racial (i.e. genetic) differences, whereas in truth the differences are due to less good care. A particularly striking example is a careful analysis of outcomes of renal transplantation in Afrocaribbean and Caucasian Americans. Although graft survival was worse in Afrocaribbean individuals, analysis of the population studied showed that these recipients received less well matched kidneys than Caucasian recipients, and if this and other factors were controlled for, then the survival of both recipient populations was more or less the same (Butkus *et al.* 1992).

Multiplicity of outcomes, and patient values

So far I have considered straightforward outcomes, such as death, or eradication of bacteria, or a reduction in blood pressure. However, a central aspect of out thinking in the measurement of outcomes, must be the multiplicity of possible outcomes, and their valuation by the individual patient.

There is often a potential conflict between the outcome valued by a patient and the outcome that the neurologist values. For example, neurologists know from epidemiological experience that those who have little use of the hand 24 days after a hemiplegic stroke stand little chance indeed of having useful function of that hand in the future (Heller *et al.* 1987). However, they know from the scientific literature that, if hypertensive, a reduction in the patient's blood pressure will reduce the chances of a subsequent stroke. Neurologists also know from experience that handicap can be successfully minimized by suitable attention to the patient's environment and the provision of appropriate aids and appliances. A neurologist's successful outcome therefore will be, with the aid of an occupational therapist, to help a hemiplegic woman back to self-care, to work or to look after her own home. The patient's perspective on outcome, however, will be that the hand has not got better, and that as far as she is concerned, treatment has been a failure. All doctors must sit down with their patients when they plan management and inform them what outcomes can be realistically expected, such disclosure being tempered by what is thought to be kind, and supportive of the individual patient. It is likely that resources are wasted upon continuing physiotherapy for stroke patients for whom there is no likelihood of useful further recovery simply because the neurological team have not had the courage to explore with the patient both what their difficulties are, and what can be realistically offered in the way of improvement.

The case of a hemiplegic stroke can be used to illustrate another point about the multiplicity of outcomes. In spite of the protestations of speech therapists, the weight of research evidence suggests that speech therapy does not much help the recovery of language after stroke. An important UK study showed that recovery, in terms of one respected measure of communication (the PORCH index), was the same whether the 'therapy' was given by speech therapists or by volunteers, who had received some basic training and supervision by a speech therapist (David *et al.* 1982). There are a number of possible interpretations of the recovery in communication. It is possible (were it not for other studies [David *et al.* 1982]) that volunteers can acquire, in a few hours training, the skills that it takes speech therapists three years to acquire. More likely, the limited recovery reflects innate spontaneous cerebral recovery. But this example would not encourage any health provider to put further resources into the training of speech therapists for the treatment of dysphasia following stroke.

Speech therapists might respond by stating that they accepted that the evidence was slight that their efforts could improve language, but that patients valued their help in *coming to terms with their difficulties, and in being taught various coping strategies.* If the words in italics are defined as the outcome, then it would be necessary to mount a new trial. Perhaps volunteers would be as effective in these domains as well. Using this example as a model, social research should discover what achievable outcomes are valued by patients, and further discover the most cost-effective way of achieving them. To switch examples, if a specially trained nurse, on a lower salary than a junior doctor, more successfully harvests saphenous vein grafts for coronary bypass surgery, then there are good arguments for moving to such a system.

The problem of outcome definition may perhaps more strikingly be brought into prominence by considering the case of a woman aged 38 years who has had bitemporal headaches for the last 2 or 3 years, worse in the evening and worse at times of menstruation, not relieved by analgesics. They occur on a background of confessed anxiety about her husband's fidelity. All clinical supposition is that she has tension headaches. Two weeks before this neurological consultation, a distant acquaintance was reputed to have a brain tumour, and the headache patient has taken it into her head that she might also have a tumour. Such anxieties amongst patients with head-aches are common, and are usually relatively easily laid at rest (Fitzpatrick & Hopkins 1981). The patient feels that she needs a scan of some sort to exclude a tumour. The outcome that both patient and neurologist will wish to achieve is reassurance about the absence of a tumour, which in itself may go some way towards encouraging the patient to cope with her headaches, even if they do not necessarily resolve. From a technical diagnostic point of view, an imaging study in this circumstance is a waste of the resources of the health care system, as the chances of it showing a tumour or some other important treatable lesion are extraordinarily low (Lavson *et al.* 1980). However, if the focus of the interaction between doctor and patient is on reassurance, rather than on the sensitivity and specificity of the investigation, then the imaging study may be an effective and an appropriate intervention. All clinical neurologists will recognize this dilemma, and hopefully most attempt to spare resources by relying upon relatively cheap counselling and supportive therapy. However, the conflict in perspective be-tween what is considered appropriate by the health care system from a population perspective, determined to husband its resources for effective technical health care, and what the patient considers to be appropriate has not been resolved (NHS Manage-ment Executive 1993). The unwritten understanding that doctors control access to investigations and procedures for safety's sake becomes strained at the edges, particularly when an investigation costs a lot of money, but, as far as we know, the procedure itself carries no conceivable risk to the patient as is the case with magnetic resonance imaging. The conclusion of Brett and McCullough (1986) that no patient in such a situation should not have the investigation if they wanted it and were prepared to pay for it is probably just, but in practice, the burden of payment is often shifted onto health care insurers, whose utilization review tends to be more directed towards interventional procedures. Furthermore, Brett and McCullough do not recognize the diversion of capital resources and the time of trained staff away from what most physicians would consider more appropriate health care.

This apparent digression into the ethics of 'unnecessary' imaging studies does, however, introduce the notion that the outcomes towards which doctors should work must be the outcomes desired by the patient. Other chapters in this book review the reliability, sensitivity to change and so on of various measures of functional status, which are certainly one important measure of the outcome of rehabilitative care. However, it may be that neurologists and physiotherapists too readily perceive disabled people from their own stance of locomotor perfection, and concentrate excessively upon functional aspects of daily living to the extent that they fail to address how best to help patients achieve their own targets and goals, which may in part be emotional.

To illustrate further the multiplicity of outcomes that must be considered in good care, consider a simple procedure from general surgical rather than neurosurgical practice, such as a herniorrhaphy. First of all, there is the unlikely event of perioperative mortality. There are potential adverse outcomes other than mortality, including wound infection and of course recurrence of the hernia at a later date. There is the outcome of freedom from dragging pain in the groin, and from an embarrassing unsightly lump. Then there is the satisfaction of the patient with postoperative pain relief, the cosmetic acceptability of the scar, with the courtesy of the surgeon who talked to him kindly before and after the operation, and with the depth of the advice that he received in relation to future activities, such as return to work, to sexual intercourse, and to lifting. All neurologists and neurosurgeons could translate such a scenario to procedures in their own practice. All of us would acknowledge that each of the dimensions just recorded in relation to herniorrhaphy were all aspects of good care. The truth of the matter is that it is very difficult to capture such data for clinical audit, with the exception of gross adverse outcomes such as perioperative mortality; even recurrence rate may be confused by case mix, such as previous herniorrhaphy, obesity, occupation, and by co-morbidities such as chronic bronchitis which, by causing repeated coughing, makes a recurrence of the hernia more likely.

Measures of quality of life

Faced with the complexities of individual patient characteristics and of real life, there have understandably been a number of attempts to record in a single number a patient's overall 'quality of life.' Some of the methods of doing this are reviewed elsewhere (Bowling 1991; Hopkins 1992) but there are two principal ways of going about it. First of all, researchers can decide, after prolonged exploration with the public, what dimensions of existence are important (mobility, freedom from pain, mood, sexuality and so on). Scales can then be derived for each of these dimensions, and standards set by applying the scales to a normative population. The Nottingham Health Profile (Bowling, 1991) and the Sickness Impact Profile (Bergnev *et al.* 1976) are both examples of these. There is no doubt that these scales are sensitive at detecting changes in health status which accord with clinical reality and patient judgement. However, their very multidimensionality militates to some extent against their easy use. For example if, after an intervention, a patient scores more favourably on freedom from pain, and less favourably on freedom of mobility, how do we judge the success of our intervention? To take another example from everyday neurological practice, trials of treatment for headache are bedevilled by patients who say sometimg along the lines that 'I have fewer headaches, but those that I do have are more severe.' Similarly, trials of drugs for migraine and epilepsy are bedevilled by whether or not one should weight the severity of headaches or seizures. Faced with these difficulties, therefore, another school of research tries to integrate all aspects of a patient's wellbeing and quality of life on a scale of 0 to 1. The original and highly imaginative work of Rachel Rosser (1978) was to ask members of the population to rate on two axes of impairment and distress various health states as briefly described. Critics of this work pointed out that the raters were unusually medically orientated, being healthy staff largely in and around one hospital, but that criticism has been laid to rest by extensive surveys of valuations of health states amongst a more representative population carried out by the Institute of Health Economics at York. From such valuations of health states, and from the duration of survival in those states, quality adjusted life years (QALYs) can be calculated. That is to say, ignoring discounting the future, a year of life in a perfect health state (value 1) is equivalent to two years of life in a health state valued at 0.5. If the costs of interventions and subsequent support are adequately calculated, then, in theory at least, league tables can be constructed to show what resources buy the most QALYs (Williams 1985). To illustrate this point, calculations purport to show that a hip replacement costs £800 per QALY gained, and a neurosurgical intervention on a malignant glioma over £100,000 (at current prices) per QALY gained.

There is growing concern about the use of such calculations, which do not take into account many research and ethical issues (Hopkins, 1992). From the research point of view, there is no evidence to suppose that the valuations by the general public of what it is like to be in a certain health state bear any relationship to what it is *really* like to be in that health state. Unfortunately, one cannot ask the patients in that health state, as they have no experience of other health states with which to compare their present situation. To give an example of the ethical concerns, what of the care given to people with learning disabilities? I know of no evidence that humane care improves cognitive function and memory in those with severe learning disabilities, but any ethical society would expect to look after those so severely handicapped in a humane and caring way.

In this sense, humane care of people with severe learning disabilities is a 'good outcome' for society as well as for the individually disabled person.

Proponents of the multidimensional measures of health status such as the Nottingham Health Profile believe that it is without common sense to compress into a single figure all the complexities of life. Proponents of single figure valuations do, however, have powerful arguments on their side: first of all, to take an economic parallel, people consider the resources at their disposal and all the available goods and services that they can consume, and do without difficulty integrate all the information to make what they consider to be the best choice – a more expensive car, compared perhaps with a cheaper car and a holiday as well. Clinicians also have some faith in the ability of their patients to integrate all the complex dimensions of health status, as their opening question in a follow-up clinic is usually something along the lines of 'Well, how are you today?' The patient replies 'better' (or worse) according to his own integration of all that has gone on since his last visit.

Conclusion

In this introductory chapter, I have underlined some of the conceptual problems relating to the measurement of outcomes. Succeeding chapters will focus upon outcome measurement in each of a number of neurological and neurosurgical disorders. The plea that I make is that the development of such measures must follow the highest standards of international biomedical research, in order to prevent manipulation and abuse for political ends. Technical issues of measurement such as validity, reliability, sensitivity to change, absence of floor and ceiling effects, and so on, necessary prerequisites of any measurement instrument in any discipline, are reviewed elsewhere in particular relation to the measurement of health status. To these one would add ease of use; even if a scale fulfils all the desirable attributes just mentioned, it would be little use if it required a trained metrologist an hour or so to record. Then there is a final problem upon which the literature hardly touches – when should the outcome measurement be made. Once one gets away from mortality, which at least occurs at a definite point in time, uncertainty prevails. Lack of clarity about this has led to some confusing results in the neurological literature. For example, the outcome of patients admitted to a special stroke unit is 'better' when measured at 6 months, in comparison with people treated in routine medical wards. However, this difference has disappeared at the end of a further 6 months (Langhorne *et al.* 1995). Should we set up special stroke units on the basis of such a study? To take another example from outside neurology and neurosurgery, the benefits of a hip replacement may not be fully apparent until some 3 months or so after the operation, when perioperative pain and discomfort has settled. Are primary care physicians going to be responsible for measuring outcomes after such an interval, and, if so, what will be their training needs, what audits of their measurement capability will be required, and how are their results fed back into the health care system for outcome audit?

The whole area of outcome measurement is potentially so important to the allocation of health care resources, and superficially so easy that there is considerable danger that the field will not be addressed with the rigour that it requires.

References

Allen, C. M. C. (1984). Predicting the outcome of acute stroke: a prognostic score. *J. Neurosurg. Psychiatry* **47**, 475–80.

Bergner, M., Bobbitt, R., Pollard, W., Martin, D. & Gilson, B. (1976). The Sickness Impact Profile: development and final revision of a health status measure. *Med. Care* **19**, 787–805.

Bowling, A. (1991). *Measuring health: a review of quality of life scales.* Milton Keynes: Open University Press.

Brett, A. S. & McCullough, L. B. (1986). When patients request specific interventions; defining the limits of the physician's obligations. *N. Engl. J. Med.* **315**, 1347–51.

Butkus, D. E., Meydrech, G. F. & Raju, S. S. (1992). Racial differences in the survival of cadaveric renal allocrafts. Overall effects of HLA matching and socioeconomic factors. *N. Engl. J. Med.* **327**, 840–5.

David R., Enderby, P. & Bainton, D. (1982). Treatment of acquired aphasia. *J. Neurol. Neurosurg. Psychiatry* **45**, 957–61.

Davies, E. A. (1997). Malignant cerebral glioma. I. Survival, disability and morbidity following radiotherapy. *Br. Med. J.* **313**, 1507–12.

Department of Health (1992). *The Health of the nation,* London: HMSO.

Fitzpatrick, R. & Hopkins, A. (1981). Patients' satisfaction with communication in neurological outpatients clinics. *Psychosomat. Res.* **25**, 329–34.

Grimley Evans, J. (1993). Health Active Life Expectancy (HALE) as an index of effectiveness of health and social services for elderly people. *Age Ageing* **22**, 297–301.

Heller, A., Wade, D. T. & Wood, V. A., Sunderland, A., Langton Hewer, R., Ward, E. (1987). Arm function after stroke: measurement and recovery after the first three months. *J. Neurol. Neurosurg. Psychiatry* **50**, 714–19.

Hopkins, A. (ed.) (1992). *Measures of the quality of life – and the uses to which they may be put.* London: RCP Publications.

Hopkins, A., Clarke, C. & Garman, A. (1988). The first seizure in adult life; value of electroencephalography and computerised scanning in prediction of seizure recurrence. *Lancet* **I**, 721–7.

The International Neonatal Network (1993). The CRIB (clinical risk index for babies) score: a tool for assessing initial neonatal risk and comparing performance of neonatal intensive care units. *Lancet* **342**, 193–8.

Krumholz, H. M., Forman, D. E., Kuntz, R. E., Baim, D. S. & Wei, J. Y. (1993). Coronary revascularization after myocardial infarction in the very elderly: outcomes and long-term follow-up. *Ann. Intern. Med.* **119**, 1084–90.

Langhorne, P., Williams, B. O. Gilchrist, W. & Howie, K. (1993) Do stroke units save lives? *Lancet* **342**, 395–8.

Larson, E. B., Omenn, G. S. & Lewis, H. (1980). Computerised scans for headache. *JAMA* **244**, 133–4.

Laupacis, A., Sackett, D. L. & Roberts, R. S. (1988). An assessment of clinically useful measures of the consequences of treatment. *N. Engl. J. Med.* **318**, 1728–33.

NHS Management Executive (1993). Report of a working group prepared for the Director of Research and Development of the NHS Management Executive. What do we mean by appropriate health care? *Qual. Health Care* **2**, 117–23.

Pickard, J. D., Bailey, S., Sanderson, H., Rees, M. & Garfield, J. S. (1990). Steps towards cost-benefit analysis of regional neurosurgical care. *Br. Med. J.* **301**, 629–35.

Rosser, R. & Kind, P. (1978). A scale for valuations of states of illness: is there a consensus? *Int. J. Epidemiol.* **7**, 347–57.

Rowan, K. M., Kerr, J. H., McPherson, K., Short, A. & Vessey, M. P. (1993). Intensive Care Society's APACHE II study in Britain and Ireland. I. Variations in case mix of adult admissions to general intensive care units and impact on outcome. *Br. Med. J.* **307**, 972–7.

Wennberg, J. E., Freeman, J. L. & Culp, W. J. (1987). Are hospital services rationed in New Haven or over-utilised in Boston? *Lancet* **I**, 1185–9.

Wilcox, R. G., Mitchell, J. R. A. & Hampton, J. R. (1986). Treatment of high blood pressure: should clinical practice be based on results of clinical trials? *Br. Med. J.* **293**, 433–7.

Williams, A. (1985). The economics of coronary by-pass grafting. *Br. Med. J.* **291**, 326–9.

2 Definition and measurement of outcome

ANN BOWLING AND CHARLES NORMAND

Donabedian (1985) defined health outcome as a change in patients' current and future health status that can be attributed to antecedent health care. Outcome indicators include information on avoidable mortality, standardized mortality ratios, hospital readmission or retreatment rates (analysed in relation to cause), other service use indicators, laboratory investigations and other diagnostic tests, morbidity, case severity, adverse reactions, complications, the technical success of the treatment where quantifiable, symptom relief, pain, cost-effectiveness, patient satisfaction, and, increasingly, broader indicators of health status or health-related quality of life. Clinical indicators of outcome are no longer sufficient, particularly in view of the debate about whether to survive in a vegetative state is no better than death, or even worse (Jennett, 1976). It is important that the research design enables a comparison to be made between the outcome of the intervention group and a control group, in order to ensure that the outcome obtained would not have occurred anyway (i.e. without the intervention). Baselines are not necessarily static and require monitoring via controls.

The term quality of life is often used but seldom defined. It is a broader concept than health status, and takes social well-being into account. Health-related quality of life can be defined as optimum levels of mental, physical, role (e.g. work, school, parent, carer, etc.) and social functioning, including relationships. It also encompasses *perceptions* of health, fitness, life satisfaction and well-being. It should also include some assessment of the patient's level of satisfaction with treatment, outcome and health status and with future prospects. It is an abstract concept, comprising diverse areas. It is distinct from quality of life as a whole, which would also include adequacy of housing, income, perceptions of the immediate environment, etc. Measures implicitly or explicitly purporting to tap health-related quality of life are usually referred to as broader measures of health status. In practice, the measurement of health-related quality of life requires the inclusion of an overall index of health status, and perceptions of health, of functional ability, pain, relevant dimensions of mental health, life satisfaction, coping ability, social support and integration. It is inevitably based on subjective feelings and attitudes.

In many cases, the inclusion of a global index of health status to supplement disease-specific items will suffice. However, this will not be enough if, for example, the outcome is expected to influence a specific domain, such as depression. In such cases a scale measuring that domain will also need to be included. There is little point in including a health status measure alone if it is unlikely to detect the effects of the treatment in question, or symptoms specific to the condition. Such measures require supplementation with disease-specific items. In addition, some measure of disease severity will also be required, although these are often fairly crude (Linn *et al.* 1968).

Measures of health-related quality of life (or health status)

The recognition of the importance of information on health outcomes for the purchasing of effective health services has culminated in the establishment by the Department of Health of a UK Clearing House on Health Outcomes, at the Nuffield Institute in Leeds (Long *et al.* 1992). This provides an information service on, among other things, health status measurement tools and their use. Information on health outcomes is essential for the assessment of need for (effective) services.

Measures of overall health status provide the researcher with a summary measure of global health status, or, in the case of the broader measures of health-related quality of life, they may encompass the dimensions of physical, mental and social health which were listed earlier.

There is now recognition that measures of health outcome should incorporate the patient's perspective, not simply in terms of whether or not the treatment was a success, but, more globally in relation to perceived mental and physical well-being as a consequence of an intervention. A person can feel ill without medical science being able to detect any apparent disease. A person's ill-health is indicated by feelings of pain and discomfort, or perceptions of change in usual functioning and feeling.

Measures of health outcome need to take both the traditional disease model (pathological abnormality indicated by a set of symptoms and signs) and the patient's perspective into account. What matters is how patients feel, not only what doctors think they ought to feel on the basis of clinical measurements. Who should be involved in measuring health-related quality of life? A number of health status scales require a health professional to complete a questionnaire on behalf of the patient, such as the rating scales of dependency, work and school performance, family and non-family relationships used by Horowitz & Cohen (1968), Taylor & Falconer (1968) and Rausch & Crandall (1982), in their studies of patients with temporal lobe seizures. Research indicates wide discrepancies between patients' and doctors' ratings of outcome after specific therapies (Orth-Gomer *et al.* 1979; Thomas & Lyttle 1980; Jachuck *et al.* 1982; Slevin *et al.* 1988). The implication is that patients should complete questionnaires about their health status themselves; health care professionals should not complete them on their behalf.

A concept of health

There are multiple influences upon patient outcome, and these require a broad model of health. The non-biological factors which may affect recovery and outcome include patient psychology, motivation, coping, adherence to therapy, socioeconomic status, availability of health care, social support networks and individual cultural beliefs and health behaviours.

A measure of health status should be based on a concept of health. Most health status indicators are based on negative definitions of health as the absence of illness and disease, and rarely reflect the global definition of the World Health Organization (1946, published in 1958) as total social, psychological and physical well-being. Scales need to be more balanced in order to reflect feelings of mental and physical well-being, full functioning, physical fitness, ability to cope, social adjustment and efficiency of mind and body. Collectively, these positive states have been referred to in the literature variously as positive health, social health and health-related quality of life, and have been described in greater detail by Bowling (1991). The difficulty in practice, is that most scales that exist are based on the negative model, and require supplementation with positive scales (such as those measuring life satisfaction, and adequate as well as inadequate social support) in order to achieve a more positive balance.

Criteria for selecting a health status indicator

In choosing a health status measure, or set of measures, key questions to consider are whether a disease-specific and/or a broad ranging instrument(s) is required. In the case of a specialty such as neurology, with a disease impact on a broad range of functioning, the instruments of choice will often be both (see earlier discussion).

Essential criteria to consider when choosing a health status measure, are the reliability (can the indicator consistently produce the same results?), and validity (does the indicator measure the underlying attribute or not?) of the instrument, and its sensitivity to change over time. As Wade (1988) argues, any assessment tools that have not had their reliability and validity tested should be discarded, and he adds that this includes almost all of the in-house assessment schedules used in most hospitals. He also argues that the number of measures of function used should be limited to one or two. He suggests that the Barthel ADL Index be used as the standard measure of physical disability (see later).

In addition, account must be taken of the type of scoring that the instrument is based on and whether it yields nominal (numbers are used simply for classification, e.g. 'died' 'survived'), ordinal (scale items stand in some kind of relation to each other, e.g. 'very difficult' through to 'not very difficult'), interval (the characteristics of an ordinal scale but the distances between any two numbers on the scale are of a known size, e.g. temperature) or ratio scale (the characteristics of an interval scale and in addition has a true – not arbitrary – zero point, e.g. weight) data. The definition of these concepts can be found in Bowling (1991) and in most research methods textbooks; their consideration is crucial because different scales are suitable for answering different types of question. In addition, interval and ratio scales are required if powerful statistical analysis is envisaged.

Clinicians also need to agree over what types of changes will be expected (outcomes) over specific time periods. For some conditions the reference periods may be from admission to hospital to 3 months later and 12 months after discharge. In the case of chronic conditions it will be necessary to consider longer time periods (Bardsley & Coles, 1992). It may be regarded as desirable to measure patient outcomes not just once, in comparison with baseline measures, but several times (e.g. at quarterly intervals), in order to document the speed of any progress or deterioration. However, repeated follow-ups do become expensive.

Some caution in the selection of scales is needed in the case of baseline data collection after the patient has been admitted to hospital, as health status scores may be raised (e.g. worsened) by admission, and thus the results contaminated (Bardsley *et al.* 1992). It is wise to avoid scales with items about 'staying in bed more than usual', for example if the baseline data are collected on admission when the patient is going to be doing so simply by virtue of being in hospital. It is also important to identify any patient characteristics or items that may affect outcome (e.g. age, co-morbidity, etc.), as well as disease severity (Krischer 1979).

Several of the issues pertinent to the decision making involved in scale selection have been summarized by Wade (1988). Finally Wade (1988), along with all methodologists in health services research, warns against reinventing the wheel by developing new measures; we should instead concentrate on improving existing measures. Given the tremendous amount of work involved in testing scales for reliability and validity, which *is* essential, this point is well worth emphasizing.

Which measure of broader health status?

Given that a subjective health indicator will be required, the issue becomes which measure to choose. There are single item questions on self-rated health, for example the widely used 'Is your health excellent, good, fair or poor (for your age)?', although as around half a random sample of the population will rate their health as 'excellent' or 'good', and most of the remainder as 'fair' its usefulness is limited (Ware 1984).

Symptom checklists are also commonly used, although questions about symptoms in research produce a high proportion of affirmative responses because trivial problems are usually included in people's replies (Dunnell & Cartwright 1972), the latter are unlikely to have much discriminatory power. Unquestionably, if time permits, the health indicator of choice will be a health status scale (see below).

Clearly different criteria for assessing outcome of care will be different for different disease syndromes within neurology. For example, the consequences of suffering from a cerebrovascular accident will be different, and affect different dimensions of functioning, than for, say head injury or epilepsy. The specific effects of care and treatment will also require specification. Beyond the identification of the specific types of patient outcomes which will require measurement for the particular disease syndrome, a general measure of health status should be selected in order to assess patients' perceptions and facilitate comparisons with other population groups. Such a tool should be selected carefully, as a wide variety, which tap different dimensions, exist (see review by Bowling 1991). A generic, widely used and well-tested measure will enable researchers to compare their results with population norms and, if necessary, with other patient populations.

Many health status scales are American in origin, and their applicability to other cultures has to be carefully assessed before use. The major problem with most existing scales is their length, which can easily reach 100 items, and partly explains their limited use by busy clinicians. More encouraging is the recent development of the Short-Form-36 (SF-36) from the RAND Medical Outcomes Survey (Stewart & Ware 1992; Brazier *et al.* 1992; Ware & Sherbourne 1992).

The SF-36 contains 36 items which tap seven dimensions of health-related quality of life: general health perceptions (5 items), energy/fatigue (4 items), social function (2 items), emotional well-being (5 items), role limitations due to emotional problems (3 items), physical function (10 items), role limitations due to physical health problems (4 items); and it also includes a two-item scale measuring pain and a single item on changes in health state. It is the result of extensive methodological development based on the RAND Medical Outcomes Study (Stewart *et al.* 1992). It is easy for people to complete, it has been adapted for use in the UK, and although initial test results are encouraging, work on its applicability is still continuing (Stewart & Ware 1992; Brazier *et al.* 1992; Ware & Sherbourne 1992). It is rapidly becoming an international health status scale. The different sections produce individual section scores; these cannot be combined to form an overall score. Some other scales, such as the Nottingham Health Profile (Hunt *et al.* 1986), do produce a score, and items are weighted, although the scores and weighting have been criticized (Kind & Carr-Hill 1987). Overall scores can be insensitive, and camouflage particularly high individual section scores.

Some of the other relevant dimensions of health status and health-related quality of life are presented below, with a selection of pertinent and commonly used measurement scales. Many others exist but space does not permit their review here. Nor is it possible within the confines of a chapter to review other important dimensions of health status which the researcher may specifically wish to include in a fuller scale form, for example social support. Interested readers are referred to a more extensive review elsewhere (Bowling 1991).

Cerebrovascular accident and epilepsy

There are numerous areas within neurology where the application of broader outcome measures would be appropriate. For example, there is a rapidly increasing psychological literature on the measurement of outcome of head injury (Brooks 1984). This is an area which has leapt from fairly crude indicators of outcome, based on subjective ratings of 'good, fair, poor, practical, worthwhile and acceptable' a decade ago, to more detailed indicators of social outcome. For example the Glasgow Outcome Scale (Jennett & Bond 1975) was developed to assess outcome after head injury and other types of acute brain damage.

For the purposes of this chapter, it was decided to concentrate on two main disease syndromes, cerebrovascular accident and epilepsy. In each of these areas progress is being made by neurologists and neurosurgeons on developing appropriate indicators of health status, or health outcome. However, the section on general measures of health status and the sections below on functional ability and mental health indicators are pertinent to all disease syndromes.

Cerebrovascular accident (stroke)

The incidence of cerebrovascular accident (CVA), or stroke as it is commonly known, increases with age, and with the projected demographic changes in the future (the ageing of the populations worldwide) stroke could be an increasing cause of mortality and morbidity. In the UK, about 75% of stroke patients are admitted to hospital, and about 12% who survive are admitted to institutional care 1 year after their stroke (see review by Freemantle et al. 1992). Over half of stroke survivors have continuing problems with mobility (Collin & Wade 1990).

The organization of services for stroke is diverse, and can include general medical wards in hospital, special stroke units, special rehabilitation units and community services. Several disciplines can be involved: doctors, nurses, physiotherapists, occupational therapists, speech therapists, social workers, counsellors, psychologists, chiropodists, etc. A review of the known effectiveness of these services in the care of stroke patients has been published by Freemantle et al. (1992). There is a continuing need to evaluate the effectivenes of services for stroke patients, hence the importance of careful selection of outcome indicators. Freemantle et al. (1992) concluded that more research, of better quality, is required to establish which aspects of rehabilitation are most effective and what form of organization it should take.

A number of fairly concise 'stroke scales' have been developed, which provide a simple and quick assessment of stroke severity (i.e. the severity of neurological deficits), sometimes encompassing a prognostic score. These vary in their prognostic accuracy and, while useful, provide only rudimentary information. Examples include the Scandinavian Stroke Scale (Scandinavian Stroke Study Group 1985, 1987; Lindenstrom et al. 1991; Boysen 1992); the NIH Stroke Scale (Brott et al. 1989; Brott, 1992); and the Canadian Neurological Scale (Cote et al. 1989; Cote & Hachinski 1992). Some of the more detailed assessment tools are described below.

The Stroke TyPE tool: for acute stroke

Stroke TyPE is a tool for the assessment of outcome of acute stroke, defined by the authors as a sudden or stepwise onset of focal neurological deficit that lasts more than 24 hours, for which there is no evidence of a non-vascular aetiology.

The Stroke TyPE tool was developed in the USA for the Health Outcomes Institute (HOI), in Boston, by Matchar and colleagues at Duke University. The HOI is also one of several organizations that act as a registration body for the use of the SF-36. It has compiled a battery of outcome indicators for a wide range of medical conditions, including stroke. The tools were constructed on the basis of analyses of longitudinal data on patients' experiences. The first principle that they applied to scale construction was to capture outcomes that were relevant to stroke, and secondly to include data that provided estimates of stroke severity, on the basis that these were early predictors of stroke outcome. The third principle was to keep the form simple. The elements of the TyPE specification were derived from a complete review of the literature, and inclusion of expert opinion (from neurologists and health services researchers). They encourage users to supplement the Stroke TyPE Specification with other scales where required, as well as basic demographic information that might affect outcome (e.g. age, sex, marital status, socioeconomic status). The tool is licensed, and for a small fee users are kept informed of any updates.

The Stroke TyPE Specification consists of four forms (the first two are for the doctor to complete). The SF-36 is also included, with the recommendation that it is administered during the period of the acute hospitalization, and at 1 and 12 months after the stroke. The pack includes a form for the assessment of pre-stroke function by the patient (or carer, if necessary) in relation to the extent of limitation in a range of activities (e.g. walking, writing, driving, speaking); a form for the doctor to complete on the severity of the patient's disability after the stroke (e.g. walking, etc., as before), including items on confusion and depression; co-morbidity, level of consciousness, complications and level of care given; a form about post-stroke function to be completed by the patient (similar to the pre-stroke function form); and a form for the doctor to complete at 12 months on 'later outcomes', which concentrates on medical diagnosis.

The authors point out in the handbook that the range of diseases pre-coded on the forms are limited deliberately, on the grounds that their research indicated few neurological findings, that can be reliably measured, or were predictive of patient outcome, beyond the patient's level of consciousness on admission. The handbook points out the problem of assessing people once they are in hospital and instructs that it is important to determine the pre-stroke level of function. Thus the SF-36 should be administered with the instruction to patients that they should reply to the question in relation to their pre- stroke health state (responses at 1 and 12 months relate to function at that time).

The tools are extremely concise. Those who require a more detailed set of assessment tools relating to functional ability will prefer the set used by Wade and his colleagues (see below), although this TyPE tool has the advantage of being a broader measure of health status by virtue of inclusion of the SF-36. It may be preferable to include the SF-36, selected items from the TyPE tool combined with the functional ability scales suggested by Wade and his colleagues (below). A measure of psychiatric morbidity may also be required. Details of the TyPE tools for a range of disease conditions are available from the HOI, 2001 Killebrew Drive, Suite 122, Bloomington, MN 55425, USA.

Functional ability

Functional ability is one specific domain of health status, or health-related quality of life. When assessing the outcome of a disabling condition, such as stroke, the areas that will require inclusion in measurement tools will include the pathology, the impairment (e.g. central nervous system, skeletal, muscular, etc.), the resulting disability (e.g. speaking, walking, etc.) and the handicap (e.g. communication, mobility, etc.) (World Health Organization 1980). These concepts lead to the concept of dependency on other people or on service providers, although they should not be equated with dependency. As with the concept of handicap, functional dependency is a social consequence – societal attitudes and expectations decide on its definition and existence.

Much effort is spent on the reduction of disability in relation to mobility in stroke patients (Collen *et al.* 1991). Difficulties which may be experienced by patients suffering a stroke include difficulties in performing activities of daily living (e.g. washing, dressing self), mobility (e.g. walking) and aphasia. These are obvious dimensions to include on an outcome instrument. Spontaneous recovery should also be included, which may occur with or without formal care. Most stroke sufferers recover rapidly within the first 3 months (this should be noted as a time reference for a follow-up assessment), regardless of rehabilitation, although it is unusual for improvement to continue beyond 1 year (another time reference for follow-up) (Freemantle *et al.* 1992).

Various functional outcome measures have been used in studies of stroke. The Clearing House for Health Outcomes at the Nuffield Institute in Leeds currently cites four frequently cited outcome measures for stroke: the Activities of Daily Living (Katz & Akpom 1976); the Barthel Index (Mahoney & Barthel 1965; revised by Granger *et al.* 1979); the Quality of Well-being Scale (Bush 1984); and the Karnofsky Performance Scale (Karnofsky *et al.* 1948). The most popular functional ability scale in this area is the Barthel Index (Mahoney & Barthel, 1965). Others include the Frenchay activities index (see Wade *et al.* 1992), the Rivermead mobility index (Collen *et al.* 1991), and the Nottingham extended activities of daily living index (Nouri & Lincoln 1987). Others exist which have also been used with stroke patients, for example, the Rankin Scale (van Swieten *et al.* 1988; Bamford *et al.* 1989; Gijn *et al.* 1991). Not all are equally well tested, and perhaps the Barthel Index is the most well used, and has also been more recently tested with good results by Collin *et al.* (1988). This was designed for use in institutions and requires supplementation with items reflecting domestic (or 'elective') activities if used in community settings. These scales have been tested for reliability and validity by Wade *et al.* (1985, 1992) and Collen *et al.* (1990) in their evaluations of therapies for stroke patients, and have been more fully described by Wade (1992). Results for reliability and validity, on the whole, are so far good, but further testing is still required.

Wade and his colleagues use this group of functional indicators, including the nine-hole test of manual dexterity, the motricity index and functional ambulation categories (Holden *et al.* 1984; Heller *et al.* 1987; Collen & Wade 1990; Collen *et al.* 1990) because no one scale taps the wide range of disabilities that stroke patients can experience, and there was concern that the measures should detect the useful benefits of therapy that might be achieved, particularly in quality of walking and gait speed. Gait speed was chosen as the primary outcome measure by these authors in their evaluation of physiotherapy with stroke patients, and they list several references which illustrate the reliability and validity of this indicator (see Wade *et al.* 1992). A further advantage of including gait speed in a battery of measures of outcome is that it achieves the criteria of a ratio scale, as well as being simple. These authors reported that gait speed was, in fact, the only outcome measure which showed improvement (an 8% improvement in gait speed associated with treatment), confirming other research that gait speed is a more sensitive measure than scales of functional ability (Stewart *et al.* 1990; Wade *et al.* 1992). Wade *et al.* (1992) also recommend including a measure of starting and stopping to 'walk outside' in future studies, although large numbers of study patients would be needed in order to detect any changes in behaviour.

Psychiatric morbidity

Psychiatric morbidity is a key component of health status and health-related quality of life. If the researcher wishes to tap this dimension of health directly, it is wise to select a specific scale, rather than rely solely on the mental health items in a health status scale.

Diagnostic measurement scales should base their categories on one of the international diagnostic classifications. The Americans generally use the Diagnostic and Statistical Manual (DSM IV) of the American Psychiatric Association (1994), while the Europeans use the World Health Organization's International Classification of Diseases (ICD). ICD-9 has been extensively used in Europe, although it does not equate well with the DSM. However, ICD-10 was published in 1992 and the psychiatric section is more closely based on the earlier DSM III, to facilitate international comparisons. These are regarded as the gold standards for psychiatric classification.

The dimension of psychiatric morbidity that is most commonly measured is depression, although scales do exist for detecting general psychiatric morbidity, such as anxiety and depression. The most commonly used international scale of general psychiatric morbidity, across a wide range of patients, is Goldberg's General Health Questionnaire (GHQ). It is probably the most extensively tested scale for reliability, validity, and sensitivity to change and results are good (Goldberg 1978; Goldberg & Williams 1988). It has been translated into several languages, and adapted for use in many cultures. There are concerns that, as the GHQ includes psychosomatic items, it may measure physical health status, not only psychiatric morbidity.

Confidence in the use of the GHQ with frail or physically ill populations has been enhanced by the validation study recently conducted by Lewis & Wessely (1990), who used the GHQ and the Hospital Anxiety and Depression Scale (HAD) (Zigmond & Snaith 1983) with a sample of dermatology patients, and compared the results with a criterion – The Clinical Interview Schedule (Goldberg *et al.* 1970). The Hospital Anxiety and Depression Scale, unlike the GHQ, does not include questions which overlap with physical illness. In this respect it is a preferable scale to most other depression scales, although it has been less extensively tested than most. No difference was found between the GHQ and the HAD in their ability to detect cases of minor psychiatric disorder among a physically ill population. The HAD has been used with stroke patients by Wade *et al.* (1992).

There are numerous, fairly brief, scales for the measurement of depression, that readers might like to consider, for example, the Beck Depression Inventory (Beck *et al.* 1961). Several of these have been reviewed by Bowling (1991). In the USA the development of the eight-item depression scale, from the Medical Outcomes Study at RAND, is a promising development (the authors are also developing a six-item scale). As with all scales developed in other countries, some minor alteration of wording will be required, and tested, before adoption elsewhere (e.g. 'blue' is used for 'feeling sad') (Burnam *et al.* 1988).

Cognitive impairment

A measure of cognitive impairment is likely to be required. These are used routinely in research among people aged 65+, in order to assess for any effects on outcome and the validity of replies to questionnaires. Among the concise indicators of cognitive impairment, the most widely used include the Mental Status Questionnaire (Kahn *et al.* 1960), the Abbreviated Mental Test Score (Hodkinson 1972), and the Mini-Mental State Examination (Folstein *et al.* 1975).

For those concerned to assess cognitive impairment fully among older people, the most extensively tested and most widely used scale is the Geriatric Mental State, with its associated AGECAT computer package (Copeland *et al.* 1976; Dewey & Copeland 1986). Assessment tools for the measurement of mental status are, however, culture specific and should be used in cultures outside the country of creation only after careful adaptation and further testing. The Geriatric Mental State has been carefully adapted for use across the world. To date, none of the existing scales are very successful at distinguishing between Alzheimer and vascular dementias, apart from an ischaemic score which has been incorporated into a newer scale developed in the UK called CAMDEX (Roth *et al.* 1986). However, the CAMDEX interview takes about an hour, and it was designed to be administered by doctors, which limits its use in large-scale research. The range of scales for the measurement of Alzheimer's disease and related disorders has been reviewed by Jorm (1990).

Life satisfaction

Life satisfaction refers to an assessment of one's life, or a comparison, reflecting some perceived discrepancy between one's aspirations and achievement. Instruments assessing life satisfaction are increasing in popularity among researchers, in order to shift the balance of health status measures from a focus on negative aspects to the more positive. Life satisfaction measures include a balance of negative and positive items. Scales of morale and well-being tap overlapping dimensions.

The most commonly used scales are the Neugarten Life Satisfaction Scales (Neugarten *et al.* 1961), the Delighted–Terrible Faces Scale (Andrews & Withey 1976), the Philadelphia Geriatric Morale Scale (Lawton 1972, 1975), the Affect-Balance Scale (Bradburn 1969), and the General Well-being Schedule (Dupuy 1978). Most of these scales were developed for use with elderly people. The most popular scale among gerontologists now is the Philadelphia Geriatric Morale Scale, on the grounds of its superior results for reliability and validity. There is insufficient space here to describe these scales and they have been reviewed more fully elsewhere (Bowling 1991). An important dimension of psychological well-being to measure is self-esteem. There are numerous, but fairly long, scales of self-esteem, some of which were reviewed by Bowling (1991). Self-image or self-esteem has been investigated successfully in neurology patients by Collings (1990) using more concise 20 seven-point semantic differential rating scales (Osgood *et al.* 1957).

A further dimension of social health that should be included in health status scales is social support. There is no space to review these here, but a review of the most commonly used scales can be found again in Bowling (1991).

Epilepsies

Treatment for epilepsy may be medical or surgical, depending on type. Hauser (1987) pointed out that a small but sizeable number of people who develop epilepsy are considered to be medically intractable and be eligible for consideration for surgical intervention. Surgery does not always stop seizures. Nor can surgery necessarily reverse any existing pattern of disability, social difficulties, impaired performance, but, by virtue of aiming to affect seizures, it aims to help. The question of whether patients are 'better' following epilepsy surgery has not been resolved, although many specialists report good results (Taylor 1987). Standardized results from throughout the world from the first International Conference on Surgical Treatment of the Epilepsies in 1987, reproduced by Spencer & Spencer (1991) show that results of respective procedures are widely discrepant. Between 26% and 80% of patients were reported to be seizure-free after temporal lobectomy, 0–73% after extratemporal resection, and 0–100% after hemispherectomy. Figures for 'worthwhile' and 'no' improvement were similarly variable. On average, 55% of patients were seizure free after temporal lobectomy, 43% after extratemporal resection, and 77% after hemispherectomy. These data were a powerful reason for further studies of patient outcome following surgery. Vickrey *et al.* (1993) report on the literature that suggests that surgery controls seizures in two-thirds of selected patients, although they point to other literature that indicates that surgery may adversely affect quality of life for some patients by imposing new problems, in particular of memory.

The assessment of outcome requires the assessment of the patients before and after the surgical intervention. As with other conditions, the retrospective collection of data on presurgical state after surgery has been performed may be unreliable due to recall bias, and may be influenced by the patients' and carers' expectations of surgery. Follow-up periods in the literature vary tremendously, from 6 months to several years. Spencer & Spencer (1991) report that some centres follow up patients at 5 years, and some for 10 or 15 years, although others have much shorter follow-ups.

The assessment of outcome

Most of the scales referred to in the previous sections can be used with patients with epilepsy (with the exception of the disease or function-specific scales), although their applicability may not be perfect. Wade (1992) notes that 'the major effects of epilepsy are probably at the level of handicap ... there are no good measures for use at this level with epilepsy'. In addition, scales to measure personality disorder, psychiatric disorder (e.g. psychosis) and suicidal tendency, intellectual impairment, social functioning, sexual problems and aggression may be required when evaluating the effects of surgical intervention (Taylor 1987; Dodrill & Wilensky 1990). Vickrey *et al.* (1993) have reviewed the international literature on assessing quality of life of epilepsy patients. Among the scales most commonly used are the Washington Psychosocial Seizure Inventory (Dodrill 1978; Dodrill *et al.* 1980), the Minnesota Multiphasic Personality Inventory (Dahlstrom *et al.* 1972; Hathaway & McKinley 1990), the Beck Depression Inventory (Beck *et al.* 1961), the Sickness Impact Profile (Deyo *et al.* 1982, 1983), the Epilepsy Surgery Inventory (Vickrey *et al.* 1992), the Quality of Well-Being Scale (Kaplan *et al.* 1976; Bush 1984), the SF-36 (Ware & Sherbourne, 1992), and the General Health Questionnaire (Goldberg 1978). Some of these scales were referred to earlier. The Health Outcomes Clearing House in Leeds cites the Epilepsy Surgery Inventory as a major reference (Vickrey *et al.* 1992).

Seizure control and other physical indicators of outcome

Outcome should be evaluated according to the aims of the intervention. At the most basic level, the aim of surgery is presumably seizure control (see above). The assessment of outcome thus necessitates the collection of data on preoperative frequency of seizures and variations in seizure patterns, duration and severity. Self-reports can be subject to recall bias and subjectivity in assessments, although adult patients are still the best source of information about seizures, and it has been suggested that they be encouraged to keep seizure diaries (Hayes *et al.* 1993).

An outcome classification relating pattern and type of seizures has been developed by the Temporal Lobe Club, and has been reproduced by Engel (1987). Hayes *et al.* (1993) report that the assessment of seizure severity is difficult, although they refer to recent attempts to develop such scales as encouraging, for example the Chalfont Seizure Severity Scale (Duncan & Sander 1991). Hayes *et al.* (1993) also report on the development of a patient-based seizure severity scale, which includes items on perception of control (Baker *et al.* 1991). These scales are reviewed by Hayes *et al.* 1993) and Vickrey (1993). The use of some such classification is essential, given that surgery does not always stop seizures, although far more development and assessment of existing measures is required.

Also to be included are details of medication, co-morbidity, adverse effects and complications. Mortality is also a pertinent indicator. Pre- and postoperative data on neurological status will be required. In addition to the results of diagnostic tests relating to neuropsychologic evaluation, data will be required on other morbidity relating to the presurgical state of the patient, early postoperative and long-term morbidity (Hauser 1987).

Functional ability

Functional ability, or disability, will require measurement because of associated disorders, or as a consequence of seizure (e.g. falls leading to fractures). However, Vickery *et al.* (1993) report that most patients who are considered for temporal lobectomy are independent in activities of daily living, although they argue that measures tapping the latter should be included in case of any disability resulting from surgical complications. The range of functional ability scales has been reviewed by Bowling (1991), although the SF-36 contains some items which tap this dimension, and which may be adequate.

Psychiatric status

The incidence of preoperative psychosis was estimated by Jensen & Larsen (1979) to be 15%, and almost all the patients they studied had evidence of some psychiatric disorder. It is not known how representative their findings are of other patients with epilepsy. Spencer & Spencer (1991) briefly reviewed the literature on outcome, and reported that there was a suggestion of some improvement in neurotic, aggressive and personality traits after respective procedures, although preoperative psychoses were unchanged. They also report that there appears to be a high rate of postoperative suicide, and of significant postoperative psychosis in 5–15% of patients after temporal lobectomy. Each of these dimensions requires measurement.

Psychological and social measurements

Most psychological scales used with epileptic patients were developed for use either with other types of patients, or for use with a population sample. Personality assessment has usually involved the Minnesota Multiphasic Personality Inventory, either the version for adults or that for adolescents and children (Welsh & Dahlstrom 1956; Dahlstrom *et al.* 1972; Hathaway & McKinley 1990).

Commonly used scales of psychiatric status include the Present State Examination (Wing *et al.* 1974), and, in the case of depression, the Hamilton (Hamilton 1967) and the Beck (Beck *et al.* 1961) Depression Scales. The most commonly used IQ test is the

Wechsler Intelligence Scale (Matazzaro 1972; Wechsler 1986). American and UK adaptations are available from the distributors. Just because scales are well known and widely used does not always imply that they are to be recommended. For example, the Wechsler Memory Scale will not necessarily distinguish between people with brain damage and those with non-psychotic functional disorders (see review by Dye 1982).

Rarely has an attempt been made to develop a single scale to evaluate psychological problems among epileptics. One attempt to develop a scale to permit a comprehensive assessment of psychosocial problems among epileptics is the Washington Psychosocial Seizure Inventory (Dodrill 1978; Dodrill *et al.* 1980).

Broader measures of health status and health-related quality of life

Outcome measurement in epilepsy surgery has traditionally focused on changes in seizure frequency and type, although the ultimate goal of surgery is to improve quality of life (Vickrey *et al.* 1993). Broader indices of outcome in relation to health-related quality of life in epilepsy have focused variously on independence in living, functional ability, psychiatric status, the quality of family and friendship relationships, social activities, sexual adjustment and performance at work or school. Hayes *et al.* (1993) reviews studies using these indicators. Social support networks; IQ, socioeconomic status and level of education have been suggested as affecting outcome and will require including in an assessment tool. In addition, dimensions of personality or social adjustment may be affected by surgery and will also require inclusion (e.g. ability to interact with others, employment, performance at work or school, or in usual main roles such as parent, sexual function and driving). Improvement in social adjustment, including improved social relationships, might also be included as an outcome measure (Taylor & Falconer, 1968). Spencer and her colleagues (personal communication) are considering the utility of including suitable scales of adaptive behaviour in the assessment of outcome, such as the Vineland Adaptive Behaviour Scales (Volkmar *et al.* 1987). This scale, which includes communication, daily living skills, socialization and motor skills (depending on age group) was developed for use with autistic children and adults, with good results for reliability and validity.

The relevant dimensions for inclusion in a health-related quality of life scale for epilepsy patients have been extensively discussed by Vickrey *et al.* (1993). They suggest the inclusion of physical symptoms (see previous discussion on severity of seizures, etc.), physical functioning (see previous section), role activities (e.g. ability to remain in employment, school or manage a household, driving), mental health, cognitive functioning (e.g. verbal memory deficits, IQ [controlling for effects of medication]), social functioning (e.g. the ability to develop and maintain relationships with friends and kin), general health perceptions, life satisfaction, energy/fatigue, sleep and rest. All scales require further development in order to incorporate specific questions on patient expectations of, and satisfaction with, the outcome.

The Washington Psychosocial Inventory

A commonly used measure to assess health-related quality of life outcome of treatment for epilepsy is The Washington Psychosocial Inventory (Dodrill 1978; Dodrill *et al.* 1980). The Washington Psychosocial Inventory provides some measure of psychological and social adjustment, specific to epilepsy, and patient satisfaction (Dodrill 1978; Dodrill *et al.* 1980). It contains 132 yes/no items and is based on self-report methods. It is easy to administer and score, and is reported by the authors to be acceptable to patients. It is suitable for people aged 16 and over. It covers family background, emotional adjustment, interpersonal adjustment, vocational adjustment, financial status, adjustment to seizures, management of medication, overall psychosocial functioning and patient satisfaction. Hayes *et al.* (1993) point out that the scale does have important omissions, particularly in relation to cognitive distress, physical functioning, energy/fatigue and overall quality of life. Vickrey *et al.* (1993) also point out that a limitation of this scale in longitudinal research is the inclusion of some items that would not be expected to change on retesting (e.g. the items asking whether something had ever occurred).

The Epilepsy Surgery Inventory

An improvement on this scale is the Epilepsy Surgery Inventory (ESI-55) which testing so far reveals to be reliable, valid and sensitive to differences in seizure status (Vickrey *et al.* 1992). This includes the increasingly popular SF-36 (see earlier) as a generic core measure (Ware & Sherbourne 1992), and supplements this with disease (epilepsy) specific items. This collection of measures contains 55 items (the 36 SF-36 items, supplemented with 19 additional items) and assesses physical health (physical function, role limitations, pain), mental health (emotional well-being, cognitive function, role limitations due to emotional problems and memory problems), and general health (health perceptions, energy/fatigue, overall quality of life, social function) as well as an item on change in health status (Vickrey *et al.* 1992; Hayes *et al.* 1993). Despite all these items, the completion time is just 15 minutes.

Conclusion

In conclusion, it is worthwhile reemphasizing that the outcome of intervention and rehabilitation can no longer be viewed solely in terms of morbidity and mortality, particularly given the debate about whether to survive in a vegetative state is no better than death, or even worse (Jennett, 1976). An important dimension of health to measure is broader health status, or health-related quality of life. This broader concept encompasses physical, psychological and social health, and encompasses the patient's subjective view of the outcome. The measurement of health-related quality of life requires the inclusion of an overall index of health status, and perceptions of health, of functional ability, pain, relevant dimensions of mental health, life satisfaction, coping ability, social support and integration. It is inevitably based on subjective feelings and attitudes. Disease-specific measures require supplementation with a broader set of indicators if they are to tap health-related quality of life.

Numerous scales of health status have been developed, and used by social scientists for many years. However, their use by clinicians has been limited due to their excessive length. Progress is now being made with the development of shorter scales. An exciting development in health status measurement are the measures developed from the RAND Medical Outcomes Study in the USA, in particular the SF-36 which is currently being tested for applicability across a wide range of conditions. Even where this broad indicator is chosen, however, a range of disease specific and function specific scales will still be required, as well as scales measuring specific dimensions of health where an improvement will be expected (e.g. depression, memory, pain, etc.). Interest among clinicians in the use of broader measures of health status is on the increase, alongside the realization that intervention and therapy have to be evaluated in relation to whether they lead to an outcome of a life worth living in social, psychological and physical terms. The obstacles in incorporating these measures into clinical practice have been discussed by Wagner and Vickery (1995).

References

American Psychiatric Association (1992). *Diagnostic and Statistical Manual of Mental Disorders*, 3rd edn, DSM-IV. Washington, DC: American Psychiatric Association.

Andrews, F. M. & Withey, S. B. (1976). *Social Indicators of Wellbeing. Americans' Perceptions of Life Quality.* New York: Plenum Press.

Baker, G. A., Smith, D. F., Dewey, M., Morrow, J., Crawford, P. M. & Chadwick, D. W. (1991). The development of a seizure severity scale as an outcome measure of epilepsy. *Epilepsy Res.* **8**, 245–51.

Bamford, J. L., Sandercock, P. A. G., Warlow, C. P. & Slatterly, J. (1989). Inter-observer agreement for the assessment of handicap in stroke patients. *Stroke* **20**, 828.

Bardsley, M. J. & Coles, J. M. (1992). Practical experiences in auditing patient outcomes. *Qual. Health Care* **1**, 124–30.

Bardsley, M. J., Venables, C. W., Watson, J., Goodfellow, J. & Wright, P. D. (1992). Evidence for validity of a health status measure in cholecystectomy. *Qual. Health Care* **1**, 10–14.

Beck, A. T., Mendelson, M., Mock, J. *et al.* (1961). Inventory for measuring depression. *Arch. Gen. Psychiatry* **4**, 561–71.

Bowling, A. (1991). *Measuring Health. A Review of Quality of Life Measurement Scales.* Milton Keynes: Open University Press.

Boysen, G. (1992). The Scandinavian Stroke Scale. Cerebrovascular diseases, *Second Eur. Stroke Conf. Issue* (abstracts) **2**, 239–40.

Bradburn, N. M. (1969). *The Structure of Psychological Wellbeing.* Chicago: Aldine Press.

Brazier, J., Harper, R., Jones, N. M. B., O'Cathain, A., Thomas, K. J., Usherwood, T. & Westlake, L. (1992). Validating the SF-36 health survey questionnaire: new outcome measure for primary care. *Br. Med. J.* **305**, 160–4.

Brooks, N. (1984). *Closed Head Injury. Psychological, Social and Family Consequences.* Oxford: Oxford University Press.

Brott, T. (1992). Utility of the NIH Stroke Scale. Cerebrovascular diseases. *Second Eur. Stroke Conf. Issue* (abstracts) **2**, 241–2.

Brott, T., Adams, H. P., Olinger, C. P., Marler, J. R., Barsan, W. G., Biller, J., Spilker, J., Holleran, R., Eberle, R., Hertzberg, V., Rorick, M., Moomaw, C. J. & Walker, M. (1989). Measurements of acute cerebral infarction. A clinical examination scale. *Stroke* **20**, 864–70.

Burnam, M. A., Wells, K. B., Leake, B. & Landsverk, J. (1988). Development of a brief screening instrument for detecting depressive disorders. *Med. Care* **26**, 775–89.

Bush, J. W. (1984). General health policy model: quality of well-being (QWB) scale. In: Wenger, N. K., Mattson, M. E., Furberg, C. D. *et al.* (eds.). *Assessment of Quality of Life in Clinical Trials of Cardiovascular Therapies.* New York: Le Jacq.

Collen, F. M., Wade, D. T. & Bradshaw, C. M. (1990). Mobility after stroke: reliability of measures of impairment and disability. *Int. Disability Stud.* **12**, 6–9.

Collen, F. M., Wade, D. T., Robb, G. F. & Bradshaw, C. M. (1991). The Rivermead Mobility Index: a further development of the Rivermead Motor assessment. *Int. Disability Stud.* **13**, 50–4.

Collin, C. & Wade, D. T. (1990). Assessing motor impairment after stroke: a pilot reliability study. *J. Neurol. Neurosurg. Psychiatry* **53**, 567–9.

Collin, C., Wade, D. T., Davis, S. *et al.* (1988). The Barthel ADL Index: a reliability study. *Int. Disability Stud.* **10**, 61–3.

Collings, J. A. (1990). Psychosocial well-being and epilepsy: an empirical study. *Epilepsia* **31**, 418–26.

Copeland, J. R. M., Kelleher, M. J., Kellet, J. M. *et al.* (1976). A semi-structured clinical interview for the assessment and diagnosis of mental state in the elderly. The Geriatric Mental State: Schedule I. Development and reliability. *Psychol. Med.* **6**, 439–49.

Cote, R., Battista, R. N., Wolfson, C., Boucher, J., Adam, J. & Hachinski, V. (1989). The Canadian Neurological Scale: validation and reliability assessment. *Neurology* **39**, 638–43.

Cote, R. & Hachinski, V. (1992). The Canadian Neurological Scale. Cerebrovascular Diseases. *Second Eur. Stroke Conf. Issue* (abstracts) **2**, 243–44.

Dahlstrom, W. G., Welsh, G. S. & Dahlstrom, L. E. (1972). *An MMPI Handbook*, vol. 1, Minneapolis: University of Minnesota Press.

Dewey, M. E. & Copeland, J. R. M. (1986). Computerised psychiatric diagnosis in the elderly: AGECAT. *J. Microcomp. Appl.* **9**, 135–40.

Deyo, R. A., Inui, T. S., Leininger, J. D. *et al.* (1982). Physical and psychological functions in rheumatoid arthritis: clinical use of a self-administered instrument. *Arch. Intern. Med.* **142**, 879–82.

Deyo, R. A., Inui, T. S., Leininger, J. D. *et al.* (1983). Measuring functional outcomes in chronic disease: a comparison of traditional scales and a self-administered health status questionnaire in patients with rheumatoid arthritis. *Med. Care,* **21**, 180–92.

Dodrill, C. B. (1978). A neuropsychological battery for epilepsy. *Epilepsia* **19**, 611–23.

Dodrill, C. B. & Wilensky, A. J. (1990). Intellectual impairment as an outcome of status epilepticus. *Neurology* **40**, 23–7.

Dodrill, C. B., Batzel, L. W., Queisser, H. R. & Temkin, N. R. (1980). An objective method for the assessment of psychological and social problems among epileptics. *Epilepsy* **21**, 123–35.

Donabedian, A. (1985). *Explorations in Quality Assessment and Monitoring*, vols. 1–3. Ann Arbor, Michigan: Health Administration Press.

Duncan, J. S. & Sander, J. W. A. S. (1991). The Chalfont Seizure Severity Scale. *J. Neurol. Neurosurg. Psychiatry* **54**, 873–6.

Dunnell, K. & Cartwright, A. (1972). *Medicine Takers, Prescribers and Horders*. London: Routledge and Kegan Paul.

Dupuy, H. J. (1978). Self-representations of general psychological well-being of American adults. Paper presented at American Public Health Association meeeting, 17 October, Los Angeles, California.

Dye, C. (1982). Intellectual functioning. In: Mangen, D. J. & Peterson, W. A. (eds.). *Research Instruments in Social Gerontology*, vol. I, *Clinical and Social Psychology*. Minneapolis: University of Minnesota Press.

Engel, J. (1987). Outcome with respect to epileptic seizures. In: Engel, J. (ed.). *Surgical Treatment of the Epilepsies*. New York: Raven Press.

Folstein, M. F., Folstein, S. E. & McHugh, P. R. (1975). Mini-mental state. A practical method for grading the cognitive state of patients for the clinician. *J. Psychiatr. Res.* **12**, 189–98.

Freemantle, N., Pollock, T. A., Sheldon, T. A., Mason, J. M., Song, F., Long, A. F. & Ibbotson, S. (1992). Formal rehabilitation after stroke. *Qual. Health Care* **1**, 134–7.

Gijn, J. van & members of the Dutch TIA Trial Study Group (1991). A comparison of two doses of aspirin (30 mg vs 283 mg a day) in patients after a transient ischaemic attack of minor ischaemic stroke. *N. Engl. J. Med.* **325**, 1261–6.

Goldberg, D. P. (1978). *Manual of the General Health Questionnaire*. Windsor: NFER-Nelson.

Goldberg, D. P. & Williams, P. (1988). *A User's Guide to the General Health Questionnaire*. Windsor: NFER-Nelson.

Goldberg, D. P., Cooper, B., Eastwood, M. R. *et al.* (1970). A standardised psychiatric interview for use in community surveys. *Br. J. Prev. Soc. Med.* **24**, 18–23.

Granger, C. V., Albrecht, G. L. & Hamilton, B. B. (1979). Outcome of comprehensive medical rehabilitation: measurement by PULSES profile and the Barthel Index. *Arch. Phys. Med. Rehabil.* **60**, 145–54.

Hamilton, M. (1967). Development of a rating scale for primary depressive illness. *Br. J. Soc. Clin. Psychol.* **6**, 278–96.

Hathaway, S. & McKinley, J. (1990). *Minnesota Multiphasic Personality Inventory*. Reference code: 0090. Windsor: NFER.

Hauser, A. (1987). Postscript: how should outcome be determined and reported? In: Engel, J. (ed.). *Surgical Treatment of the Epilepsies*. New York: Raven Press.

Hayes, R. D., Vickrey, B. G. & Engel, J. (1993). Postscript: epilepsy surgery outcome assessment. In Engel, J. (ed.). *Surgical Treatment of the Epilepsies*, 2nd edn. New York: Raven Press.

Heller, A., Wade, D. T., Wood, V. A., Sunderland, A., Langton-Hewer, R. & Ward, E. (1987). Arm function after stroke: measurement and recovery over the first three months. *J. Neurol. Neurosurg. Psychiatry* **50**, 714–19.

Hodkinson, H. M. (1972). Evaluation of a mental test score for the assessment of mental impairment in the elderly. *Age Ageing* **1**, 233–8.

Holden, M. K., Gill, K. M., Magliozzi, M. R., Nathan, J. & Piehl-Baker, L. (1984). Clinical gait assessment in the neurologically impaired: reliability and meaningfulness. *Phys. Therapy.* **64**, 35–40.

Horowitz, M. J. & Cohen, F. M. (1968). Temporal lobe epilepsy: effect of a lobectomy on psychosocial functioning. *Epilepsia* **9**, 23–41.

Hunt, S. M., McEwan, J. & McKenna, S. P. (1986). *Measuring Health Status*. London: Croom Helm.

Jachuck, S. J., Brierly, H., Jachuk, S. *et al.* (1982). The effect of hypotensive drugs on the quality of life. *J. R. Coll. Gen. Pract.* **32**, 103–5.

Jennett, B. (1976). Resource allocation for the severely brain damaged. *Arch. Neurol.* **33**, 595–7.

Jennett, B. & Bond, M. (1975). Assessment of outcome after severe brain damage. *Lancet* I, 734–7.

Jensen, I. & Larsen, K. (1979). Mental aspects of temporal lobe epilepsy. *J. Neurol. Neurosurg. Psychiatry* **42**, 256–65.

Jorm, A. F. (1990). *The Epidemiology of Alzeheimer's Disease Related Disorders.* London: Chapman and Hall.

Kahn, R. L., Goldfarb, A. I., Pollack, M. *et al.* (1960). Brief objective measures for the determination of mental status in the aged. *Am. J. Psychiatry* **117**, 326–8.

Kaplan, R. M., Bush, J. W. & Berry, C. C. (1976). Health status: types of validity and the Index of Wellbeing. *Health Serv. Res.* **11**, 478–507.

Karnofsky, D. A., Abelmann, W. H., Craver, L. F. *et al.* (1948). The use of nitrogen mustards in the palliative treatment of carcinoma. *Cancer,* **1**, 634–56.

Katz, S. & Akpom, C. A. (1976). Index of ADL. *Med. Care* **14**, 116–18.

Kind, P. & Carr-Hill, R. (1987). The Nottingham Health Profile: a useful tool for epidemiologists? *Soc. Sci. Med.* **25**, 905–10.

Krischer, J. P. (1979). Indexes of severity: conceptual development. *Health Serv. Res.* **14**, 56–67.

Lawton, M. P. (1972). The dimensions of morale. In: Kent, D., Kastenbaum, R. & Sherwood, S. (eds.). *Research, Planning and Action for the Elderly.* New York: Behavioural Publications.

Lawton, M. P. (1975). The Philadelphia Geriatric Center Morale Scale: a revision. *J. Gerontol.* **30**, 85–9.

Lewis, G. & Wessely, S. (1990). Comparison of the General Health Questionnaire and the Hospital Anxiety and Depression Scale. *Br. J. Psychiatry* **157**, 860–4.

Lindenstrom, E., Boysen, G., Christiansen, L. W., Rogvi-Hansen, B. & Nielsen, P. W. (1991). Reliability of Scandinavian neurological stroke scale. *Cerebrovasc. Dis.* **1**, 103–7.

Linn, B. S., Linn, M. W. & Gurel, L. (1968). Cumulative illness rating scale. *J. Am. Geriatr. Soc.* **16**, 622–6.

Long, A. F., Bate, L. & Sheldon, T. A. (1992). Establishment of UK clearing house for assessing health services outcomes. *Qual. Health Care* **1**, 131–3.

Mahoney, F. I. & Barthel, D. W. (1965). Functional evaluation: the Barthel Index. *Maryland State Med. J.* **14**, 61–5.

Matazzaro, J. D. (1972). Wechsler's measurement and appraisal of intelligence. Baltimore: Williams and Wilkins.

Neugarten, B. L., Havighurst, R. J. & Tobin, S. S. (1961). The measurement of life satisfaction. *J. Gerontol.* **16**, 134–43.

Nouri, F. M. & Lincoln, N. B. (1987). An extended activities of daily living scale for stroke patients. *Clin. Rehabil.* **1**, 301–5.

Orth-Gomer, K., Britton, M. & Rehnqvist, N. (1979). Quality of care in an out-patient department: the patient's view. *Soc. Sci. Med.* **13A**, 347–57.

Osgood, C. E., Suci, G. T. & Tannenbaum, P. H. (1957). *The Measurement of Meaning.* Urbaba, Illinois: University of Illinois Press.

Rausch, R. & Crandall, P. H. (1982). Psychological status related to surgical control of temporal lobe seizures. *Epilepsia* **23**, 191–202.

Roth, M., Tym, E., Mountjoy, C. Q. *et al.* (1986). CAMDEX: a standardised instrument for the diagnosis of mental disorder in the elderly with special reference to the early detection of dementia. *Br. J. Psychiatry* **149**, 698–709.

Scandinavian Stroke Study Group (1985). Multicentre trial of hemodilution in ischemic stroke. Background and study protocol. *Stroke* **16**, 885–90.

Scandinavian Stroke Study Group (1987). Multicentre trial of hemodilution in ischemic stroke. *Stroke* **18**, 691–9.

Slevin, M. L., Plant, H., Lynch, D. *et al.* (1988). Who should measure quality of life, the doctor or the patient? *Br. J. Cancer* **57**, 109–12.

Spencer, S. S. & Spencer, D. D. (1991). Dogma, data and directions. In: Spencer, S. S. & Spencer, D. D. *Surgery for Epilepsy.* Oxford: Blackwell Scientific Publications.

Stewart, A. L. & Ware, J. E. (eds.). (1992). *Measuring Functioning and Wellbeing. The Medical Outcomes Study Approach.* Durham, North Carolina: Duke University Press.

Stewart, A. L., Sherbourne, C., Hays, R. D. *et al.* (1992). Summary and discussion of MOS measures. In: Stewart, A. L. & Ware, J. E. (eds.). *Measuring Functioning and Wellbeing. The Medical Outcomes Study Approach.* Durham, North Carolina: Duke University Press.

Stewart, D. A., Burns, J. M. A., Dunn, S. G. & Roberts, M. A. (1990). The two-minute walking test: a sensitive index of mobility in the rehabilitation of elderly patients. *Clin. Rehabil.* **4**, 273–6.

Taylor, D. C. (1987). Psychiatric and social issues in measuring the input and outcome of epilepsy surgery. In: Engel, J. (ed.). *Surgical treatment of the Epilepsies.* New York: Raven Press.

Taylor, D. C. & Falconer, M. A. (1968). Clinical, socio-economic and psychological changes after temporal lobectomy for epilepsy. *Br. J. Psychiatry* **114**, 1247–61.

Thomas, M. R. & Lyttle, D. (1980). Patient expectations about success of treatment and reported relief from low back pain. *J. Psychosom. Res.* **24**, 297–301.

van Swieten, J. C., Koudstaal, P. J., Visser, M. C., Schouten, H. J. A. & van Gijn, J. (1988). Inter-observer agreement for the assessment of handicap in stroke patients. *Stroke* **19**, 604–7.

Vickrey, B. G., Hays, R. D., Graber, J., Rausch, R., Engel, J. & Brook, R. H. (1992). A health-related quality of life instrument for patients evaluated for epilepsy surgrery. *Med. Care* **30**, 299–319.

Vickrey, B. G., Hays, R. D., Hermann, B., Bladin, P. F. & Batzel, L. (1993). Quality of life outcomes. In Engel, J. (ed.). *Surgical Treatment of the Epilepsies*, 2nd edn. New York: Raven Press.

Volkmar, F. R., Sparrow, S. S., Goudreau, D., Cicchetti, D. V., Paul, R. & Cohen, D. (1987). Social deficit in autism: operational approach using the Vineland Adaptive Behaviour Scales. *J. Am. Acad. Child Adolesc. Psychiatry* **26**, 156–61.

Wade, D. T. (1988). Measurement in rehabilitation. *Age Ageing* **17**, 289–92.

Wade, D. T. (1992). *Measurement in Neurological Rehabilitation.* Oxford: Oxford University Press.

Wade, D. T., Legh-Smith, G. L. & Langton-Hewer, R. (1985). Social activities after stroke: measurement and natural history using the Frenchay Activities Index. *Int. Rehabil. Med.* **7**, 175–81.

Wade, D. T., Collen, F. M., Robb, G. F. & Warlow, C. P. (1992). Physiotherapy intervention late after stroke and mobility. *Br. Med. J.* **304**, 609–13.

Wagner, A. K. & Vickery, B. G. (1995). The routine use of health-related quality of life measures in the care of patients with epilepsy: rationale and research agenda. *Quanlity of Life Research* **4**, 169–71.

Ware, J. E. (1984). Methodological considerations in the selection of health status assessment procedures. In: Wenger, N. K., Mattson, M. E., Furberg, C. D. *et al.* (eds.). *Assessment of Quality of Life in Clinical Trials of Cardiovascular Therapies.* New York: Le Jacq.

Ware, J. E. & Sherbourne, C. D. (1992). The MOS 36-item Short Form Health Survey (SF-36). I. Conceptual framework and items selection. *Med. Care* **30**, 473–83.

Wechsler, D. (1986). *Wechsler Adult Intelligence Scale*, revised UK edn, (WAIS-R UK), reference code 9000GC. Sidcup: Psychological Corporation (Harcourt, Brace, Jovanovich).

Welsh, G. S. & Dahlstrom, W. G. (1956). *Basic Readings on the MMPI in Psychology and Medicine.* Minneapolis: University of Minnesota Press.

Wing, J. K., Cooper, J. E. & Sartorius, N. (1974). *The Measurement and Classification of Psychiatric*

Symptoms: An Instruction Manual for the PSE and Catego Programme. Cambridge: Cambridge University Press.

World Health Organization (1958). *The First Ten Years. The Health Organization.* Geneva: World Health Organization.

World Health Organization (1980). *International Classification of Impairments, Disabilities and Handicaps.* Geneva: World Health Organization.

World Health Organization (1992). *International Classification of Diseases*, 10th edn. Geneva: World Health Organization.

Zigmond, A. S. & Snaith, R. P. (1983). The Hospital Anxiety and Depression Scale. *Acta Psychiatr. Scand.* **67**, 361–70.

3 Cost-benefit analysis

CHARLES NORMAND AND ANN BOWLING

Introduction

When applied to health and health services, the purpose of cost-benefit analysis is to identify and provide those services that have the largest effects on health (Drummond 1980; Drummond *et al.* 1997; Mooney *et al.* 1986; Le Grand *et al.* 1992). This means that we should not provide services that have no useful effects, or those that are likely to be damaging to health. Many services can do good, but there is also a risk that they will do harm. One important criterion is that the expected benefit exceeds the expected harm by a sufficient margin to justify taking the risk.

Applying cost-benefit analysis also means that we need to avoid those interventions that do some good, *but not enough to justify inclusion in the programme.* This is where the difficult decisions lie, since we know that services that are medically useful will be denied to patients. However, the justification for the cost-benefit approach is that it allows us to choose to spend the health service resource to better effect.

Cost-benefit analysis provides a framework for choices. It is not a set of rules that makes choices. There are two reasons for this. First, the techniques are not sufficiently developed for simple decision rules to be applied. Second, cost-benefit analysis can only be as good as the data that are used. Often these data are not complete, and assumptions and estimates have to be used. It is better to see cost-benefit analysis as a useful way of thinking about problems rather than as a set of decision rules.

Cost-benefit analysis is about health. It is not really about money, although it is about using the available money to generate the largest possible improvement in health. There should be no conflict between the objectives of medical and nursing staff, who want to see the best outcomes for patients, and the cost-benefit approach that tries to focus services where the impact is greatest. It is important to understand the practical significance of the difference between the objectives of cost-benefit analysis and minimizing costs. In the former case costs are minimized *for any level of benefits*, but there is no prejudice in favour of lower costs if this is associated with lower benefits (Drummond *et al.* 1987). It is hard to argue for waste and extravagance (not least because this means that people who could be offered treatment are denied it), but small savings with large losses of benefit cannot easily be justified.

The problem of scarcity

As with all other services, health care provision is always constrained by resources. The advent of new (but often costly) technologies has made this fact more visible, but there has never been a time when resources were adequate to provide all treatment and care that does some good. For practical purposes we can assume that need for health care (in the sense of a capacity to benefit from treatment or care) is infinite (Normand 1991), but much of the need is for services that have quite little effect. More resource can be helpful in extending the range of needs that can be met, but cannot (and indeed should not) ensure that all needs are met. Better funding of health services may be very desirable, but there will always be a need to limit health services, and for priorities to be set.

Choices in neurology and neurosurgery

Cost-benefit analysis is concerned with identifying priorities. It attempts to help answer questions such as 'should computed tomography (CT) scans be given to all patients following stroke?' or 'should magnetic resonance (MR) scans be offered to patients with suspected multiple sclerosis (MS)?' (Hutton & Maisey 1991; Hutton *et al.* 1990). It can also help in decisions about treatment options. Many people are offered rehabilitation services following stroke, and this might be extended to all patients, but such a policy should depend on being able to show that the services is cost-effective (Freemantle *et al.* 1992). Similarly there are choices of some treatments being performed in inpatient, outpatient or primary care settings, and whether or not certain treatments should be provided at all.

Health care professionals often identify the best ways for providing services. For example, it is sometimes argued that work currently carried out by general medicine specialists should be transferred to neurologists or vice versa. Whether or not this should happen depends on the effects of such a change on the health of patients, and the knock-on effects on other services if extra resources are needed. The aim of cost-benefit analysis is to ensure that such choices are made on the basis of costs and outcomes.

The cost-benefit framework

Cost-benefit analysis has its origins in welfare economics, which is the branch of economic theory concerned with answering normative (what should be) questions. In terms of ethical principles it is utilitarian (Gillon 1986), that is it is concerned with attempting to increase the overall level of welfare by increasing the welfare of individuals. This is sometimes described as seeking the greatest happiness for the greatest number.

The challenge is how to measure costs and benefits. This section is concerned with the measurement of costs, the measurement of benefits and the problems when the two are brought together.

Measuring costs

Health services are very diverse. Different services are provided by different professionals in different combinations to different people. One of the most difficult things in measuring costs is the definition of the service that is being costed.

At one time in centrally managed and funded health care systems the measurement of cost of individual items or episodes of care was considered unimportant. Managers and health care professionals worked within a fixed budget to provide those services that they perceived to be the highest priorities. The trend in most countries towards more decentralized management of the provision of care, and the more explicit use of cost-benefit approaches to setting priorities for services, has led to a need to be more explicit in identifying the costs of individual services. This need had separately been identified in health care systems in which services are funded by insurance (such as the USA), where the insurance organizations have become concerned about the overall cost of services, and the lack of mechanisms to control costs.

Methods of classifying cases have existed for many years, such as the disease classification systems, for example ICD-9 and ICD-10 (WHO 1978, 1992) and systems of surgical codes. The problem is that there are thousands of different categories, and each of these can occur in many different circumstances. What was needed was a simpler system, taking into account the disease, the treatment and the type of patient. The best-known system of classifying cases is Diagnosis Related Groups (DRGs), which aim to put together classes of treatment and patients that have similar treatment costs. Four hundred and eighty five categories were originally identified. Examples of DRGs in neurology are DRG 25 (seizure and headache, age over 17, no complications) and DRG 13 (Multiple sclerosis and cerebellar) (HSI 1988).

The desire for simplicity led to the merging of a range of cases or types of patients into a single group. There is a range of expected costs for treating patients within a group. Providers of health care became skilled at identifying cases where the costs were relatively low, and chose only to treat those. This practice, known as "cream-skimming", allowed hospitals to be more profitable. A result of this is that the new systems of classification, including DRGs, are introducing additional categories.

A further problem in obtaining clear classification of cases is that there is some genuine uncertainty and difference of opinion as to which category is correct for some individuals. Where cases are classified as moderate or severe, or where the presence or absence of co-morbidity is important, then there is scope for judgement as to the appropriate category. When in doubt, and where fees for higher DRGs are greater than those for lower ones, then there is a strong incentive to choose the higher. The trend for cases to be classified in higher categories is known as DRG creep.

Research is continuing on methods of case classification, and rival systems of defining case-mix are available. All aim to provide a more definitive way of describing the required work, which in turn allows costs to be calculated. Failure to account for case-mix makes comparison of costs meaningless. A stroke unit with a predominantly elderly mix of patients will have different costs for treatment and different lengths of stay than one with a higher proportion of younger patients. There are continued arguments about the reasons for higher costs in teaching hospitals and tertiary referral centres. Part of these arguments concerns the mix of cases being treated.

To the economist there is only one sensible way to describe a cost: it is an opportunity foregone. For example, the cost of a day of training is the time and other inputs by the trainers (which could otherwise provide training for other people), the work that would otherwise have been done, or the leisure time lost for the trainees. The cost of a surgical procedure is the decision not to offer the same resources to another patient or provide this patient another procedure. Economists call this notion *opportunity cost* (Le Grand *et al.* 1992). Whenever costs are being measured, the attempt is to get as close as possible to opportunity costs.

Opportunity cost is often very different from expenditure. Equipment provided by a charity is not paid for by the hospital, but nevertheless has an opportunity cost since it could be used to treat other patients. Opportunity cost is sometimes less than the expenditure. Surplus buildings may have a very low opportunity cost, since they may have no alternative use, but still attract rent or capital charges.

An easy way for a health care provider to reduce cost to itself is to pass on the cost. For example, if patients are discharged earlier from hospital (whether for good or bad reasons), some of the cost will be transferred to the primary care services, to relatives and friends and to patients themselves. From the point of view of cost-benefit analysis, there is no particular advantage in savings to one party that are offset by costs to another. Cost shifting is often undesirable, since there is no benefit in terms of better care, and no overall savings. Centralization of services can have this effect. It may be possible to lower the cost of direct provision of care by using fewer staff and making better use of facilities and equipment, but there can be offsetting costs in terms of higher ambulance and private transport costs.

Costing must be carried out in full knowledge of the service provided, and the ways in which the pattern of services will change with changing scale. There is no simple answer to the question 'what is the cost of this service?'. Depending on the problem being addressed, the appropriate estimate will vary. For example, if the problem is to discover the cost of an expansion of the service, or to identify savings from bed closures, the need is to identify the change in cost (marginal cost), which will contain little or no overheads. An interesting example of this has come in the studies of the process of closure of continuing care hospitals.

Traditional hospital facilities for people with mental health problems, learning difficulties and physical disabilities have been reduced in size and in some places closed altogether. It is common for funds to be withdrawn from the hospital as the numbers of patients in them decline, but the question is, how much money should be withdrawn and made available to the new providers in the community? (Normand & Taylor 1987; Korman & Glennerster 1990).

There are two problems. First, it is not possible to save all the fixed costs, so that the removal of average cost (that is the total cost divided by the number of patients) has the effect of cutting the resources available for those patients remaining in hospital. Second, and often more important, the care needs of those selected to be the first to leave hospital are often quite different from those of the people who remain in hospital, who are usually more dependent. It is usually easier to provide alternatives to hospital care for people who are fairly independent. Evidence shows that the cost of continuing care in hospital can be as low as £5000 and as high as £80 000 per person per year (Dockrell *et al.* 1993). It is therefore important to know about the care needs of individual patients before coming to conclusions about costs.

The point of the discussion above is to emphasize that cost is difficult to measure even when overall expenditure is known. Costing requires knowledge of what service is provided for whom and how. It is too difficult a task to pass on to the accountants. Cost may be quite different from observed expenditure, and the correct estimate of cost should reflect the opportunity cost of the resources used.

An illustration of the importance of interdisciplinary assessment of costs and benefits is the way in which extra-contractual referrals (ECRs) are controlled in the British NHS. Joint decisions between those concerned with finance and public health doctors about the criteria for ECRs are, in effect, exercises in cost-benefit analysis, that are seen as particularly important for high-cost treatments.

In cost-benefit analysis, costs and benefits are measured for an intervention and compared with the costs and benefits had the intervention not taken place. It is seldom the case that the alternative to a treatment is simply no involvement with health and other caring services. For example, a person whose disability leads to a need for residential or nursing care may be treated to restore physical functioning, and eliminate the need for expensive care. Equally a person may be successfully treated for coronary heart disease, but survive to require expensive dementia services.

In principle the cost of an intervention should be measured in terms of all the additional costs falling on all parties as a result of the intervention, net of all the savings. There are a few treatments that can clearly be shown to save resources by eliminating future care needs. Successful screening for congenital dislocation of the hip, with relatively inexpensive non-invasive treatment is such a case (Kernohan *et al.* 1990). Many other treatments can lead to reductions in the need for treatment and care, but this will only occur some of the time. For example, some interventions to diagnose an untreatable condition can be justified through eliminating expensive (and sometimes dangerous) treatments for other diseases with similar symptoms.

Looking at the costs in this way means that an apparently cheap treatment turns out in fact to be quite expensive once the consequences are considered. For example, earlier discharge from hospital saves resources, but can increase community care costs, and may lead to higher readmission rates. It is only cheaper if these knock-on cost effects are smaller than the original savings. However, if a more expensive treatment is chosen, it may be justified, but this must be done in terms of subsequent savings, longer life or better health.

Measuring benefits

The benefit of a health care intervention is the difference between the outcome and the outcome in the absence of the intervention. It is therefore important to assess the most likely outcome without treatment if we are to obtain an accurate measure of success. This is often difficult. For many common diseases and well-established treatments, there is no chance to observe the natural history, and therefore we have only limited knowledge of the effectiveness of the treatment. Proper randomized controlled trials are often ruled out on ethical grounds since there is a belief that patients would be refused effective treatment. The ethics of providing treatments that have not been fully assessed may also be seen to be doubtful (Smith 1993).

The significance of a successful intervention depends on circumstances. A full cure may have a large impact, or may be of minor consequence when other diseases are present. It is often disappointing to observe an apparently successful intervention that does little or nothing to change morbidity or mortality in the population. This is often because the patient quickly develops other health problems, especially when the successful treatment is for elderly people (Langham *et al.* 1992).

Health care produces benefits of longer life and improvements in the quality of life (QOL). Especially in treatment of chronic conditions, it is important to consider the quality of the process (the experience of being a patient), since treatment and care may persist for the rest of the life of the patient.

It is important to focus on *extending* rather than *saving* life. A treatment that extends life by many years is likely to be a higher priority than one that does so for only a few weeks, although this will depend also on the effects on quality of life. The results of medical research often give only a poor guide to the extent of life-extending effects. It is difficult and expensive to follow up patients to calculate the full effects. It is easy to overestimate the effects of treatment, since those successfully made free of a particular disease may die early as a result of a related or unrelated problem.

In addition there is always a danger that an apparent effect on life expectancy is really a change in the lead time. For example, in earlier detection of disease through screening, the time from diagnosis to death can lengthen even if the time of death is unchanged. Naïve comparison of life expectancy following diagnosis and treatment can therefore exaggerate the benefit. Life-extending effects should be measured in comparison with what would have been the case in the absence of an intervention.

Some treatments do not aim to extend life, but rather to improve the quality of life. Economists have normally confined their interest to those elements of quality of life that are related to health status, so that what are described as quality of life measures are often more properly seen as health status indicators. They have also tended to take the view that a benefit of longer life or better quality of life should not take into account the age or circumstances of patients. The value of a treatment for an old person might be less because that person will enjoy the benefits for only a few years, but a year of full-quality life is considered the same for all.

Full health-related quality of life is where a person is in good health, and can therefore do all the things that would be expected of someone of that age. This leads to some difficulties in making comparisons. It might be argued that treatment for younger people restores a greater range of physical functioning, and therefore produces more health gain than that for older people.

People's expectations of what is good health varies, as does the importance of good health to different people. For some, physical fitness is necessary to pursue sporting interests, but for others there is less need for this. At the level of the overall priority for the use of resources this is not a very great problem, since it is the average that matters. However, at the level of the individual patient, it is important to consider the aspirations of that person, and not to assume gains to all will always be the same.

There is sometimes a trade-off between extending life and the quality of life for the patient. There is always a trade-off between using resources to extend life and using them to improve the quality of life. For example, there is clear evidence that expansion of haemodialysis in the UK could extend life for some people (albeit not by very long, and some people would have poor health), but interventions that improve the quality of life may be a higher priority.

The fact that treatment can affect both life expectancy and quality of life means that we need to be able to compare the effects of each. If the dilemma is between devoting resources to expanding dialysis, carrying out more heart surgery or doing more hip replacements (Williams 1985), the choice is between a life-extending and a quality of life-enhancing treatment. To make this comparison more explicitly, researchers have attempted to elicit the views of the population on the relative merits of life-extending and life-enhancing improvements. The aim of the research has been to explore the possibility of a single index of benefit, combining life extension and improvements in the quality of life (e.g. EuroQol[c] Group 1990). The result has been the Quality Adjusted Life Year, or QALY. A QALY is defined as a year in good health. If a treatment extends life by 1 year with full health, then the output is 1 QALY. Equally, if the treatment does nothing to lengthen life, but improves quality of life from two-thirds to full quality for 3 years, that is also a gain of 1 QALY.

In considering the debate around the use of QALYs, it is important to distinguish between the arguments about the idea and an aspiration to calculate and use QALYs, and the issues raised in the early attempt to make the idea operational. If we accept that health care resources need to be limited, as we must, then comparisons will be made between interventions that are mainly life extending and those that mainly improve health-related quality of life. In this sense, a comparison of the importance of improvements on both dimensions is made. It is possible to argue that the decision is political, and should be made through political processes, but there remains the difficulty that inconsistent decisions will be made. If an agreed trade-off between extending life and effecting improvement in health-related quality of life can be defined, then consistent decisions could be taken, taking into account the opinions of the population about each.

This leads to the conclusion that QALYs would be a good thing (Normand 1991). Separate judgements are needed as to the feasibility of deriving QALYs, and whether the progress so far justifies their use. Reasons for caution are the problems with single index outcome measures (and QALYs need a single health status/QOL index to combine with life extension to form an overall measure), small sample sizes in some of the existing studies, problems in determining whose opinions should be taken into account and some evidence of inconsistency in the responses received (Carr-Hill 1991).

Since health is multidimensional, many measures of health status (e.g. SF-36, Ware & Sherbourne 1992) provide a profile of health, with no predetermined importance for each dimension. It is always possible to impose weighting for each dimension and define a single index score, but many instruments were not designed for this purpose, and there is significant doubt about the reliability and validity of such indices. Single scores are available for some health status indicators, such as the Rosser Matrix (Rosser & Kind 1978) or the EuroQol[c], but neither of these has had the necessary validation work completed.

The argument between single index measures and profile measures will not be resolved quickly, but is based in part on the very different objectives in the attempts to measure health-related quality of life. For some purposes it is important to keep the dimensions of health gain separate (Cairns *et al.* 1991; Donaldson *et al.* 1988). People working on stroke rehabilitation have particular concerns with mobility, self-care and communication. Using a health status index with a strong emphasis on pain may not be appropriate, since the gains will appear diluted. Some profile measures are designed to be disease-specific, and lack dimensions required for a full index measure. There are therefore good reasons why some people who design or use profile measures object to their use in calculating index measures. However, for resource allocation purposes implicit or explicit combining of dimensions is unavoidable.

The arguments above concern the need for, but difficulty in obtaining, a single index measure of outcome, combining agreed changes in life expectancy and quality of life. A further set of problems relate to who should decide on the valuation given to different changes in life years and quality of life. A simple question is whether those with more experience of distress or disability (for example former or current sufferers from a disease) should have more say, since they have the necessary knowledge. However, we know that such people differ systematically in their views from those who have no experience. It is too early to know whether the current research will demonstrate a degree of consensus on the valuation of health status, but it may be difficult to detect one.

One reason for interest in disease-specific measures is the probable importance of context in determining the effect on a patient of a given level of disability. For example, disability resulting from MS may be similar in terms of ability to perform tasks as some spinal injuries, but the patient's knowledge of the disease process can be important in determining the attitude to it (McGuire *et al.* 1988). Temporary disability for 1 month may be borne for that month more cheerfully than a permanent restriction. On the other hand, people develop strategies for coping with disabilities, so that the impact of context may be complex.

Although there are many difficulties with the measurement of benefits, and much criticism of the use of QALYs, the problem of scarcity, the need to make choices, and the consequent need to compare different interventions on the same basis means that attempts will continue to derive acceptable ways of combining life-extending and quality of life-enhancing benefits in a single index.

Applying cost-benefit analysis to neurology and neurosurgery interventions

Cost-benefit analysis is both a set of techniques and a way of thinking. It can be applied to questions of what diseases should be treated, which patients with these diseases should be treated and which treatment should be offered. It can in principle be used in the decision to treat or not to treat a particular patient, but this conflicts with the normal objective of clinicians to provide the best treatment for the individual currently needing help. It is therefore more common to apply cost-benefit analysis formally in the context of making available facilities and services. However, this may lead to decisions not to offer treatment to categories of patients who would benefit, but not enough to justify the use of the scarce resources.

Neurology and neurosurgery cover a wide range of diagnostic, treatment, rehabilitation and continuing care services. Attempts have been made to apply cost-benefit analysis in all these areas, with different approaches being compared, and some attempt to compare interventions to other medical and surgical services. Here, some of the issues and results arising from these studies, and some of the implications for the application of cost-benefit analysis will be considered.

Diagnostic services present particular challenges for cost-benefit studies, since the justification of interventions must be to provide better treatment and care. Better diagnosis is cost-effective if the resources used lead to longer life being possible or better quality of life. It can be particularly difficult to justify additional tests when the answer is certain or highly probable. In the case of stroke, the evidence suggests that clinical diagnosis (without the use of scanning) is seldom wrong (Wade 1992). The use of magnetic resonance imaging (MRI) has been considered in a cost-benefit framework (Hutton *et al.* 1990).

MRI has applications in conforming the diagnosis of MS. However, there is no established cure for MS. The question is whether there are sufficient benefits in terms of avoiding other inappropriate treatment, better care or important psychological advantages that justify the use of MRI. In some of its applications (for example in replacing myelography) MRI may be justified on the ground of reducing pain, risk and suffering by patients. In others it can lower costs (as in investigation of knees). In MS the certainty of diagnosis is aided by MRI, producing patient and physician benefits, but the effect on treatment and management, at present, is, perhaps, not so large.

There are interesting arguments on some of the applications of MRI to scanning heads. Surgeons may operate with slightly better knowledge, and may sometimes make a different decision about the treatment. Again it is important to consider what would otherwise have happened. To an extent scanning using X-ray tomography is a cheaper substitute, and it must be established that there are sufficient benefits to justify the additional cost. Lower levels of ionizing radiation have been used as an argument, but the risk associated with X-ray scanning can be shown to be slight (Hutton *et al.* 1990). Despite the apparent advantages over alternatives, MRI can be shown to be a cost-effective tool for diagnosis in only some neurological and neurosurgical work. This does not deny its usefulness in research, and the superiority over other diagnostic equipment, but simply that the additional benefit cannot justify the additional costs. It could also be argued that the instrument used to measure benefit in the clinical application of MRI in comparison with other imaging techniques does not yet capture the perceived medical and surgical benefit in patient management. Similarly, reviews of studies on the effectiveness and cost-effectiveness of stroke rehabilitation show that there is currently very little good evidence (Freemantle *et al.* 1982). Most of the inputs to rehabilitation have never been systematically evaluated (McKenna *et al.* 1992) Physiotherapy and occupational therapy services seem to make a useful contribution (although it is not clear whether this improvement is long-lasting), and there is conflicting evidence on the effectiveness of speech therapy for aphasia. For evidence of cost-effectiveness there is first a need to demonstrate effectiveness. Thus, there may be very significant benefits from rehabilitation (Wade 1992), the problem being the lack of well-designed studies that can demonstrate the existence of such benefits. However, this requires randomizing patients to what are believed to be less effective treatments or to receive no rehabilitation service in a full prospective trial.

The main justification of additional resources for continuing care is the improvement in quality of life. It may be possible to support people in their own homes, even when it would be cheaper to provide residential care. Within residential care additional resources can provide more privacy, independence and choice (Dockrell *et al.* 1993).

In making comparisons between neurological and neurosurgical services and other health care it is important to remember that many other well-established services have never been subjected to rigorous trials, and the evidence supporting their use is correspondingly often weak. Many 'life-saving' treatments do little to extend life, and there are questions about the usefulness of some common treatments for advanced cancers.

Cost-benefit analysis can lead to questioning the priority of existing services, especially where costs are high and effectiveness has not been demonstrated. It can also lead to a higher priority to be given to some undramatic but useful services. It is particularly important to retain a focus on the outcome in terms of longer life and a better quality of life, since this may help to justify services that do nothing to prevent premature death, but can be very helpful in improving the quality of the remaining life.

References

Cairns, J., Johnston, K. & McKenzie, L. (1991). *Developing QALYs from Condition Specific Measures*. Aberdeen: University of Aberdeen, HERU discussion paper 91–114.

Carr-Hill, R. A. (1991). Current practice in obtaining the 'Q' in QALYs: a cautionary note. *Br. Med. J.* **305**, 699–701.

Dockrell, J. E., Gaskell, G., Normand, C. & Rehman, H. (1993). Service provision for people with mild learning difficulty and challenging behaviour: the MIETS evaluation. In Kiernan, C. (ed.) *Research to Practice? Implications of Research on the Challenging Behaviour of People with Learning Disabilities*. London: BIMH.

Donaldson, C., Atkinson, A., Bond, J. & Wright, K. (1988). Should QALYs be programme specific? *J. Health Econ.* **7**, 47–57.

Drummond, M. F. (1980). *Principles of Economic Appraisal in Health Care*. Oxford: Oxford University Press.

Drummond, M. F., O'Brien B., Stoddart, G. L. & Torrance, G. W. (1997). *Methods for the Economic Evaluation of Health Care Programmes*, 2nd Edition. Oxford: Oxford University Press.

EuroQol Group (1990). EuroQol^c: a new facility for the measurement of health-related quality of life. *Health Policy* **16**, 199–208.

Freemantle, N., Ibbotson, S., London, A. *et al.* (1992). *Effective Health Care – Stroke Rehabilitation*. Leeds: University of Leeds.

Gillon, R. (1986). *Philosophical Medical Ethics*. Chichester: Wiley.

HSI (1988). *Diagnosis Related Groups, 5th revision, Definitions Manual*. New Haven: Health Systems International.

Le Grand, J., Propper, C. & Robinson, R. (1992). *The Economics of Social Problems*, 3rd edn. Basingstoke: Macmillan.

Hutton, J. & Maisey, M. N. (1991). *Guidelines for the Evaluation of Radiological Technologies*, BIR Working Party Report. London: British Institute of Radiology.

Hutton, J., Leese, B., Williams, A. & Burton, H. (1990). *Economic Evaluation of the Clinical Application of MR Imaging*. York: University of York, Centre for Health Economics.

Kernohan, W. G., Trainor, B. P., Mollan, R. A. B. *et al.* (1990). Cost-benefit appraisal of screening for congenital dislocation of the hip. *Management Med.* **4**, 230–5.

Korman, N. & Glennerster, H. (1990). *Hospital Closure*. Milton Keynes: Open University Press.

Langham, S., Piercy, J., Normand, C. & Rose, G. (1992). *Epidemiologically Based Needs Assessment – Coronary Heart Disease*. Leeds: NHS Management Executive.

McGuire, A., Henderson, J. & Mooney, G. (1988). *The Economics of Health Care*. London: Routledge and Kegan Paul.

McKenna, M., Maynard, A. & Wright, K. (1992). *Is Rehabilitation Cost-effective?* CHE/HEC Discussion Paper 101. York: University of York.

Mooney, G. H., Russell, E. & Weir, R. (1986). *Choices for Health Care*. Bassingstoke: Macmillan.

Normand, C. (1991). Economics, health and the economics of health. *Br. Med. J.* **303**, 1572–7.

Normand, C. & Taylor, P. (1987). *The Decline in Patient Numbers in Mental Handicap Hospitals: How The Cost Savings Should be Calculated*. CHE/HEC Discussion Paper 26. York: University of York.

Rosser, R. & Kind, P. (1978). A scale of valuations of states of illness: is there a consensus? *Int. J. Epidemiol.* **7**, 347–58.

Smith, R. (1993). GMC in the dock again. *Br. Med. J.* **306**, 82.

Wade, D. T. (1992). Epidemiologically based needs assessment: stroke (acute cerebrovascular disease). Leeds: NHS Management Executive.

Ware, J. E. & Sherbourne, C. D. (1992). The SF-36 Short-Form health status survey. I. Conceptual framework and items selection. *Med. Care* **30**, 473–83.

Williams, A. (1985). The economics of coronary artery bypass grafting. *Br. Med. J.* **249**, 326–9.

World Health Organization (1978). *International Classification of Disease*, 9th revision. Geneva: WHO.

World Health Organization (1992). *International Classification of Disease*, 10th Revision. Geneva: WHO.

4 Imaging of the nervous system

B. SCHUKNECHT AND A. VALAVANIS

Outcome research in neuroradiology is focused on two mainstays: diagnostic and interventional neuroradiology. The objective of diagnostic neuroradiology is to establish an accurate diagnosis and reveal criteria with respect to prognosis and optimal patient treatment. Adequate and rational utilization of the 'instrumentarium' of imaging techniques is mandatory. This has witnessed a dramatic change since the development of ventriculography and pneumencephalography in 1918–19 by W. E. Dandy, the introduction of myelography in 1922 by Sicard and the advent of cerebral angiography in 1927 by E. Moniz (Taveras 1990). However, the introduction of computed tomography (CT) and magnetic resonance imaging (MRI) have exerted the greatest impact on the development of neuroradiology as a specialty within the 'neurosciences' (Bucci 1991). The use of ionizing radiation by CT, myelography, angiography on the one hand, and the use of ultrasound and radiowaves of particular frequency by Doppler sonography and MRI respectively, result in differing diagnostic capabilities available for a broad spectrum of physiological and pathological conditions. PET, magnetic resonance angiography and functional imaging, and Doppler sonography, have extended the information provided from a mere morphological to a functional level. With interventional neuroradiology a rapidly developing specialty is providing a therapeutic alternative to surgery in many vascular pathologies. Tables 4.1–4.7 conceptualize our experience by attributing a specific diagnostic modality to the most frequent pathologies. Taking into account that access to hardware and software even among university hospitals differs, the potential of the currently used imaging devices is discussed with particular emphasis on criteria affecting patient prognosis and improving our ability to forecast outcomes.

Computed tomography

Rapid access, easy repeatability of individual CT slices and facilitated patient surveillance have attributed to CT the role of a primary imaging modality in emergency as well as non-emergency situations (Table 4.1a,b). This holds particularly true in the management of trauma patients, where the presence of epidural and subdural haematomas, a midline shift and shearing injuries in central locations have severe adverse effects on

Table 4.1a. *Computed tomography emergency diagnostic evaluation*

Head and neck, orbital, temporal bone trauma
Spinal trauma
Acute cervical or lumbar radicular syndrome
Space-occupying lesions: neoplastic, inflammatory, vascular
Decompensated hydrocephalus
Subarachnoid haemorrhage
Dural and venous sinus thrombosis
Post-therapeutic/postoperative complications
Orbital/labyrinthine complications of adjacent inflammation

Table 4.1b. *Computed tomography elective diagnostic evaluation*

Neoplastic, inflammatory, vascular lesions
Follow-up after trauma, surgery, conservative treatment
Epilepsy, dementia, psychiatric disorders
Radicular and non-radicular spinal symptomatology
3D-reconstruction in dental, maxillofacial and spinal surgery
3D-angio CT to characterize intracranial aneurysms
Xenon-CT in cerebrovascular disease, arteriovenous malformations
CT-cisternography in CSF-rhinorrhoea
CT-guided stereotaxic lesion localization

patient survival (Levi *et al.* 1990). Peripherally located cerebral shearing injuries and the extent of cortical and subcortical contusions are relevant with respect to functional prognosis and the likelihood of post-traumatic epilepsy (Berger *et al.* 1985). However CT compared with MRI is more likely to miss bland contusions than haemorrhagic ones (Gentry *et al.* 1988). Early post-traumatic and postoperative complications are delineated to better advantage by CT. Recognition of subarachnoid haemorrhage is time-dependent with a significant loss of sensitivity between the first and fourth day after haemorrhage. The location of the subarachnoid clot within the interpeduncular cistern correlates with a frequently negative angiogram and good prognosis (Rinkel *et al.* 1991). Conversely, subarachnoid blood exceeding 5 mm in thickness in the sylvian cistern accounts for a high proportion of delayed vasospasm and a high secondary morbidity (Kistler *et al.* 1983).

In stroke, exclusion of primary haemorrhage is readily performed by CT. Recognition of subtle signs like the 'dense artery sign' indicates major cerebral artery thromboembolism in the middle cerebral or vertebrobasilar territory and subsequent ischaemia (Schuknecht *et al.* 1990). The application of stable xenon-CT not only allows early recognition of infarction but a functional evaluation of the cerebral circulatory reserve capacity in patients with proximal cerebral artery stenosis or occlusion (Johnson *et al.* 1991). The degree of mass effect within 5 to 6 days after middle cerebral artery infarction correlates with a negative effect on patient prognosis as opposed to the often incidental finding of a partial haemorrhagic transformation of an ischaemic infarct.

The hallmark of venous sinus thrombosis is a combination of signs like the 'empty triangle' or 'delta sign', the 'cord' sign, haemorrhagic infarction or oedema (Wodarz *et al*. 1982). Recognition of these signs leading to early diagnosis and institution of therapy are particularly dependent on a high degree of suspicion and a meticulous examination technique. Visibility of hypodense striatal lesions within 6 hours and the presence of the acute 'reversal sign' are indicators of a severe cerebral hypoxia with early mortality of 80% and 50% respectively (Han *et al*. 1990; Huber & Schuknecht 1991). Since the introduction of CT in the mid-1970s mortality has significantly declined in patients with cerebral abscess and subdural empyema (Schuknecht *et al*. 1988). This also holds true for earlier recognition and therapy of herpes simplex encephalitis (Ketonen & Koskiniemi 1980).

In traumatic, neoplastic and inflammatory lesions affecting the osseous structures of the skull base, temporal bone and spinal column CT has proved to be superior in delineating detailed morphology but at the expense of reduced sensitivity as compared with scintigraphy and MRI. Refinements of hardware and software have extended the application of high-resolution CT so that functional and cosmetic postoperative results benefit from the ability of CT volumetric calculations and 3D reconstructions particularly in traumatic midface reconstructive surgery (Manson *et al*. 1986; Levy *et al*. 1992).

Application of intravenous and, in case of traumatic and non-traumatic CSF rhinorrhoea, intrathecal contrast media, increase the diagnostic sensitivity and specificity of CT examinations.

Non-stochastic effects of radiation exposure have to be taken into account in examinations effecting the lens (Fridrich 1991), where exposure in dental CT examinations was measured to be 0.7 mGy for 10 slices (Schuller *et al*. 1992). Gantry angulation modifications in brain and petrous bone examinations avoiding the lens reduce the dose applied by 90% (Torizuka *et al*. 1992; Yeoman *et al*. 1992).

Magnetic resonance imaging

High sensitivity, multiplanar imaging capability, superior soft tissue resolution and the lack of ionizing radiation render magnetic resonance the imaging modality of choice in a wide number of applications summarized in Table 4.2. The superiority of MRI over CT is evident with respect to intra-axial lesion detection, delineation and characterization. This holds true in patients with epilepsy, where symptomatic lesions such as mesial temporal lobe sclerosis, neoplasia, infection and vascular lesions e.g. cavernomas are detected with superior sensitivity. Furthermore, criteria for potential surgical therapy are provided. The superior sensitivity of MRI allows the early institution of therapy in patients with intra- and extra-axial manifestation of primary and secondary central nervous system malignancy, infectious diseases and inflammatory conditions (Lester *et al*. 1988; Haimes *et al*. 1989). Recognition and anatomical delineation of central nervous system malignancy and the effects of surgery, radiotherapy and chemotherapy are monitored to better advantage by MRI (Hudgins *et al.* 1991). Better delineation of low-grade glioma with histological recognition of tumour cells in areas of increased T2 signal intensity lead to a more precise definition of tumour boundaries by MRI compared with CT (Kelly *et al.* 1987). Delineation of extra-axial space-occupying lesions in the posterior and anterior cranial fossae with respect to the course of cranial nerves and the dural coverings contribute to improved surgical results and earlier recognition of recurrence. After radio- and/or chemotherapy early warning identification of toxic side effects on the white matter is provided (Ball *et al.* 1992), but differentiation of radionecrosis from recurrent tumour occasionally is difficult.

Superiority of MRI compared with CT is evident in certain anatomic locations such as the apex orbitae, sella, cerebellopontine angle, parotid and parapharyngeal space (Curtin 1987; Hansberger & Osborne 1991), where recognition of infection or small tumors is often feasible. The application of contrast media is mandatory in these locations as it is required to differentiate cystic intra-axial lesions. Intramedullary, intra- and extradural spinal lesions are rendered visible to better advantage by MRI. MRI not only demonstrates earlier manifestations of leptomeningeal neoplastic and inflammatory disease but allows visualization of paravertebral extension, of osseous involvement and recognition of spinal cord compression occurring between areas of myelographic block. Higher sensitivity renders MRI the primary imaging modality in the recognition and follow-up of spontaneous or post-traumatic diskitis. The sequelae of trauma to the spinal cord (Silberstein *et al.* 1992), to the basal frontal and temporal lobe and the corpus callosum (Hesselink *et al.* 1988) are delineated to better advantage by MRI. In patients with multiple sclerosis MRI not only serves diagnostic purposes, but provides information as to the time course of disease and therapy effects (Kappos & Radü 1991).

With MRI paediatric neuroimaging has undergone a dramatic change. Recognition of heterotopias is facilitated as well as demyelinating and dysmyelinating conditions (Valk 1991). Patients with dysraphic conditions and their complications benefit with respect to the less invasive and more accurate character of the diagnostic procedure and therefore potentially improve surgical results.

Due to its non-invasive character MR-angiography has begun to supersede some indications for cerebral angiography. Investigations of the patency of major cerebral arteries and dural sinuses, pre- and post-therapeutic evaluation of patients with arteriovenous malformations and fistulas can be performed with MR angiography.

The potential of functional and metabolic imaging exerted by magnetic resonance imaging and proton spectroscopy is directed towards tumor and myelin metabolism and in multiple sclerosis is under intensive investigation (Grossman *et al.* 1992; Posse *et al.* 1993).

Adverse effects exerted by the static magnetic field rule out the examination of patients with cardiac stimulators and ferric iron implants. The biological effects of local heat transmission due to closely applied surface coils are reduced with adequate patient and coil positioning within the magnetic bore. Perfusion studies with intra-

Table 4.2. *Magnetic resonance diagnostic evaluation*

Intra- and extra-axial neoplastic, inflammatory disease of brain
Vertebral column neoplastic, inflammatory, degenerative disease
Post-traumatic, posthypoxic sequelae
Vascular malformations, dissections, venous anomalies
Epilepsy, neurodegenerative diseases
Development of myelination
White matter demyelinating and dysmyelinating disease
Dysgraphic conditions, neuronal migration disorders
Neurovascular compression syndromes
MR-angiography in vascular pathology, vascular compromise
MR-spectroscopy in brain tumours, white matter disease
Functional MRI in order to localize visual/motor function

venous contrast agents have extended the information gained to the capillary level (Edelman *et al.* 1990).

Myelography

In the presence of magnetic resonance imaging the indications for lumbar and cervical myelography have significantly declined (Table 4.3). CT or MRI will frequently be diagnostic in cases with radiculopathy, low back pain and myelopathy due to disc herniation or the presence of a narrow spinal canal. Where available MRI has replaced myelography in the evaluation of extra- or intradural malignancy avoiding the potential for clinical deterioration observed in up to 10% of patients with myelographic block. Headache is the most frequent side effect of myelography. The need therefore to admit patients to hospital for at least one night increased the cost for myelography to twice the cost of MRI in a recent British evaluation (Du Boulay *et al.* 1990). The incidence of headache is known to correlate with the size of the needle employed, the location of puncture – headache being less frequent in cervical punctures – and the normality of the myelogram (Lee *et al.* 1990). The incidence has been noted to be reduced to 10% in patients with cervical myelography via direct lateral cervical puncture and the use of non-ionic monomeric contrast media (Volle *et al.* 1991).

Contrast media

The characteristics of an ideal contrast medium are maximum positive contrast enhancement, chemical and biological inertness and complete elimination from the body. While ionic high-osmolar compounds are sufficiently water soluble due to excellent hydrophilicity, they exhibit the negative effects of high osmalality such as bradycardia and negative cardiac inotropism. General side effects such as nausea and vomiting, and allergy-like reactions are three to eight times more frequent than in non-ionic agents. Non-ionic compounds have less pronounced haemodynamic effects and are better tolerated in intra-arterial injections. Still the antithrombotic effect is lower for non-ionic compared with ionic substances with at least a theoretically higher risk of thromboembolic events (Fritzsch *et al.* 1992). In patients with limited kidney function a dose-dependent further impairment is likely to occur, adequate hydration being one of the most important precautions to be taken. Isotonicity has been achieved with the dimeric substance iotrolan, which is particularly advantageous for application in myelography supported by its moderate viscosity. Superior tolerance has been achieved for the first contrast agents that received approval for magnetic resonance application, Gd-DTPA and Gd-DOTA. Both are hydrophilic, inert substances, being distributed in the interstitium after intravenous application.

Applications of 0.1–0.3 mmol/kg body weight have proved to be well tolerated with very few side effects such as headache, dizziness and nausea and a transient increase in serum iron and bilirubin. The use of Gadolinium as a contrast agent may reveal lesions not recognized on the unenhanced scan particularly in extra-axial locations, and in multiple sclerosis, will reveal additional lesions in a significant proportion of patients and result in a substantially increased diagnostic confidence of the examination. The recent introduction of stable air microbubbles bound to a galactose carrier represents significant progress in the evaluation of the intracranial circulation patients with insufficient signal in transcranial doppler ultrasound.

Doppler ultrasound

Doppler sonography has gained increasing recognition due to a broad spectrum of potential applications, listed in Table 4.4. Non-invasiveness, mobility of the examination device, easy repeatability, low costs and the ability for extra- and transcranial evaluation are the main advantages of this technique. Still the information gained relies very much on the experience of the examiner. Doppler sonography may be performed as pulse wave Doppler sonography or colour-coded Doppler sonography. Colour-coded Doppler sonography provides visual information as to the velocity of flow, the presence of turbulence and, with a B-mode image, gives additional evidence of pathological alterations of the extracranial vessel wall. Evaluation of cerebrovascular disease, diagnosis and follow up of vasospasm after subarachnoid haemorrhage are well-recognized indications. Pre- and post-therapeutic evaluation of patients prior to and after angioplasty of arteriovenous malformations or fistulas before and after embolization, is being increasingly recognized as a valuable adjunct to angiography in interventional neuroradiology.

PET

Positron emission tomography (Table 4.5) provides maps of the quantitative cerebral distribution of a tracer identified by evaluating the emission of isotopes. Different tracers are available, that serve as markers of cerebral blood flow, of neuroreceptors

Table 4.3. *Diagnostic evaluation by myelography*

Mono- and oligoradicular symptoms
Traumatic nerve root avulsion
Radicular or cord compromise after stabilization procedures

Table 4.4. *Doppler ultrasound evaluation*

Cerebrovascular disease
Assessment of arteriovenous malformations, fistulas
Postembolization control and follow-up in AVMs and AVFs
Assessment of vasospasm
Assessment of intracranial circulatory arrest

(Baron 1991), tumor metabolism (Fulham 1991) and blood–brain barrier disruption. The functional information provided may differentiate viable from ischaemic tissue in cerebrovascular disease (Brooks 1991) and may be utilized to distinguish high- from low-grade glioma (Di Chiro 1991; Frackowiak 1991). In the evaluation of epilepsy, dementia and movement disorders PET is gaining increasing importance not only with respect to the differential diagnosis among these diseases but in order to evaluate therapeutic effects and monitor the course of a disease.

Angiography

Angiography is the key investigatory device to detect, localize and quantify the extent of cerebrovascular disease (Table 4.6). Patients examined by angiography were noticed to have a better prognosis, when stenoses or occlusions were restricted to the verte-brobasilar system compared with those located within the carotid territory (Asplund *et al.* 1981). In many centres angiography is mandatory to select patients for reconstructive vascular surgery (Caplan & Wolpert 1991).

In the evaluation of patients suspected of harbouring an aneurysm angiography assumes a leading role. Knowledge of the aneurysm location, size, configuration of its neck, relation to the parent vessel and adjacent perforating arteries is required in order to decide on subsequent treatment – either surgical or interventional. Recognition of vasospasm by angiography may institute early therapy. Angiography assumes a leading role in the diagnosis, evaluation and therapy of arteriovenous malformations (AVM) and fistulas. Criteria for the timing and mode of treatment are derived from a meticulous analysis of the angioarchitecture (Valavanis 1997).

Prognostic factors comprise the presence of fistulas and related aneurysms, recognition of obstruction of the venous drainage in patients with AVM, and the presence of cortical venous drainage in dural AVM respectively.

Neurological complications in the course of or subsequent to cerebral angiography depend particularly on the duration of the examination. The rate of transient and

Table 4.5. *Indications for positron emission tomography (PET)*

Cerebrovascular disease
Brain tumours
Epilepsy, dementias
Neuroreceptor studies

Table 4.6. *Angiographic diagnostic evaluation*

Subarachnoid, intracerebral haemorrhage
Carotid, vertebral, cerebral artery dissection
Cerebral circulatory arrest
Cerebrovascular disease
Arteriovenous malformations, fistulas
Cervicofacial haemangiomas
Intractable epistaxis

permanent complications after cerebral angiography varies from 0.54% to 3.5% and 0.09% to 0.36% respectively (Grzyska *et al.* 1990). Fluoroscopy time is the major contributor to the patient's dose with an average proportion of 67% (Feygelman *et al.* 1992). Again the age of the patient examined and the experience of the neuroradiologist determine the duration of the examination and the dose applied. However, digital subtraction angiography reduces the dose to the orbit by a factor of four in intracranial examinations, and by a factor of 10 in cervical series (Gilgenbach *et al.* 1990).

Interventional neuroradiology

In an increasing number of vascular lesions diagnostic angiography is followed by endovascular therapy. The objective of endovascular therapy is to recanalize an occluded or stenotic vessel (recanalizing endovascular therapy) or to occlude a vascular lesion (occluding endovascular therapy).

Intra-arterial thrombolysis has been proposed as the therapy of choice in acute vertebrobasilar thrombosis. However, thrombolysis in the carotid territory – in the past a matter of debate – is gaining increasing acceptance as well. Recanalization rates of 80% in the middle cerebral artery territory appear to foster this strategy (Zeumer & Zenella 1993). But despite the fact that a proportion of vessels can be recanalized after urokinase or rTPA therapy, treatment in a significant number of patients even begun within 6 hours will be instituted too late to reach satisfactory functional recovery. Still, in an increasing proportion of patients superselective intravascular thrombolysis offers the only possibility for survival in acute major cerebral arterial thrombembolism. This therapy requires formal evaluation.

Transluminal angioplasty revealed excellent results in patients with haemodynamically significant stenosis in the vertebral and basilar arteries with clinical improvement found in 92.9% of cases treated (Higashida *et al.* 1993). Restenosis was recognized in 7%

after 1 year but was found in 16% after treatment of the carotid arteries (Monari *et al.* 1992). Permanent neurological deficit occurred in 7.1% and 6.8% of patients respectively.

Endovascular therapy has particularly gained benefit from the development of coaxial microcatheters, balloons and the introduction of smaller particulate and better fluid embolic materials. Increased selectivity of catheterization has rendered therapy of skull base and head and neck tumours feasible with improved procedural and subsequent surgical safety. This holds true for preoperative embolization of meningiomas, glomus tumours, angiofibromas and palliative embolization of neoplasms in patients considered poor candidates for surgery (Valavanis 1993). Due to superselectivity of deposition of embolic material in sphenopalatine septal branches the long-term success rate in patients treated for intractable epistaxis was increased to over 80%.

Due to the availability of microcatheters superselective embolization of the nidus of an arteriovenous malformation is feasible. The objective is to eliminate particular vascular components within or associated with the AVM that expose the patient to an increased risk of spontaneous haemorrhage. This is known to occur in 2 to 4% per year with an annual risk of mortality of 7% and morbidity of 13% (Valavanis 1991). Analysis of the angioarchitecture by angiography may predict the features of an increased risk of haemorrhage. These comprise associated aneurysms present in 10–15% of cases, high-degree stenoses or varices of draining veins and the presence of cortical venous drainage in cases of dural AVM. Therapy is primarily directed towards elimination of these components (Fox 1991). With increased experience, technical refinement and improved pre- and post-therapeutic evaluation by MRI and Doppler ultrasound the degree of embolization of the AVM and the safety of the procedure has significantly increased. Evaluation of intracranial vascular malformations by MRI and superselective angiography has provided a classification that is based on topography, angio architecture and haemodynamics leading to a concise endovascular therapeutic concept (Valavanis 1997).

Total occlusion of carotid-cavernous fistulas type A by balloon embolization is possible in 98% of patents with preservation of the internal carotid artery in 95%. Dural arteriovenous fistulas of the cavernous sinus (carotid cavernous fistulas type B) treated by different procedures are feasible in 94% of cases (Berenstein 1990).

Saccular aneurysms with a small neck and difficult surgical access are amenable to endovascular therapy. As opposed to endosaccular balloon therapy the application of detachable platinum coils (Guglielmi detachable coils, GDC) is promising. The rate of thrombosis was 100% in locations filled by the coil, with definite occlusion of the aneurysm being achieved in most of the cases treated (Guglielmi 1993). The GDC coils have found rapid acceptance in many centres in the world with the expectation of revolutionizing endovascular aneurysm therapy and significantly reduced morbidity. After aneurysm surgery a significant proportion of morbidity is related to vasospasm of the supraclinoid internal carotid, and the proximal middle and anterior cerebral arteries. The rapid inflation and deflation of a non-detachable balloon in segments of spasm in combination with heparin and/or papaverine might offer a chance to reverse vasospasm and vasospasm-related symptoms (Brothers & Holgate 1990; Eskridge 1991).

Non-vascular interventional techniques such as percutaneous diskectomy and intradiskal chemonucleolysis (Leonardi *et al.* 1993) have been developed. Strict application of clinical as well as radiological criteria have contributed to the development of these techniques as alternatives to surgery, potentially available on an outpatient basis. Morbidity and costs are potentially significantly reduced.

References

Asplund, K., Liliequist, B., Fodstad, H. & Ester, P. O. (1981). Long-term outcome in cerebrovascular disease in relation to findings at aortocervical angiography. A 12-year follow-up. *Stroke* **12**, 307–13.

Ball, W., Prenger, E. C. & Ballard, E. T. (1992). Neurotoxicity of radio/chemotherapy in children: pathologic and MR correlation. *AJNR* **13**, 761–76.

Baron, J. C. (1991). Neurotransmitter-receptor studies with PET. *Neuroradiology* **33** (Suppl.), 105.

Belliveau, D. W., Kennedy, D. N., McHinstry, R. C. *et al.* (1991). Functional mapping of the human visual cortex by magnetic resonance imaging. *Science* **254**, 716–19.

Berenstein, A. (1990). Cerebral arteriovenous malformations. Abstracts of the Seventh Annual Stonwin Medical Conference: Endovascular interventional neuroradiology. *AJNR* **11**, 217–28.

Berger, M. S., Pitts, L. H., Lovely, M., Edwards, M. S. & Bartkowski, H. M. (1985). Outcome from severe head injury in children and adolescents. *J. Neurosurg.* **62**, 194–9.

Brooks, D. J. (1991). PET in the evaluation of cerebrovascular disease. *Neuroradiology* **33** (Suppl.), 104.

Brothers, M. F. & Holgate, R. C. (1990). Intracranial angioplasty for treatment of vasospasm after subarachnoid hemorrhage. Technique and modifications to improve branch access. *AJNR* **11**, 239–47.

Bucci, V. A. (1991). Health outcomes research: its influence on clinical decision making and the development of new imaging technologies. *AJNR* **12**, 397–9.

Caplan, L. R. & Wolpert, S. M. (1991). Angiography in patients with occlusive cerebrovascular disease: views of a stroke neurologist and neuroradiologist. *AJNR* **12**, 593–601.

Curtin, H. D. (1987). Separation of the masticator space from the parapharyngeal space. *Radiology* **163**, 195–204.

Di Chiro, G. (1991). PET and the neuroradiologists. *Neuroradiology* **33** (Suppl.), 103.

Du Boulay, G. H., Hawkes, S., Lee, C.-C., Teather, B. A. & Teather, D. (1990). Comparing the cost of spinal MR with conventional myelography and radiculopathy. *Neuroradiology* **32**, 124–36.

Eddelman, R. R., Mattle, H. P., Atkinson, D. J. *et al.* (1990). Cerebral blood flow assessment with dynamic contrast-enhanced T2-weighted MR imaging. *Radiology* **176**, 211–20.

Eskridge, J. (1991). Angioplasty for cerebral vasospasm. *Neuroradiology* **33** (Suppl.), 137–8.

Feygelman, V. M., Huda, W. & Peters, K. R. (1992). Effective dose equivalents to patients undergoing cerebral angiography. *AJNR* **13**, 845–9.

Fox, A. J. (1991). Working group in interventional neuroradiology: 11th annual meeting. *AJNR* **12**, 798–804.

Fridrich, R. (1991). Zur Prolematik der Risikobewertung von diagnostischen Strahlendosen. *Schweiz. Med Wochenschr.* **121**, 1595–600.

Frackowiak, R. S. J. (1991). The role of PET in neuroradiology. *Neuroradiology* **33**(Suppl.), 103 4.

Fritzsch, T., Krause, W. & Weinmann, H. J. (1992). Status of contrast media research in MRI, ultrasound and X-ray. *Eur. Radiol.* **2**, 2–13.

Fulham, M. J. (1991). PET in brain tumors. *Neuroradiology* **33** (Suppl.), 104–5.

Gentry, L. R., Godersky, J. C., Thompson, B. & Dunn, V. D. (1988). Prospective comparative study of intermediate-field MR and CT in the evaluation of closed head trauma. *AJNR* **9**, 91–100.

Gilgenbach, R., Schröder, U. & Heuser, L. (1990). Strahlenexposition bei der Angiographie der hirnversorgenden Arterien. Ein Vergleich zwischen intrarterielller DSA und Blattfilmtechnik. *Fortschr. Röntgenstr.* **153**, 418–22.

Grossman, R. I., Lenkinski, R. E., Ramer, K. N., Gonzalez-Scarano, F. & Cohen, J. A. (1992). MR proton spectroscopy in multiple sclerosis. *AJNR* **13**, 1535–43.

Grzyska, U., Freitag, J. & Zeumer, H. (1990). Selective cerebral intraarterial DSA. Complication rate and control of risk factors. *Neuroradiology* **32**, 296–9.

Guglielmi, G. (1993). Endovascular treatment of intracranial aneurysms with detachable coils and electrothrombosis. In: Valavanis, A. (ed.). *Interventional Neuroradiology*, pp. 111–22. Berlin: Springer-Verlag.

Haimes, A. B., Zimmerman, R. D., Morgello, S., Weingarten, K., Becker, R. D., Jennis, R. & Deck, M. F. D. (1989). MR imaging of brain abscesses. *AJNR* **10**, 279–91.

Han, B.K., Towbin, R. B., De Courten-Myers, G., McLaurin, R. L. & Ball, W. S. (1990). Reversal sign on CT: effect of anoxic-ischemic cerebral injury in children. *AJNR* **10**, 1191–8.

Harnsberger, H. R. & Osborne, A. G. (1991). Differential diagnosis of head and neck lesions based on their space of origin. I. The suprahyoid part of the neck. *AJR* **157**, 147–54.

Hesselink, J. R., Dowd, C. F., Healy, M. E., Hajek, P., Baker, L. L. & Luerssen, T. G. (1988). MR imaging of brain contusions: a comparative study with CT. *AJNR* **9**, 269–78.

Higashida, R. T., Tsai, F. Y., Van Halbach, V., Dowd, C. F., Smith, T., Fraser, K. & Hieshima, G. B. (1993). Transluminal angioplasty for atheroslerotic disease of the vertebral and basilar arteries. *J. Neurosurg.* **78**, 192–8.

Huber, P. & Schuknecht, B. (1991). CT-Befunde und klinische Verläufe bei schwerer zerebraler Hypoxie. *Klin. Neuroradiol.* **1**, 212–17.

Hudgins, P. A., Davis, P. C. & Hoffman, J. C. (1991). Gadopentetaste dimeglumine-enhanced MR imaging in children following surgery for brain tumor: spectrum of meningeal findings. *AJNR* **12**, 301–7.

Johnson, D. W., Stringer, W. A., Marks, M. P., Yonas, H., Good, W. F. & Gur, D. (1991). Stable xenon CT cerebral blood flow imaging: rationale for and role in clinical decision making. *AJNR* **12**, 201–13.

Kappos, L. & Radü, E. W. (1991). Magnetische Resonanztomographie bei multipler Sklerose: eine Bestandsaufnahme. *Klin. Neuroradiol.* **2**, 110–26.

Kelly, P. J., Daumas-Duport, C., Scheithauer, B. W., Kall, B. A. & Kispert, D. B. (1987). Stereotactic histologic correlations of computed tomography- and magnetic resonance imaging-defined abnormalities in patients with glial neoplasms. *Mayo Clin. Proc.* **62**, 450–9.

Ketonen, L. & Koskiniemi, M. L. (1980). Computed tomography appearance of herpes simplex encephalitis. *Clin. Radiol.* **31**, 161–5.

Kistler, J. P., Crowell, R. M., Davis, K. R., Heros, R., Ojemann, R. G., Zervas, T. & Fisher, C. M. (1983). The relation of cerebral vasospasm to the extent and location of subarachnoid blood visualized by CT scan: a prospective study. *Neurology* **33**, 424–36.

Lee, T., Maynard, N., Anslow, P., Briggs, M. & Northover, J. (1990). Postmyelogram headache – physiological or psychological? *Neuroradiology* **33**, 155–8.

Leonardi, M., Fabris, G. & Lavaroni, A. (1993). Percutaneous diskectomy and chemonucleolysis. In: Valavanis, A. (ed.) *International Neuroradiology*, pp. 173–90. Berlin: Springer-Verlag.

Lester, J. W., Carter, M. P. & Reynolds, T. L. (1988). Herpes encephalitis: MR monitoring of response to acyclovir therapy. *JCAT* **12**, 941–3.

Levi, A., Guilburd, J. N., Lemberger, A., Soustiel, J. F. & Feinsod, M. (1990). Diffuse axonal injury: analysis of 100 patients with radiological signs. *Neurosurgery* **27**, 429–32.

Levy, R. A., Edwards, W. T., Meyer, J. R. & Rosenbaum, A. E. (1993). Facial trauma and 3D reconstructive imaging: insufficiencies and correctives. *AJNR* **13**, 885–92.

Manson, P. N., Grivas, A., Rosenbaum, A., Vannier, M., Zinreich, J. & Iliff, N. (1986). Studies on enophthalmos. II. The measurement of orbital injuries and their treatment by quantitative computed tomography. *Plast. Reconstr. Surg.* **77**, 203–14.

Munari, L. M., Belloni, G., Perreti, A., Ghia, F., Moschini, L. & Porta, M. (1992). Carotid percutaneous angioplasty. *Neurol. Res.* **14**, 156–8.

Ondra, S. L., Troupp, I. J., George, E. D. *et al.* (1990). The natural history of symptomatic arteriovenous malformations of the brain: a 24-year follow-up assessment. *J. Neurosurg.* **73**, 387–91.

Posse, S., Schuknecht, B., Smith, M. E., van Zijl, P. C. M., Herschkowitz, N. & Moonen, C. T. W. (1993). Short echo time proton MR spectroscopic imaging. *J. Comput. Assist. Tomogr.* **17**, 1–14.

Rao, S. V., Binder, J. R., Bandestini, P. A. *et al.* (1993). Functional magnetic resonance imaging of complex human movements. *Neurology* **43**, 2311–18.

Ries, F., Honisch, C., Lambertz, U. & Schlief, R. (1993). A transpulmonary contrast medium enhances the transcranial Doppler signal in humans. *Stroke* **24**, 1903–9.

Rinkel, G. J., Wijdicks, E. F. M., Vermeulen, M., Ramos, L. M. P., Tanghe, H. L. J., Hasan, D., Meiners, L. C. & van Gijn, J. (1991). Nonaneurysmal perimesencephalic subarachnoid hemorrhage: CT and MR patterns that differ from aneurysmal rupture. *AJNR* **12**, 829–34.

Schüller, H., Köster, O. & Ewen, K. (1992). Untersuchung zur Strahlenbelastung der Augenlinse und Schilddrüse bei der hochauflösenden Computertomographie der Zähne. *Fortschr. Röntgenstr.* **156**, 189–92.

Schuknecht, B. F., Ratzka, M. & Nadji, M. (1988). Aussagekraft neuer bildgebender Verfahren in der Diagnostik bakterieller Infektionen des Gehirns. *Röntgen-Berichte* **17**, 93–114.

Schuknecht, B. F., Ratzka, M. & Hofmann, E. (1990). The "dense artery sign" – major cerebral artery thromboembolism demonstrated by computed tomography. *Neuroradiology* **32**, 98–103.

Silberstein, M., Tress, B. M. & Hennessy, O. (1992). Delayed neurologic deterioration in the patient with spinal trauma: Role of MR imaging. *AJNR* **13**, 1373–81.

Taveras, J. M. (1990). Neuroradiology: past, present, future. *Radiology* **175**, 593–602.

Torizuka, T., Hayakawa, K., Tanaka, F., Saitoh, H., Okuno, Y., Ogura, A., Nakayama, Y. & Konishi, J. (1992). High-resolution CT of the temporal bone: a modified baseline. *Radiology* **184**, 109–11.

Valavanis, A. (1993). Embolization of intracranial and skull base tumors. In: Valavanis, A. (ed.) *International Neuroradiology*, pp. 63–91. Berlin: Springer-Verlag.

Valavanis, A. (1997). The role of angiography in the evaluation of cerebral vesicular malformations. *Neuroimaging Clin. North Am.* **6**, 679–707.

Valk, J. (1991). Pediatric neuroimaging: what's new? *Klin. Neuroradiol.* **1**, 237–67.

Volle, E., Hedde, J. P. & Gormanns, R. (1991). Die direkte zervikale Myelographie mit Iotrolan 300. *Fortschr. Röntgenstr.* **154**, 197–201.

Wodarz, R., Ratzka, M. & Nadjmi, M. (1982). Zur Sicherheit der CT-Diagnose bei zerebralen Sinusthrombosen. *Radiologie* **22**, 383–8.

Yeoman, L. J., Howarth, L., Britten, A., Cotterill, A. & Adam, E. J. (1992). Gantry angulation in brain CT: dosage implications, effect on posterior fossa artifacts, and current international practice. *Radiology* 184, 113–16.

Zeumer, H. & Zanella, F. (1993). Local intraarterial fibrinolysis in the vertebrobasilar and carotid territories. In: Valavanis, A. (ed.) *Interventional Neuroradiology*, pp. 159–72. Berlin: Springer-Verlag.

5 Stroke

JULIEN BOGOUSSLAVSKY, MARC HOMMEL AND
CLAUDIO BASSETTI

In most countries of the Western world, stroke is the commonest disease of the central nervous system to warrant admission of a patient to hospital. Although fatality rates and, in some studies, even incidence rates have been reported to decrease over the last few decades (Mas & Zuber 1991), stroke remains one of the major challenges of medicine at the end of the second millenium, because of its frequency, mortality, and the risk of disabling sequelae in survivors.

Definitions

Stroke is a focal neurological deficit of acute onset of a presumed vascular origin. This definition implies a clinical event, with a focal dysfunction (usually a persisting lesion) of the central nervous system (usually the brain), which is likely (though often unproven) to be secondary to a primary disease involving the vessels and circulation. Stroke can be ischaemic or haemorrhagic. Pure subarachnoid haemorrhage is usually considered separately, because of the initial lack of focal cerebral involvement.

Ischaemic stroke is the most common type (85%–90%) (Oxfordshire Community Stroke Project 1983; Bogousslavsky *et al.* 1988c). It corresponds to transient or persisting interruption or decrease of blood flow in a focal area of the brain, usually in a partial or complete territory of a cerebral artery. The cause is usually an occlusion of the corresponding artery, but rather from embolism than from *in situ* disease, except in the very small branches which perforate the parenchyma (50–300 μm in diameter) (Fisher 1965). The lack of local (global cerebral ischaemia is not stroke) blood supply triggers a bioelectric and metabolic cascade which ultimately results in tissue necrosis (*cerebral infarct*), if blood flow is not restored during the very first minutes or hours. If the occluded artery reopens early, with subsequent improvement or normalization of blood supply, tissue lesion will be small or absent, and its clinical expression will be a *transient ischaemic attack* (TIA). By international, but arbitrary, convention, a TIA is defined as a focal neurological deficit with symptoms and signs lasting no longer than 24 hours. TIAs constitute about 10% of all strokes. About one-third of TIAs precede the development of a permanent stroke, and about one-third of permanent strokes have been preceded by TIA(s). There are two problems with the definition of TIAs. First, it cannot be verified that signs were not present after 24 hours but resolved thereafter when patients are seen a few days or a few weeks later, which is far from being uncommon. Second, it should be remembered that most TIAs last only a few minutes (15 to 30), not a few hours. Moreover, it has been shown that when the deficit lasts longer than 1 hour, the rate of underlying infarct may be as high as 75% (Bogousslavsky & Regli 1985); in this situation, though it still fits with the international definition, the term TIA can be misleading, and *cerebral infarct with transient signs* (CITS) has been proposed (Toole 1991). Other terms (prolonged TIA, reversible ischaemic neurological deficit [RIND], etc.) have been proposed in patients with deficits lasting more than 24 hours but less than 2 or 3 weeks, but these subdivisions may not be warranted in that prognosis of patients with TIA or cerebral infarct with minor deficit (minor stroke) is remarkably similar (Koudstaal *et al.* 1992; Carolei *et al.* 1992). We recommend a descriptive approach to the severity and duration of symptoms, recognizing that it will probably be impossible to modify the international usage of the term TIA. However, it may be important to specify the presence or absence of a visible infarct (on CT or MRI) in patients with a short-lasting event, because there is evidence that, if an infarct is present, a second stroke can be associated with more severe and long-lasting dysfunction (Besson *et al.* 1991).

Cerebral haemorrhage accounts for no more than 15% of strokes (Oxfordshire Community Stroke Project 1983; Bogousslavsky *et al.* 1988a), except in non-White populations (Mas & Zuber 1991). It is due to the irruption of blood into the brain parenchyma, with laceration, oedema, and subsequent necrosis, usually from rupture of a small perforating artery. Though the bleeding is primarily intraparenchymatous, extension to the subarachnoid space, less often directly to the ventricular system, is not uncommon. Intraventricular bleeding influences negatively the prognosis of intraparenchymatous haemorrhage (Young *et al.* 1990).

A *haemorrhagic infarct* corresponds to bleeding into an area of infarction. In fact, at autopsy, most infarcts show extravasation of blood and haemorrhagic zones, but in clinical practice the term is restricted to visible haemorrhage on CT (or MRI). Sequential CT studies show that over one-third of infarcts may show visible haemorrhage within 1 month of stroke onset (Hornig *et al.* 1986). The appearance is typical, with heterogeneous and gyriform areas of bleeding within a well-demonstrated infarct. However, in some patients, the bleeding may take the aspect of a frank haematoma within the infarct, which becomes invisible (*intra-infarct haematoma*) (Bogousslavsky *et al.* 1991b), so that differentiation of a primary ischaemic process with secondary bleeding from a primary cerebral haemorrhage can be exceedingly difficult. This can be supported by a previous CT scan done early after stroke with no haemorrhage and the presence of a triggering factor such as anticoagulant therapy, but there is evidence that intra-infarct haematoma can develop as early as a few hours after stroke onset and without anticoagulation, so that it is not impossible that many of these patients have been classified into the group with primary haemorrhage. The presence of a potential cardiac source of embolism in a patient with so-called primary cerebral haemorrhage should suggest this diagnosis of intra-infarct haematoma (Bogousslavsky *et al.* 1991a).

The two most widely used *stroke classifications* are (1) topographic and; (2) aetiologic. This is legitimate, since recognition of one of the subtypes can alter the patient management, and because there are significant links between the topography and aetiology of a stroke. Other useful categorizations can also consider age (0–15, 16–45, 46–75, > 75 years, for example), or stroke features such as type of onset. *Non-progressive*, *progressive* and *fluctuating* are the three main types of onset which are usually considered, though there is no universal definition available (Asplund 1992), especially with reference to the duration of symptom evolution in progressing versus non-progressing stroke.

Epidemiology

Incidence and secular trends

Stroke incidence varies between 1.7 and 17.9/1000 per year (Bonita *et al.* 1990). Mortality of stroke is particularly high in Asia and Eastern Europe, lower in Western Europe and North America (Bonita *et al.* 1990; Zuber & Mas 1992) and still lower in some developing countries because of the low mean age of the general population (Beaglehole 1992). Several surveys suggest that stroke mortality has decreased over the last decades in most countries, in women more than in men and more so than coronary heart disease (CHD) (Bonita *et al.* 1990). This trend could reflect a decline in stroke incidence, a decline in stroke mortality or better diagnosis of milder forms of stroke (mainly since the CT era). However, some studies have reported increasing (Terént 1988; Broderick *et al.* 1989; Jörgensen *et al.* 1992) or unchanging (Harmsen *et al.* 1992) rates of stroke incidence. Better survival after stroke may also be attributed to better management of risk factors with decreased stroke severity at onset, lower incidence of stroke subtypes with high fatality rates and improvement in patient management in the acute phase. Even in studies which reported a decreased incidence of stroke, the rate of decline of stroke seems to have slowed considerably since the late 1970s (Cooper *et al.* 1990), probably because of an increasingly ageing population and improved detection of minor strokes.

Risk factors

The concept of risk factors for stroke is important in assessing the most appropriate therapy both in patients presenting with stroke (Table 5.1) and in those without stroke (Table 5.1, and 5.2).

Inherent biological traits

Age is the most important risk factor of stroke: less than 15% of stroke patients are less than age 45 and at least two-thirds are older than 60 (Mas & Zuber, 1991). The older

Table 5.1. *Increased risk of stroke*

Risk factor	Relative risk
Hypertension	4–5
Cigarette smoking	1.5–3
Atrial fibrillation	5–7
Diabetes mellitus	1.5–2
Alcohol abuse	1–4

Table 5.2. *Stroke rates in high-risk patients*

Group	Stroke rate (%/year)
General population, aged > 70 years	0.6
Asymptomatic bruit	1.5
Asymptomatic carotid stenosis	2.0
Lone atrial fibrillation	5
After TIA or minor stroke	12
TIA[a]	6
With carotid stenosis > 70%	13
Previous ischaemic stroke	9

[a] After TIA the stroke risk is 12% in the first year, and 30% in the first 5 years.

population has a higher mortality rate, probably related in part to a more severe neurological deficit at onset (Asplund *et al.* 1992). A positive *family history* may represent a risk factor not only for CHD but also for stroke (Brass *et al.*, 1992). *Women* have a 2–3 times lower incidence of stroke, a difference which decreases with age and is not present in those over 85 years (Malmgren *et al.* 1987). An influence of *race* has been postulated but differences in diet and psychosocial stress may also play a role (Mas & Zuber, 1991).

Physiological characteristics

Hypertension is the major treatable risk factor of stroke. It is present in half to three-quarters of patients (Sandercock *et al.* 1989). The relative risk of stroke increases parallel to blood pressure values (even within normal levels) and exceeds 4 for values above 160/90 (Wolf *et al.* 1991b). This risk is substantially increased by an association with additional risk factors. Both systolic and diastolic hypertension increase the risk of stroke (Collins *et al.* 1990; SHEP Cooperative Research Group 1991). A benefit of lowering the blood pressure has been suggested also for normotensive subjects with additional risk factors (Fletcher & Bulpitt, 1992). *Cholesterol* levels above 220 mg% increase the relative risk of stroke by 2.9 (Quizilbash *et al.* 1992), but an inverse relationship has been postulated for intracerebral haemorrhage (ICH) (Iso *et al.* 1989). *Diabetes* increases the relative risk of coronary heart disease (CHD) and stroke (Mas & Zuber 1991; Barret-Connor & Khaw 1988). A higher risk of stroke has been found also for subjects with increased blood levels of *fibrinogen* and *elevated haematocrit,* but other haematological factors probably also predispose to stroke (Mas & Zuber 1991).

Behaviours

Cigarette smoking predisposes not only to CHD but also to stroke (Abbott *et al.* 1986; Colditz *et al.* 1988; Shinton & Beevers 1989). The risk is present also for passive smokers and is higher in heavy and young smokers, but decreases considerably as early as 2–5 years after cessation of smoking. Excess *alcohol consumption* increases the risk of both ischaemic and haemorrhagic stroke (Gill *et al.* 1986, Stampfer *et al.* 1988) whereas moderate alcohol consumption (< 60 g ethanol per day) might exert a protective effect, as in CHD (Bogousslavsky *et al.* 1990). *Estrogens* in oral contraceptives (Mas & Zuber 1991) are associated with a slightly higher risk of stroke, particularly in women over 35 years presenting other risk factors. For hormone replacement therapy, increased (Wilson *et al.* 1985), decreased (Hunt *et al.* 1987; Paganini-Hill *et al.* 1988) or unchanged (Stampfer *et al.* 1991) incidence of stroke has been reported. The risk of stroke is affected by *diet* through the independent influence of sodium, potassium and alcohol intake as well as by the effect of body weight on blood pressure (Stamler *et al.* 1989). A few reports have suggested an independent protective effect of high potassium (Khaw & Barret-Connor, 1987), calcium and animal protein diet (Lee *et al.* 1988).

Socioenvironmental features

More data are needed to assess the role of physical activity (Salonen *et al.* 1982), socioeconomic status and psychosocial stress (Harmsen *et al.* 1992; James & Kleibaum 1976) on stroke. Stroke seems to be more common during cold months (Malmgren *et al.* 1987).

Risk of stroke with cardiovascular disease

The general prevalence of *carotid bruits* ranges (depending on age) between 4% and 13% (Van Ruiswyk *et al.* 1990) and is associated with a 1-year risk of stroke of 1–2%. In 1–2% of the population, the bruit is due to a 'significant' (> 70%) *carotid stenosis,* corresponding to a 1-year stroke rate of 5–6% (Norris 1992; Bogousslavsky *et al.* 1986a). For *an already symptomatic severe carotid stenosis,* the 1 year stroke rate is higher, reaching 10–20% (NASCET Collaborators 1991). Patients who have experienced a TIA have a 1 year stroke rate of 6–16% (Norris 1992; Dennis *et al.* 1990). Recurrence rate of stroke probably exceeds 10% in the first year. *Ischaemic heart disease* and *cardiac failure* are associated with an increased incidence of first stroke and of recurrent stroke (Dexter *et al.* 1987). *Atrial fibrillation* is present in 5–10% of subjects over 50 years of age and probably represents an independent risk factor of stroke (Wolf *et al.* 1991a). This risk is very low (< 1%) for patients under 60 years of age with 'lone' fibrillation (Kopecky *et al.* 1987), but increases considerably in older patients and in association with other risk factors (Wolf *et al.* 1991a). *Intermittent claudication* is a risk indicator of CHD and stroke

(Mas & Zuber 1991). An increase of stroke risk has been shown in subjects with *snoring* (Waller & Bhopal 1989).

Stroke prevention

The role of prevention is exemplified by the decline of stroke mortality over the last decades, by the estimation that up to 50% of cerebrovascular deaths in patients under 70 years could be prevented and by the observation that the most important prognostic factors in acute stroke presently cannot be modified after stroke onset (Marmot & Poulter, 1992). *Primary prevention* can be accomplished through management of risk factors. The positive effect on stroke risk is accepted, while that of lowering cholesteol level awaits confirmation. Warfarin anticoagulation is effective in the primary prevention of stroke in patients with non-rheumatic atrial fibrillation (Singer 1992). In *secondary prevention* (Barnett 1992), while risk factors must still be addressed, other measures may include carotid endarterectomy in severe carotid stenosis (NASCET Collaborators 1991; ECST Collaborative Group 1991) and aspirin, ticlopidine or anticoagulant therapy in subsets of patients (Barnett 1992; Hass *et al.* 1989).

Causes of cerebral infarcts

In the Western world, most cerebral infarcts are linked to atherosclerosis in the cardiovascular system, though usually through an indirect mechanism (embolism). Early and sequential angiography has shown that distal intracerebral occlusions are present in most patients within the first 24 hours and disappear thereafter. Actually, local disease of intracranial arteries is an uncommon cause of stroke, except in Asians and to a lesser extent in Blacks, and apart from small-artery disease associated with hypertension and diabetes which leads to lacunar infarction (Oxfordshire Community Stroke Project 1983; Bogousslavsky *et al.* 1987a). Thus, it is legitimate that the term cerebral thrombosis be deleted from the usual medical vocabulary. Overall, the three leading causes of cerebral infarcts are:

(1) *Extracranial large-artery disease* (40%), usually with *artery-to-artery embolic occlusion* of intracerebral artery(ies). The embolic material can be either fibrinoplatelet or from a thrombus which usually occludes the extracranial artery (for example embolic middle cerebral artery trunk occlusion from ipsilateral internal carotid artery occlusion: *occlusio supra occlusionem*). Haemodynamic mechanisms may play a role in large-artery occlusion or severe stenosis, but they are usually not prominent.

(2) *Cardioembolism* is the presumed cause of infarct in at least 25% of infarcts, though definite proof of embolization from the heart is usually lacking. Less than 5% to 10% of the patients with stroke and a potential cardiac source of embolism actually show a *direct* source of embolism (intracardiac thrombus or tumour) (Urbinati *et al.* 1992). The most common potential cardiac sources of embolism include (a) dysrhythmias: atrial fibrillation, sick-sinus syndrome; (b) structural changes: rheumatic heart

disease, acute myocardial infarct, left ventricular akinetic segment or aneurysm, dilated cardiomyopathy (Cardiac Embolism Task Force 1989). Haemodynamic phenomena associated with decreased cardiac output are only uncommonly a cause of stroke, but they are also commonly overlooked as a potentially contributing or aggravating factor (Bogousslavsky *et al.* 1991a).

(3) Small-artery disease (microangiopathy) accounts for about 15% of cerebral infarcts. It corresponds to *in situ* stenosis and occlusion of deep perforating branches of the hemispheres and brainstem. Contrary to pial arterial branches, these perforators lack significant anastomoses so that collateral supply is not available when occlusion develops, leading to a small infarct (⩽ 15 mm in diameter) limited to the territory of the occluded perforator (*lacunar infarct*) (Fisher 1965). Hypertension is the main risk factor for small-artery disease, and diabetes may also contribute (Ghika *et al.* 1989).

Between 5% and 25% of the patients may have coexistence of these three leading causes, and it may be difficult to determine the precise aetiology in them. Other potential causes of cerebral infarct are innumerable but much more uncommon (Bogousslavsky *et al.* 1988b), the main groups being non-atheromatous arterial diseases, venous thromboses, etc. Many of these more uncommon causes of cerebral infarct become important in the *younger patients* (⩽ 45 years). In this age group, the three most commonly determined causes of ischaemic stroke are (Bogousslavsky & Pierre 1992):

(1) *Cardioembolism* (25–30%). Up to 40–50% of the patients may demonstrate a *patent foramen ovale*, compared with 15–20% in age and sex-matched controls (Lechat *et al.* 1988; Webster *et al.* 1988). Though paradoxical embolism is difficult to prove in most instances, even with systematic phlebography for demonstrating deep venous thrombosis, it is often suspected on the basis of triggering factors with Valsava manoeuvre. Also, the recent finding of an association with *interatrial septal aneurysm* suggests that a paradoxical embolism may occur without a venous source (Nater *et al.* 1992). *Mitral valve prolapse* has been an overused diagnosis in young stroke patients, but, with strict echocardiographic criteria, its frequency has dropped below 10% (Cerebral Embolism Task Force 1989).

(2) *Arterial dissection* (20%), mainly in the carotid circulation (Bogousslavsky *et al.* 1987a). Although it is classically divided into spontaneous and traumatic types, it seems more likely that there is a continuum between these two extremes. Cerebral infarction develops when the arterial lumen is severely narrowed or occluded, with the development of local thrombosis and subsequent embolization.

(3) *Migraine stroke* (10%) remains controversial. It may be a specific entity but it should be diagnosed only with strict criteria, which underscore the temporal relationship between a prolonged attack of migraine with aura ending in cerebral infarction (Bogousslavsky *et al.* 1988b).

Changing patterns of the aetiology of ischaemic stroke in the young may appear in the near future, as suggested in recent studies emphasizing the role of inherited mitochondrial dysfunction in familial and sporadic cases (Tournier-Lasserve *et al.* 1991; Mas *et al.* 1992).

The main similarity between stroke in the young and *stroke in the elderly* (> 75 years) is the importance of cardioembolic sources (Ferrazzini *et al.* 1988; Asplund *et al.* 1992), while large-artery atheroma and small-vessel disease are less prominent than in the intermediate age groups (probably because these latter patients will have died from vascular disease before the age of 75). Also, the proportion of women exceeds that of men above 75 years, and below 30 years (Bogousslavsky *et al.* 1988c).

Cerebral infarcts: analysis by vascular territory

Middle cerebral artery (MCA) pial (superficial) territory infarcts

The main characteristic of this territory is its extensive collateral system, so that multiple embolism is usually necessary to cause infarction. The cause of embolism is artery-to-artery in at least one-third of the patients and cardiac in a quarter, the latter being especially common in infarcts in the territory of the lower division of the MCA (Bogousslavsky *et al.* 1989).

Anterior cerebral artery (ACA) territory infarcts

These are at least 20 times less common than MCA territory infarcts, but their aetiologic patterns do not differ (Bogousslavsky & Regli 1989).

Subcortical infarcts in the anterior circulation

Arterial supply to the basal ganglia and white matter is through perforating branches, which originate either from the trunk of large arteries at the level of the circle of Willis (internal carotid artery, MCA, ACA, anterior choroidal artery) (*deep perforators*), or from the pial branches which course in the cortical sulci (*superficial perforators* or white matter medullary branches) (Bogousslavsky & Regli 1992).

Infarction limited to the territory of one single perforator has been called *lacunar* (ischaemic lacunes), and is usually associated with *in situ* small-artery disease linked to chronic hypertension or diabetes (Fisher 1965, 1991; Ghika *et al.* 1989). These lacunar infarcts are small (diameter < 15 mm, usually 3–5 mm) and most of them are not associated with a stroke syndrome, being often asymptomatic (Fisher 1965). On the other hand, *larger infarcts* encompassing the territory of several perforators are usually symptomatic and they are not associated with small-vessel disease. Artery-to-artery embolism, cardioembolism and intracranial large-artery stenosis occluding the mouth of perforating branches are the most common aetiologies (Weiller *et al.* 1991; Bogousslavsky *et al.* 1991b; Donnan *et al.* 1992). The best known of these larger subcortical infarcts are the striatocapsular infarcts (lenticulostriate branches of the MCA trunk), the large infarcts in the anterior choroidal artery territory, and the large centrum ovale infarcts (white matter medullary branches).

Thus, classification of the subtypes of cortical infarcts depends upon their size, potential aetiology, and clinical manifestations. The term *lacunar syndrome* was initially introduced to report *any* possible manifestation of lacunar infarcts (Fisher 1991), but its commonly accepted meaning is at present syndromes which are *suggestive* of lacunar infarcts. Confusion between these two definitions has lead to innumerable misleading assumptions on subcortical infarcts. According to recent studies, syndromes suggestive of lacunar infarction are few, and strict criteria of the distribution of motor or sensory deficits must be used (in particular, combined involvement of face, upper limbs and lower limb in 'pure motor hemiparesis', 'pure sensory stroke', 'ataxic hemiparesis', and 'sensorimotor stroke') (Melo *et al.* 1992.)

The topographic classification of subcortical infarcts in the anterior circulation is the following:

1. Infarcts in the territory of deep perforators (from MCA, ACA, anterior choroidal artery, posterior communicating artery)
2. Infarcts in the territory of superficial perforators (white matter medullary branches)
3. Borderzone infarcts between 1 and 2 (they are associated with ipsilateral severe carotid disease, as are large infarcts from group 2)
4. Combined infarcts.

Superficial posterior cerebral artery (PCA) territory infarcts

As in the posterior MCA infarcts, the frequency of embolic sources is high, which may explain why bilateral infarcts occur in up to 5% of cases.

Thalamic infarcts

These develop in four main arterial territories: paramedian (first segment of PCA), thalamogeniculate, posterior choroidal (second segment of PCA), tuberothalamic (posterior communicating artery) (Bogousslavsky *et al.* 1988a). These branches are deep perforators but, as they may show anastomoses and collaterals, the aetiology of infarction is biased towards embolic causes, as the occlusion of more than one perforator may be necessary to yield infarction, contrary to other subcortical infarcts.

Borderzone infarcts

There are two main types: (1) watershed infarcts developing at the level of the most distal anastomoses between two main branch territories; and (2) other borderzone infarcts occurring in the area between the terminal territory of deep and superficial perforators (subcortical borderzone infarcts). They are associated with ipsilateral severe carotid disease, usually occlusion (Bogousslavsky & Regli 1986).

Large hemispheric infarcts

These combine the superficial and deep territory of MCA or PCA, or correspond to MCA with PCA or ACA territory involvement. Extensive subcortical infarcts sparing the cortical ribbon are associated with ipsilateral severe carotid disease (Levine *et al.* 1988).

Brainstem infarcts

These can be limited to the medulla, pons or midbrain, or combined. Partial infarcts involve either the paramedian or the lateral territory. These infarcts may not uncommonly be associated with severe local disease of the basilar artery or distal vertebral artery, which may occlude the origin of perforating or short circumferential branches. Dorsolateral infarcts are usually associated with cerebellar infarcts, as this part of the brainstem is supplied by the cerebellar arteries (long circumferential branches).

Cerebellar infarcts

Posterior inferior cerebellar artery (PICA) territory infarcts are often associated with atheromatous disease of the vertebral artery, while superior cerebellar artery (SCA) territory infarcts are associated with cardioembolic sources. Anterior inferior cerebellar artery (AICA) territory infarcts are uncommon (Amarenco & Hauw 1990).

Transient ischaemic attacks

TIAs accounted for 21% of all stroke events in the Framingham study (Wolf *et al.* 1992a). Their incidence is about 2.2–8/1000 per year, with higher rates in the older and male population. Cardiovascular risk profile for TIAs and minor ischaemic stroke are similar (Dennis *et al.* 1989).

Clinical manifestations

Two-thirds of TIAs involve the carotid system, with transient monocular blindness (TMB) or transient hemispheral attack (THA). In the remaining the vertebrobasilar system is involved. In a significant percentage of cases (isolated hemianopia, dysarthria, etc.), the involved territory cannot be determined.

TMB (or amaurosis fugax) consists in a monocular, total or partial, visual obscuration (described as a curtain, shading or blurring) or loss appearing within seconds, occasionally with positive visual phenomena (The Amaurosis Fugax Study Group 1990). TMB disappears progressively within 1–15 minutes but can recur. Sudden exposure to bright light can rarely provoke uni- or bilateral TMB (Furlan *et al.* 1979). Intravascular material in the retinal circulation can occasionally be seen during attacks. THAs consists of one, few, rarely over 20 attacks (Pessin *et al.* 1977); unilateral neurological deficit is usually limited to one or two parts of the body (face, arm, leg), visual field deficits, speech or other neuropsychological dysfunctions, alone or in combination. Rare forms of carotid TIAs include limb shaking (Baquis *et al.* 1985) and simultaneous onset of TMB and THA (Bogousslavsky *et al.* 1987b). *Lacunar TIAs* (Hankey & Warlow 1991; Kappelle *et al.* 1991) have been defined as transient lacunar syndromes corresponding to ('pure') motor or sensory symptoms involving face, arm and leg. *Verte-*

brobasilar TIAs are suggested by the simultaneous onset of bilateral sensorimotor deficits or blindness, vertigo, diplopia, dysphagia, ataxia and gait disturbances, but in practice, their diagnosis is not easy.

Aetiology

Artery-to-artery *embolism of carotid origin* is often assumed as the cause of most TIAs, but only 20–50% of patients have an appropriate carotid stenosis (Bogousslavsky *et al.* 1986b). This mechanism is particularly plausible in patients with recurrent stereotyped episodes of TMB, THA, or both. A *haemodynamic mechanism* should be evoked in limb-shaking TIAs or simultaneous TMB and THA associated to haemodynamic stress (change of posture, hypotensive treatment). Uni- or bilateral visual loss on bright light is also suggestive of severe carotid disease. Cardioembolism is a possible cause of TIAs in patients with a potential cardiac source of embolism, alternating THA, longer duration of episodes (Pessin *et al.* 1977) and in the young. In this latter group, *hyper-coagulable states* and *non-atherosclerotic vasculopathies* (dissection, vasculitis, drug-induced vasospasm) should also be considered.

Diagnosis and differential diagnosis

A TIA is diagnosed on the basis of history and normal neurological examination. Completed stroke, non-focal cerebral symptoms (confusion, syncope, amnesia, etc.) and transient, non-vascular neurological deficits (isolated episodes of vertigo, imbalance, drop attacks, diplopia, dysphagia, dysarthria, etc.) have to be excluded. In up to one-third of patients, the diagnosis of TIA may remain uncertain (Calanchini *et al.* 1977) and agreement between two neurologists may be at best about 65–77% for diagnosis and 31–65% for territory involved (Koudstaal *et al.* 1986). However, the actual criteria for TIAs are probably too strict and the true incidence may be underestimated (Toole 1991). The differential diagnosis of cerebral TIAs includes focal seizures and migraine – both with the characteristic march of neurological symptoms (lasting seconds in seizures and minutes in migraine) – hypoglycaemia, 'transient tumour attacks' (Weisberg & Nice 1977), 'cardiac spells' (with bilateral visual disturbances, dizziness, syncope) (De Bono *et al.* 1982) and hyperventilation. The median duration of TIAs is 8 minutes in the vertebrobasilar and 14 minutes in the carotid system (Dyken *et al.* 1977) with more than 50% of TIAs resolving within 1 hour (Werdelin & Juhler 1988; Levy 1988). With increasing duration, the risk of underlying cerebral infarct increases (Toole 1991; Scott & Miller 1985; Bogousslavsky & Reglia 1985). Up to 48% of those patients examined by CT and even more of those studied by MRI show an infarct. In such instances, the correct diagnosis is that of a 'cerebral infarction with transient symptoms' (CITS). The differential diagnosis of TMB includes glaucoma, papilloedema, migraine, optic neuritis and optic nerve compression (The Amaurosis Fugax Study Group 1990).

Prognosis and treatment

The risk of stroke is higher in the first months after a TIA and reaches an overall rate of about 30% (range 7–48%) (Carolei *et al.* 1992). This risk does not seem to depend on duration or severity of TIAs (Dennis *et al.* 1989; Carolei *et al.* 1992) but is lower for TMB than for THA. Recurrent TIAs, the combination of carotid and vertebrobasilar TIAs, increasing age, associated risk factors and cardiovascular disease are thought to in-crease the risk of stroke (Carolei *et al.* 1992). TIAs associated with normal investigations (including angiography, echocardiography and Holter monitoring) may have a better prognosis (Shaib & Hachinski 1990). Cardiac morbidity and mortality in patients with TIA is high, particularly with coexisting cardiac disease (Heyman *et al.* 1984). Manage-ment of patients with TIA should start as early as possible and should associate a lesion-specific treatment strategy with the management of risk factors (Caplan 1988b). For patients with severe (> 70%) carotid stenosis appropriate to TIA, surgery should be considered (NASCET Collaborators 1991; ECST Collaborative Group 1991). Anticoagula-tion is indicated in cardioembolic TIAs and perhaps in patients with recurrent TIAs on antiplatelet treatment and in whom surgery is contraindicated or not feasible (intra-cranial or vertebrobasilar disease). In the remaining patients, aspirin is the mainstay of treatment. Though its optimal dose is still a matter of debate (Dyken *et al.* 1992), 325 mg per day are probably sufficient; lower doses do not prevent the major unwanted effects (Antiplatelet Trialists' Collaboration 1988). For patients with aspirin allergy or intoler-ance, the new antiplatelet agent ticlopidine hydrochloride seems to offer at least as good a protective effect (Hass *et al.* 1989).

Intracerebral haemorrhage

Intracerebral haemorrhage (ICH) has an incidence of 6–23/100 000 per year (Schütz 1992) with higher rates in the population over 60 years of age, in men and in certain races (Blacks and Orientals). Advanced age, hypertension, alcohol abuse and cigarette smoking are the most common risk factors of ICH.

Aetiology

Chronic hypertension is the most common aetiology of ICH but its role is declining, and only about 50% of cases are now attributed to it (Bogousslavsky *et al.* 1988c; Schütz 1992). Bleeding occurs at the level of small penetrating arteries, which may develop microaneurysmal changes (Charcot–Bouchard aneurysms).

Acute hypertension causes ICH not only in the setting of chronic hypertension but also, independently, in association with alcohol or drug abuse (amphetamine, cocaine, phenyl-propanolamine, other sympathomimetic agents) (Kase *et al.* 1987), exposure to extreme cold, trigeminal nerve stimulation, after carotid endarterectomy and heart surgery (Caplan 1988a). The proportion of non-hypertensive causes of ICH is variable and depends on age and site of bleeding, exceeding 50% in patients below 40 years.

Cerebral amyloid angiopathy, a sporadic condition characterized by deposits of amyloid in the media and adventitia of small and medium sized arteries, is responsible for 7–17% of cases of ICH. This diagnosis should be assumed in non-hypertensive patients over 60 years, with recurrent subcortical lobar haemorrhages with or without Alzheimer's type of dementia.

Ten per cent of ICH cases are related to *anticoagulation/thrombolysis* (Caplan, 1988a). The location of bleeding is often lobar or cerebellar, the onset is characteristically slowly progressive, and prognosis is particularly poor (mortality > 50%). The risk of ICH during anticoagulation/thrombolysis is about 0.3–3.3% (Forsting *et al.* 1991; Sloan & Price 1991). It depends upon the type and dose of treatment, age of patients and concomitant hypertension. The role of preceding cerebral infarction, trauma and duration of treatment remains debated.

Congenital or *acquired coagulopathies* are uncommon but should be considered in patients with both systemic and cerebral haemorrhages (Samuels & Thalinger 1991). *Vascular malformations* are responsible for about 5% of ICHs but are more frequent (up to 29% of cases) in adults below 45 years (Toffol *et al.* 1987). ICH occurs in about 1% of intracranial tumours. A tumour (usually pituitary adenoma, glioblastoma or metastases) may be found conversely in up to 5–10% of patients with ICH (Bogousslavsky & Regli 1993). Together with acute hypertension and vasospasm, *arteritis* is supposed to be the mechanism of ICH associated with drug abuse (Caplan, 1988a). ICH due to mycotic aneurysm and systemic or cerebral vasculitis are rare. ICH may complicate *cerebral venous thrombosis* in 10–50% of cases. *Traumatic* ICH is typically multiple, located basally in the frontal and temporal lobes. *Aneurysmal* bleeding can rarely be complicated by meningocerebral haemorrhages. Finally, up to one-fifth of cases of ICH may remain of *unknown origin* after extensive investigation.

Clinical presentation

TIA(s) may precede ICH in 5–10% of the patients. Two-thirds of haemorrhages stabilize rapidly, while one-third have a progressive course over hours or even days (Giroud *et al.* 1991). ICH occurs usually during daytime and develops during physical activity, and the clinical picture includes classically headache and vomiting (40–50% of cases), decreased alertness (60%), systolic hypertension (90%) and meningeal signs. On the other hand, up to 10% of ICHs may produce a 'lacunar syndrome' (Bogousslavsky *et al.* 1988c; Groothuis *et al.* 1977). ICH can also mimic ischaemic stroke with short-lasting neurological symptoms without headache or clouding of consciousness (Scott & Miller 1985). It can also occur in a pseudotumoral form with seizures and a focal deficit progressing over weeks (Pozzati *et al.* 1986). Overall seizures are not common (10%) in ICH, but in stroke a seizure at onset may suggest an ICH. Multiple haemorrhages are found in 2% of cases, being often associated with hypertension (Weisberg 1981). Intraventricular bleeding may present with a 'subarachnoid bleeding-like' picture (headache, meningismus, confusion). Bleeding into the ventricles occurs in one-third of cases of ICH, but primary intraventricular bleeding is rare (Moya-Moya disease, angiomas, anticoagulation and bilateral carotid disease) (Gates *et al.* 1986).

Deep supratentorial ICH

About 50% of ICHs involve deep supratentorial structures (Hier *et al.* 1977; Walshe *et al.* 1977; Pedrazzi *et al.* 1990; Trouillat *et al.* 1990; Massaro *et al.* 1991) and among them most (> 70%) are due to chronic hypertension. *Putaminal haemorrhages* are the most common forms. They present with hemiparesis, decreased alertness and ipsilateral conjugate eye deviation. In larger lesions, hemisensory disturbances, neuropsychological defects, hemianopia and coma can be found. Smaller lesions can present with 'lacunar syndromes' or paroxysmal movement disorders. *Thalamic haemorrhages* account for 5–15% of ICHs. They should be suspected in patients with hemisensory (-motor) dysfunction, vertical eye movement disturbances, bilateral miosis and behavioural abnormalities following decreased alertness. *Haemorrhages* of the *head* of the *caudate nucleus* represent 3–7% of ICHs. They are characterized by 'subarachnoid bleeding-like' features or by a slight hemiparesis with prominent behavioural changes (mainly apathy, confusion and memory dysfunction).

Lobar ICH

Superficial (lobar) structures (Ropper & Davis, 1980; Lipton *et al.* 1987; Trouillat *et al.* 1990; Massaro *et al.* 1991; Wakai *et al.* 1992) are involved in 21–59% of ICH cases. A non-hypertensive origin is common (50–70% of cases). Headache, vomiting, meningism and seizures are more frequent than in deeply situated haemorrhage, but decreased alertness, severe hemiparesis and death are less frequent. The neurological manifestations depend on the lobe involved.

Brainstem ICH

Between 5 and 10% of ICHs are located in the brainstem (Weisberg 1981; Caplan & Goodwin 1982; Kilpatrick *et al.* 1991; Weisberg 1986a; Neumann *et al.* 1985). The most common form involves the *basis of the pons*. It is usually of hypertensive origin, prognosis is commonly poor. The clinical picture includes coma, pinpoint pupils, tetraparesis and eye movement disorders. More circumscribed bleeding of the *tegmentum pontis* can present with more limited dysfunction. In these forms and in the rarer cases of *midbrain* or *medullary haemorrhages*, non-hypertensive causes must be considered.

Cerebellar ICH

Five to fifteen per cent of ICHs involve the cerebellum (Ott *et al.* 1974; Labauge *et al.* 1983). Bleeding usually develops in the vicinity of the dentate nucleus. It is often due to chronic hypertension. It presents with headache, vomiting, dizziness and inability to walk. Gait and limb ataxia, dysarthria, gaze palsy and clouding of consciousness are common. Pseudolacunar and pseudotumoral clinical forms are occasionally encountered. The clinical course is often unpredictable, but prognosis is poor if coma develops. Bleeding involving the vermis is rare in practice because of intraventricular extension and early death.

Diagnosis

Diagnosis of ICH on clinical grounds is not always possible (Sandercock *et al.* 1985) and must therefore rely on neuroimaging. However, on early CT spontaneous haematoma in cerebral infarct may mimic primary haemorrhage, so that this eventually should always be kept in mind (Bogousslavsky *et al.* 1991c). Early recognition of haemorrhage may be difficult on MRI which, on the other hand, can determine the age and often the origin of ICH. Angiography should be considered in young patients, in lobar ICH and in haemorrhages of unusual topography.

Prognosis

Overall mortality of ICH (Tuhrim *et al.* 1988; Francke *et al.* 1992) is about 30–40% (Giroud *et al.* 1991b), but it varies depending on location and size of bleeding, and severity and progression of clinical signs. Patients with supratentorial haematomas over 3–4 cm in diameter, pontine haematomas (unless below 1 cm in diameter), and coma have a bad prognosis. Early recurrent bleeding is suggestive of a non-hypertensive cause of ICH.

Treatment

Treatment probably influences the course of medium-sized but not of small and large ICH (Caplan 1992). Hypertension in the acute phase should be corrected if values are high (systolic > 180–200 mmHg). Oedema is sometimes treated by hyperventilation and hyperosmotic agents, while steroids are not recommended (Poungvarin *et al.* 1987). Bleeding related to anticoagulation/thrombolysis and coagulopathies should be treated with fresh frozen plasma, vitamin K, protamine and platelet transfusions. Routine use of anticonvulsants is not recommended. Surgery is indicated mainly in cerebellar ICH and acute occlusive hydrocephalus, but it may be considered for other accessible haemorrhages (lobar and putaminal) in non-comatose patients showing rapid deterioration despite conservative treatment, although this issue remains controversial.

Natural history of stroke

The mortality of stroke has been addressed in the preceding part of this chapter.

Functional and social consequences of stroke

After a stroke, there is often a reduction of mobility, and in independence in daily activities, participation in household duties and socialization, interest in previous activities and leisure, and of professional activities. These reductions are mostly related to the stroke itself and not to previous co-morbidity (Gresham *et al.* 1979). Recovery after a stroke is almost always achieved within the first 3 months. After 6 months, the remaining signs usually persist as permanent sequelae.

Disability

Consequences of stroke in all daily activities: 45–66% of stroke survivors are independent in all daily activities 6 months after the stroke, as assessed for example with the Barthel index (Gresham, 1986; Wade & Langton Hewer 1987). Wade & Langton Hewer (1987) reported the rate of recovery of activities in daily living. They showed, for example, that the recovery of walking alone or with help was achieved for 70–85% of the survivors (Wade & Langton Hewer 1987).

Returning home with or without help (nursing, speech therapists, physiotherapists, etc.) occurs in about 80% of the stroke survivors. However, returning home is not only dependent on the medical state and functional abilities of the patient but mostly rests on familial and social circumstances (Henley *et al.* 1985).

Returning to work is only possible for about 20% of stroke patients. Here also the influence of social factors is critical (Howard *et al.* 1985).

Predictors of recovery

Disability In completed stroke, many of the predictors of recovery are present from the onset of the stroke. Wade & Langton Hewer (1987) have modelled predictors of the functional state at 6 months as assessed with the Barthel index. The best predictors present at 7 days were urinary incontinence, the Barthel scale at day 7, age, and sitting balance. The predictors of disability were the same as the predictors of death. This finding suggests that a treatment which would be able to reduce mortality is also likely to reduce disability. The predictors of disability are reported in Table 5.3.

Age Age is a negative marker of functional recovery (Allen 1984). However, the role of age alone is not clear because ageing is also related to more frequent co-morbidity which hinders recovery (Jongbloed 1986).

Stroke topography and size Vertebrobasilar strokes may have a better functional prognosis than hemispheric strokes. Middle cerebral artery occlusions may have slower functional recovery than carotid artery occlusions. Small (by size) strokes may have a better prognosis than large strokes (Marquardsen 1983).

Table 5.3. *Predictors of disability*

Age
Motor deficit, when affecting the lower limb
Head and eye deviation
Sitting balance
Impaired consciousness
Urinary incontinence
Size and topography of the stroke
Ischaemic or haemorrhagic nature of the stroke
Speed of recovery
Hemianopia
Neuropsychological deficit

Intracranial haemorrhages These have a poor early prognosis for life. However, the survivors of haemorrhage may have a better functional prognosis than the survivors of infarction (Marquardsen 1983).

Stroke subtypes After a lacunar infarct, residual disability is often slight, 64% of patients being independent in all of a day's activities, 21% needing some help, and 15% remaining bedridden in a French study (Giroud *et al.* 1991c). In the Oxfordshire Stroke Community Project, the patients were more dependent, probably in relation to co-morbidity (Bamford *et al.* 1987). Within lacunar infarcts the disability depends on the clinical subtype: about 80% of the patients with a motor deficit being dependent in some activities (Gandolfo *et al.* 1986). The disability may be more severe in patients with leukoaraiosis on CT (Mikayo *et al.* 1992). Libman *et al.* (1992) compared pure motor strokes with other strokes. The lacunar infarcts had a quicker and better recovery, as soon as 10 days after the stroke. When long-term disability was compared, lacunar infarcts had a better functional prognosis than the other infarcts (Libman *et al.* 1992).

Speed of recovery Recovery of urinary continence, mobility, ability to dress, feeding, and ability to transfer from bed to chair occurs mainly within the first 2 weeks, by which time at least 50% of recovery has occurred (Wade *et al.* 1985). However, after 3 weeks and 6 months, there was still some further recovery (Wade & Langton Hewer 1987). If the speed of recovery is high, functional prognosis is better (Marquardsen 1983).

Urinary incontinence This (mainly between day 7 to 10 after the stroke) is one of the most adverse prognostic factors both for long-term survival and for recovery of function (Wade *et al.* 1985).

The combination of the different predictors is a key point in the prediction of disability. Hemianopia and neuropsychological disturbances are predictors of poor prognosis when associated with the other poor outcome predictors, especially motor deficits (Marquardsen 1983).

Returning home

Previous independence, living with a partner, a high frequency of social contacts before the stroke, a mild stroke and a positive mood are favourable predictors of returning home (Marquardsen 1983; Henley *et al.* 1985). The contribution of the family is critical. On the other hand, loose family interactions are associated with iterative hospital admissions, and a stronger predictor of long stays in hospitals and nursing homes than disability itself (Evans *et al.* 1987).

Returning to work

Returning to work depends on age, functional status, aphasia, and the type of profession practised before the stroke. Unskilled workers may have major difficulties in returning to work (Howard *et al.* 1985).

Quality of life and handicap

A handicap is defined as 'a disadvantage for a given individual, resulting from impairment or disability, that limits or prevents the fulfilment of a role that is normal (depending upon age, sex, and social and cultural factors) for that individual'. According to this definition, there are different axes that constitute the quality of life: orientation, physical independence, mobility, occupation of time, social integration, and economic self-sufficiency. Obviously there is no gold standard with which to compare handicap, and this makes measurement of quality of life in stroke difficult. Moreover, it is necessary to compare measured performance with expected performance. One of the major limitations in the study of quality of life in stroke patients consists in the cognitive deficits which hinder the self-assessment (Wade 1992). This important problem in methodology probably explains why so few studies have evaluated quality of life after stroke.

The quality of life before and after stroke was assessed in 96 patients: 6 months after the stroke 70% reported a decrease in their quality of life compared with their pre-stroke status. No improvement was observed after 2 years. There was a strong correlation between the quality of life, anxiety, depression and functional state (Ahlsiö *et al.* 1984). Aström *et al.* (1992) reported the living conditions and life satisfaction in 80 patients before and after stroke and compared the results with a general elderly population. Even before stroke, stroke patients had more health problems, a lower functional ability, longer inactive periods, and a lower life satisfaction than the control subjects. However, the economic resources, the social network, and the psychiatric morbidity were identical. This result suggests that some of the disabilities pre-exist stroke. Half of the patients reported a reduction in their quality of life. Depression and functional disability were related to the quality of life. Four years after stroke, 83% of the survivors reported a decrease in their quality of life as assessed on professional and household activities, family relations, sexual activity and leisure. Motor deficits, dependence and depression were related to the decrease in quality of life (Niemi *et al.* 1988). While the reduction in quality of life after stroke is clear, it must be stressed that the strain on the family and caregivers also has to be taken into account (Schultz, Tompkins & Rau 1988; Wade 1992).

Many difficulties still remain in the assessment of quality of life after stroke. Major methodological impovements are needed before we shall be able to assess more reliably the quality of life concept and to use it in the allocation of resources.

Cost-effectiveness

There is, to our knowledge, no cost-effectiveness study of the need for hospital admission, of the need for precise stroke subtype diagnosis, or of the comparison of different stroke treatments. However, technological costs are only a small part of the medical care costs in stroke, and several investigations can sometimes be done on an outpatient basis. Moreover, the personal and economic costs of a wrong diagnosis can also be considered as outweighing the expenses linked to medical care.

Long-term prognosis, stroke recurrence

Up to 15 to 40% of the patients will have a recurrence of stroke. Stroke recurrence occurs at a constant rate of about 9% per year (Marquardsen 1986). The severity of the initial sroke is not an indicator of the risk of recurrence. In a study of TIA and minor strokes, the risk of recurrence was higher for all the subtypes of stroke in patients with leukoaraiosis on CT. The authors considered that leukoaraiosis could be an independent risk factor for stroke recurrence (Van Swieten *et al.* 1992).

Kappelle *et al.* (1994) studied the outcome of stroke in 296 consecutive patients aged 15–44 years referred to the University of Iowa Hospitals between 1977 and 1992. The mortality from death due to vascular causes was 1.7%/year. The mortality was twice as great in those with large vessel disease. In those without risk factors for stroke the mortality was only about a tenth of this figure. More than a half of the survivors had serious social or personal problems, and only 40% were employed.

Treatment

Hospital admission: why admit?

Hospital admission of stroke patients has been questioned by several authors, and a better organization of rehabilitation services has been advocated (Wade & Langton Hewer 1983). In this debate it has been stressed that about 15% of patients with suspected stroke may not have an acute stroke, but had a previous stroke, seizures, dementia, or a tumour (Norris & Hachinski 1982). Moreover, diagnostic reliability is far better related to the clinical skills of the doctors than to the availability of laboratory data. Also, hospital admission has been proposed because trained doctors assessing many stroke patients would probably make a better diagnosis than general practitioners, who see only 2–6 acute strokes per year, and because nursing hemiplegic patients is difficult, especially at home with aged relatives (Hugget 1983; Steiner 1983).

Where to admit: stroke units?

In the early 1970s, the efficiency criterion for an 'acute care unit' was reduction in the mortality. However, this was very difficult to demonstrate, because most of the studies were open and the controls were historical (Kennedy *et al.* 1970; Carpenter & Reed, 1972; Cooper *et al.* 1972; Pitner & Mance 1973; Drake *et al.* 1973). The efficiency of stroke units was not evident. Recently, a randomized and controlled study was conducted between a stroke unit and general medical wards. This study showed an identical mortality rate within the first 5 days of stay. However, the mortality was thereafter reduced for the patients admitted to the stroke unit compared with the patients admitted to other medical wards (Indredavik *et al.* 1991). Moreover, there was a decrease in the occurrence of complications (deep venous thrombosis, pneumonia, etc.) in stroke units, probably related to the training of the team (Cooper *et al.* 1972; Norris & Hachinski 1976; Woimant *et al.* 1984). The result of this better care probably also explains the improvement in disability (Strand *et al.* 1985, 1986), reduced rate of patients discharged to nursing homes (Indredavik *et al.* 1991), and reduction of the length of stay for the patients admitted to stroke units (Strand *et al.* 1985).

Medical treatment

Medical treatment of acute stroke

In acute stroke, the ischaemic area can be schematically separated into a central core that will rapidly evolve toward necrosis and a peripheral area in which the neurons are potentially viable (the ischaemic penumbra). Treatments mainly focus on the protection of viable ischaemic neurons in the penumbra, and can be described as (1) restoration of perfusion; and (2) protection of the neurons.

Treatments aimed at improvement of cerebral blood flow

Fibrinolytics and defibrinating agents have been tried in acute stroke. Their aim is to restore arterial patency. Wardlaw & Warlow (1992) conducted a meta-analysis of thrombolytic trials. In the small number of patients treated in randomized trials with a CT scan, there was a 37% reduction of the odds of death and a significant 56% reduction in the odds of death and deterioration. The tolerance appeared to be acceptable, the risk of symptomatic haemorrhagic transformation and severe oedema formation being not excessive.

The role of endovascular stenting, balloon dilation, and other procedures in patients with stenosis of major vessels inaccessible to conventional surgical approaches is not yet resolved. Similarly, attempts to treat strokes within hours of the onset by intravascular thrombolytic therapy, or by systemic thrombolysis, have not so far demonstrated a benefit in relation to the incidence of unwanted effects of treatments (see Coull 1996).

Asplund (1991) reviewed the effect of haemodilution on mortality and disability. He did not report any significant effect on the outcome.

Neuroprotective treatments

Calcium antagonists have been used in many studies of acute stroke. An overview of the trials using nimodipine has shown that there could be an improvement in mortality and functional state with nimodipine if given in the first few hours after stroke onset (Orgogozo *et al.* 1992). However, this finding should be confirmed in a prospective trial.

Trials with new drugs, such as excitatory amino acid inhibitors or free radical scavengers are awaited.

Heparin is sometimes used in acute stroke. There is evidence for its effect on prevention of deep venous thrombosis and pulmonary embolism. However, data supporting its efficacy in mortality and functional state are controversial. Two very large studies are ongoing in order to test this (Sandercock & Huub 1992).

In the conduct of clinical trials in acute stroke, the time schedule of therapy may be of first importance. Hospital admission in the first few hours after a stroke in centres involved in multicentre trials is crucial for improving our knowledge in acute stroke treatments.

Stroke prevention: anticoagulants, antiplatelet agents

There are various sources of cardiac embolism to the brain (Hart 1992). Atrial fibrillation carries an increased risk of stroke. Oral anticoagulants have proved to be efficient in primary stroke prevention in five trials (Hart 1992). They reduced the risk of arterial thromboembolism by 70%. The effect of aspirin was not uniform in the different studies: a 42% reduction was reported in the Stroke Prevention in Atrial Fibrillation study (Stroke Prevention in Atrial Fibrillation Investigators 1991), but there was no significant effect in another trial (Hart 1992). In secondary prevention, the results of the large European Atrial Fibrillation Trial were also positive.

In stroke prevention, aspirin is a mainstay. Its efficacy in stroke reduction is about 25% (Antiplatelet Trialist's Collaboration 1988). The dose of aspirin is still a matter of debate. In the earliest studies, a dosage of 1 g per day or more was given. In more recent studies, very low doses (75 or 30 mg per day) were also effective (Dutch TIA Trial Study Group 1991; SALT Collaborative Group 1991). Ticlopidine has also proved to be efficient in a study against placebo in reducing vascular death, non-fatal stroke, or non-fatal myocardial inarction by 30% (Gent *et al.* 1989), and in a trial against aspirin by reducing the risk of non-fatal or fatal stroke by 21% (Hass *et al.* 1989).

A meta-analysis (Anti-platelet Triallists' Collaboration 1994) of 101 302 patients with cerebral, coronary or peripheral vascular disease, or in other high-risk categories (Table 5.4), entering clinical trials of aspirin showed a 23% reduction in the risk of non-fatal stroke in those with a history of TIA or previous stroke. The reduction in risk of stroke in

Table 5.4. *Reduction in risk of stroke with antiplatelet drug treatment*

Category	Event rate (controls) %/year	Event rate (drugs) %/year	Odds reduction (% ± SD)
Stroke and TIA	10.2	8.2	23 ± 6
Acute MI	0.6	0.4	40 ± 17
Chronic MI	1.5	1.0	39 ± 11
Other high-risk patients[a]	1.9	1.1	49 ± 6
All high-risk patients	2.9	2.1	31 ± 5
Low-risk patients	0.95	1.15	− 21 ± 1

[a] Stable or unstable angina, vascular surgery, angioplasty, atrial fibrillation, valvular heart disease, peripheral vascular disease.

those with coronary or peripheral vascular disease was of similar magnitude. This reduction in risk was independent of age, hypertension or diabetes mellitus.

The use of aspirin in primary stroke prevention in people without risk factors is not supported by the evidence available (Barnett, Eliasziw & Meldrum 1995). In people in whom aspirin cannot be tolerated ticlopidine can be considered, although this therapy carries a small risk of serious neutropenia, or even marrow asplasia. Dipyridamole has been disappointingly ineffective in clinical trials and has no place in the management of stroke prevention. The risk of stroke in patients with atrial fibrillation can be reduced by about 70% (Table 5.4) with warfarin therapy in patients older than 65 years. However, warfarin is probably not indicated in people older than 75 years, since the beneficial effect is equalled by the increased risk of cerebral haemorrhage in this age group (Atrial Fibrillation Investigators 1994). In people with a history of stroke associated with valvular heart disease, or some other cardiac source of embolism, warfarin is effective (66% reduction in stroke risk) compared with aspirin therapy (European Atrial Fibrillation Study Group 1993).

Surgical treatment

The first carotid endarterectomy for atheromatous stenosis was performed in 1954. However, in 1991 two studies, the European Carotid Surgery Trial (ECST) and the North American Symptomatic Carotid Endarterectomy Trial (NASCET) reported preliminary results demonstrating the efficacy of carotid endarterectomy for secondary prevention in symptomatic carotid stenosis (MRC European Carotid Surgery Trial 1991; North American Symptomatic Carotid Endarterectomy Trial Collaborators 1991). This efficacy was obtained in the subgroup with stenosis equal to or higher than 70% for ipsilateral srokes (14% absolute risk reduction in 3 years for the ECST; 17% absolute risk reduction in 2 years for the NASCET) and for all strokes and death (10% absolute risk reduction in 3 years in the ECST; 10% absolute risk reduction in 2 years in the NASCET). For the subgroup with stenosis less than 30%, the ECST showed no benefit of surgery. The difference in efficacy betwccn these trials may be related to differences in the inclusion criteria, and in the method used for measuring the stenosis. The risk of stroke is strongly related to the degree of stenosis, and the NASCET method may underrate the degree of stenosis when compared with the ECST method. Thus, the group of patients with more than 70% stenosis may have a lesser degree of stenosis in the ECST, carrying a lower spontaneous risk, making the demonstration of the efficacy of surgery less impressive (Bousser 1992; Warlow, 1992). The rate of surgery-related deaths and severe stroke was 3.7% in ECST and 2.7% in NASCET. The difference is not significant and may be related to the differences in the choice of the centres participating in the trials. Both trials contained randomization for patients with stenosis between 30% and 70%.

In primary stroke prevention, carotid endarterectomy has been recommended in the management of asymptomatic carotid stenosis (Executive Committee for the Asymptomatic Carotid Atherosclerosis Study 1995) in people with stenosis > 60%, provided that the operation is carried out in centres in which the combined mortality and morbidity of the procedure is < 3%. The absolute reduction in risk of stroke in this group of people with this operation is only 1% per year, and this needs to be considered in recommending the procedure to any individual. In half the cases the complications of the procedure resulted from the angiography rather than from the operation itself, a matter that indicated the need for safer arterial investigation. A further caveat in considering the role of this operation in primary stroke prevention is that this study did not demonstrate any graded benefit in relation to increasing degrees of stenosis, and that the benefit in women was only 16%, much less than in men.

Conclusion

Improving stroke outcome is one of the major challenges in medicine. We are entering a phase in which recent improvements in stroke prevention are likely to be followed by significant results in the acute phase of stroke. Because the efficacy of new drugs and treatments is likely to be limited to the very first hours of stroke, and may also vary according to the different stroke subtypes, very early admission to hospitals with acute care and investigation units may be one of the critical steps in this progress.

References

Abott, R. D., Yin Yin, M. A., Reed, D. M. & Yano, K. (1986). Risk of stroke in male cigarette smokers. *N. Engl. J. Med.* **315**, 717–20.

Ahlsiö, B., Britton, M., Murray, V. & Theorell, T. (1984). Disablement and quality of life after stroke. *Stroke* **15**, 886–90.

Allen, C. M. C. (1984). Predicting the outcome of acute stroke: a prognostic score. *J. Neurol. Neurosurg. Psychiatry* **47**, 475–80.

Amarenco, P. & Hauw, J.-J. (1990). Cerebellar infarction in the territory of the anterior and inferior cerebellar artery. *Brain* **113**, 139–55.

Antiplatelet Triallists' Collaboration (1988). Secondary prevention of vascular disease by prolonged antiplatelet treatment. *Br. Med. J.* **296**, 320–31.

Anti-platelet Triallists' Collaboration (1994). Collaborative overview of randomized trials of antiplatelet therapy. I. Prevention of death, myocardial infarction and stroke by prolonged antiplatelet therapy in various categories of patients. *Br. Med. J.* **308**, 81–106.

Asplund, K. (1991). Hemodilution in acute stroke. *Cerebrovasc. Dis.* **1** (Suppl. 1), 129–38.

Asplund, K. (1992). Any progress on progressing stroke? *Cerebrovasc. Dis.* **2**, 317–19.

Asplund, K., Carlberg, B. & Sundström, G. (1992). Stroke in the elderly. *Cerebrovasc. Dis.* **2**, 152–7.

Aström, M., Adolfson, R., Asplund, K. & Aström, T. (1992). Life before and after stroke. Living conditions and life satisfaction in relation to a general elderly population. *Cerebrovasc. Dis.* **2**, 28–34.

Atrial Fibrillation Investigators (1994). Risk factors for stroke and efficacy of antithrombotic therapy in atrial fibrillation: analysis of pooled data from five randomized trials. *Arch. Intern. Med.* **154**, 1449–57.

Bamford, J., Sandercock, P., Jones, L. & Warlow, C. (1987). The natural history of lacunar infarction: the Oxfordshire community Stroke Project. *Stroke* **18**, 545–51.

Barnett, H. J. M. (1992). 35 years of stroke prevention: challenges, disappointments and successes. *Cerebrovasc. Dis.* **1**, 61–70.

Barnett, H. J., Eliasziw, Meldrum, H. E. (1995). Drugs and surgery in the prevention of ischaemic stroke. *N. Engl. J. Med.* **332**, 238–48.

Barret-Connor, E. & Khaw, K. T. (1988). Diabetes mellitus: an independent risk factor for stroke? *Am. J. Epidemiol.* **128**, 116–23.

Baquis, G. D., Pessin, M. S. & Scott, R. M. (1985). Limb shaking; a carotid TIA. *Stroke* **16**, 444–8.

Besson, G., Bogousslavsky, J., Regli, F. & Maeder, P. (1991). Acute pseudobulbar or suprabulbar palsy. *Arch. Neurol.* **48**, 501–7.

Bogousslavsky, J. & Pierre, P. (1992). Ischemic stroke in patients under age 45. *Neurol. Clin.* **10**, 113–24.

Bogousslavsky, J. & Regli, F. (1985). Cerebral infarct in apparent transient ischaemic attack. *Neurology* **35**, 1501–3.

Bogousslavsky, J. & Regli, F. (1986). Unilateral watershed cerebral infarcts. *Neurology* **36**, 373–7.

Bogousslavsky, J. & Regli, F. (1989). Anterior cerebral artery territory infarction in the Lausanne Stroke Registry: clinical and etiological patterns. *Arch. Neurol.* **47**, 144–50.

Bogousslavsky, J. & Regli, F. (1992). Centrum ovale infarcts: Subcortical infarction in the superficial territory of the middle cerebral artery. *Neurology* **42**, 1992–8.

Bogousslavsky, J., Despland, P. A. & Regli, F. (1986a). Asymptomatic tight stenosis of the internal carotid artery: long-term prognosis. *Neurology* **36**, 861–3.

Bogousslavsky, J., Hachinski, V., Boughner, D. R. *et al.* (1986b). Cardiac and arterial lesions in carotid transient ischaemic attack. *Arch. Neurol.* **43**, 223–8.

Bogousslavsky, J., Despland, P. A. & Regli, F. (1987a). Spontaneous carotid dissection with acute stroke. *Arch. Neurol.* **44**, 137–40.

Bogousslavsky, J., Regli, F., Zografos, L. & Uské, A. (1987b). Opticocerebral syndrome. Simultaneous hemodynamic infarction of optic nerve and brain. *Neurology* **37**, 263–8.

Bogousslavsky, J., Regli, F. & Uské, A. (1988a). Thalamic infarcts: clinical syndromes, etiology and prognosis. *Neurology* **38**, 837–48.

Bogousslavsky, J., Regli, F., Van Melle, G., Payot, M. & Uské, A. (1988b). Migraine stroke. *Neurology* **38**, 223–7.

Bogousslavsky, J., Van Melle, G. & Regli, F. (1988c). The Lausanne Stroke Registry Group: analysis of 1000 consecutive patients with first stroke. *Stroke* **19**, 1083–92.

Bogousslavsky, J., Van Melle, G. & Regli, F. (1989). Middle cerebral pial territory infarcts: a study of the Lausanne Stroke Registry. *Ann. Neurol.* **25**, 555–60.

Bogousslavsky, J., Van Melle, G., Despland, P. R. & Regli, F. (1990). Alcohol consumption and carotid atherosclorosis in the Lausanne Stroke Registry. *Stroke* **21**, 715–20.

Bogousslavsky, J., Cachin, C., Regli, F., Despland, P. A., Van Melle, G. & Kappenberger, L. for the Lausanne Stroke Registry Group. (1991a). Cardiac sources of embolism and cerebral infarction. Clinical consequences and vascular concomitants. *Neurology* **41**, 855–9.

Bogousslavsky, J., Regli, F. & Maeder, P. (1991b). Intracranial large-artery disease and "lacunar" infarction. *Cerebrovasc. Dis.* **1**, 154–9.

Bogousslavsky, J., Regli, F., Uské, A. & Maeder, P. (1991c). Early spontaneous hematoma in cerebral infarct: is primary cerebral hemorrhage overdiagnosed? *Neurology* **41**, 837–40.

Bogousslavsky, J. & Regli, F. (1993). Klinik der intrazerebralen Blutung. In: Poeck, K., Schliack, M. & Hopf, H. C. (eds.) Klinische Neurologie. Heidelberg: Springer-Verlag.

Bonita, R., Stewart, A. W. & Beaglehole, R. (1990). International trends in stroke mortality: 1975–1985. *Stroke* **32**, 989–92.

Brass, L. M., Isaacsohn, J. L., Merikangas, K. R. & Robinette, C. D. (1992). A study of twins and stroke. *Stroke* **23**, 221–3.

Broderick, J. P., Philipps, S. J., Whisnant, J. P., O'Fallon, W. M. & Bergstrahl, E. J. (1989). Incidence rates of stroke in the eighties: the end of the decline in stroke? *Stroke* **20**, 577–82.

Calanchini, P. R., Swanson, P. D. & Gotshall, R. A. (1977). Cooperative study of hospital frequency and criteria of transient ischaemic attacks. IV. The reliability of diagnosis. *JAMA* **338**, 2029–33.

Caplan, L. R. (1988a). Intracerebral hemorrhage revisited. *Neurology,* **38**, 624–7.

Caplan, L. R. (1988b). TIAs: we need to return to the question, 'What is wrong with Mr Jones?' *Neurology* **38**, 791–3.

Caplan, L. R. (1992). Intracerebral hemorrhage. *Lancet* **339**, 656–8.

Caplan, L. R. & Goodwin, J. A. (1982). Lateral tegmental brainstem hemorrhages. *Neurology* **32**, 252–60.

Cardiac Embolism Task Force (1989). Cardiogenic brain embolism. The second report of the Cerebral Embolism Task Force. *Arch. Neurol.* **46**, 727–43.

Carolei, A., Candelise, L., Fiorelli, M. *et al.* (1992). Long-term prognosis of transient ischemic attacks and reversible neurologic deficits: a hospital-based study. *Cerebrovasc. Dis.* **2**, 266–72.

Carpenter, R. R. & Reed, D. E. (1972). The outcome for patients with cerebrovascular disease in university and community hospitals. *Stroke* **3**, 747–58.

Colditz, G. A., Bonita, R. & Stampfer, M. J. (1988). Cigarette smoking and risk of stroke in middle-aged women. *N. Engl. J. Med.* **318**, 937–41.

Collins, R., Peto, R., McMahon, S. *et al.* (1990). Blood pressure, stroke and coronary heart disease. II. Short-term reductions in blood pressure: overview of randomized drug trials in their epidemiological context. *Lancet* **335**, 827–8.

Cooper, S. W., Olivet, J. A. & Woolsey, F. M. Jr (1972). Establishment and operation of combined intensive care unit. *NY State J. Med.* **72**, 2215–20.

Cooper, R., Sempos, C., Hsieh, S. C. & Kovar, M. G. (1990). Slowdown in the decline of stroke mortality in the United States, 1978–1986. *Stroke* **21**, 1274–9.

Coull, B. M. (1996). The many windows of therapeutic opportunities in stroke. *Curr. Opin. Neurol.* **9**, 43–5.

De Bono, D. P., Warlow, C. P. & Hyman, N. M. (1982). Cardiac rhythm abnormalities in patients presenting with transient non-focal neurologic symptoms: a diagnostic gray area? *Br. J. Med.* **284**, 1437–9.

Dennis, M. S., Bamford, J. M., Sandercock, P. A. G. *et al.* (1989). A comparison of risk factors and prognosis for transient ischemic attacks and minor ischemic strokes. The Oxfordshire Community Stroke Project. *Stroke* **20**, 1494–9.

Dennis, M. S., Bamford, J. M., Sandercock, P. A. G. & Warlow, C. (1990). Prognosis of transient ischemic attacks in the Oxfordshire Community Stroke Project. *Stroke* **21**, 848–53.

Dexter, D. D., Whisnant, J. P., Connoly, D. C. & O'Fallon, W. M. (1987). The association of stroke and coronary artery disease. A population study. *Mayo Clin. Proc.* **62**, 1077–83.

Donnan, G. A., Bladin, P. F., Berkovic, S. F., Longley, W. A. & Saling, M. M. (1992). The stroke syndrome of striatocapsular infarction. *Brain* **114**, 51–70.

Drake, W. E., Hamilton, M. J., Carlson, M. & Blumenkrantz, J. (1973). Acute stroke management and patient outcome: the value of neurovascular care units. *Stroke* **4**, 933–45.

Dyken, J. L., Conneally, M., Haerer, A. *et al.* (1977). Cooperative study of hospital frequency and criteria of transient ischemic attacks. IV. The reliability of diagnosis. *JAMA* **237**, 882–6.

Dyken, M. L., Barnett, H. J. M., Easton, J. D. *et al.* (1992). Low-dose aspirin and stroke. 'It ain't necessarily so'. *Stroke* **23**, 1395–9.

European Atrial Fibrillation Study Group (1993). Secondary prevention in non-rheumatic atrial fibrillation after transient ischaemic attack or minor stroke. *Lancet* **342**, 1255–62.

European Carotid Surgery Triallists's Collaborative Group. (1991). MRC European Carotid Surgery Trial: interim results for symptomatic patients with severe (70–99%) or with mild (0–29%) carotid stenosis. *Lancet* **337**, 1235–43.

Executive Committee for the Asymptomatic Carotid Atherosclerosis Group (1995). Endarterectomy for asymptomatic carotid artery stenosis. *JAMA* **273**, 1421–8.

Ferrazzini, M., Regli, F. & Bogousslavsky, J. (1988). Pathogenèse des accidents cérébrovasculaires dans une population âgée. Etude de 62 patients âgés de plus de 75 ans. *Schweiz. Med. Wochenschr.* **118**, 462–6.

Fisher, C. M. (1965). Lacunes: small deep cerebral infarcts. *Neurology* **15**, 774–84.

Fisher, C. M. (1991). Lacunar infarcts. A review. *Cerebrovasc. Dis.* **1**, 311–20.

Fletcher, A. E. & Bulpitt, C. J. (1992). How far should blood pressure be lowered? *N. Engl. J. Med.* **326**, 251–4.

Forsting, M., Mattle, H. P. & Huber, P. (1991). Anticoagulation-related intracerebral hemorrhage. *Cerebrovasc. Dis.* **1**, 97–102.

Francke, C. L., van Swieten, J. C., Algra, A. & van Gijn, J. (1992). Prognostic factors in patients with intracerebral hematoma. *J. Neurol. Neurosurg. Psychiatry* **55**, 653–7.

Furlan, A. J., Whisnant, J. P. & Kearns, T. P. (1979). Unilateral visual loss in bright light. An unusual symptom of carotid artery occlusive disease. *Arch. Neurol* **36**, 675–6.

Gandolfo, C., Moretti, C., Dall Agata, D., Primavera, A., Brusca, G. & Loeb, C. (1986). Long-term prognosis of patients with lacunar syndromes. *Acta Neurol. Scand.* **74**, 224–9.

Gates, P. C., Barnett, H. J. M., Vinters, H. V. *et al.* (1986). Primary intraventricular hemorrhage in adults. *Stroke* **17**, 872–7.

Gent, M., Blakely, J. A., Easton, J. D., Ellis, D. J., Hachinski, V. C., Harbison, J. W., Panak, E., Roberts, R. S., Sicurella, J., Turpie, A. G. G. & the CATS Group. (1989). The Canadian–American Ticlopidine Study (CATS) in thromboembolic stroke (1989). *Lancet* **I**, 1215–20.

Ghika, J., Bogousslavsky, J. & Regli, F. (1989). Infarcts in the territory of the deep perforators from the carotid system. *Neurology* **39**, 507–12.

Gill, J. S., Zezulka, V. & Shipley, M. J. (1986). Stroke and alcohol consumption. *N. Engl. J. Med.* **315**, 1041–6.

Giroud, M., Gras, P., Chadan, N. *et al.* (1991a). Cerebral hemorrhage in a French prospective population study. *J. Neurol. Neurosurg. Psychiatry* **54**, 595–8.

Giroud, M., Milan, C., Beuriat, P., Gras, P., Essayagh, E., Arveux, P. & Dumas, R. (1991b). Incidence and survival rates during a two-year period of intracerebral and subarachnoid haemorrhage, cortical infarcts, lacunes, and transient attacks. The Stroke Registry of Dijon: 1985–1989. *Int. J. Epidemiol.* **20**, 892–9.

Giroud, M., Gras, P., Milan, C., Arveux, P., Beuriat, P., Vion, Ph. & Dumas, R. (1991c). Histoire naturelle des syndromes lacunaires. Apport du registre Dijonais des accidents vasculaires cérébraux. *Rev. Neurol.* **147**, 566–72.

Gresham, G. E. (1986). The rehabilitation of the stroke survivor. *Stroke* **17**, 358–60.

Gresham, G. E., Phillips, T. F., Wolf, P. A., McNamara, P., Kannel, W. B. & Dawber, T. R. (1979). Epidemiologic profile of long-term stroke disability: the Framingham Study. *Arch. Phys. Med. Rehabil.* **60**, 487–91.

Groothuis, D. R., Duncan, G. W., Fisher, C. M. (1977). The human thalamocortical sensory path in the internal capsule: anatomic evidence from a small capsular hemorrhage causing a pure sensory stroke. *Ann. Neurol.* **2**, 328–31.

Hankey, G. L. & Warlow, C. P. (1991). Transient ischemic lacunar attacks: a useful clinical concept? *Lancet* **337**, 335–8.

Harmsen, P., Tsipogianni, A. & Wilhelmsen, L. (1992). Stroke incidence rates were unchanged while fatality rates declined, during 1971–1987 in Göteborg, Sweden. *Stroke* **23**, 1410–15.

Hart, R. G. (1992). Cardiogenic embolism to the brain. *Lancet* I, 589–94.

Hass, W. K., Easton, J. D., Adams, H. P. Jr., Pryse-Phillips, W., Molony, B. A., Anderson, S., Kamm, B. (1989). For the Ticlopidine Aspirin Stroke Study Group: a randomized trial comparing ticlopidine hydrochloride with aspirin for the prevention of stroke in high-risk patients. *N. Engl. J. Med.* **321**, 501–17.

Henley, S., Pettit, S., Todd-Pokropek, A. & Tupper, A. M. (1985). Who goes home? Predictive factors in stroke recovery. *J. Neurol. Neurosurg. Psychiatry* **48**, 1–6.

Heyman, A., Wilkinson, W. E., Hurwitz, B. J. *et al.* (1984). Risk of ischemic heart disease in patients with TIA. *Neurology* **34**, 626–30.

Hier, D. B., Davis, K. R., Richardson, E. P. & Mohr, J. P. (1977). Hypertensive putaminal hemorrhage. *Ann. Neurol.* **1**, 152–9.

Horning, C. R., Dorndorf, W. & Agnoli, A. L. (1986). Hemorrhagic cerebral infarction. A prospective study. *Stroke* **17**, 179–85.

Howard, G., Till, J. S., Toole, J. F., Matthews, C. & Truscott, B. L. (1985). Factors influencing return to work following cerebral infarction. *JAMA* **253**, 226–32.

Hugget, I. O. (1983). Why admit stroke patients to hospital? *Lancet* I, 1165–6.

Hunt, K., Vessey, M., MacPherson, K. & Coleman, M. (1987). Long-term surveillance of mortality and cancer incidence in women receiving hormone replacement therapy. *Br. J. Obstet. Gynaecol.* **94**, 620–35.

Indedravik, B., Bakke, F., Solberg, R., Roikseth, R., Haaheim, L. L. & Holme, I. (1991). Benefit of a stroke unit: a randomized controlled trial. *Stroke* **22**, 1026–31.

Iso, H., Jacobs, D. R. & Wentworth, D. (1989). Serum cholesterol levels and six-year mortality from stroke in 350 977 men screened for multiple risk factors intervention. *N. Engl. J. Med.* **320**, 904–10.

Jongbloed, L. (1986). Prediction of function after stroke: a critical review. *Stroke* **17**, 765–76.

Jörgensen, H. S., Plesner, A. M., Hübbe, P. & Larsen, K. (1992). Marked increase of stroke incidence in men between 1972 and 1990 in Frederiksberg, Denmark. *Stroke* **23**, 1701–4.

Kappelle, L. J., van Latum, J. C., Koudstaal, P. J. & van Gijn, J. (1991). Transient ischemic attacks and small vessel disease. *Lancet* **337**, 339–41.

Kase, C. S., Forster, T. E., Reed, J. E. *et al.* (1987). Intracerebral hemorrhage and phenylpropanolamine use. *Neurology* **37**, 309–14.

Kennedy, F. B., Pozen, T. J. & Gabelman, E. H. (1970). Stroke intensive care. An appraisal. *Am. Heart J.* **80**, 188–96.

Khaw, K. T. & Barrett-Connor, E. (1987). Dietary potassium and stroke-associated mortality. *N. Engl. J. Med.* **316**, 1041–6.

Kilpatrick, T. J., Davis, S. M., Tress, B. M. & Rosenfeld, J. V. (1991). Lateral tegmental pontine hemorrhage due to vascular malformations. *Cerebrovasc. Dis.* **1**, 108–12.

Kopecky, S. L., Gersh, B. J., McGoon, M. D. & Whisnant, J. P. (1987). The natural history of lone atrial fibrillation. A population-based study over three decades. *N. Engl. J. Med.* **317**, 669–74.

Koudstaal, P. J., van Gijn, J. & Staal, A. (1986). Diagnosis of transient ischemic attacks: improvement of interobserver agreement by a check-list in ordinary language. *Stroke* **17**, 723–8.

Koudstaal, P. J., Van Gijn, J., Frenken, C. W. G., Hijdra, A., Loddler, J., Vermeulen, M., Bulens, C. & Franke, C. L. (1992). TIA, RIND, minor stroke: a continuum, or different subgroups. *J. Neurol. Neurosurg. Psychiatry* **55**, 95–7.

Labauge, R., Boukobza, M., Zinszner, J. *et al.* (1983). Hématomes spontanés du cervelet. 28 observations personnelles. *Rev. Neurol.* **139**, 193–204.

Lechat, P., Mas, J. L., Lascault, G., Loron, P., Theard, M., Klivuczac, M., Drobinski, Thomas, G. & Grosgogeat, Y. (1988). Prevalence of patent foramen ovale in patients with stroke. *N. Engl. J. Med.* **318**, 1148–52.

Lee, C. N., Reed, D. M., MacLean, C. J., Yano, K. & Chiu, D. (1988). Dietary potassium and stroke. *N. Engl. J. Med.* **318**, 995.

Levine, R. L., Lagreze, H. L., Dobkin, J. A. & Turski, P. A. (1988). Large subcortical hemispheric infarctions: presentation and prognosis. *Arch. Neurol.* **45**, 1074–7.

Levy, D. E. (1988). How transient are transient ischemic attacks. *Neurology* **38**, 674–7.

Libman, R. B., Sacco, R. L., Shi, T., Tatemichi, T. K. & Mohr, J. P. (1992). Neurologic improvement in pure motor hemiparesis: implications for clinical trials. *Neurology* **42**, 1713–16.

Lipton, R. B., Berger, A. R., Lesser, M. L. *et al.* (1987). Lobar vs thalamic and basal ganglionic hemorrhage: clinical and radiographic features. *J. Neurol.* **234**, 86–90.

Malmgren, M., Warlow, C., Bamford, J. & Sandercock, P. (1987). Geographical and secular trends in stroke incidence. *Lancet* **II**, 1196–2000.

Marmot, M. G. & Poulter, N. R. (1992). Primary prevention of Stroke. *Lancet* **339**, 344–6.

Marquersden, J. (1983). Natural history and prognosis of cerebrovascular disease. In: Ross Russel, R. W. (ed.) *Vascular Disease of the Central Nervous System*, 2nd edn. pp. 25–40. New York: Churchill Livingstone.

Marquersden, J. (1986). Epidemiology of strokes in Europe. In: Barnett, H. J. M., Stein, B. M., Mohr, J. P., Yatsu, F. M. (eds.), *Stroke Pathophysiology, Diagnosis and Management*, pp. 31–43. New York: Churchill Livingstone.

Mas, J. L. & Zuber, M. (1991). Epidemiology of ischemic stroke. *Cerebrovasc. Dis.* **1** (Suppl. 1), 36–44.

Mas, J. L., Dilonya, A. & de Recondo, J. (1992). A familial disorder with subcortical ischemic strokes, dementia and leucoencephalopathy. *Neurology* **42**, 1015–19.

Massaro, A. R., Sacco, R. L., Mohr, J. P. *et al.* (1991). Clinical discriminators of lobar and deep hemorrhages. The stroke data bank. *Neurology* **41**, 1881–5.

Melo, T. P., Bogousslavsky, J., Van Melle, G. & Regli, F. (1992). Pure motor stroke: a reappraisal. *Neurology* **42**, 789–98.

Mikayo, S., Takano, A., Teramoto, J., Takahashi, A. (1992). Leukoaraiosis in relation to prognosis for patients with lacunar infarction. *Stroke* **23**, 1434–8.

MRC European Carotid Surgery Trial (1991). Interim results for symptomatic patients with severe (70–99%) or very mild (0–29%) carotid stenosis. *Lancet* **337**, 1235–43.

Nater, B., Bogousslavsky, J., Regli, F. & Stauffer, J. C. (1992). Stroke patterns with atrial septal aneurysm. *Cerebrovasc. Dis.* **2**, 342–46.

Neumann, P. E., Mehler, M. F. & Horoupian, D. S. (1985). Primary medullary hypertensive hemorrhage. *Neurology* **35**, 925–8.

Niemi, M. L., Laaksonen, R., Kotila, M. & Waltimo, O. (1988). Quality of life 4 years after stroke. Stroke 1988, **19**, 1101–7.

Norris, J. W. (1992). Risk of cerebral infarction, myocardial infarction and vascular death in patients with asymptomatic carotid disease, transient ischemic attack and stroke. *Cerebrovasc. Dis.* **2** (Suppl. 1), 2–5.

Norris, J. W. & Hachinski, V. C. (1976). Intensive care management of stroke patients. *Stroke* **7**, 573–7.

Norris, J. W. & Hachinski, V. C. (1982). Misdiagnosis of stroke. *Lancet* I, 328–31.

North American Symptomatic Carotid Endarterectomy Trial Collaborators (1991). Beneficial effect of carotid endarectomy in symptomatic patients with high-grade carotid stenosis. *N. Engl. J. Med.* **325**, 445–53.

Orgogozo, J. M., Mohr, J. P., Harrison, M., Hennerici, M., Wahlgren, N., Gelmers, H. J., Martinez-Vila, E., Dycha, J. & Tettenborn, D. (1992). An overview of acute stroke trials with oral nimodipine (abstract). *Cerebrovasc. Dis.* **2**, 198.

Ott, K. H., Kase, C. S., Ojemann, R. G. & Mohr, J. P. (1974). Cerebellar hemorrhage: diagnosis and treatment. *Arch. Neurol.* **31**, 160–7.

Oxfordshire Community Stroke Project (1983). Incidence of stroke in Oxfordshire: first year's experience of a community stroke register. *Br. Med. J.* **287**, 713–17.

Paganini-Hill, A., Ross, R., Henderson, B. E. (1988). Postmenopausal oestrogen treatment and stroke. A prospective study. *Br. Med. J.* **298**, 519–22.

Pedrazzi, P., Bogousslavsky, J. & Regli, F. (1990). Hématomes limités à la tête du noyau caudé. *Rev. Neurol.* **146**, 726–38.

Pessin, M. S., Duncan, G. W., Mohr, J. P. & Poszanker, D. C. (1977). Clinical and angiographic features of carotid transient ischemic attacks. *N. Engl. J. Med.* **296**, 358–62.

Pitner, S. E. & Mance, C. J. (1973). An evaluation of stroke intensive care: results in a municipal hospital. *Stroke* **4**, 737–41.

Poungvarin, N., Bhoopat, W., Viriyavejakul, A. *et al.* (1987). Effects of dexamethason in primary supratentorial hemorrhage. *N. Engl. J. Med.* **316**, 1199–233.

Pozzati, E., Giuliani, G., Gaist, G. *et al.* (1986). Chronic expanding intracerebral hematoma. *J. Neurosurg.* **65**, 611–14.

Quizilbash, N., Duffy, S. W. & Warlow, C. (1992). Lipids are risk factors for ischaemic stroke: overview and review. *Cerebrovasc. Dis.* **2**, 127–36.

Ropper, A. H., Davis, K. R. (1980). Lobar cerebral hemorrhages: acute clinical syndrome in 26 cases. *Ann. Neurol.* **8**, 141–7.

Salonen, J., Puska, P. & Tuomilehto, J. (1982). Physical activity and risk of myocardial infarction, cerebral stroke and death. A longitudinal study in eastern Finland. *Am. J. Epidemiol.* **115**, 526–37.

Samuels, M. A. & Thalinger, K. (1991). Cerebrovascular manifestations of selected hematological diseases. *Semin. Neurol.* **11**, 411–18.

Sandercock, P. A. G. & Huub, W. (1992). Medical treatment of acute ischemic stroke. *Lancet* I, 537–9.

Sandercock, P. A. G., Allen, C. R. C., Corston, R. N. *et al.* (1985). Clinical diagnosis of intracranial hemorrhage using Guy's Hospital score. *Br. Med. J.* **291**, 1675–7.

Sandercock, P. A. G., Warlow, C. P., Jones, L. N. & Starkey, I. R. (1989). Predisposing factors for cerebral infarction: the Oxfordshire community project. *Br. Med. J.* **298**, 75–9.

Schultz, R., Tompkins, C. A. & Rau, M. T. (1988). A longitudinal study of the psychosocial impact of stroke on primary support persons. *Psychol. Aging* **3**, 131–41.

Schütz, H. (1992). Spontane intrazerebrale Blutungen. Eine Erkrankung im Wandel. *Nervenarzt* **63**, 63–73.

Scott, W. R. & Miller, B. R. (1985). Intracerebral hemorrhage with rapid recovery. *Arch. Neurol.* **42**, 133–6.

SHEP Cooperative Research Group (1991). Prevention of stroke by antihypertensive drug treatment in older persons with isolated Systolic Hypertension in the Elderly Program (SHEP). *JAMA* **265**, 3255–64.

Shinton, R. & Beevers, G. (1989). Meta-analysis of relation between cigarette smoking and stroke. *Br. Med. J.* **298**, 789–94.

Shaib, A. & Hachinski, V. (1990). Carotid transient ischemic attacks and normal investigations: a follow-up study. *Stroke* **21**, 525–7.

Singer, D. E. (1992). Randomized trials of warfarin for atrial fibrillation (editorial). *N. Engl. J. Med.* **327**, 1451–2.

Sloan, M. S. & Price, T. R. (1991). Intracranial hemorrhage following coronary thrombolytic therapy for acute myocardial infarction. *Semin. Neurol.* **11**, 385–99.

Stamler, J., Rose, Stamler, R. & Elliott, P. (1989). INTERSALT study findings: public health and medical care implications. *Hypertension* **14**, 570–7.

Stampfer, M. J., Colditz, G. A. & Willet, W. C. (1988). A retrospective study of moderate alcohol consumption and risk of coronary disease and stroke in women. *N. Engl. J. Med.* **320**, 1611–26.

Stampfer, M. J., Colditz, G. A., Willett, W. & Manson, J. E. (1991). Postmenopausal estrogen therapy and cardiovascular disease. Ten year follow-up from the Nurse's Health Study. *N. Engl. J. Med.* **325**, 756–62.

Steiner, T. J. (1983). Why admit stroke patients to hospital? *Lancet* I, 1379.

Strand, T., Asplund, K., Eriksson, S., Hägg, E., Lithner, F. & Weester, P. O. (1985). A non-intensive stroke unit reduces functional disability and the need for long-term hospitalization. *Stroke* **16**, 29–34.

Strand, T., Asplund, K., Eriksson, S., Hägg, E., Lithner, F. & Weester, P. O. (1986). Stroke unit care. Who benefits? Comparison with general care in relation to prognostic indicators on admission. *Stroke* **17**, 377–81.

Stroke Prevention in Atrial Fibrillation Investigators (1991). The Stroke Prevention in Atrial Fibrillation Study: final results. *Circulation* **84**, 527–39.

Terént, A. (1988). Increasing rate of stroke among Swedish women. *Stroke* **19**, 598–603.

The Amaurosis Fugax Study Group (1990). Current management of amaurosis fugax. *Stroke* **21**, 201–8.

The Dutch TIA Trial Study Group. (1991). A comparison of two doses of aspirin (30 mg vs 283 mg a day) in patients after a transient ischemic attach or minor ischemic stroke. *N. Engl. J. Med.* **325**, 1261–6.

The SALT Collaborative Group (1991). Swedish aspirin low-dose trial (SALT) of 75 mg aspirin as secondary prophylaxis after cerebrovascular ischaemic events. *Lancet* **338**, 1345–9.

Toffol, G. J., Biller, J. & Adams, J. P. (1987). Nontraumatic intracerebral hemorrhage in young adults. *Arch. Neurol.* **44**, 483–5.

Toole, J. F. (1991). The Willis Lecture: transient ischemic attacks, scientific method and new realities. *Stroke* **22**, 99–104.

Tournier-Lasserve, E., Iba-Zizen, M. T., Romero, N., Bousser, M. G. (1991). Autosomal dominant syndrome with stroke-like episodes and leukoencephalopathy. *Stroke* **22**, 1277–302.

Trouillat, R., Bogousslavsky, J., Regli, F. & Uské, A. (1990). Hémorragies intracérébrales supratentorielles. *Schweiz Med. Woschenschr.* **120**, 1056–63.

Tuhrim, S., Dambrosia, J. M., Price, T. R. *et al.* (1988). Prediction of intracerebral hemorrhage survival. *Ann. Neurol.* **24**, 258–63.

Urbinati, S., Di Pasquale, G., Andreoli, A., Lusa, A. M., Manini, G., Lanzino, G., Grazi, P., Ruffini, M. & Pinelli, G. (1992). Role and indication of two-dimensional echocardiography in young adults with cerebral ischemia: a prospective study in 125 patients. *Cerebrovasc. Dis.* **2**, 14–21.

Van Ruiswyk, J., Noble, H., Sigmann, P. (1990). The natural history of carotid bruits in elderly persons. *Ann. Intern. Med.* **112**, 340–3.

Van Swieteo, J. C., Kappelle, L. J., Algra, A., van Latum, J. C., Koudstaal, P. J. & van Gijn, J. for the Dutch TIA Study Group (1992). Hypodensity of the cerebral white matter in patients with transient ischemic attack or minor stroke: influence on the rate of subsequent stroke. *Ann. Neurol.* **32**, 177–83.

Wade, D. T. & Langton Hewer, R. (1983). Why admit stroke patients to hospital? *Lancet* **I**, 807–9.

Wade, D. T. & Langton Hewer, R. (1987). Functional abilities after stroke: measurement, natural history and prognosis. *J. Neurol. Neurosurg. Psychiatry* **50**, 177–82.

Wade, D. T., Wood, V. A. & Langton Hewer, R. (1985). Recovery after stroke – the first 3 months. *J. Neurol. Neurosurg. Psychiatry* **48**, 7–13.

Wakai, S., Kumakura & Nagai, M. (1992). Lobar intracerebral hemorrhage. A clinical, radiographic, and pathological study of 29 consecutive operated cases with negative angiography. *J. Neurosurg.* **76**, 231–8.

Waller, P. C. & Bhopal, R. S. (1989). Is snoring a cause of vascular disease. An epidemiological review. *Lancet* **II**, 143–5.

Walshe, T. M., David, K. D. & Fisher, C. (1977). Thalamic hemorrhage. A computed tomographic-clinical correlation. *Neurology* **27**, 217–22.

Warlow, C. (1992). Carotid endarterectomy. *Cerebrovasc. Dis.* **2**, 121.

Wardlaw, J. M. & Warlow, C. P. (1992). Thrombolysis in acute ischemic stroke: does it work? *Stroke* **23**, 1826–39.

Webster, M. W. I., Chancellor, A. M., Smith, H. J. *et al.* (1988). Patent foramen ovale in young stroke patients. *Lancet* **II**, 11–12.

Weiller, C., Ringelstein, E. B., Reiche, W., Thron, A. & Buell, U. (1990). The large striatocapsular infarct. A clinical and pathophysiological entity. *Arch. Neurol.* **47**, 1085–91.

Weisberg, L. A. (1981). Multiple spontaneous intracerebral hematomas: clinical and CT correlations. *Neurology* **31**, 897–900.

Weisberg, L. A. (1986a). Mesencephalic hemorrhages: clinical and CT correlations. *Neurology* **36**, 713–16.

Weisberg, L. A. (1986b). Primary pontine hemorrhage: clinical and CT correlations. *J. Neurol. Neurosurg. Psychiatry* **49**, 346–52.

Weisberg, L. A. & Nice, C. N. (1977). Intracranial tumors simulating the presentation of cerebrovascular syndromes. Early detection with cerebral computed tomography. *Am. J. Med.* **63**, 517–24.

Werdelin, L. & Juhler, M. (1988). The course of transient ischemic attacks. *Neurology* **38**, 677–80.

Wilson, P. W. F., Garrison, R. J. & Castelli, W. P. (1985). Postmenopausal oestrogen use, cigarette smoking, and cardiovascular morbidity in women over 50. The Framingham Study. *N. Engl. J. Med.* **313**, 1038–43.

Woimant, F., de Liège, P., Dupuy, M., Haguenau, M. & Pépin, B. (1984). Traitement des accidents vasculaires cérébraux dans une unité de soins intensifs. *Press Méd.* **13**, 2121–4.

Wolf, P. A., Abbott, R. D. & Kannel, W. B. (1991a). Atrial fibrillation, an independent risk factor for stroke in the elderly: the Framingham study. *Stroke* **22**, 983.

Wolf, P. A., D'Agostino, R. B., Belanger, A. J. & Kannel, W. B. (1991b). Probability of stroke: a risk profile from the Framingham study. *Stroke* **22**, 312–18.

Wolf, P. A., Cobb, J. L. & D'Agostino, R. B. (1992a). Epidemiology of stroke. In: Barnett, J. M., Mohr, J. P., Stein, B. M., Yatsu, F. M. (eds.) *Stroke. Pathophysiology, Diagnosis and Management*, 2nd edn, pp. 3–28. New York: Churchill Livingstone.

Wolf, P. A., D'Agostino, R. B., O'Neal, M. A. & Sytkowski, P. (1992b). Secular trends in stroke incidence and mortality. The Framingham study. *Stroke* **23**, 1551–5.

Young, W. B., Lee, K. P., Pessin, M. S., Kwan, E. S., Rand, W. M. & Caplan, L. R. (1990). Prognostic significance of ventricular blood in supratentorial hemorrhage: a volumetric study. *Neurology* **40**, 616–19.

6 Intracranial aneurysms and subarachnoid haemorrhage

AKIO MORITA, MICHAEL R. PUUMALA AND FREDRIC B. MEYER

Introduction

Subarachnoid haemorrhage (SAH) and intracranial aneurysms have been a condition of humans for thousands of years. An Egyptian skull dating back to the fifth or sixth century AD contained erosive bony lesions referable to a probable aneurysm of the internal carotid artery (Sundt 1990). Annotations to cerebral aneurysms can be found in Egyptian, Greek, and Arabic literary antiquities (de Moulin 1961; Al-Rodhan 1986).

The modern history of the study and treatment of SAH and intracranial aneurysms parallels the history of development of neurosurgery. From the anatomists of the 1700s, to the first successful ligation by Cooper in 1808 (Schorstein 1940), to Horsley's confirmation of an intracranial aneurysm at craniotomy (Beadles 1907), to the introduction of angiography by Moniz in 1927 (Moniz *et al.* 1928), to Dott's wrapping of an intracranial aneurysm in 1931 (Dott 1969), and to Dandy's clipping of an intracranial internal carotid artery aneurysm (Cushing 1911; Dandy 1938), the advances in neurosurgery have often been designed better to treat patients suffering from SAH. Perhaps the greatest advance in the treatment of aneurysms was the introduction of the operating microscope and microsurgical techniques in the 1960s. Despite these great technical advances, the treatment of cerebral aneurysms and subarachnoid hemorrhage remains a formidable challenge. The purpose of this chapter is to examine SAH in terms of its incidence, aetiology, clinical features, natural history and surgical outcomes.

The incidence of intracranial aneurysms is estimated at 1–8% of the general population according to autopsy and angiographic series (McCormick & Nofzinger 1965; Pakarinen 1967; Stehbens 1972; Sekhar & Hevos 1981; Atkinson *et al.* 1989). The most common presentation is SAH with an incidence of 10–15 per 100 000 population each year (Pakarinen 1967; Philips *et al.* 1980) or 1–1.4% per year of known aneurysm patients (Jane *et al.* 1985; Juvela *et al.* 1993). The outcome from a SAH is disappointing, with 8–60% of patients dying before reaching the hospital (Freytag 1966; Pakarinen 1967; Phillips *et al.* 1980; Kiyohara *et al.* 1989). After admission to hospital, the mortality is 37% and the severe disability is 17% with a favourable outcome achieved in only 47% of patients assessed 3 months postoperatively according to the Cooperative Study (Sahs *et al.* 1981). In addition, two-thirds of patients who are treated successfully never return to the same quality of life as prior to the SAH (Drake 1981). Despite tremendous effort to improve the outcome following SAH, the overall mortality has not been significantly reduced over the past 30 years because of the difficulty in reducing both the number of deaths prior to hospitalization and the number of poor-grade patients who have suffered severe brain injury from the initial haemorrhage (Phillips *et al.* 1980). Despite these pessimistic facts, aggressive management can salvage many patients with severe neurological injury following the SAH by preventing rerupture of the aneurysm, attenuating the severity and sequela of vasospasm, and reducing surgical complications (Storey 1967; Ljunggren *et al.* 1985).

Aetiology and classification of intracranial aneurysms

Aetiology

Since the incidence of idiopathic intracranial aneurysms is age dependent (Sahs 1969) and there are reports of de novo development of aneurysms and the growth of aneurysms (Hashimoto *et al.* 1978; Handa *et al.* 1983; Dyske & Beck 1989; Schievink *et al.* 1992; Rinne & Harnesniemi 1993), intracranial aneurysms can be considered acquired lesions (Stehbens 1963; 1922; Juvela *et al.* 1993). Supporting this acquired theory is the observation that aneurysms typically develop at branching points of major arteries where the haemodynamic stress forces are greatest. It is also probable that there are genetic influences which contribute to the development of intracranial aneurysms as evidenced by some familial cases of inracranial aneurysms (Kak *et al.* 1970; Lozano & Le Blanc 1987) and the association with certain pathologies such as polycystic kidney disease (Levey *et al.* 1983). In addition, Type III collagen deficiency is noted to have a strong relationship with aneurysm formation (Neil-Dwyer *et al.* 1983). Therefore, the aetiology of idiopathic aneurysms should be considered multifactorial with the following factors contributing to their evolution: (1) developmental defects of the arterial wall which may be affected by genetic factors; (2) hypertension or haemodynamic stress; and (3) atherosclerosis, especially in the development of fusiform or giant ectatic aneurysms (Crawford 1959).

There are several medical conditions which are associated with intracranial aneurysms. Approximately 10–30% of patients with polycystic kidney disease have an intracranial aneurysm (Levey *et al.* 1983). Abnormalities in the arterial wall are known to accompany this disease, along with a high incidence of hypertension. Fibromuscular dysplasia is also associated with intracerebral aneurysms. Haemodynamic stress can be a major aetiology of aneurysms in cases with intracranial arteriovenous malformations, moyamoya disease (Kodama & Suzuki 1978; Waga & Tochio 1985); unilateral carotid occlusion or agenesis (Kunishio *et al.* 1987); or coarctation of the aorta. Diseases which have defects in the arterial wall may also have cerebral aneurysms such as Ehlers–Danlos and Marfan syndromes, and pseudoxanthoma elasticum (Weir 1987).

Other acquired pathologies which damage the arterial wall such as infection, neoplasm, or trauma can lead to the development of cerebral aneurysms. These aetiologies usually result in aneurysms in the periphery of a major cerebral artery as opposed to the typical location along the circle of Willis. Though rare, severe trauma associated with a skull base fracture can result in development of an aneurysm in the petrous segment of the internal carotid artery (Benoit & Wortzman 1973).

Classification of intracranial aneurysms

Intracranial aneurysms are classified in several different ways by: (1) aetiology, (2) size, (3) location, and (4) shape. All of these factors are important in deciding the appropriate treatment.

Aetiological classification of aneurysms

As reviewed in the preceding paragraphs on pathogenesis, aneurysms can be caused by multiple aetiologies and classified accordingly.

Idiopathic These aneurysms are related in some way to a combination of abnormalities in the arterial wall, perhaps influenced by both genetic factors and haemodynamic stresses. The patient's age, hypertension, and smoking can be risk factors for the development of aneurysms.

Aneurysms associated with specific medical conditions Polycystic kidney disease, fibromuscular dysplasia, coarctation of aorta, connective tissue diseases, arteriovenous malformations, moyamoya disease, and unilateral carotid or vertebral occlusion or agenesis can be associated with intracranial aneurysms. These aneurysms are at similar locations to those of idiopathic aneurysms.

Miscellaneous causes which affect the arterial wall Trauma, metastatic neoplasms, or septicaemia can induce aneurysm formation. These aneurysms are typically located in peripheral arteries and are fusiform in shape. At surgery, there is often no neck which can be clipped and therefore the diseased segment of artery with aneurysm must be resected and possibly reconstructed.

Aneurysm size

Aneurysm size is categorized by the largest diameter of the dome as: (a) *saccular (small)*, less than 1.5 cm; (b) *globular (large)*, 1.5–2.5 cm; and (c) *giant*, greater than 2.5 cm (Sundt 1990). The size of an aneurysm is important in the decision to consider treatment of unruptured aneurysms since there is some evidence that small aneurysms are at decreased risk for haemorrhage. Alternatively, giant aneurysms require special surgical considerations due to factors such as the presence of a calcified neck, thrombus, and the location of major arteries and perforators in relationship to the aneurysm neck.

Location of aneurysms

Intracranial aneurysms are usually located at the bifurcation of major circle of Willis arteries because of haemodynamic stresses. The location of aneurysms from major cooperative studies are as follows: internal carotid artery (ICA) in 41%, anterior communicating/anterior cerebral artery (AComA/ACA) in 34%, middle cerebral artery (MCA) in 20%, vertebrobasilar artery (VBA) in 4%, and other locations in 1% (Sahs *et al.* 1981). Autopsy studies have noted locations as ICA in 24%, AComA/ACA in 30%, MCA in 33%, and VBA in 12% (Stehbens 1972). Multiple cerebral aneurysms are seen in approximately 20% of patients (Stehbens 1972; Ostergaard & Hog 1985).

Shape of aneurysms

This classification is strongly related to the aetiology of the aneurysm and has important implications regarding surgical accessibility.

Saccular aneurysm This shape is the most common observed in clinical practice. By definition, this type of aneurysm should have a well-defined neck and aneurysm dome. However, in some situations, especially with giant aneurysms, the neck may be obscured and sometimes involve the parent artery (Yasargil 1987; Sundt 1990). Most idiopathic aneurysms are of the saccular type.

Fusiform aneurysm These are primarily caused by atherosclerosis similar to that observed in aortic aneurysms. Trauma, infection, or tumour can occasionally result in the development of a fusiform aneurysm.

Saccular and fusiform aneurysms comprise the majority of aneurysms which are approached surgically. However, the following two categories may also occur and have important surgical implications.

Dissecting aneurysms These are intraluminal dissections of arteries and are quite rare in the intracranial vasculature. Typically, dissecting aneurysms are seen in the extracranial internal carotid or vertebral arteries and usually present with ischaemic events. There are some rare reports of intracranial dissecting aneurysms. They appear to be more common in the posterior circulation as opposed to the anterior circulation. They often present with haemorrhage. At surgery, these aneurysms are purplish, fusiform dilatations of the parent artery (Friedamn & Drake 1984).

False aneurysm Although this is not a category by shape, it may be included in this classification. Except for some dissecting aneurysms, the three shapes mentioned above are usually true aneurysms which involve some component of the arterial wall in the aneurysm dome. However, in false aneurysms, there is no definite wall except for reactive connective tissue or blood clot. False aneurysms are usually due to trauma but occasionally occur from infection or tumour. Special care is required at surgery since these aneurysms can rupture easily and also are difficult to repair without sacrificing or reconstructing the parent artery.

Clinical presentations of intracranial aneurysms

Incranial aneurysms can present in many different ways. Aneurysms without any presenting symptoms are termed asymptomatic aneurysms. Notably, asymptomatic aneurysms should be differentiated from unruptured aneurysms, since aneurysms can cause symptoms without rupture and those symptoms are important warning signs which can be useful in the detection of an aneurysm prior to a disastrous haemorrhage. The rate of rupture is higher in aneurysms which are symptomatic. In one study with a 5-year follow-up, 26% of patients with symptomatic unruptured aneurysms died of SAH, compared with 2.6% of patients with asymptomatic aneurysms (Sahs *et al.* 1981). The clinical presentations of cerebral aneurysms are summarized below.

Subarachnoid haemorrhage or other intracranial haemorrhage

The most common presentation of an intracranial aneurysm is SAH, which is the first manifestation in 90% of cases (Lindsey *et al.* 1991). In addition, most (> 80%) nontraumatic SAH is caused by aneurysmal rupture. Patients typically complain of 'the worst headache of my life', which may or may not be associated with nausea and vomiting. Patients with a severe SAH rapidly deteriorate to a comatose state or have a respiratory arrest from extremely high intracranial pressure which induces a profound reduction in cerebral perfusion pressure. Of note, approximately 40–50% of patients have been reported to experience warning signs caused by a minor leak or expansion of the aneurysm prior to rupture (Okawara 1973; Le Blanc 1987). These warning signs are often followed by aneurysm rupture in 10–20 days.

Other types of haemorrhage associated with aneurysms include intracerebral or intraventricular haemorrhage. These haemorrhages can be decompressed by surgery or ventricular drainage and the use of tissue plasminogen activator (tPA) or urokinase irrigation (Todo *et al.* 1991) with greater ease than a pure SAH. The damage to the brain from a cerebral haemorrhage may be reversible depending on its location and size. In fact, surgical removal of an intracerebral clot or placement of an external ventricular drain may lead to dramatic improvement in the clinical grade.

Mass effect

A secondary common presentation of intracranial aneurysms is mass effect which occurs in approximately 10% of patients. The aneurysm which presents with mass effect it typically large; however, even small aneurysms can exert pressure against the adjacent neural structures (Sahs *et al.* 1981). The symptoms may include retro-orbital pain, a third nerve palsy, cavernous sinus syndromes, hydrocephalus, visual field deficits, mild to moderate hemiparesis, or hypothalamic–pituitary dysfunction. If the aneurysm enlarges rapidly over a short period of time, it can cause pain by stretching the arterial wall or adjacent dura. Although these signs can be a significant problem in themselves for the patient, they also forewarn that there is an increased risk for rupture in the near future (Sundt 1990). Accordingly, immediate surgical intervention is indicated.

Embolus

Incranial aneurysms, especially partially thrombosed giant or fusiform aneurysms, can occasionally be the source of a cerebral embolus (Fisher *et al.* 1980; Sakaki *et al.* 1980). Treatment in this situation is difficult since anticoagulation, although the primary treatment for a cerebral embolus, is contraindicated in a cerebral aneurysm. In addition, treatment of a fusiform or partially thrombosed giant aneurysm is difficult and rarely straightforward. Often they require bypass surgery with trapping of the aneurysm.

Grading system of subarachnoid haemorrhage

The prognosis of SAH is quite dependent on the presenting clinical status (consciousness and neurological deficit) which is a good indicator of the severity of the initial brain injury. Damage to brain by SAH is not caused by mass effect but rather by the initial impact of high intracranial pressure. Therefore, dramatic improvement after removing pure subarachnoid clot or decompression is rare. There have been many approaches to grading severity of SAH on a clinical basis. For example, grading systems such as the World Federation of Neurologic Surgeons (WFNS) (Drake 1988), Hunt and Hess (1968), or Boterell systems (Botterell *et al.* 1956) have correlated well with outcome (Table 6.1). According to Phillips *et al.* (1980), in the Olmsted County, Rochester, Minnesota group of patients who present to the Mayo Clinic, approximately 48% will be Hunt and Hess clinical grades 1 and 2, 20% will be grade 3, and 30% will be grades 4 and 5. Each hospital or referral centre may have a different percentage of clinical grades depending on that institution's referral pattern (Whisnant *et al.* 1993).

Other complicating factors which influence the outcome following a SAH include delayed cerebral arterial vasospasm, hydrocephalus, and aneurysm rerupture. There have been several reports which have classified SAH on computed tomography (CT) appearance in an attempt to predict the incidence of cerebral vasospasm (Table 6.2) (Fisher *et al.* 1980). The Fisher group 3 has a statistically significant higher risk (96%) of developing symptomatic vasospasm compared with the other groups.

These clinical and CT grading systems are useful in the decision as to the indications and timing of surgery. Other factors which are considered in this decision include the location and size of the aneurysm, and the patient's age and overall general medical condition.

Table 6.1. *Subarachnoid haemorrhage (SAH) grading systems*

Clinical grade (modified Botterell)

0   Nonruptured or no SAH in past 30 days
1   With or without mild headache, alert, oriented, no motor or sensory deficits
2   Severe headache and major meningeal signs, mild alteration in sensorium or focal deficits
3   Major alteration in sensorium or a major focal deficit
4   Semi-comatose or comatose, with or without major lateralizing findings

Clinical grade (Hunt and Hess)

0   Nonruptured
1   Asymptomatic or minimal headache and slight nuchal rigidity
2   Moderate to severe headache, nuchal rigidity, no neurological deficit (other than cranial
    nerve palsy)
3   Drowsiness, confusion, or mild focal deficit
4   Stupor, moderate to severe hemiparesis, possibly early decerebrate rigidity and vegetative
    disturbances
5   Deep coma, decerebrate rigidity, moribund appearance

Clinical grade (World Federation of Neurologic Surgeons: WFNS)

	Glasgow coma scale	Motor deficit
1	15	Absent
2	13–14	Absent
3	13–14	Present
4	7–12	Absent or present
5	3–6	Absent or present

Medical versus surgical treatment

There are many factors which are important to consider when determining if an aneurysm should be surgically treated. Currently, the most important issue is whether the aneurysm has ruptured or whether it is asymptomatic. Natural history of each scenario and surgical risks of each case should be weighed. Other important factors include accessibility of the aneurysm for surgical repair, configuration and size of the aneurysm neck, the presence of thrombus, and the relationship of the neck of the aneurysm to the parent artery and perforators. The patient's age and general medical condition are also important considerations.

Ruptured aneurysms

According to the Cooperative Study of the natural history of subarachnoid haemorrhage overall mortality after SAH in 20 years was 66.8% and the majority (44%) of these deaths were due to recurrent haemorrhage or strokes. Mortality due to recurrent haemorrhage was 78% (Nishioka *et al.* 1984). These data cannot be compared with surgical group data because poor grade or more complex (posterior circulation) aneurysms are managed conservatively. Obviously, however, in better grade patients such as WFNS grades 1–3, surgery is strongly indicated since the risk of rebleed with

Table 6.2. *Fisher CT scan classification for SAH*[a]

Group 1	No blood detected
Group 2	Diffuse deposition on thin layer with all vertical layers of blood (interhemispheric fissure, insular cistern, ambient cistern) less than 1 mm
Group 3	Localized clot and/or vertical layers of blood 1 mm or greater in thickness
Group 4	Diffuse or no subarachnoid blood, but with intracerebral or intraventricular clots

[a] Fisher *et al.* (1980).

associated morbidity and mortality is exceedingly high compared with the surgical risks. In poor grade patients, some clinicians question the value of surgical intervention since the patient's outcome is poor regardless of treatment. In our institution, poor grade patients are not excluded from surgery unless they are brain dead. It is important to emphasize that although a patient may arrive in the emergency room in a comatose, moribund state, they may benefit dramatically with significant improvement in their clinical grade after placement of an external ventricular drain if the CT scan shows acute hydrocephalus.

Unruptured symptomatic aneurysms

Surgery for this type of aneurysm is typically recommended since, as mentioned earlier, these symptoms are often disabling and are a warning sign for rupture in the near future. However, most of these aneurysms are large or giant in size and the risk of surgery is accordingly higher than that for a small saccular aneurysm. This increased risk of surgery needs to be recognized both by the surgeon and the patient in order to make the appropriate therapeutic decision.

Asymptomatic aneurysms

Surgery for this group of patients has been controversial for decades (Wiebers *et al.* 1981, 1987; Juvela *et al.* 1993). The comparison between risks of surgery versus the natural history of unruptured aneurysms is critical in making the appropriate decision for this group. Unruptured aneurysms are reported to rupture at approximately 1–1.4% rate per year (Jane *et al.* 1985; Juvela *et al.* 1993). The risk of aneurysm rupture also increases with size, although a critical size in relationship to increased risk of rupture is still unknown. The consensus thus far is that the risk of rupture for aneurysms larger than 1.0 cm is greater than the risk of surgery, if the surgery is performed in patients under the age of 65 years (Wiebers *et al.* 1987). Although some natural history studies suggest that the risk for rupture of an aneurysm under 1.0 cm is small, many surgeons do operate on small aneurysms based on the intraoperative observation that most aneurysms which have ruptured are under 1.0 cm in size.

Subarachnoid haemorrhage of unknown aetiology

Initial radiological studies fail to show a cause in 13–28% of cases with spontaneous SAH (Nishioka *et al.* 1984). In about 10% of these patients, repeated angiogram or autopsy showed lesions. Rebleeding occurred in 9–16% of patients in 20 years. Prognosis of these patients compared favourably to a matched United States population except for patients with high blood pressure. Recently some surgeons advocated surgical exploration of the area of suspected aneurysms without angiographic proof (Di Lorenzo & Guidetti 1988; Jafor & Weiner 1993). While their outcome is satisfactory, their experience is small and real expected positive exploration rate should be low according to autopsy series (4 of 35 cases showed lesion) (Nishioka *et al.* 1984). The authors believe that surgical exploration could be justified only if subarachnoid clot is located in inter-hemispheric fissure or unilateral sylvian fissure in multiple episodes and if the patient is young.

Surgical options and outcome

Outcome from our Mayo Clinic experience is based on the data obtained from the group of 1947 patients who underwent surgery at the Mayo Clinic from 1969 to 1990. The mean age was 51.4 years (range 3 months to 88 years) with a male/female ratio of 2 to 3. Because of referral patterns, there were more better clinical grade patients, posterior circulation aneurysms (17% compared with the usual 5–10%), and giant aneurysms (21% compared with the usual 5%). Most patients were considered modified Botterell grade 0 (39%) or grade 1 (32%) and only 3% were Botterell grade 4. The aneurysms were saccular in 59%, globular in 20%, and giant in 21%. There were 1196 patients who suffered from SAH. The time from SAH to surgery for the group showed a trend favouring later surgery with only 21% of patients receiving surgery in the first 3 days and 58% undergoing surgery after the first week. This reflects both the prevailing surgical practice of the study period as well as referral patterns. In this series, there was also a disproportionate number of patients with posterior circulation aneurysms (19%) when compared with other series of aneurysms (10%), which again reflects referral patterns. For the patients in this subgroup, there was a mean follow-up of 25.5 months.

   The outcomes are scaled by Sundt's classification which is similar to the Glasgow outcome scale (GOS) as follows:

> *Excellent*: Normal employment with normal neurological examination (GOS 5)
> *Good*: Neurological deficit, but normal mentation and employment (GOS 4)
> *Poor*: Anything less than full activity (GOS 2–3)
> *Death*: Mortality within 6 months of SAH (GOS 1)

Direct clipping

Currently, direct clipping is the most routine and definitive treatment for an intra-

Table 6.3. *Admission grade and surgical results*

Results	Admission grade (modified Botterell and Hunt and Hess)					Total	Total (SAH)
	0	1	2	3	4		
Excellent	623(83%)	534(86%)	221(64%)	58(35%)	9(14%)	1445(74%)	822(69%)
Good	69(9%)	52(8%)	57(17%)	41(25%)	12(19%)	231(12%)	162(13%)
Poor	31(4%)	25(4%)	47(14%)	40(24%)	28(44%)	171(9%)	140(12%)
Death	28(4%)	14(2.3%)	18(5%)	26(16%)	14(22%)	100(5%)	72(6%)
Total	751	625	343	165	63	1947	1196

cranial aneurysm and the results in this aneurysm series usually reflect the surgical outcome. With direct clipping the aneurysm neck is obliterated by application of a aneurysm clip whose strength, shape, and size prevents blood flow into the aneurysm dome but preserves the parent artery and perforating arteries.

Outcome of optimum surgical procedures

The Cooperative Study for Aneurysmal Subarachnoid Hemorrhage (Sahs *et al.* 1981) reported on 274 patients with a single intracranial aneurysm treated surgically between 1963 and 1970. For this group there was an overall mortality of 37%. Most patients (74%) were Hunt and Hess grade 1 or 2, and the mortality for this group was 35%, whereas for the smaller group of patients who were Hunt and Hess grade 4 or 5 (14%) the mortality rate was 50%.

The International Cooperative Study on the Timing of Aneurysm Surgery (Kassell *et al.* 1990a,b) examined the medical and surgical management of 3521 patients treated between 1980 and 1983. Most of these patients (75%) were in good neurological condition and 83% underwent surgery. The 6 month mortality was 26% and only 58% had a complete recovery.

In one study (Saveland *et al.* 1992), 80% of all Swedish aneurysmal SAH over a 1 year period (1989) were followed and treated with a uniform protocol which favoured surgery within 72 hours. This study group had more patients with worse Hunt and Hess grades at admission, reflecting referral and inclusion patterns. Overall outcomes were good in 56% of the total group and mortality was 21%.

In the Mayo experience of the patient group comprising 1196 SAH patients, most patients (69%) had an excellent outcome and only 6% died (Table 6.3).

The results for grade 1 (*n* = 606) and grade 2 (*n* = 303) patients were similar, both with excellent results (Fig. 6.1a,b). The grade 1 group had slightly more excellent outcomes as compared with the grade 2 group (86% as compared with 64%), and the grade 2 group had a corresponding increased number of good outcomes (17% compared with 8%). Excellent or good outcomes were seen in 94% of grade 1 patients and 87% of grade 2 patients. There was no significant difference in outcome in either group with respect to the timing of surgery. For the 221 patients who were clinical grade 3, the timing of surgry did have an effect on outcome (Fig. 6.1c). Patients in this group having surgery within the first week had a higher mortality rate, and a correspondingly lower number of patients with poor outcomes. Grade 3 patients having surgery after the first week, however, had a lower mortality and a correspondingly higher number of poor outcomes. The number of patients with excellent and good results were approximately equal irrespective of the timing of surgery. The 63 patients in the group with admission clinical grade 4 had increasingly more mortality and poor outcomes with increasing time to surgery, especially when surgery was delayed until after day 12 from SAH (Fig. 6.1d). For the grade 4 patients the number of good and excellent outcomes increased with time up to the group with surgery past the 11th day. The grade 4 patients who received surgery days 4–7 from haemorrhage had the highest percentage of excellent outcomes as well as the highest percentage of deaths.

In our review of all aneurysm cases including non-SAH patients, overall 1445 patients (75%) had an excellent outcome, 231 (12%) had a good outcome, 171 (9%) had a poor outcome, and 100 (5%) died. There were certain trends related with outcome (Table 6.3). Younger patients had a better outcome while in the older age group between the sixth and eighth decades good and poor outcomes increased as excellent outcomes reduced. The mortality did not increase significantly until the ninth decade (Table 6.4).

Timing of surgery for ruptured intracranial aneurysms

The timing of surgery after SAH has been a debated issue over the last three decades (Kassell & Drake 1982; Kassell *et al.* 1982; 1990a,b). Currently, the decision to operate should be based on the clinical grade of SAH, the location of the aneurysm, and the patient's medical condition. The advantages and disadvantages of early versus delayed surgery are listed in Table 6.5.

For better grade patients (WFNS grades 1–2), several early cooperative studies demonstrated a superior outcome for delayed surgery (Sahs *et al.* 1981). Although the surgical outcome in these preceding studies was better with late surgery, approximately 30% of patients did not survive to surgery (Kassell 1990a,b). In prospective studies from Sweden, early surgery offered the best opportunity for a good recovery (81%) in better grade patients (Hunt and Hess grades 1–3) (Saveland *et al.* 1992).

For intermediate grade patients (WFNS grade 3) this timing of surgery is controversial. Data from our institution did not show any difference in mortality or morbidity between early or delayed surgery for this group of patients. A recent report from a group in Japan demonstrated a benefit of early surgery in grade 3–4 patients (Miyaoka *et al.* 1993).

For poor grade patients (WFNS grades 4–5), it is difficult to decide if and when surgery should be performed since the overall outcome is poor, with or without surgical intervention. If a patient in a poor grade improves with conservative treatment, then a more aggressive approach would be pursued. In addition, if the patient has an in-

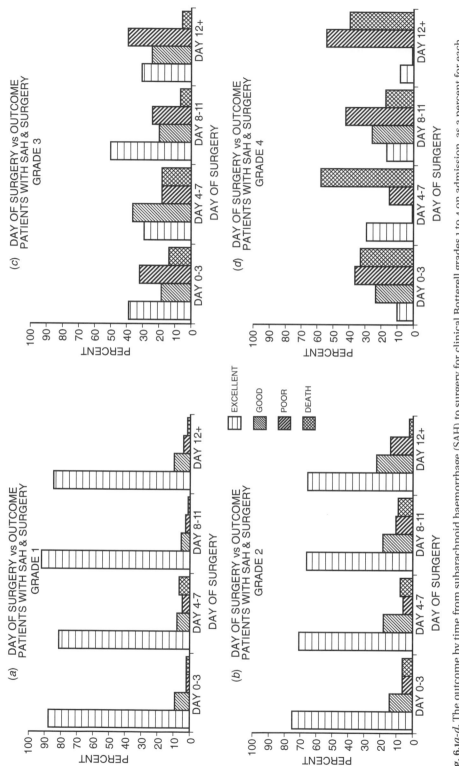

Fig. 6.1*a–d.* The outcome by time from subarachnoid haemorrhage (SAH) to surgery for clinical Botterell grades 1 to 4 on admission, as a percent for each time period. The day of SAH is considered Day 0.

Table 6.4. *Age and surgical outcome*

Result	Age by decade								Total
	10s	20s	30s	40s	50s	60s	70s	80s	
Excellent	37	68	208	358	420	289	57	8	1445(74%)
Good	2	8	24	52	62	54	28	1	231(12%)
Poor	1	7	15	15	46	57	26	4	171(9%)
Death	1	2	8	18	25	30	12	5	101(5%)
Total	41	85	255	443	553	430	123	18	

Table 6.5. *Timing of surgery: advantages and disadvantages*

Early operation (within 3 days)
Advantage
1. Prevention of rebleeding
2. Amelioration of vasospasm by removal of subarachnoid clot
3. Prevention and treatment of ischaemic complications
4. Prevention of medical complication
5. Psychological factors
6. Shorter hospitalization
Disadvantage
1. Brain is tight and swollen
2. High risk for intraoperative rupture

Delayed operation (after 11 days)
Advantage
1. Brain slackness
2. Ease of dissection
3. Opportunity to monitor patients
4. Flexibility of scheduling
Disadvantage
1. Rerupture
2. Difficult to manage if spasm developed
3. Adhesions around aneurysm

traparenchymal or intraventricular haemorrhage which is causing mass effect, then early surgical decompression, aneurysm clipping, and placement of a ventricular drain should be considered. Although the overall prognosis for this group of patients is poor, surgery does appear to salvage some patients and therefore, until proven otherwise, an aggressive approach should be adopted. There has been a trend towards earlier surgery. Improved understanding of the natural history of SAH and the pathogenesis and treatment of vasospasm have facilitated better medical management and made early surgical treatment of ruptured cerebral aneurysms preferable. Early clipping of the aneurysm allowed the patient to be treated with the necessary volume expansion and blood pressure support needed for the prevention and treatment of delayed ischaemia.

In our experience, as indicated earlier, the timing of surgery after SAH and outcome were assessed for patients who underwent surgery (total of 1196 cases) (Fig. 6.1a–d).

Early surgery (days 0–3) was performed in 21% and delayed surgery after the first week was done in 59% of patients. Although previous reports (Kassell 1990a,b) have indicated that surgery during the vasospasm period (days 4–11) has a poorer prognosis, our results did not show any difference except for those in grade 1 with surgery performed between days 4 and 7. The best outcome in grade 4 patients was achieved with early surgery (30%) (days 0–3). Therefore, our current approach is to operate on all patients in good grades as soon as possible irrespective of the date from haemorrhage. The one exception to this general rule is posterior circulation aneurysms, especially those of the basilar tip. Surgery for aneurysms in this location often requires significant brain retraction for exposure. It may be advantageous to delay surgery for several days to allow for the initial edema after the SAH to decrease. However, some surgeons recommend early surgery in some of these posterior circulation aneurysms (Peerless *et al.* 1994).

Alternative surgical approaches

Interventional neuroradiological treatment

This type of treatment is evolving rapidly and over the next several years the indications for this procedure will become more clearcut. It is reasonable to predict that endovascular treatment will play an important role in the treatment of cerebral aneurysms (Nichols 1993). Since the development of balloons to obliterate aneurysms by Romodanov *et al.* (1982) and Serbinenko (1974), there has been a rapid evolution in techniques including the placement of platinum coils into the aneurysm dome (Guglielmi coil). Higashida *et al.* (1991) recently reported the outcome in 215 cerebral aneurysm cases treated by detachable balloon. Parent vessel occlusion was performed in 59.1% and primary aneurysm obliteration was achieved in 40.9%. The mortality was 9.8% and the stroke rate was 7.4%. More recently, Guglielmi *et al.* (1991a,b) introduced a platinum coil electrothermocoagulation method. Although the clinical results with these Guglielmi detachable coils (GDC) are still preliminary, our clinical experience suggests that they will have a significant impact on the treatment of aneurysms. Balloons have the disadvantage of deflation, rupture, parent artery compromise, and a water hammer effect (Higashida *et al.* 1990, 1991; Hodes *et al.* 1990; Halbach *et al.* 1991; Kwan *et al.* 1991). Alternatively, Guglielmi coils eliminate some of these problems since they are soft, flexible, and induce thrombosis within the aneurysm dome. These coils can be applied or contoured to fit the configuration of the aneurysm. They have proved to be effective in the treatment of small to large size aneurysms with a definitive neck (Guglielmi *et al.* 1992a). A recent report on coil (non-Guglielmi type) embolization of aneurysms showed an excellent outcome in 84.5% of cases at 1-year follow-up with a morbidity of 4.2% and mortality of 11.3% (Casasco *et al.* 1993). The introduction of these new treatments may affect the decision for treatment irrespective of the timing or grade of the patient. Disadvantages of endovascular treatment include the risk of stroke or haemorrhage (Swann *et al.* 1986; Hodes *et al.* 1990; Halbach *et al.* 1991). Also, endovascular therapy may have a limited role in giant aneurysms or aneurysms with a wide neck for fear of embolization of coils and thrombus out of the aneurysm into the parent artery (Guglielmi *et al.* 1992b). Since endovascular treatment with detachable coils is a relatively new technique, it will be necessary to await long-term follow-up before a decision can be made regarding its role for the treatment of cerebral aneurysms (Hilal & Solomon 1992; Heilman *et al.* 1992).

Occasionally, the combination of endovascular and surgical approaches is useful in achieving the optimum results in complex cases. Accordingly, the future treatment of cerebral aneurysms will evolve into a team approach in which the surgeon and inter-ventional neuroradiologist analyze each case to determine the optimum treatment.

Another indication for endovascular treatment is planned occlusion of the parent vessel which can be useful in cases such as fusiform carotid cavernous aneurysms (Fox *et al.* 1987). Prior to the occlusion, a trial balloon occlusion is performed to determine whether parent vessel occlusion will be tolerated. During this trial balloon occlusion, in addition to a neurological examination, blood flow studies including SPECT scan (Mathews *et al.* 1993) can be performed to provide useful data. In complex aneurysms in which a temporary parent vessel occlusion is anticipated, a preoperative trial balloon occlusion provides important data.

One further radiological technique useful in the management of cerebral aneurysm patients is balloon dilatation of arteries in spasm (Zubkov *et al.* 1984). This technique can produce dramatic improvement in a patient suffering from ischaemic deficits. Higashida reported neurological improvement in 69% of patients who were deteriora-ting (Higashida *et al.* 1989). Balloon dilatation of an artery in spasm should be per-formed with caution since it can cause rupture of a vessel or embolic stroke (Linskey *et al.* 1991). Therefore, currently balloon dilatation should not be performed for *asympto-matic* angiographic vasospasm.

Proximal ligation or trapping of aneurysms with or without bypass

If the neck of an aneurysm is poorly defined, one option is proximal ligation of the parent vessel or trapping of the aneurysm either with surgery or through endovascular techniques. Proximal ligation has been used since the 1800s (Sundt 1990). A cooperative study demonstrated a failure rate of 6–8% (Sahs *et al.* 1981) in ruptured aneurysms. However, proximal ligation appears to be an effective treatment for giant aneurysms in the cavernous sinus and possibly other locations by facilitating thrombosis (Tindall *et al.* 1966; Swearingen & Heros 1987; Steinberg *et al.* 1993). Drake has successfully treated giant basilar artery aneurysms with a tourniquet technique (Drake 1975, 1979).

Trapping is a relatively definitive treatment for aneurysms since there is minimal perfusion to the vessel which has been trapped. In cases with cavernous or ophthalmic aneurysms, there can be collateral blood flow to the aneurysm through the ophthalmic artery. Rarely, aneurysms in other locations recruit retrograde blood supply from back flow through perforators. Failure of trapping can occur through this collateral blood flow.

In performing a trapping procedure, the major concern is the risk of ischaemia to the territory of the parent vessels which will be occluded. Ligation of the internal carotid artery has been reported to cause ischaemic complications in 49% of patients and 28% in common carotid ligation (30% overall) (Nishioka *et al.* 1984). Hashi & Nin (1984) reported that external carotid–internal carotid (EC–IC) bypass using the superficial temporal artery did not improve this rate of ischaemic complications (25% in their experience). They also found that gradual ligation using the Selverstone clamp or other techniques had an ischaemic complication rate as great as that with abrupt ligation. Currently, endovascular techniques allow a trial balloon occlusion to predict the risk of early ischaemic complications. By using preoperative trial balloon occlusion for assessment, the surgeon can determine which patient might need a bypass graft to prevent ischaemic complications. If a patient successfully passes a trial balloon occlusion, the requirement for a bypass during the trapping procedure is unlikely although this decision must be based on each individual case. For example, if there is a small aneurysm on the contralateral side or other vessel territory which may have increased haemodynamic stress by occlusion of one vessel, bypass might be indicated to prevent enlargement or rupture of this aneurysm (Dyste & Beck 1989). In addition, even despite a successful trial balloon occlusion, there is the risk of late ischaemic complications (Roski *et al.* 1981). The ischaemic complication rate by balloon occlusion after a negative trial occlusion test has been reported to be 4–22% (Higashi *et al.* 1981; Osguthorpe & Hungerford 1984; Origitano *et al.* 1994).

Fox *et al.* (1987) reported their results of balloon occlusion of proximal vessels after a trial balloon occlusion test. In 18 cases, an extracranial-intracranial (EC–IC) bypass was performed prior to permanent occlusion. Delayed ischaemia was seen in 13.2% and permanent morbidity (major stroke) was seen in only one case. Eighty-five per cent of internal carotid and 65% of VB aneurysms were thrombosed following the balloon occlusion.

With regard to bypass surgery during balloon occlusion, we typically prefer a saphenous vein interposition graft and rarely use a superficial temporal artery bypass pedicle because of its insufficient blood supply (Diaz *et al.* 1982). However, the STA–MCA bypass still has use in cases of marginal ischaemia secondary to the loss of a single arterial branch. Currently, our results with vein bypass have been satisfactory in preventing ischaemia with good long-term patency rates. Specifically, the patency rate at a follow-up of 1 year has been 86% in a total of 132 grafts. The long-term follow-up patency rate at 5 years was 82% and at 13 years was 73% (L. Regli and D. Piepgras, personal communication). An excellent or good result was achieved in 80% of patients with anterior circulation giant aneurysms and in 44% of patients with posterior circulation giant aneurysms. Some problems associated with a vein bypass include multiple incisions and the length of surgery which is approximately 7–8 hours compared with an STA–MCA bypass which requires only about 3–4 hours. The complication rate is higher in a vein bypass, however, this reflects the fact that these are difficult, complicated problems. Some of the specific complications associated with a vein bypass compared with STA–MCA bypass include thrombosis at either the proximal or distal anastomosis or haemorrhage from a high-flow bypass graft. Internal carotid artery aneurysms can be bypassed from either the cervical or petrous carotid artery distal to the aneurysm in the supraclinoid carotid artery (Sundt *et al.* 1986; Sundt 1990; Fukushima *et al.* 1993). If the aneurysm involves the C2 segment of the internal carotid artery, our current choice is to perform a EC–MCA bypass to the proximal MCA–M2 segment. In some cases, multiple bypasses are necessary to supply all major branches of the MCA. In these circumstances, the STA can be an important donor vessel. In the posterior circulation, the surgical options are more limited since there are only three vessels which are available for bypass. The occipital artery to posterior inferior cerebral artery bypass is an option for vertebral artery aneurysms although the blood supply is comparable to that achieved through an STA–MCA bypass. More often, we will perform vein bypass from the external carotid to either the posterior cerebral artery (PCA) or a superior cerebral artery as a treatment for giant basilar, vertebral, or PCA aneurysms (Sundt *et al.* 1986; Sundt 1990).

Wrapping or coating aneurysm

In some rare cases with fusiform or dissecting aneurysms, wrapping or coating might be the only option available (Bederson *et al.* 1992). Coating of an aneurysm will not prevent enlargement of the aneurysm or eventual rerupture. In addition, it makes exploration of the aneurysm extremely difficult by obscuring planes and perforators. Occasionally, when there is a small remnant of aneurysm neck after clipping, place-ment of some cotton or Teflon around the neck will induce fibrosis and decrease enlargement of the neck (Wilson & Spetzler 1978). However, wrapping of an aneurysm is the only treatment that should be excluded.

Complications after subarachnoid haemorrhage: their significance for prognosis and treatment

Post-SAH complications include: (a) rerupture (b) hydrocephalus, (c) delayed cerebral arterial vasospasm with ischaemic neurological deficits.

Rerupture

Rerupture is the most dreaded complication in the early phase of SAH management. The greatest risk for rerupture is in the first 24 hours (4.1%) and then decreases to 1.5% per day for the next 13 days. The cumulative risk of rerupture is 19% in 14 days, 40–50% overall at 6 months, and then 3% per year thereafter (Kassell & Torner 1983; Jane *et al.* 1985). The reported mortality from rerupture is as high as 78% (Nishioka *et al.* 1984; Lindsey *et al.* 1991).

The fear of early rerupture is the primary motivation for considering early surgical intervention. The patient should be kept in a quiet room and the blood pressure should be maintained no greater than 140 mmHg. Poor grade patients have probable increased intracranial pressure. In these patients, the blood pressure will most likely be high, but should be kept less than 150 mmHg systolic. This will help ensure adequate perfusion pressure. If the patient is agitated, sedation with mild analgesics or narcotics may be considered. However, it is important not to oversedate, so a full neurological assessment can be performed on a regular basis.

Hydrocephalus

Hydrocephalus occurs in the acute phase as well as in the chronic phase following SAH. Hydrocephalus in the acute phase is caused by blockage of the ventricular system or cisterns by blood clot (Graff-Radford et al. 1989). It is seen in 10–30% of patients with SAH by CT scan; 30–40% of those are symptomatic (Vassilouthis & Richardson 1979; van Gijn et al. 1985). Acute hydrocephalus can be the cause of progressive neurological deterioration. A poor-grade patient has a greater tendency to develop hydrocephalus because of the increased amount of blood in the basal cisterns (Graff-Radford et al. 1989). Drainage of CSF through a ventricular catheter is indicated if the hydrocephalus is causing neurological impairment or deterioration. In fact, a poor-grade patient can improve significantly upon placement of a ventricular drain on an emergency basis. Milhorat (1987) reported that two-thirds of their patients after SAH had significant improvement after placement of a ventricular drain. However, since acute decompression can be associated with rerupture of an aneurysm, the amount of CSF removed should be carefully controlled (Pare et al. 1992). Intermittent ventricular drainage when the ICP increases is preferred as opposed to continuous drainage which tends to have a greater risk of accidental excessive drainage.

Hydrocephalus in the chronic phase following SAH is caused by scarring of the arachnoid granules with disturbances in CSF absorption (Vassilouthis & Richardson 1979; Hayashi et al. 1982; Vasilouthis 1984). These patients may present with a normal pressure hydrocephalus syndrome including incontinence, gait instability, and cognitive deterioration. The CT or magnetic resonance imaging (MRI) scan will typically show enlarged ventricles including the 4th ventricle and probable transependymal CSF absorption. The treatment for chronic post-SAH hydrocephalus is placement of a permanent ventricular shunt (Vassilouthis 1984; Black et al. 1985).

Delayed cerebral arterial vasospasm

Delayed cerebral arterial vasospasm is a phenomenon in which major cerebral vessels constrict 3–9 days after the SAH (Ecker & Riemenschneider 1951; Weir et al. 1978). The pathophysiology of post-SAH vasospasm is still not well defined despite intensive investigation for over three decades (Wilkins 1980a,b, 1986; Kassell et al. 1985). The instigators of vasospasm are the products of blood clot lysis in the subarachnoid space including oxyhaemoglobin, leukotrienes and arachidonic acid. Nutritional deficits of

Table 6.6. *Management of delayed arterial vasospasm*

1. Early detection of clinical signs of vasospasm
2. Maintain normal physiological status such as euvolaemia, normothermia, normal natraemia and normal oxygenation.
3. Nimodipine 60 mg p.o./iv 4 hourly or other calcium antagonist
4. Surgical clot removal: tPA application, cisternal drainage, brain shaker, etc.
5. Hypervolaemia using packed red blood cells, colloid, albumin solution, fludocortisone 2 mg/day or desoxycortisone 20 mg/day. Pitressin may be indicated to keep urine output low.
   Support central venous pressure 10 mmHg, pulmonary artery wedge pressure 19 –20 mmHg
6. Induced hypertension with dopamine, dobutamine
7. Balloon angioplasty
8. Topical or intra-arterial papaverine injection

the arterial wall in the basal cisterns (Kim *et al.* 1992), involvement of protein kinase C chain (Maksui *et al.* 1992) have also been proposed to be a trigger of vasospasm. From the surgical perspective, the incidence and severity of vasospasm is clearly related to the amount of subarachnoid or periarterial blood as demonstrated by Fisher *et al.* (1977, 1980).

The incidence of this phenomenon by angiogram is reported to be 30–70% and is symptomatic in 20–30% with a permanent morbidity of 10–20% (mortality 7%, severe morbidity 7%) (Kassell *et al.* 1985).

Prevention of vasospasm would be the ideal treatment (Wilkins 1980a,b, 1996) (Table 6.6). There is some evidence which indicates that clot removal, especially that achieved through the intrathecal administration of tPA, may significantly decrease the risk of delayed arterial spasm (Saito *et al.* 1977; Taneda 1982; Findlay *et al.* 1988, 1991; Zabramski *et al.* 1991; Mizoi *et al.* 1993). The calcium antagonist, nimodipine, has been reported to decrease significantly the morbidity and mortality in patients of all grades who suffer a SAH (Allen *et al.* 1983; Petruk *et al.* 1988). Therefore, nimodipine at a dose of 60 mg p.o. 4 hourly should be routinely administered. Although high-dose steroids have been suggested by some to be of benefit, this is not universally accepted and remains controversial (Chyatte *et al.* 1987). Optimum general care including maintenance of a euvolaemic, eunatraemic condition may retard the development of symptomatic vasospasm.

If vasospasm becomes symptomatic an early response is critical. Clinically symptomatic changes need to be closely monitored in the intensive care unit. Volume expansion is indicated and is achieved by the infusion of colloid and occasionally blood (Kassell & Drake 1982; Kassell *et al.* 1982, 1985). If clinically significant vasospasm does not respond to these conventional treatments, a cerebral angiogram should be performed for consideration of balloon angioplasty. Higashida *et al.* (1989) reported that this technique significantly improved neurological symptoms in 70% of patients suffering from vasospasm. Recently intra-arterial injection of papaverine has been reported to be beneficial (Kaku *et al.* 1992). Transcranial Doppler is a useful noninvasive tech-

Table 6.7. *Anterior circulation versus posterior circulation*

Surgical result	Circulation	
	Anterior	Posterior
Excellent	76%	65%
Good	10%	18%
Poor and death	14%	17%

nique for monitoring the success of treatments, including volume expansion, in reversing vasospasm (Aaslid *et al.* 1984).

Factors affecting surgical outcome

In addition to post-SAH complications, there are several factors which influence surgical outcome. Patient's age, presenting grade of SAH and volume of haemorrhage detected by CT scan significantly affect outcome of patients as discussed earlier. Also location and size of the aneurysm are very important points affecting surgical risks.

Patients with aneurysms in the anterior circulation had a better outcome than patients with posterior circulation lesions (Table 6.7). According to the Mayo Clinic experience, most patients with anterior circulation aneurysms had an excellent outcome (75%), compared with 65% of cases with posterior circulation aneurysms. Basilar caput aneurysms had the highest incidence of poor outcome (poor and death 30%).

In examining the aneurysm size in relationship to outcome, saccular and globular aneurysms had similar outcomes, while giant aneurysms had a higher death (10%) rate (Table 6.8a). However, an excellent outcome was achieved in 293 patients (69%) with giant aneurysms and in 75% of those who did not have a SAH (Table 6.8b).

There are several types of aneurysms which require special surgical consideration because of anatomical complexity.

Aneurysms of the intracavernous and ophthalmic internal carotid artery

Until recently, direct surgical repair of aneurysms in this location was thought to be associated with high risk. However, with the contributions of surgeons like Parkinson (1965, 1973) and Dolenc (1983, 1985) along with other pioneer skull base surgeons (Sekhar *et al.* 1989; Fukushima *et al.* 1993), increased knowledge of surgical anatomy in this region along with improvement in technical skills has led to a dramatic decrease in the surgical risk for intracavernous aneurysms. Currently, the risk of permanent injury to the cranial nerves during direct cavernous sinus surgery is approximately 10% in experienced hands (Fukushima *et al.* 1993). Some of the aneurysms in this region are giant in size and require an intracranial bypass procedure (Fukushima bypass). In our

Table 6.8a. *Aneurysm size and surgical outcome (all grades)*

Result	Size of aneurysm			
	Saccular	Globular	Giant	Unknown
Excellent	872(75%)	213(75%)	293(69%)	67(82%)
Good	130(11%)	35(12%)	60(14%)	6(7%)
Poor	105(9%)	30(10.5%)	28(7%)	8(10%)
Death	51(4%)	7(2.5%)	41(10%)	1(1%)
Total	1158	285	422	82

Table 6.8b. *Aneurysm size and surgical outcome (grade 0/nonruptured aneurysm)*

Result	Size of aneurysm		
	Saccular	Globular	Giant
Excellent	89%	88%	75%
Good	7%	8%	12%
Poor	2.5%	2%	6%
Death	1.5%	2%	7%

experience, about half the aneurysms in this location have an acceptable neck and can be directly clipped, with a good result achieved in approximately 90% of patients (Al–Rodhan *et al.* 1993).

Endovascular treatment of these aneurysms may be a good alternative to surgery. Specifically, in one report of 87 cases, endovascular detachable balloon occlusion of the parent carotid artery was performed in 78%, and primary aneurysm obliteration was achieved in 22%. Bypass surgery was required in only 2% of patients. Transient ischaemia was seen in 10.3% and permanent morbidity (strokes) was seen in only 4.6% of cases (Higashida *et al.* 1990). By comparison, Fukushima *et al.* (1993) reported their experience in 79 cases which included cranial nerve deficits in six, optic nerve injury in five, cochlear damage in two, temporary hemiparesis or hemiplegia in three, and CSF leak in two patients. Their overall morbidity was 17% with a mortality of 0. It should be noted that the case material between these two series was different and therefore not directly comparable.

The natural history of aneurysms of the cavernous carotid artery which are completely within the cavernous sinus is relatively benign (Linskey *et al.* 1990). Since both surgical and endovascular treatments have a high complication rate, they should be reserved for cavernous carotid aneurysms which extend into the subarachnoid space or present with significant mass effect including pain or ophthalmoplegia. The small asymptomatic cavernous carotid artery aneurysm should be observed.

Posterior circulation aneurysms

The largest surgical series of posterior circulation aneurysms has been reported by Drake (1979) and Peerless *et al.* (1985). In 1055 aneurysms, 76% had an excellent or good outcome, while 18% had a poor result and 6% died. Giant aneurysms had an especially poor outcome (Peerless *et al.* 1985). At our institution, comparable surgical results for posterior circulation aneurysms have been achieved with the same observation regarding giant lesions. The results of proximal basilar or vertebral artery ligation for the treatment of 201 unclippable posterior circulation aneurysms was recently reported from Drake's group (Steinberg *et al.* 1993). In 78%, successful aneurysm thrombosis was induced. The overall outcome was excellent in 68%, good in 5%, poor in 3%, and 24% died. Partial thrombosis of the aneurysm was associated with early or late neurological deterioration in 67% of cases by either SAH or thromboembolic complications. Both of these resulted in a high mortality rate. Considering the high complexity of these selected cases, reported results for proximal arterial ligation are quite good and emphasize that the surgeon should consider this treatment if an aneurysm of the posterior circulation appears to be unclippable.

Endovascular treatment of 25 posterior circulation aneurysms using a detachable balloon technique was recently reported by Higashida *et al.* (1989). They achieved primary aneurysm obliteration in 65% and parent vessel occlusion in 35% of patients. Three patients had strokes and five patients died (20%) of immediate or delayed rupture of the aneurysm. Treatment of 43 vertebrobasilar aneurysms by GDC coils was reported by Guglielmi (1992a,b) with good results. Complete occlusion of the aneurysm was achieved in 81% of those with a small neck but in only 15% with a wide neck. The overall morbidity was 4.8% and the mortality was 2.4% including ischaemia and rupture of the aneurysm during the precedure. Therefore, in posterior circulation aneurysms which have a well defined small neck, GDC coils may prove to be a good alternative treatment to direct surgical repair.

Giant aneurysms

Giant aneurysms present certain unique considerations in treatment (Kadon & Stein 1979; Heros 1984). They are seen in approximately 5% of all patients with aneurysms. At our institution, the incidence is approximately 20% because of referral patterns. These aneurysms often present with mass effect, although SAH occurs in 35% (Pia & Zierski 1982). Giant aneurysms are quite difficult, not only because of their size but also because of their different pathogenesis. Some of these aneurysms are comparable to atherosclerotic aneurysms which occur in the aorta or extracranial carotid artery with a thick calcified wall, intraluminal thrombus, and a poorly defined neck (Sundt & Pipegvas 1979).

The outcome of our surgical experience with giant aneurysms is depicted in Table 6.9. For the giant aneurysms in this series, the overall trend of outcomes was similar to

Table 6.9. *Result of 416 giant aneurysms (all grades, with and without subarachnoid haemorrhage)*

Procedure (n)	Excellent	Good	Poor	Death
Proximal ligation (34)	24	4	1	5
	71%	12%	3%	15%
Simple trapping (29)	18	8	2	1
	62%	28%	7%	3%
Direct clipping with or without	128	39	24	17
thrombectomy (208)	61.5%	19%	11.5%	8%
Bypass surgery with proximal ligation or	67	19	11	10
clipping or trapping (107)	63%	18%	10%	9%
Direct repair with vessel reconstruction (29)	18	6	3	2
	62%	21%	10%	7%
Mycotic aneurysm, excision of aneurysm (3)	1	2	—	—
Exploration only, no repair of aneurysm (2)	—	—	—	2
Wrapping (4)	4	—	—	—
Total	260	78	41	37
	62.5%	19%	10%	9%
	81.5%			

that of the entire group (Table 6.8a,b). Of 416 patients with giant aneurysms, 260 (62.5%) had excellent outcomes. There was more morbidity and mortality in this group as compared with the overall series, with a 9% mortality for giant aneurysms as opposed to a 5% overall mortality. Whereas surgical treatment of smaller aneurysms almost always involves clipping of the aneurysm, giant aneurysms may be difficult to clip directly. Other surgical treatment options must therefore be considered for giant aneurysms. Variables such as size, location and shape of the aneurysm, and the configuration of its neck influence the treatment plan.

Interventional endovascular treatment may have a role in the treatment of giant aneurysms (Debrun *et al.* 1981; Taki *et al.* 1992). However, because of the irregular shape and poorly defined neck in many of these cases, successful obliteration is difficult to achieve (Taki *et al.* 1992). We have two cases in which there was significant morbidity due to partial occlusion of a giant aneurysm with GDC coils. Following treatment, the aneurysms continued to enlarge, possibly due to a water-hammer effect, necessitating surgical resection of the coils followed by aneurysm clipping. Removing the GDC coils can be extremely difficult since they become entangled in a thick fibrotic mass within the aneurysm. During removal, these coils become miniature gigli saws and can easily sever any adjacent neurovascular structures. At present, the use of GDC coils for giant aneurysms needs further clinical investigation before their use can be confirmed.

Acknowledgment

The authors acknowledge expert assistance from Ms Mary Soper in the preparation of this manuscript.

References

Aaslid, R., Huber, P. & Nornes, H. (1984). Evaluation of cerebrovascular spasm with transcranial Doppler ultrasound. *J. Neurosurg.* **60**, 37–41.

Allen, G. S., Ahn, H. S., Preziosi, T. J. *et al.* (1983). Cerebral arterial spasm – a controlled trial of nimodipine in patients with subarachnoid hemorrhage. *N. Engl. J. Med.* **308**, 619–24.

Al-Rodhan, N. R. F. & Fox, J. L. (1986). Al-Zahrawi and Arabian neurosurgery AD 936–1013. *Surg. Neurol.* **26**, 92–5.

Al-Rodhan, N. R. F., Piepgras, D. G. & Sundt, T. M. Jr. (1993). Transitional cavernous aneurysms of the internal carotid artery. *Neurosurgery* **33**, 993–8.

Atkinson, J. L. D., Sundt, T. M. Jr., Houser, O. W. & Whisnant, J. P. (1989). Angiographic frequency of anterior circulation intracranial aneurysms. *J. Neurosurg.* **70**, 551–5.

Beadles, C. F. (1907). Aneurysms of the larger cerebral arteries. *Brain* **30**, 285–336.

Bederson, J. B., Zabranski, J. M. & Spetzler, R. F. (1992). Treatment of fusiform intracranial aneurysms by circumferential wrapping with slip reinforcement. Technical note. *J. Neurosurg.* **77**, 478–80.

Benoit, B. G. & Wortzman, G. (1973). Traumatic cerebral aneurysms. Clinical features and natural history. *J. Neurol. Neurosurg. Psychiatry* **36**, 127–38.

Black, P. M., Ojemann, R. G. & Tzouras, A. (1985). CSF shunts for dementia, incontinence, and gait disturbance. *Clin. Neurosurg.* **32**, 632–51.

Botterell, E. H., Lougheed, W. M., Scott, J. W. & Vandewater, S. L. (1956). Hypothermia, and interruption of carotid, or carotid and vertebral circulation, in the surgical management of intracranial aneurysms. *J. Neurosurg.* **13**, 1–42.

Casasco, A. E., Aymard, A., Gobin, Y. P. *et al.* (1993). Selective endovascular treatment of 71 intracranial aneurysms with platinum coils. *J. Neurosurg.* **79**, 3–10.

Chyatte, D., Fode, N. C., Nichols, D. A. & Sundt, T. M. Jr (1987). A preliminary report: effects of high-dose methylprednisolone on delayed cerebral ischemia in patients at high risk for vasospasm after aneurysmal subarachnoid hemorrhage. *Neurosurgery* **21**, 157–60.

Crawford, T. (1959). Some observations on the pathogenesis and natural history of intracranial aneurysms. *J. Neurol. Neurosurg. Psychiatry* **22**, 259–66.

Cushing, H. (1911). The control of bleeding in operations for brain tumors. With the description of silver "clips" for the occlusion of vessels inaccessible to the ligature. *Ann. Surg.* **54**, 1–19.

Dandy, W. E. (1938). Intracranial aneurysm of internal carotid artery, cured by operation. *Ann. Surg.* **107**, 654–9.

Debrun, G., Fox, A., Drake, G. G., Peerless, S., Girvin, J. & Ferguson, G. (1981). Giant unclippable aneurysms: treatment with detachable balloons. *AJNR* **2**, 167–73.

de Moulin, D. (1961). Aneurysms in antiquity. *Arch. Chir. Neerl.* **13**, 49–63.

Diaz, F. G., Ausman, J. I. & Pearce, J. E. (1982). Ischemic complications after combined internal carotid artery occlusion and extracranial-intracranial anastomosis. *Neurosurgery* **10**, 563–70.

Di Lorenzo, N. & Guidetti, G. (1988). Anterior communicating aneurysm missed at angiography: report of two cases treated surgically. *Neurosurgery* **23**, 494–7.

Dolenc, V. (1983). Direct microsurgical repair of intracavernous vascular lesions. *J. Neurosurg.* **58**, 824–31.

Dolenc, V. (1985). A combined epi- and subdural direct approach to carotid-ophthalmic artery aneurysms. *J. Neurosurg.* **62**, 667–72.

Dott, N. M. (1969). Intracranial aneurysmal formation. *Clin. Neurosurg.* **16**, 1–15.

Drake, C. G. (1975). Ligation of the vertebral (unilateral or bilateral) or basilar artery in the treatment of large intracranial aneurysms. *J. Neurosurg.* **43**, 255–74.

Drake, C. G. (1979). The treatment of aneurysms of the posterior circulation. *Clin. Neurosurg.* **26**, 96–144.

Drake, C. G. (1981). Progress in cerebrovascular disease. Management of cerebral aneurysms. *Stroke* **12**, 273–83.

Drake, C. G. (1988). Report of World Federation of Neurological Surgeons Committee on a universal subarachnoid hemorrhage grading scale. *J. Neurosurg.* **68**, 985–6.

Dyste, G. N. & Beck, D. W. (1989). De novo aneurysm formation following carotid ligation: case report and review of the literature. *Neurosurgery* **24**, 88–92.

Ecker, A. & Riemenschneider, P. (1951). Arteriographic demonstration of spasm of the intra cranial arteries: with special reference to saccular arterial aneurysms. *J. Neurosurg.* **8**, 660–7.

Findlay, J. M., Weir, B. K. A., Steinke, D., Tanabe, T., Gordon, P. & Grace, M. (1988). Effect of intrathecal thrombolytic therapy on subarachnoid clot and chronic vasospasm in a primate model of SAH. *J. Neurosrg.* **69**, 723–35.

Findlay, J. M., Weir, B. K. A., Kassell, N. F., Disney, L. B. & Grace, M. G. A. (1991). Intracisternal recombinant tissue plasminogen activator after aneurysmal subarachnoid hemorrhage. *J. Neurosurg.* **75**, 181–8.

Fisher, C. M., Roberson, G. H. & Ojemann, R. G. (1977). Cerebral vasospasm with ruptured saccular aneurysm: the clinical manifestations. *Neurosurgery* **1**, 245–8.

Fisher, C. M., Kistler, J. P. & Davis, J. M. (1980). Relation of cerebral vasospasm to subarachnoid hemorrhage visualized by computerized tomographic scanning. *Neurosurgery* **6**, 1–9.

Fisher, M., Davidson, R. I. & Marcus, E. M. (1980). Transient focal cerebral ischemia as a presenting manifestation of unruptured cerebral aneurysms. *Ann. Neurol.* **8**, 367–72.

Fox, A. J., Vinuela, F., Pelz, D. M. *et al.* (1987). Use of detachable balloons for proximal artery occlusion in the treatment of unclippable cerebral aneurysms. *J. Neurosurg.* **66**, 40–6.

Freytag, E. (1966). Fatal rupture of intracranial aneurysms. *Arch. Pathol.* **81**, 418–24.

Friedamn, A. H. & Drake, C. G. (1984). Subarachnoid hemorrhage from intracranial dissecting aneurysm. *J. Neurosurg.* **60**, 325–34.

Fukushima, T., Day, J. & Tung, H. (1993). Intracavernous carotid artery aneurysms. In: Apuzzo, M. L. J. (ed.) *Brain Surgery. Complication Avoidance and Management*, vol. 1, pp. 925–44. New York: Churchill Livingstone.

Graff-Radford, N. R., Torner, J., Adams, H. P. Jr. & Kassell, N. F. (1989). Factors associated with hydrocephalus after subarachnoid hemorrhage. *Arch. Neurol.* **46**, 744–52.

Guglielmi, G., Vinuela, F., Sepetka, I. & Macellari, V. (1991a). Elecrothrombosis of saccular aneurysms via endovascular approach, part 1, electrochemical basis, technique, and experimental results. *J. Neurosurg.* **75**, 1–7.

Guglielmi, G., Vinuela, F., Dion, J. & Duckwiler, G. (1991b). Electrothrombosis of saccular aneurysms via endovascular approach, part 2, preliminary clinical experience. *J. Neurosurg.* **75**, 8–14.

Guglielmi, G., Vinuela, F., Duckwiler, G. *et al.* (1992a). Endovascular treatment of posterior circulation aneurysms by electrothrombosis using electrically detachable coils. *J. Neurosurg.* **77**, 515–24.

Guglielmi, G., Vinuela, F., Dion, J. & Duckwiler, G. (1992b). Response to S. K. Hilal & R. A. Solomon: Endovascular treatment of aneurysms with coils. *J. Neurosurg.* **76**, 338–9.

Halbach, V. V., Higashida, R. T., Dowd, C. F., Barnwell, S. L. & Hieshima, G. B. (1991). Management of vascular perforations that occur during neurointerventional procedures. *AJNR* **12**, 319–27.

Handa, H., Hashimoto, N., Nagata, I. & Hazama, F. (1983). Saccular cerebral aneurysms in rats: a newly developed animal model of the disease. *Stroke* **14**, 857–86.

Hashi, K. & Nin, K. (1984). Complications following carotid ligation combined with EC–IC bypass. *Neurosurgeon* **4**, 359–66.

Hashimoto, N., Handa, H. & Hazama, F. (1978). Experimentally induced cerebral aneurysms in rats. *Surg. Neurol.* **10**, 3–8.

Hayashi, M., Kobayashi, H., Munemoto, S. *et al.* (1982). An analysis of time course of intracranial pressure in patients with communicating hydrocephalus following subarachnoid hemorrhage due to ruptured intracranial aneurysms. *Brain Nerve* **34**, 653–60.

Heilman, C. B., Kwan, E. S. K. & Wu, J. l. (1992). Aneurysm recurrence following endovascular balloon occlusion. *J. Neurosurg.* **77**, 260–4.

Heros, R. C. (1984). Thromboembolic complications after combined internal carotid ligation and extra-to-intracranial bypass. *Surg. Neurol.* **21**, 75–9.

Higashida, R. T., Halbach, V. V., Cahan, L. D., Hieshima, G. B. & Konishi, Y. (1989a). Detachable balloon embolization therapy of posterior circulation intracranial aneurysms. *J. Neurosurg.* **71**, 512–19.

Higashida, R. T., Halbach, V. V., Cahan, L. D. *et al.* (1989b). Transluminal angioplasty for treatment of intracranial arterial vasospasm. *J. Neurosurg.* **71**, 648–53.

Higashida, R. T., Halbach, V. V., Dormandy, B., Bell, J. D. & Hieshima, G. B. (1990a). Endovascular treatment of intracranial aneurysms with a new silicone microballoon device: technical considerations and indications for therapy. *Radiology* **174**, 687–91.

Higashida, R. T., Halbach, V. V., Dowd, C. *et al.* (1990b). Endovascular detachable balloon embolization therapy of cavernous carotid artery aneurysms: results in 87 cases. *J. Neurosurg.* **72**, 857–63.

Higashida, R. T., Halbach, V. V., Dowd, C., Barnwell, S. L. & Hishima, G. B. (1991). Intracranial aneurysms: interventional neurovascular treatment with detachable balloons – results in 215 cases. *Radiology* **178**, 663–70.

Hilal, S. K. & Solomon, R. A. (1992). Endovascular treatment of aneurysms with coils. *J. Neurosurg.* **76**, 337–8.

Hodes, J. E., Fox, A. J., Pelz, D. M. & Peerless, S. J. (1990). Rupture of aneurysms following balloon embolization: *J. Neurosurg.* **72**, 567–71.

Hunt, W. E. & Hess, R. M. (1968). Surgical risk as related to time of intervention in the repair of intracranial aneurysms. *J. Neurosurg.* **28**, 14–20.

Jafar, J. J. & Weiner, H. L. (1993). Surgery for angiographically occult cerebral aneurysms. *J. Neurosurg.* **79**, 674–9.

Jane, J. A., Kassell, N. F., Torner, J. C. & Winn, H. R. (1985). The natural history of aneurysms and arteriovenous malformations. *J. Neurosurg.* **62**, 321–3.

Juvela, S., Porras, M. & Heiskanen, O. (1993). Natural history of unruptured intracranial aneurysms: a long-term follow-up study. *J. Neurosurg.* **79**, 174–82.

Kak, V. K., Gleadhill, C. A. & Baily, I. C. (1970). The familial incidence of intracranial aneurysms. *J. Neurol. Neurosurg. Psychiatry* **33**, 29–33.

Kaku, Y., Yonekawa, Y., Tsukahara, T. & Kazekawa, K. (1992). Superselective intra-arterial infusion of papaverine for the treatment of cerebral vasospasm after subarachnoid hemorrhage. *J. Neurosurg.* **77**, 842–7.

Kasdon, D. L. & Stein, B. M. (1979). Combined supratentorial and infratentorial exposure for low-lying basilar aneurysms. *Neurosurgery* **4**, 422–6.

Kassell, N. F. & Drake, C. G. (1982). Timing of aneurysm surgery. *Neurosurgery* **10**, 514–19.

Kassell, N. F. & Torner, J. C. (1983). Aneurysmal rebleeding: a preliminary report from the cooperative aneurysm study. *Neurosurgery* **13**, 479–81.

Kassell, N. F., Peerless, S. J., Durward, Q. J., Beck, D. W., Drake, C. G. & Adams, H. P. (1982). Treatment of ischemic deficits from vasospasm with intravascular volume expansion and induced arterial hypertension. *Neurosurgery* **11**, 337–43.

Kassell, N. F., Sasaki, T., Colohan, A. R. T. & Nazar, G. (1985). Cerebral vasospasm following aneurysmal subarachnoid hemorrhage: progress reviews. *Stroke* **16**, 562–72.

Kassell, N. F., Torner, J. C., Haley, E. C. Jr, Jane, J. A., Adams, H. P., Kongable, G. L. *et al.* (1990a). The international cooperative study on the timing of aneurysm surgery, part 1, overall management result. *J. Neurosurg.* **73**, 18–36.

Kassell, N. F., Torner, J. C., Jane, J. A., Haley, E. C. Jr, Adams, H. P. *et al.* (1990b). The international cooperative study on the timing of aneurysm surgery, part 2, surgical results. *J. Neurosurg.* **73**, 37–47.

Kim, P., Jones, J. D. & Sundt, T. M. Jr (1992). High-energy phosphate levels in the cerebral artery during chronic vasospasm after subarachnoid hemorrhage. *J. Neurosurg.* **76**, 991–6.

Kiyohara, Y., Ueda, K., Hasuo, Y. *et al.* (1989). Incidence and prognosis of subarachnoid hemorrhage in a Japanese rural community. *Stroke* **20**, 1150–5.

Kodama, N. & Suzuki, J. (1978). Moyamoya disease associated with aneurysm. *J. Neurosurg.* **48**, 565–9.

Kunishio, K., Yamamoto, Y., Sunami, N. & Asari, S. (1987). Agenesis of the left internal carotid artery, common carotid artery, and main trunk of the external carotid artery associated with multiple cerebral aneurysms. *Surg. Neurol.* **27**, 177–81.

Kwan, E. S. K., Heilman, C. B., Shucart, W. A. & Klucznik, R. P. (1991). Enlargement of basilar artery aneurysms following balloon occlusion – "water-hammer effect". *J. Neurosurg.* **75**, 963–8.

LeBlanc, R. (1987). The minor leak preceding subarachnoid hemorrhage. *J. Neurosurg.* **66**, 35–9.

Levey, A. S., Pauker, S. G. & Kassirer, J. P. (1983). Occult intracranial aneurysms in polycystic kidney disease: when is the cerebral arteriography indicated? *N. Engl. J. Med.* **308**, 986–94.

Lindsey, K. W., Bone, I. & Callander, R. (1991). *Neurology and Neurosurgery Illustrated*, 2nd edn. Edinburgh: Churchill Livingstone.

Linskey, M. E., Sekhar, L. N., Hirsch, W. L., Jr, Yonas, H. & Horton, J. A. (1990). Aneurysms of the intracavernous carotid artery: natural history and indications for treatment. *Neurosurgery* **26**, 933–8.

Linskey, M. E., Horton, J. A., Rao, G. R. & Yonas, H. (1991). Fatal rupture of the intracranial carotid artery during transluminal angioplasty for vasospasm induced by subarachnoid hemorrhage. Case report. *J. Neurosurg.* **74**, 985–90.

Ljunggren, B., Sonesson, B., Saveland, H. & Brandt, L. (1985). Cognitive impairment and adjustment in patients without neurological deficits after aneurysmal SAH and early operation. *J. Neurosurg.* **62**, 673–9.

Lozano, A. M. & LeBlanc, R. (1987). Familial intracranial aneurysms. *J. Neurosurg.* **66**, 522–8.

Mathews, D., Walker, B. S., Purdy, P. D. *et al.* (1993). Brain blood flow SPECT in temporary balloon occlusion of carotid and intracerebral arteries. *J. Nucl. Med.* **34**, 1239–43.

Matsui, T., Takuwa, Y., Johshita, H., Yamashita, K. & Asano, T. (1992). Erratum: possible role of protein kinase C-dependent smooth muscle contraction in the pathogenesis of chronic cerebral vasospasm. *J. Cereb. Blood. Flow. Metab.* **12**, 707.

McCormick, W. F. & Nofzinger, J. D. (1965). Saccular intracranial aneurysm: An autopsy study. *J. Neurosurg.* **23**, 155–9.

Milhorat, T. H. (1987). Acute hydrocephalus after aneurysmal subarachnoid hemorrhage. *Neurosurgery* **20**, 15–20.

Miyaoka, M., Sato, K. & Ishii, S. (1993). A clinical study of the relationship of timing to outcome of surgery for ruptured cerebral aneurysms. A retrospective analysis of 1622 cases. *J. Neurosurg.* **79**, 373–8.

Mizoi, K., Yoshimoto, T., Takahashi, A., Fijuwara, S., Koshu, K. & Sugawara, T. (1993). Prospective study on the prevention of cerebral vasospasm by intrathecal fibrinolytic therapy with tissue-type plasminogen activator. *J. Neurosurg.* **78**, 430–7.

Moniz, E., Dias, A. & Lima, A. (1928). La radio-arteriograhie et la topagraphie cranio-encephalique. *J. Radiol.* **12**, 72–82.

Neil-Dwyer, G., Bartlett, J. R., Nicholls, A. C., Narcis, P. & Pope, F. M. (1983). Collagen deficiency and ruptured cerebral aneurysms. *J. Neurosurg.* **59**, 16–20.

Nichols, D. A. (1993). Endovascular treatment of the acutely ruptured intracranial aneurysm. *J. Neurosurg.* **79**, 1–2.

Nishioka, H., Torner, J. C., Graf, C. J., Kassell, N. F., Sahs, A. L. & Goettler, L. C. (1984). Cooperative study of intracranial aneurysms and subarachnoid hemorrhage: a long-term prognostic study. II. Ruptured intracranial aneurysms managed conservatively. *Arch. Neurol.* **41**, 1142–6.

Nishioka, H., Torner, J. C., Graf, C. J., Kassel, N. F., Sahs, A. L. & Goettler, L. C. (1984). Cooperative study of intracranial aneurysms and subarachnoid hemorrhage: a long-term prognostic study. III. Subarachnoid hemorrhage of unknown etiology. *Arch. Neurol.* **41**, 1147–51.

Okawara, S.-H. (1973). Warning signs prior to rupture of an intracranial aneurysm. *J. Neurosurg.* **38**, 575–80.

Origitano, T. C., Al-Mefty, O., Leonetti, J. P., DeMonte, F. & Reichman, O. H. (1994). Vascular considerations and complications in cranial base surgery. *Neurosurgery* **35**, 351–63.

Osguthorpe, J. D. & Hungerford, G. D. (1984). Transarterial carotid occlusion. *Arch. Otolaryngol.* **110**, 694–6.

Ostergaard, J. R. & Hog, E. (1985). Incidence of multiple intracranial aneurysms. Influence of arterial hypertension and gender. *J. Neurosurg.* **63**, 49–55.

Pakarinen, S. (1967). Incidence, aetiology, and prognosis of primary subarachnoid haemorrhage: a study based on 589 cases diagnosed in a defined urban population during a defined period. *Acta Neurol. Scand.* **43** (Suppl. 29), 1–128.

Pare, L., Delfino, R. & Leblanc, R. (1992). The relationship of ventricular drainage to aneurysmal rebleeding. *J. Neurosurg.* **76**, 422–7.

Parkinson, D. (1965). A surgical approach to the cavernous portion of the carotid artery. Anatomical studies and case report. *J. Neurosurg.* **23**, 474–83.

Parkinson, D. (1973). Carotid cavernous fistula: direct repair with preservation of the carotid artery. Technical note. *J. Neurosurg.* **38**, 99–106.

Peerless, S. J. & Drake, C. G. (1985). Posterior circulation aneurysms. In Wilkins, R. H. & Rengachary, S. S. (eds.) *Neurosurgery*, vol. 2, pp. 1422–37. New York: McGraw-Hill.

Peerless, S. J., Hernesniemi, J. A., Gutman, F. B. & Drake, C. G. (1994). Early surgery for ruptured vertebrobasilar aneurysms. *J. Neurosurg.* **80**, 643–9.

Petruk, K. C., West, M., Mohr, G. *et al.* (1988). Nimodipine treatment in poor-grade aneurysm patients. Results of a multicenter double-blind placebo-controlled trial. *J. Neurosurg.* **68**, 505–17.

Phillips, L. H. II, Whisnant, J. P., O'Fallon, W. M. & Sundt, T. M. Jr. (1980). The unchanging pattern of subarachnoid hemorrhage in a community. *Neurology* **30**, 1034–40.

Pia, H. W. & Zierski, J. (1982). Giant cerebral aneurysms. *Neurosurg. Rev.* **5**, 117–48.

Rinne, J. K. & Hernesniemi, J. A. (1993). De novo aneurysms: special multiple intracranial aneurysms. *Neurosurgery* **33**, 981–5.

Romodanov, A. P. & Shcheglov, V. I. (1982). Intravascular occlusion of saccular aneurysms of the cerebral arteries by means of a detachable balloon catheter. In: Krayenbuhl, H. (ed.). *Advances and Technical Standards in Neurosurgery*, pp. 25–49. New York: Springer-Verlag.

Roski, R. A., Spetzler, R. F. & Nulsen, F. E. (1981). Late complications of carotid ligation in the treatment of intracranial aneurysms. *J. Neurosurg.* **54**, 583–7.

Sahs, A. L. (1969). Observation on the pathology of saccular aneurysms. In: *Intracranial Aneurysms and Subarachnoid Hemorrhage: A Cooperative Study*, pp. 22–36. Philadelphia: Lippincott.

Sahs, A. L., Nibbelink, D. W. & Torner, J. C. (1981). *Aneurysmal Subarachnoid Hemorrhage: Report of the Cooperative Study*. Baltimore: Urban & Schwarzenberg.

Saito, I., Ueda, Y. & Sano, K. (1977). Significance of vasospasm in the treatment of ruptured intracranial aneurysms. *J. Neurosurg.* **47**, 412–29.

Sakaki, T., Kinugawa, K., Tanigake, T., Miyamoto, S., Kyoi, K. & Utsumi, S. (1980). Embolism from intracranial aneurysms. *J. Neurosurg.* **53**, 300–4.

Saveland, H., Hillman, J., Brandt, L., Edner, G., Jakobsson, K.-E. & Algers, G. (1992). Overall outcome in aneurysmal subarachnoid hemorrhage. A prospective study from neurosurgical units in Sweden during a 1-year period. *J. Neurosurg.* **76**, 729–34.

Schievink, W. I., Piepgras, D. G. & Wirth, F. P. (1992). Rupture of previously documented small asymptomatic saccular intracranial aneurysms. *J. Neurosurg.* **76**, 1019–24.

Schorstein, J. (1940). Carotid ligation in saccular intracranial aneurysms. *Br. J. Surg.* **28**, 50–70.

Sekhar, L. N. & Heros, R. C. (1981). Origin, growth, and rupture of saccular aneurysms: a review. *Neurosurgery* **8**, 248–60.

Sekhar, L. N., Sen, C. N., Jho, H. D. & Janecka, I. P. (1989). Surgical treatment of intracavernous neoplasms: a four-year experience. *Neurosurgery* **24**, 18–30.

Serbinenko, F. A. (1974). Balloon catheterization and occlusion of major cerebral vessels. *J. Neurosurg.* **41**, 125–45.

Stehbens, W. (1963). Aneurysms and anatomical variations of cerebral arteries. *Arch. Pathol.* **75**, 45–64.

Stehbens, W. E. (1972). Intracranial arterial aneurysms. In: *Pathology of the Cerebral Blood Vessels*, pp. 351–470. Saint Louis: Mosby.

Steinberg, G. K., Drake, C. G. & Peerless, S. J. (1993). Deliberate basilar or vertebral artery occlusion in the treatment of intracranial aneurysms. Immediate results and long-term outcome in 201 patients. *J. Neurosurg.* **79**, 161–73.

Storey, P. B. (1967). Psychiatric sequelae of subarachnoid hemorrhage. *Br. Med. J.* **3**, 261–6.

Sundt, T. M. Jr (1990). *Surgical Techniques for Saccular and Giant Intracranial Aneurysms*. Baltimore: Williams and Wilkins.

Sundt, T. M. Jr & Piepgras, D. G. (1979). Surgical approach to giant intracranial aneurysms. Operative experience with 80 cases. *J. Neurosurg.* **51**, 731–42.

Sundt, T. M. Jr, Piepgras, D. G., Marsh, R. W. & Fode, N. C. (1986). Saphenous vein bypass graft for giant aneurysms and intracranial occlusive disease. *J. Neurosurg.* **65**, 439–50.

Swann, K. W., Heros, R. C., Debrun, G. & Nelson, C. (1986). Inadvertent middle cerebral artery embolism by a detachable balloon: management by embolectomy. Case report. *J. Neurosurg.* **64**, 309–12.

Swearingen, B. & Heros, R. C. (1987). Common carotid occlusion for unclippable carotid aneurysms: an old but still effective operation. *Neurosurgery* **21**, 288–95.

Taki, W., Nishi, S., Yamashita, K. *et al.* (1992). Selection and combination of various endovascular techniques in the treatment of giant aneurysms. *J. Neurosurg.* **77**, 37–42.

Taneda, M. (1982). Effect of early operation for ruptured aneurysms on prevention of delayed ischemic symptoms. *J. Neurosurg.* **57**, 622–8.

Tindall, G. T., Goree, J. A., Lee, J. F. & Odom, G. L. (1966). Effect of common carotid ligation on size of internal carotid aneurysms and distal intracarotid and retinal artery pressure. *J. Neurosurg.* **25**, 503–11.

Todo, T., Usui, M. & Takakura, K. (1991). Treatment of severe intraventricular hemorrhage by intraventricular infusion of urokinase. *J. Neurosurg.* **74**, 81–6.

van Gijn, J., Hijdra, A., Wijdicks, E. F. M., Vermeulen, M. & van Crevel, H. (1985). Acute hydrocephalus after aneurysmal subarachnoid hemorrhage. *J. Neurosurg.* **63**, 355–62.

Vassilouthis, J. (1984). The syndrome of normal-pressure hydrocephalus. *J. Neurosurg.* **61**, 501–9.

Vassilouthis, J. & Richardson, A. E. (1979). Ventricular dilatation and communicating hydrocephalus following spontaneous subarachnoid hemorrhage. *J. Neurosurg.* **51**, 341–51.

Waga, S. & Tochio, H. (1985). Intracranial aneurysm associated with moyamoya disease in childhood. *Surg. Neurol.* **23**, 237–43.

Weir, B. (1987). *Aneurysms Affecting the Nervous System*. Baltimore: Williams & Wilkins.

Weir, B., Grace, M., Hansen, J. & Rothberg, C. (1978). Time course of vasospasm in man. *J. Neurosurg.* **48**, 173–8.

Whisnant, J. P., Sacco, S. E., O'Fallon, W. M., Fode, N. C. & Sundt, T. M. Jr (1973). Referral bias in aneurysmal subarachnoid hemorrhage. *J. Neurosurg.* **78**, 726–32.

Wiebers, D. O., Whisnant, J. P. & O'Fallon, W. M. (1981). The natural history of unruptured intracranial aneurysms. *N. Engl. J. Med.* **304**, 696–8.

Wiebers, D. O., Whisnant, J. P., Sundt, T. M. Jr & O'Fallon, W. M. (1987). The significance of unruptured intracranial saccular aneurysms. *J. Neurosurg.* **66**, 23–9.

Wilkins, R. H. (1980). Attempted prevention or treatment of intracranial arterial spasm: a survey. *Neurosurgery* **6**, 198–210.

Wilkins, R. H. (ed.) (1980). *Cerebral Arterial Spasm*. Proceedings of the second international workshop. Baltimore: Williams & Wilkins.

Wilkins, R. H. (1986). Attempts at prevention or treatment of intracranial arterial spasm: an update. *Neurosurgery* **18**, 808–25.

Wilson, C. B. & Spetzler, R. F. (1978). Operative approaches to aneurysms. *Clin. Neurosurg.* **26**, 232–47.

Yasargil, M. G. (ed.) (1987). *Microneurosurgery*, vol. II. *Clinical Considerations, Surgery of Intracranial Aneurysms and Results*. Stuttgart: George Thieme.

Zabramski, J. M., Spetzler, R. F., Lee, K. S. *et al.* (1991). Phase I trial of tissue plasminogen activator for the prevention of vasospasm in patients with aneurysmal subarachnoid hemorrhage. *J. Neurosurg.* **75**, 189–96.

Zubkov, Y. N., Nikiforov, B. M. & Shustin, V. A. (1984). Balloon catheter technique for dilatation of constricted cerebral arteries after aneurysmal SAH. *Acta Neurochir.* **70**, 65–79.

7 Cerebral arteriovenous malformations

MARK G. HAMILTON AND ROBERT F. SPETZLER

Cerebral arteriovenous malformations (AVMs) represent one type of vascular malformation found within the central nervous system. Others include cavernous haemangiomas, venous angiomas and capillary telangiectasia (Golfinos *et al.* 1992). Although each of these lesions possesses a distinct natural history that is worthy of review (Wilkins 1985), this chapter will focus upon cerebral AVMs. Arteriovenous malformations are vascular anomalies, frequently congenital, that consist of direct connections between the arterial and venous systems. These lesions exist because a capillary bed is missing. The topic of cerebral AVMs will be divided into (1) true cerebral AVMs, (2) dural AVMs, and (3) vein of Galen AVMs, with review of natural history, treatment methods and patient outcome presented for each. The majority of this review will focus upon true cerebral AVMs.

Cerebral arteriovenous malformations

Natural history

The malformations in this category, representing the most common of the three general categories of AVMs, consist of those AVMs directly involving the cerebral hemispheres, cerebellar hemispheres or brain stem (Fig. 7.1). Cerebral AVMs are about one-seventh to one-tenth as common as intracranial aneurysms (Wilkins 1985). These AVMs have a congenital origin and can manifest symptoms early in life, with the majority becoming symptomatic before the end of the third decade (Wilkins 1985). The most frequent mode of presentation for patients with cerebral AVMs is haemorrhage (50–60%) or seizures (25–30%), although a small number of patients will present with headache or progressive neurological deficit unrelated to haemorrhage (Stein & Wolpert 1980; Graf *et al.* 1983; Wilkins 1985; Crawford *et al.* 1986; Heros & Tu 1987; Itoyama *et al.* 1989; Ondra *et al.* 1990; Samson & Batjer 1991; Golfinos *et al.* 1992). Recently, a significant number of asymptomatic AVMs are being discovered because of the widespread use of computed tomography (CT) and magnetic resonance (MR) imaging.

AVM haemorrhage is the most significant risk patients face, accounting for the majority of mortality and morbidity. Approximately two-thirds of haemorrhage is intracerebral, 30% subarachnoid and the remainder intraventricular. In 1985 Wilkins,

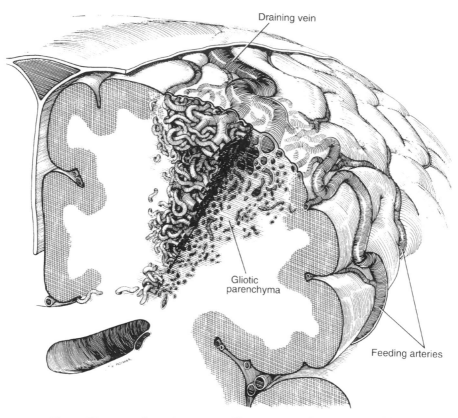

Fig. 7.1. Unruptured arteriovenous malformation. (With permission of the Barrow Neurological Institute.)

reviewing the medical literature, estimated the risk of haemorrhage for an unruptured AVM at 2–3% per year, increasing during the first year after a haemorrhage to about 6%, then decreasing to a baseline of about 2–3% per year. Furthermore, a patient with an unruptured cerebral AVM who presents with seizures has the same risk for haemorrhage as a patient with an AVM that haemorrhaged 1 year previously. The mortality associated with the first haemorrhage is estimated to be about 10%, increasing to about 13–15% for each subsequent haemorrhage. However, when the combined mortality and morbidity for AVM haemorrhage is considered, the figure is a staggering 40% for each event (Heros & Tu 1987). Samson & Batjer (1991) recently summarized the estimated risk for a patient with an cerebral AVM: (1) haemorrhage 3–4% per year or 30–40% per decade; (2) serious morbidity 2–3% per year or 30–40% per decade; and (3) death 1–1.5% per year or 10–15% per decade. In addition, a number of efforts have been directed at identifying subsets of patients with AVMs that may have a propensity for haemorrhage. Risk factors that have been implicated include the venous drainage system (Miyasaka *et al*. 1992), the presence of associated aneurysms (Brown *et al*. 1990), and the size of the AVM (Spetzler *et al*. 1992). Miyasaka *et al*. (1992) found a correlation between AVM haemorrhage rate and the pattern of venous drainage. Haemorrhage was a greater risk in those with only one draining vein, severe impairment of the draining veins (venous stenosis or occlusion), or venous dranage limited to the deep venous system. Brown *et al.* (1990) determined the annual risk of haemorrhage for patients with a coexisting aneurysm and AVM to be 7% per year at 5 years, compared with only 1.7% per year for patients with an AVM alone. Spetzler *et al.* (1992) identified a higher risk of haemorrhage, with larger haematomas, for AVMs with a diameter of less than 3 cm, and attributed this to arterial pressures which were significantly higher in small compared with larger AVMs. However, while all these observations are intriguing, they have not been subjected to a large prospective clinical evaluation.

A smaller yet significant number of patients will present with seizures, progressive neurologic deficit, or headaches (Stein & Wolpert 1980). The frequency of seizures does not correlate significantly with AVM size or hemispheric location (with the exception of low frequency with deep hemispheric, cerebellar and brainstem location) and can be partial (focal) or generalized. Seizures can occur in patients with no evidence of haemorrhage or can be triggered by intraparenchymal haemorrhage. Almost two-thirds of patients with AVMs will experience seizures at some point. Progressive neurological deficit has been reported to account for the presenting symptom in about 4–12% of patients with cerebral AVMs. This is frequently referred to as 'cerebral steal' and is typically associated with large high-flow AVMs. The current theory concerning steal is that blood is shunted preferentially through the AVM, creating a relative and absolute state of hypoperfusion in adjacent brain regions. These patients may report intermittent symptoms (frequently associated with transient hypotension or physical exertion) superimposed upon a background of chronic progressive deterioration. Chronic headaches may be a significant if not sole symptom in patients with AVMs that possess a meningeal supply from the external carotid artery or are located in the occipital lobe with a primary blood supply from the posterior cerebral artery (Troost & Newton 1956). Other rare clinical manifestations of cerebral AVMs include hydrocephalus (although most commonly related to intraventricular haemorrhage) and cranial nerve compression (trigeminal neuralgia, hemifacial spasm).

Treatment

The collected evidence supports the conclusion that the natural history for patients with cerebral AVMs is poor, with the majority of the mortality and morbidity related to AVM haemorrhage. The 'gold standard' of AVM treatment is the complete obliteration of the AVM to eliminate the risk of future haemorrhage. To determine the risk/benefit ratio for treatment requires the ability to define treatment difficulty for AVMs of different complexity. In other words, comparing the risks or outcome of treatment for a 1 cm frontal-polar AVM with a 6 cm frontoparietal AVM with deep venous drainage would not be reasonable given the obvious differences in complexity between the two lesions. To this end, a number of different grading schemes have been proposed for cerebral AVMs (Steinmeier *et al.* 1989). In 1986 Spetzler & Martin proposed a grading

Table 7.1. *Determination of arteriovenous malformation (AVM) grade[a]*

Grade features	Points assigned
Size of AVM	
Small (< 3 cm)	1
Medium (3–6 cm)	2
Large (> 6 cm)	3
Eloquence of adjacent brain	
Noneloquent	0
Eloquent	1
Pattern of venous drainage	
Superficial only	0
Deep	1

[a] Grade = [size] + [eloquence] + [venous drainage]; i.e. (1, 2, or 3) + (0 or 1) + (0 or 1).
From Spetzler & Martin (1986) with permission of the *Journal of Neurosurgery.*

system based upon three variables: (1) AVM size, (2) location of the AVM within eloquent brain (e.g., motor gyrus, internal capsule, etc.), and (3) presence of deep venous drainage (Table 7.1). There are five grades of AVM: grade I lesions are small, superficial and located in noneloquent cortex; grade V lesions are large, deep and situated in neurologically critical areas. Grade V AVMs are considered unresectable because they are either too massive and diffusely involve critical structures such as the internal capsule or brainstem. This grading system is simple to use and successfully predicts treatment difficulty and treatment risk as demonstrated by the recent prospective assessment in 120 consecutive patients undergoing complete AVM resection (Table 7.2) (Hamilton & Spetzler 1994). AVM grading systems do not deal with other important variables such as the surgeon's skill or the patient's physical condition (cardiorespiratory status) or neurological status. Further, Steinmeier *et al.* (1989) compared five grading systems in a retrospective review of 48 patients and determined that the Spetzler & Martin system provided the best prediction of surgical risks.

Treatment modalities that are available for cerebral AVMs include microsurgery, transfemoral embolization, intraoperative embolization and radiosurgery. The management of cerebral AVMs requires a multidisciplinary approach involving the neurosurgeon, interventional neuroradiologist and radiotherapist. The role for each of these different treatment modalities in the treatment of patients with cerebral AVMs is gradually being defined. Microsurgical treatment is considered the current mainstay of AVM treatment in that it is the truest method for rapid achievement of the 'gold standard' of treatment and has undergone the most comprehensive assessment. Complete and permanent obliteration of an AVM with endovascular techniques is seldom possible except for very simple lesions (Livingston & Hopkins 1992). Radiosurgery is

Table 7.2. *Early and late[a] results in relation to pretreatment status of patients with arteriovenous malformations*

Grade	Six-week outcome (%)			Late outcome (%)	
	Unchanged or improved	New deficit	Comment[b]	Unchanged or improved	New deficit
I	16 (100)	0	—	16 (100)	0
II	23 (95.8)	1 (4.2)	Surgical	24 (100)	0
III	35 (97.2)	1 (2.8)	Surgical	35 (97.2)	1 (2.8)[c]
IV	22 (00.0)	10 (31.2)	Surgical, 7 Embolization, 3	25 (78.1)	7 (21.9)[d]
V	6 (50.0)	6 (50.0)	Surgical, 2 Embolization, 4	10 (83.3)	2 (16.7)[e]

[a] Late outcome with mean follow-up of 1 year.
[b] Deficits were classified according to primary cause: related either to preoperative or intraoperative embolization or related to the microsurgical resection of the arteriovenous malformation.
[c] Late death from esophageal haemorrhage secondary to pretreatment cirrhosis. No new treatment-associated deficits occurred in this patient.
[d] All seven patients deteriorated one grade on the Glasgow Outcome Scale (Jennett & Bond 1975).
[e] One patient deteriorated one grade and one patient deteriorated two grades on the Glasgow Outcome Scale.
From Hamilton & Spetzler (1994).

maximally successful with small (< 3 cm diameter) AVMs and has an estimated 80% treatment success that requires up to 2 years for AVM obliteration to occur (Lunsford *et al.* 1991; Steiner *et al.* 1992; Lunsford 1993). AVM embolization and radiosurgery are therefore most frequently used as adjuvant therapies in concert with microsurgery. The results of treatment in 220 patients undergoing complete AVM resection (frequently with adjuvant embolization for higher grade AVMs) demonstrate that patients with grades I or II can be treated with minimal morbidity (Spetzler & Martin 1986; Hamilton & Spetzler 1994), while complete resection in patients with grade IV and V AVMs can only be accomplished with a morbidity approaching approximately 20% (Hamilton & Spetzler 1994). These findings have also been substantiated by Heros *et al.* (1990) in a review of 153 patients undergoing complete AVM resection.

An understanding of the natural history and extensive experience managing patients with cerebral AVMs have resulted in the following treatment recommendations aimed primarily at elimination of future risk of haemorrhage, although seizure control should also be a significant treatment ambition. Obviously, patient factors such as age, cardiovascular status, or neurological status can significantly influence the decision process. Furthermore, as with most neurological disorders, prognosis for neurological outcome is heavily dependent upon the baseline neurological status of the patient; once function is lost the chances of recovery begin to diminish significantly. With these factors in mind, all patients with grade I and grade II cerebral AVMs should undergo surgical resection. Endovascular techniques (Livingston & Hopkins 1992) or radiosurgery (Steiner *et al.* 1992) are not routinely required for low-grade AVM treatment, although a vast experience with radiosurgery has been published (Troost & Newton 1956; Betti *et al.* 1989; Ogilvy 1990; Lunsford *et al.* 1991; Friedman & Bora 1992; Lunsford 1993). Patients with grade III AVMs are managed on a case-by-case basis. All symptomatic patients should be offered definitive treatment, while asymptomatic patients should be carefully reviewed with regard to a risk-benefit analysis. Patients with grade IV and grade V AVMs should only be considered for complete resection when they have sustained a significant haemorrhage or repeated haemorrhages, or suffer from a significant progressive neurological deficit. Patients with grade IV and grade V AVMs face a substantial treatment risk and should demonstrate that their natural history warrants a 20% risk of serious morbidity. Endovascular techniques and radiosurgery can play a very significant role in the management of patients with grade III through V AVMs (Spetzler *et al.* 1987; Dawson *et al.* 1990; Heros *et al.* 1990; Pasqualin *et al.* 1991; Viñuela *et al.* 1991; Hamilton & Spetzler 1994). Finally, in certain situations, the 'gold standard' treatment of complete resection may not be suitable for a patient with a high-grade AVM presenting with seizures or progressive neurological deficit. Limited transfemoral or intraoperative embolization of the AVM may significantly reduce patient symptoms (Fox *et al.* 1986; Wade 1986).

Long-term follow-up of treated patients has not yet been adequately accomplished. The report from Hamilton and Spetzler (1994) had a mean follow-up of 1 year, Heros *et al.* (1990) 3.8 years, Piepgras *et al.* (1993) 7.5 years, and Lunsford *et al.* (1991) 14 months. Much longer clinical and angiographic follow-up, for all treatment modalities, is required to define not just the rate of angiographic success, but more importantly to determine the long-term results for prevention of haemorrhage and seizures. A number of recent studies have examined the results of AVM surgery for seizure control (Piepgras *et al.* 1993; Yeh *et al.* 1993). The general conclusions in these studies are that with complete AVM resection there is about a 90% chance of resolution or significant improvement in control of existing seizures, with a low incidence of new seizure activity following surgery.

Dural arteriovenous malformations

Dural AVMs are uncommon lesions that can have protean manifestations and cause significant morbidity and mortality (Awad *et al.* 1990; Rambo *et al.* 1992). The nidus of the dural AVM (or shunt) is, by definition, located within the dura mater (Fig. 7.2) (Awad *et al.* 1990; Martin *et al.* 1990; Golfinos *et al.* 1992; Rambo *et al.* 1992). The arterial supply to dural AVMs is typically from dural arteries, and the venous drainage is directed into an adjoining dural sinus or through collateral pial veins. These lesions are suspected to have primarily an acquired aetiology, most likely resulting from trauma. Dural AVMs can include carotid cavernous fistula, although the majority of reported lesions (63%) have involved the transverse–sigmoid sinus junction (Awad *et al.* 1990).

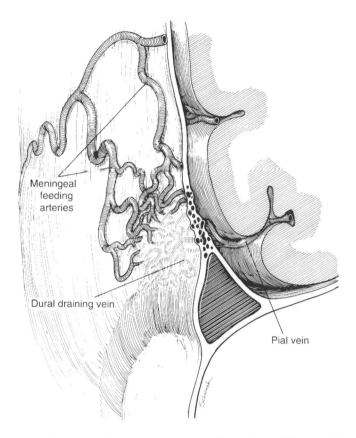

Fig. 7.2. Unruptured dural arteriovenous malformation. (With permission of the Barrow Neurological Institute.)

Little is known about the untreated natural history of patients with dural AVMs. Some dural AVMs will spontaneously thrombose and resolve, while others will have a much more malignant course. Patients with dural AVMs may present with many different symptoms ranging from headache to coma resulting from haemorrhage. A number of angiographic features have been correlated with an aggressive neurological course: leptomeningeal venous drainage, variceal or aneurysmal venous dilations, and galenic drainage (Awad *et al.* 1990). Dural AVMs of the anterior cranial fossa and those involving the tentorial incisura appear to have a great propensity for haemorrhage, and a review of the AVMs at these locations typically identifies the angiographic risk factors that have been discussed. Leptomeningeal venous drainage occurs as the venous congestion increases and collateral drainage channels develop through the leptomeningeal veins. This can result in variceal dilatation of these newly recruited drainage vessels. This results in a weakening of the vessel wall thereby predisposing the AVM to rupture.

Given that our understanding of the natural history is limited, the recommendations for treatment are somewhat less structured. As with cranial AVMs, other patient factors

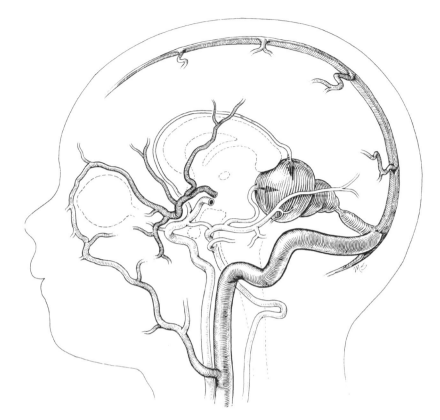

Fig. 7.3. True vein of Galen aneurysm with fistulas originating from posterior cerebral artery and pericallosal artery branches. (With permission of the Barrow Neurological Institute.)

such as cardiorespiratory status, patient age, neurological disability, etc., should be considered. The treatment options that are available for dural AVMs are the same as those for cranial AVMs; however, these lesions can be very complex and difficult to treat. Patients with high-risk angiographic features should be considered for treatment. Patients presenting with haemorrhage or other intolerable symptoms should also be considered for treatment. Few data are available regarding treatment risk factors or patient outcome.

Vein of Galen arteriovenous malformations

Vein of Galen malformations are relatively uncommon, if not rare lesions that are midline arteriovenous fistulas with single or multiple arterial feeders associated with aneurysmal dilatation of the vein of Galen. A number of classification systems have been proposed for these lesions, but the most simple is based upon anatomical features and is practical: 'true' (congenital) vein of Galen malformations and 'secondary' malformations, the latter representing vein of Galen dilatation caused by an adjacent dural or true cerebral (parenchymatous) AVM (Wilkins 1985; Mickle & Quisling 1986; Las-

Table 7.3. *Natural history of vein of Galen malformations compared with different modes of treatment*

	Normal	Impaired	Dead	Reference
Natural history (n = 166)	7%	9%	73%	Hoffman *et al.* (1982); Johnston *et al.* (1987)[a]
Open surgery (n = 54)	48%	22%	30%	Hoffman *et al.* (1982)
Endovascular (arterial) (n = 34)	6%	52%	32%	Lasjaunias *et al.* (1991)[a]
Endovascular (venous) (n = 7)	71%	29%	0	Casasco *et al.* (1991)
Transtorcular embolization (n = 15)	80%	0	21%	Hanner *et al.* (1988)

[a] In these two reviews 11% of untreated patients were lost to follow-up.

jaunias *et al.* 1989) (Figure 7.3). Patients with a vein of Galen malformation typically have different clinical presentations (Hoffman *et al.* 1982) depending upon the age of onset: (1) newborns tend to present with congestive heart failure, less frequently with head enlargement secondary to ventriculomegaly, and rarely with haemorrhage; (2) infants present with head enlargement secondary to ventriculomegaly, and much less commonly with congestive heart failure or haemorrhage; and (3) older children and adults have the most varied modes of presentation including subarachnoid haemorrhage, hydrocephalus, progressive neurological deficit secondary to the 'steal' phenomenon or mass effect, venous hypertension, and only rarely with congestive heart failure. The natural history of an untreated vein of Galen malformation is generally poor: in reviews by Johnston *et al.* (1987) and Hoffman *et al.* (1982) of 166 untreated patients, the reported mortality was 73% (Table 7.3). Treatment for vein of Galen malformations is still evolving. Treatment methods include direct surgical, arterial endovascular and venous endovascular, either alone or in combination. Unfortunately, while the results of these various treatment modalities have considerably improved outcome in relationship to natural history, marked room for improvement is still evident with mortality still ranging around 40% and significant morbidity in 30% of patients (Table 7.3).

References

Awad, I. A., Little, J. R., Akrawi, W. P. & Ahl, J. (1990). Intracranial dural arteriovenous malformations: factors predisposing to an aggressive neurological course. *J. Neurosurg.* **72**, 839–50.

Betti, O. O., Munari, C. & Roslcr, R. (1989). Stereotactic radiosurgery with the linear accelerator: treatment of arteriovenous malformations. *Neurosurgery* **24**, 311–21.

Brown, R. D., Wiebers, D. O. & Forbes, G. S. (1990). Unruptured intracranial aneurysms and arteriovenous malformations: frequency of intracranial hemorrhage and relationship of lesions. *J. Neurosurg.* **73**, 859–63.

Casasco, A., Lylyk, P., Hodes, J. E., Aymard, A. & Merland, J.-J. (1991). Percutaneous transvenous catheterization and embolization of vein of Galen aneurysms. *Neurosurgery* **28**, 260–6.

Crawford, P. M., West, C. R., Chadwick, D. W. & Shaw, M. D. M. (1986). Arteriovenous malformations of the brain: natural history in unoperated patients. *J. Neurol. Neurosurg. Psychiatry* **49**, 1–10.

Dawson, III, R. C., Tarr, R. W., Hecht, S. T., Jungreis, C. A., Lunsford, L. D., Coffey, R. & Horton, J. A. (1990). Treatment of arteriovenous malformations of the brain with combined embolization and stereotactic radiosurgery: results after 1 and 2 years. *AJNR* **11**, 857–64.

Fox, A. J. & Viñuela, F. (1986). Neurological deficit from an inoperable arteriovenous malformation. An indication for therapeutic embolization? *Arch. Neurol.* **43**, 510–11.

Friedman, W. A. & Bova, F. J. (1992). Linear accelerator radiosurgery for arteriovenous malformations. *J. Neurosurg.* **77**, 832–41.

Golfinos, J. G., Wascher, T. M., Zabramski, J. M. & Spetzler, R. F. (1992). The management of unruptured intracranial vascular malformations. *Barrow Neurol. Inst. Q.* **8**(3), 2–11.

Graf, C. J., Perret, G. E. & Torner, J. C. (1983). Bleeding from cerebral arteriovenous malformations as part of their natural history. *J. Neurosurg.* **58**, 331–7.

Hamilton, M. G. & Spetzler, R. F. (1994). The prospective application of a grading system for arteriovenous malformations. *Neurosurgery* **34**, 2–7.

Hanner, J. S., Quisling, R. G., Mickle, J. P. & Hawkins, J. S. (1988). Gianturco coil embolization of vein of Galen aneurysms: technical aspects. *Radiographics* **8**, 935–46.

Heros, R. C. & Tu, Y.-K. (1987). Is surgical therapy needed for unruptured arteriovenous malformations? *Neurology* **37**, 279–86.

Heros, R. C., Korosue, K. & Diebold, P. M. (1990). Surgical excision of cerebral arteriovenous malformations: late results. *Neurosurgery* **26**, 570–8.

Hoffman, H. J., Chuang, S., Hendrick, E. B. & Humphreys, R. P. (1982). Aneurysms of the vein of Galen: experience at The Hospital for Sick Children. Toronto. *J. Neurosurg.* **57**, 316–22.

Itoyama, Y., Uemura, S., Ushio, Y., Kuratsu, J., Nonaka, N., Wada, H., Sano, Y., Fukumura, A., Yoshida, K. & Yano, T. (1989). Natural course of unoperated intracranial arteriovenous malformations: study of 50 cases. *J. Neurosurg.* **71**, 805–9.

Jennett, B. & Bond, M. (1975). Assessment of outcome after severe brain damage. A practical scale. *Lancet* **I**, 480–4.

Johnston, I. H., Whittle, I. R., Besser, M. & Morgan, M. K. (1987). Vein of Galen malformation: diagnosis and management. *Neurosurgery* **20**, 747–58.

Lasjaunias, P., Radesch, G., Pruvost, P., Laroche, F. G. & Landrieu, P. (1989). Treatment of vein of Galen aneurysmal malformation. *J. Neurosurg.* **70**, 746–50.

Lasjaunias, P., Garcia-Monaco, R., Radesch, G., Terbrugge, K., Zerah, M., Tardieu, M. & de Victor, D. (1991). Vein of Galen malformation. Endovascular management of 43 cases. *Child's Nerv. Syst.* **7**, 360–7.

Livingston, K. & Hopkins, L. N. (1992). Endovascular treatment of intracerebral arteriovenous malformations. *Contemp. Neurosurg.* **14**(13), 1–6.

Lunsford, L. D. (1993). Stereotactic radiosurgery: at the threshold or at the crossroads? *Neurosurgery* **32**, 799–804.

Lunsford, L. D., Kondziolka, D., Flickinger, J. C., Bissonette, D. J., Jungreis, C. A., Maitz, A. H., Horton, J. A. & Coffey, R. J. (1991). Stereotactic radiosurgery for arteriovenous malformations of the brain. *J. Neurosurg.* **75**, 512–24.

Martin, N. A., King, W. A., Wilson, C. B., Nutik, S., Carter, L. P. & Spetzler, R. F. (1990). Management of dural arteriovenous malformations of the anterior cranial fossa. *J. Neurosurg.* **72**, 692–7.

Mickle, J. P. & Quislin, R. G. (1986). The vein of Galen malformations. *Neurosurgery: State of the Art Rev.* **1**: 117–31.

Miyasaka, Y., Yada, K., Ohwada, T., Kitahara, T., Kurata, A. & Irikura, K. (1992). An analysis of the venous drainage system as a factor in hemorrhage from arteriovenous malformations. *J. Neurosurg.* **76**, 239–43.

Ogilvy, C. S. (1990). Radiation therapy for arteriovenous malformations: a review. *Neurosurgery* **26**, 725–35.

Ondra, S. L., Troupp, H., George, E. D. & Schwab, K. (1990). The natural history of symptomatic arteriovenous malformations of the brain: a 24-year follow-up assessment. *J. Neurosurg.* **73**, 307–91.

Pasqualin, A., Scienza, R., Cioffi, F., Barone, G., Benati, A., Beltramello, A. & Pian, R. D. (1991). Treatment of cerebral arteriovenous malformations with a combination of preoperative embolization and surgery. *Neurosurgery* **29**, 358–68.

Piepgras, D. G., Sundt Jr, T. M., Ragoowansi, A. T. & Stevens, L. (1993). Seizure outcome in patients with surgically treated cerebral arteriovenous malformations. *J. Neurosurg.* **78**, 5–11.

Rambo Jr, W. M., Narayan, R. K. & Mawad, M. E. (1992). Cranial dural arteriovenous malformations. *Contemp. Neurosurg.* **14**(3), 1–6.

Samson, D. S. & Batjer, H. H. (1991). Preoperative evaluation of the risk/benefit ratio for arteriovenous malformations of the brain. In: Wilkins, R. H. & Rengachary, S. S. (eds.) *Neurosurgery Update II*, pp. 119–25. New York: McGraw-Hill.

Spetzler, R. F. & Martin, N. A. (1986). A proposed grading system for arteriovenous malformations. *J. Neurosurg.* **65**, 476–83.

Spetzler, R. F., Martin, N. A., Carter, L. P., Flom, R. A., Raudzens, P. A. & Wilkinson, E. (1987). Surgical management of large AVMs by staged embolization and operative excision. *J. Neurosurg.* **67** , 17–28.

Spetzler, R. F., Hargraves, R. W., McCormick, P. W., Zambramski, J. M., Flom, R. A. & Zimmerman, R. S. (1992). Relationship of perfusion pressure and size to risk of hemorrhage from arteriovenous malformations. *J. Neurosurg.* **76**, 918–23.

Steinmeier, R., Schramm, J., Müller, H.-G. & Fahlbusch, R. (1989). Evaluation of prognostic factors in cerebral arteriovenous malformations. *Neurosurgery* **24**, 193–200.

Stein, B. M. & Wolpert, S. M. (1980). Arteriovenous malformations of the brain. I. Current concepts and treatment. *Arch. Neurol.* **37**, 1–5.

Steiner, L., Lindquist, C. & Steiner, M. (1992). Radiosurgery. *Adv. Tech. Standards Neurosurg.* **19**, 19–102.

Troost, B. T. & Newton, T. H. (1956). Occipital lobe arteriovenous malformations. Clinical and radiological features in 26 cases with comment on differentiation and migraine. *Arch. Opthalmol.* **93**, 250–6.

Viñuela, F., Dion, J. E., Duckwiler, G., Martin, N. A., Lylyk, P., Fox, A., Pelz, D., Drake, C. G., Girvin, J. J. & Debrun, G. (1991). Combined endovascular embolization and surgery in the management of cerebral arteriovenous malformations: experience with 101 cases. *J. Neurosurg.* **75**, 856–64.

Wade, J. P. H. (1986). Neurological deficit from an inoperable arteriovenous malformation. An indication for therapeutic embolization? *Arch. Neurol.* **43**, 508–9.

Wilkins, R. H. (1985). Natural history of intracranial vascular malformations: a review. *Neurosurgery* **16**, 421–30.

Yeh, H.-S., Tew Jr, J. M. & Gartner, M. (1993). Seizure control after surgery on cerebral arteriovenous malformations. *J. Neurosurg.* **78**, 12–18.

8 Spinal vascular malformations

EDWARD H. OLDFIELD

Patients with spinal arteriovenous malformations (AVMs) may have an insidious, subacute or acute onset of symptoms, depending on the type of AVM and the mechanism of cord injury. Before recommending treatment, one must consider the expected clinical course based on knowledge of the natural history of the specific type of vascular abnormality affecting the patient and the risks and potential benefits of the proposed treatment. However, knowledge of the natural history of patients with spinal vascular abnormalities is incomplete. As with other rare disorders for which therapy is attempted, it is known only from retrospective studies. Furthermore, additional factors mitigate the usefulness of the previous studies. Most information on the natural history of spinal AVMs was acquired when they were all considered to be congenital AVMs of the spinal cord. Only in the past decade has it been generally recognized that the spinal vascular abnormalities are not a single entity, but are comprised of several biologically distinct forms. Based on origin, epidemiology, anatomy, pathophysiology, clinical presentation, and prognosis, three main types of spinal vascular abnormalities are now recognized: dural arteriovenous fistulas (AVFs), intradural vascular malformations and cavernous angiomas of the spinal cord (Table 8.1) (Oldfield & Doppman 1988; Oldfield 1991).

Since each type of vascular abnormality appears to be a biologically distinct entity (Rosenblum *et al.* 1987; Oldfield & Doppman 1988), the natural history and the influence of treatment of each type must be considered separately. As the dural AVMs are by far the most common type, have similar pathophysiology of cord injury from patient to patient, have a relatively stereotypic clinical course, permitting reasonable prediction about the patient's prognosis, in contrast to the other types of AVMs, which are less common, have a more sporadic, less predictable, clinical course, and in which the pathophysiology of cord injury varies from patient to patient (haemorrhage, venous congestion, aneurysm formation with cord compression, vascular steal), I emphasize the dural AVFs here.

Ideal scales for assessing the severity of neurological impairment and the outcome of treatment should be simple enough to be widely used without variance from centre to centre and they must stratify meaningful levels of function clearly. For spinal AVMs the important elements for grading are whether the patient can walk normally or with

Table 8.1. *Classification of spinal vascular malformations*

A. Dural arteriovenous fistulas (AVFs)
B. Intradural arteriovenous malformations (AVMs)
    1. Juvenile AVMs
    2. Glomus AVMs
    3. Intradural (perimedullary) AVFs
C. Cavernous angiomas

Dural AVFs are embedded in a spinal nerve root sleeve and
the surrounding spinal dura. In intradural AVMs the nidus of
the arterial-to-venous transition is either buried in the
substance of the cord or is in the pia. The intradural vascular
malformations are also further classified into three
subgroups: juvenile and glomus type AVMs, and direct AVFs
(perimedullary AVFs).

Table 8.2. *Functional grading scale of Aminoff & Logue*

Motor function	
Grade 0	No motor disturbance
Grade 1	Disturbance of gait, leg weakness, abnormal stance or gait, no restriction of locomotor activity
Grade 2	Restricted exercise tolerance
Grade 3	Requires one stick or other support for walking
Grade 4	Requires crutches or two sticks for walking
Grade 5	Unable to stand, confined to bed or wheelchair
Micturition	
Grade 0	No disturbance
Grade 1	Hesitancy, urgency or frequency
Grade 2	Occasional urinary incontinence or retention
Grade 3	Total urinary incontinence or persistent retention

From Aminoff & Logue (1974a).

minimal support, if they have normal bladder and bowel continence, and whether they
suffer chronic or disabling pain. With the exception that it does not address pain, the
classification scheme proposed by Aminoff and Logue in 1974 satisfies these requirements. (Aminoff & Logue 1974a,b). It is the functional grading scale used most often in
reports of the natural history and outcome of treatment of patients with spinal AVMs
(Table 8.2).

Dural AV fistulas

Clinical presentation and pathophysiology

Dural AVFs have a strong male predilection and present late in life: 85% of patients with
dural AVFs are male, and 80% have the onset of symptoms after the age of 40 years

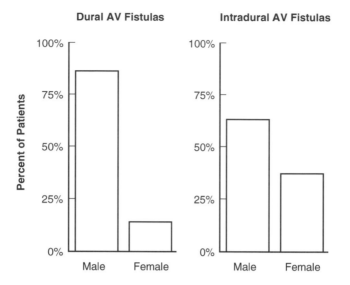

Fig. 8.1. Distribution by gender of dural arteriovenous (AV) fistulas and intradural arteriovenous malformations (AVMs). Dural AV fistulas compiled from Hurth, *et al.* (1978), Benhaiem *et al.* (1983), Symon *et al.* (1984), Merland *et al.* (1985), Rosenblum *et al.* (1987), Morgan & Marsh (1989). Intradural AVMs compiled from Symon *et al.* (1984), Yasargil *et al.* (1984), Rosenblum *et al.* (1987), Biondi *et al.* (1990).

(Figs. 8.1, 8.2). The nidus of dural AVFs is almost always in the lower half of the spinal column (Fig. 8.3). Thus, patients with dural AVFs usually present with gradual onset of paraparesis and/or sphincter dysfunction associated with back pain or radiculopathy. Most patients have exacerbation of symptoms during physical exertion or with certain postures (Rosenblum *et al.* 1987; Oldfield & Doppman 1988). Unlike intramedullary AVMs, in which the incidence of haemorrhage is 50–80%, dural AVFs rarely haemorrhage (Aminoff & Logue, 1974a,b; Tobin & Layton 1976; Logue 1979; Merland *et al.* 1980; Oldfield *et al.* 1983; Symon *et al.* 1984; Yasargil *et al.* 1984; Rosenblum *et al.* 1987; Morgan & Marsh, 1989).

The pathophysiology of the gradually progressive myelopathy that occurs with these lesions is now clear. Dural AVFs are low-flow AV shunts that cause venous hypertension of the cord (Oldfield *et al.* 1983; Oldfield & Doppman, 1988; Hassler *et al.* 1989), which reduces the arterial perfusion pressure of the spinal cord to 25–30% of normal, resulting in ischaemia and progressive cord injury.

Natural history

There are no studies of the natural history of patients with dural AVFs. The first report describing them was not published until 1977 (Kendall & Logue 1977). With that report it became apparent that treatment of AVFs was simple, safe and effective. Thus, a prospective study of the natural history of AVFs without treatment has not been possible and cannot be justified now or in the future. However, surprisingly, the natural

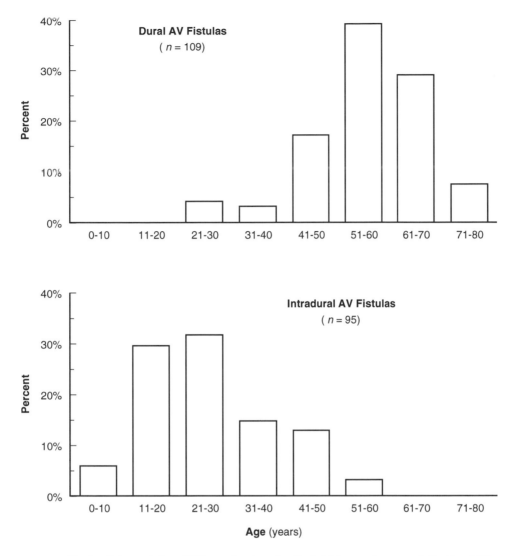

Fig. 8.2. Intramedullary AVMs predominantly affect children and young adults. Dural AV fistulas usually present in adults over 40 years old. Dural AV fistulas compiled from Symon *et al.* (1984), Merland *et al.* (1985), Rosenblum *et al.* (1987), Morgan & Marsh (1989). Intramedullary AVMs compiled from Yasargil *et al.* (1984), Rosenblum *et al.* (1987).

history of AVFs can be deduced from studies performed before the recognition of their existence and from studies of the condition of patients at treatment. This opportunity is based on (1) their high prevalence among patients with spinal AVMs, of which they comprise about 80–90% of all spinal vascular abnormalities (Aminoff & Logue 1974a,b); (2) their distinguishing epidemiological and clinical features (Rosenblum *et al.* 1987; Oldfield & Doppman 1988), features distinct enough to permit them to be identified with reasonable accuracy in prior studies (Aminoff & Logue 1974a,b; Tobin & Layton

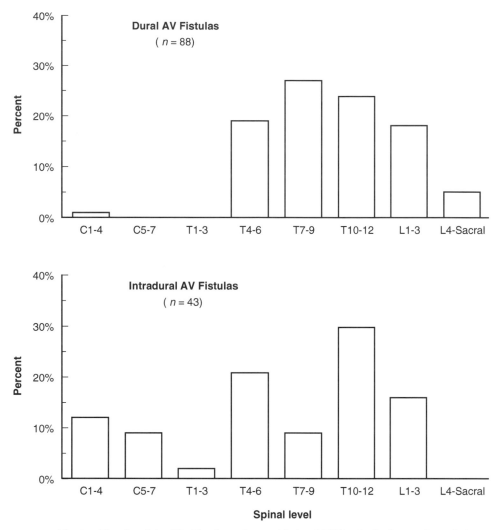

Fig. 8.3. The site of the AV nidus in patients with dural AV fistulas is almost always below the midthoracic level. Intramedullary AVMs are dispersed more uniformly along the longitudinal axis of the cord, although they also more commonly affect the lower segments. Dural AV fistulas compiled from Symon *et al.* (1984), Merland *et al.* (1985), Rosenblum *et al.* (1987). Data for intramedullary AVMs from Rosenblum *et al.* (1987).

1976; Hurth *et al.* 1978); and (3) the consistency of their clinical course. The information available to examine the natural history of AVFs comes principally from a retrospective analysis performed by Aminoff and Logue (1974a,b). Although their study began before the introduction of selective spinal arteriography, it clearly reveals the natural history of patients with dural AVFs, since it was comprised predominantly of adult males (88%) with thoracolumbar lesions (49 of the 60 patients were ≥ 41 years old, 43 of those 49 were males, and 55 of the 60 lesions (92%) were in the thoracic or lumbar spinal segments), (Aminoff & Logue 1974a) that had never haemorrhaged (90%) – features that distinguish patients with dural AVFs from the other types of spinal AVMs (Figs. 8.1–8.3).The course of the disease, as defined by their study, was one of progressive neurological decline and functional disability. One-fifth of the 60 patients required crutches or were non-ambulatory by 6 months after the onset of symptoms other than pain. Half of all patients were severely disabled (confined to a wheelchair or bed) within 3 years of the onset of gait impairment and 91% had restricted activity within 3 years of the onset of symptoms (Fig. 8.4). (Aminoff & Logue 1974a,b). Similarly, in their 1976 report, which included 23 patients with 'type I AVMs' (now known to be dural AVFs) Tobin and Layton (1976) noted 'There seems to be a distinct natural history for patients who have the angiographic type I arteriovenous malformation. These usually have a slowly progressive course, evolving over 2 to 3 years, leading to nearly complete paraplegia and bowel or bladder incontinence. Few of these patients seem to have other modes of presentation.'

Although in most patients the clinical course of progressive loss of cord function from venous hypertension is a gradual, slowly progressive decline in motor and sensory function over 2 to 3 years (Aminoff *et al.* 1974; Kendall & Logue 1977; Logue 1979; Symon *et al.* 1984; Rosenblum *et al.* 1987; Tobin & Layton 1976; Oldfield & Doppman 1988), about 15% of patients with dural AVFs have more rapid, subacute neurological worsening (the Foix–Alajouanine syndrome). This deterioration is unpredictable and seems to indicate particularly severe venous congestion, which, unless treated immediately, will lead to venous thrombosis and irreversible loss of neurological function (Foix & Alajouanine 1926; Criscuolo *et al.* 1989).

Effect of treatment

Treatment of dural AVFs is directed at the nidus of the AVF. Simple surgical excision of the dural nidus, interruption of the intrathecal drainage of the arteriovenous fistula, which results in retrograde thrombosis and fibrosis of the fistula and permanent obliteration of it, or embolic occlusion of the AVF relieves venous congestion and promptly halts the progress of myelopathy (Logue 1979; Oldfield *et al.* 1983; Symon *et al.* 1984; Yasargil *et al.* 1984; Rosenblum *et al.*1987; Oldfield & Doppman 1988).

A two-level laminectomy and simple intradural interruption of the vein draining the AVF intradurally almost universally provides lasting and effective treatment. In the series of Symon *et al.* (1984) progressive gait disturbance was arrested in 39 of 46 patients (85%). When the relatively larger series from the National Hospital for Nervous Disease (Symon *et al.* 1984) and the NIH (Rosenblum *et al.* 1987) are combined (total of 76 patients), 37 of the 49 severely disabled (Aminoff & Logue grades 3–5) patients (76%) had improved gait (Fig. 8.5). Further, 26 of 27 patients (96%) with disability, but unaided locomotion, retained independent ambulation, and 17 of the 27 (63%) improved. Of the 76 patients 70 (92%) either stabilized or improved. The only patient known to have recanalization of an AVF after surgical treatment is a rare patient who had intradural and extradural drainage from the dural AVF (Afshar *et al.* 1995).

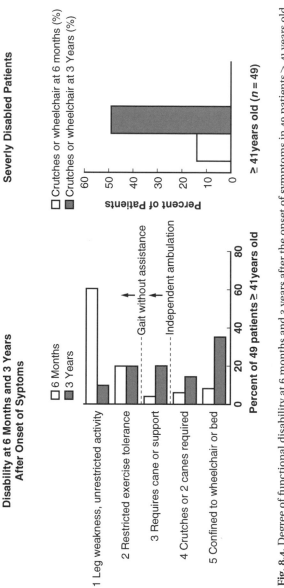

Fig. 8.4. Degree of functional disability at 6 months and 3 years after the onset of symptoms in 49 patients ≥ 41 years old reported by Aminoff & Logue (1974a,b). All, or almost all, of these patients had spinal dural AV fistulas. Note that the greatest redistribution between 6 months and 3 years is from patients with minimal neurologic deficit to severe functional disability and that by 3 years most patients are confined to a wheelchair or crutches. Functional grading scale is same as in Table 8.2.

Embolic therapy has become more popular in recent years as experience has been gained and the catheters have become smaller and more manoeuvreable. However, with embolic occlusion with particulate material (polyvinyl alcohol, Ivalon) symptomatic improvement is usually transient, lasting only a few weeks or months, as the embolized dural AVF recanalizes and causes recurrent myelopathy (Hall *et al.* 1989; Morgan & Marsh 1989).

Embolization with liquid polymerizing agents (isobutyl-2-cyanoacrylate, IBCA) is being used at some centres as primary treatment of patients with spinal dural AVFs (Merland *et al.* 1980). It has been proposed that embolization with liquid agents will pass more distally into the feeding artery, reach the vessels of the nidus of the fistula, and provide permanent obliteration of the fistula. However, embolic occlusion with these agents does not consistently provide complete or permanent occlusion of other types of vascular malformations of the CNS. Moreover, Merland and colleagues noted persistent flow through the dural AVF in 14 of 45 patients embolized with IBC, requiring immediate surgery (Merland *et al.* 1985). The frequency with which patients will require additional therapy later because of recanalization of the fistula is unknown, since minimal clinical and no arteriographic follow-up has been performed in patients with spinal dural AVFs occluded with the liquid agents. Also, haemorrhage (Djindjian 1975) and delayed paraplegia (Merland *et al.* 1980; Yasargil *et al.* 1984) after embolization of spinal dural AVFs with IBCA have been reported. The latter occurrence suggests either the possibility of propagation of venous thrombosis into the coronal venous plexus or the potential of the embolic material passing through the AVF to enter the coronal venous plexus and exacerabate the venous hypertension, leading to haemorrhage or venous infarction. Further, unpublished studies in laboratory animals implicate IBCA as a potential carcinogen, which has limited its clinical use in the United States.

Embolization cannot safely be utilized in patients in whom the same segmental artery supplies the dural AVF and a medullary artery, as occurs in about 15% of patients with dural AVFs (Doppman *et al.* 1985; Clavier *et al.* 1986; Rosenblum *et al.* 1987; Oldfield & Doppman 1988). One clear indication for embolization is the treatment of patients with the Foix–Alajouanine syndrome and incipient venous thrombosis and cord infarction. A patient with an untreated dural AVF and rapid symptomatic progression probably has perilously high venous hypertension and is at risk for irreversible cord injury. In these patients transarterial embolization of the fistula provides immediate reduction in venous congestion until definitive surgical treatment can be performed (Criscuolo *et al.* 1989).

Summary

Patients with dural AVFs have inexorable progression to severe neurological impairment. Therapy with surgery or embolization is safe, simple, and effective. In those patients who are treated early, before irreversible neurological injury occurs, the outcome after treatment of dural AVFs, with surgery or embolization, is quite good

Results of Surgery for Dural AV Fistulas

		Function After Surgery						
		Normal	Minor Weakness	Restricted Activity	Cane or Support	Crutches or 2 Canes	Wheelchair or bed	No. of Patients
Function Before Surgery	Normal	0						0
	Minor Weakness	2	2				1	5
	Restricted Activity	2	13	6				22
	Cane or Support	1	4	7	2	3		17
	Crutches or 2 Canes			4	13	3	2	22
	Wheelchair or bed					8	2	10
		← Better Worse →						Total 76

(a)

Fig. 8.5a. Relationship of preoperative functional state and postoperative outcome in patients with dural AV fistulas. *b* Relationship of preoperative functional state and postoperative outcome in patients with intramedullary AVMs. In patients with dural AV fistulas and intradural AVMs, the outcome after surgery is directly related to the neurologic status preoperatively. Generally, patients who walk independently before treatment do so after treatment, in contrast to those who cannot walk at treament. Early diagnosis and therapy offer the best outcome for patients in both groups. Note, however, that most patients were not treated until they had acquired severe functional disability. Functional grading scale is same as in Table 8.2. Stippled areas indicate patients with greater disability after surgery. Area contained within heavy outline includes patients with severe disability. Data for dural AV fistulas from Symon, *et al.* (1984) and Rosenblum *et al.* (1987); data for intramedullary AVMs from Yasargil *et al.* (1984) and Rosenblum *et al.* (1987).

(Kendall & Logue 1977; Logue 1979; Oldfield *et al.* 1983; Symon *et al.* 1984; Rosenblum *et al.* 1987; Oldfield & Doppman 1988; Muraszko & Oldfield 1990). Neurological outcome is directly related to the neurological function of the patient at treatment (Fig. 8.5) (Symon *et al.* 1984; Yasargil *et al.* 1984; Rosenblum *et al.* 1987; Oldfield & Doppman 1988). Patients who are diagnosed and treated early, before sustaining severe neurological impairment, almost always retain their pretreatment neurological function or improve. Patients with more severe preoperative disability are stabilized and are occasionally appreciably improved after treatment (Kendall & Logue 1977; Logue 1979; Merland *et al.*

Results of Surgery for Intramedullary AVMs

		Function After Surgery					
		Normal	Minor Weakness	Restricted Activity	Cane or Support	Crutches or 2 Canes	Wheelchair or bed	No. of Patients
Function Before Surgery	Normal	2	1	1				4
	Minor Weakness	2	7		1	3		13
	Restricted Activity	2	5	2	1	1		11
	Cane or Support		2	6	4	2		14
	Crutches or 2 Canes			4	9	3	8	24
	Wheelchair or bed				1	8	9	18

Better ←——— ———→ Worse

Total 84

(b)

1980; Oldfield *et al.* 1983; Symon *et al.* 1984; Yasargil *et al.* 1984; Rosenblum *et al.* 1987). Generally, patients who walk and have intact autonomic function before treatment, walk and retain continence and sexual function after treatment. Improvement or stabilization of independent ambulation and control of micturition are achieved in most patients (Kendall & Logue 1977; Logue 1979; Merland *et al.* 1980; Oldfield *et al.* 1983; Symon *et al.* 1984; Yasargil *et al.* 1984; Rosenblum *et al.* 1987). Thus, the key to successful management of these patients is early diagnosis and early treatment that permanently eliminates flow through the AVF.

Intradural AVMs

The nidus of intradural AVMs (Table 8.1) is embedded in the cord, in the pia on the surface of the cord, or partially intra- and extramedullary. The AVM is supplied by one or more enlarged medullary arteries that provide the blood supply to the spinal cord as well as the AVM. Unlike dural AVFs, these are high-flow lesions. The juvenile-type intradural AVMs have a voluminous arteriovenous nidus which typically has neural tissue within its interstices. These AVMs occasionally also involve the vertebral column and the paraspinous soft tissues. The nidus in the glomus type AVM is a tightly packed compact mass of blood vessels that is confined to a short segment of cord. These lesions typically occur in the anterior half of the cord and are usually supplied via the

Table 8.3. *Intradural arteriovenous malformations*

Reference[a]	Patients (n)	Presentation		At diagnosis or treatment	Evolution		Associated with deterioration
		Age at onset of symptoms	Initial symptoms		Progressive evolution		
Hurth et al. 1978	90	86% < 40 years	SAH in 36%	SAH in 39%; SAH in 55% of patients < 15 years old	Recurrent SAH (1 fatal) in 39% of patients with SAH; 'stepwise progression' in 69%		SAH with 'violent physical efforts', pregnancy, minor trauma
Riche et al. 1982[b]	32	All < 15 years	Acute onset in 84%, associated with sudden motor impairment in 19 of the 32 patients (59%)	SAH in 55%	71% with successive acute attack(s); 17% with gradually progressing evolution		Exertion
Rosenblum et al. 1987	54	Mean, 27 years	Acute onset in 50% of the 54 patients; SAH in 10 of 14 patients (71%) with glomus AVMs	At diagnosis paresis in 93%, sensory loss in 74%, bladder dysfunction in 74%, haemorrhage in 52%. At treatment 74% were moderately or severely disabled (cane, crutches or wheelchair); only 26% had unaided ambulation			Posture (17%), activity (15%), pregnancy (6%), Valsalva (13%), injury (13%)
Biondi et al. 1990	40	Mean, 20 years	SAH in 58%	SAH in 68%; 75% moderately or severely disabled	31% had relapse with worsening between treatments during 6 years (mean) follow-up		
Yasargil et al. 1984	41	76% < 41 years	SAH in 59%	SAH in 76%; 63% moderately or severely disabled	'Stepwise progression' in 40%		

SAH, subarachnoid haemorrhage.

[a] All series include patients with intradural AVFs, except Yasargil *et al.*, who include only patients with intramedullary AVMs, and Biondi *et al.* who include only thoracic, intramedullary AVMs.

[b] Riche *et al.* only include patients < 15 years old.

anterior spinal artery. The intradural AVF is a direct communication between an intradural spinal artery and a vein. The absence of an intervening nidus (i.e. a glomus) at the site of the AVF defines the lesion. The fistula is usually in the lower portion of the spinal cord and commonly involves the anterior spinal artery (Djindjian *et al.* 1977; Riche *et al.* 1983a; Heros *et al.* 1986; Gueguen *et al.* 1987; Rosenblum *et al.* 1987). Intradural AVFs and the glomus type AVMs are often accompanied by arterial aneurysms or venous varices. Although these three subtypes of intradural AVMs appear to have distinct anatomy and certain features of the clinical presentation and natural history of one type may differ from the others, existing studies either do not distinguish the subtypes or do not report a sufficient number of patients to provide meaningful information about the natural history or clinical presentation of the specific type addressed. Experience with the direct AVFs has been reported separately (Djindjian *et al.* 1977; Riche *et al.* 1983a; Heros *et al.* 1986; Gueguen *et al.* 1987), but the numbers are small and what little is known about their presentation and natural history suggests that it is similar to that of the intramedullary AVMs. For these reasons, I summarize the intradural AVMs here as a group.

Pathophysiology and clinical presentation

Patients with intradural spinal vascular malformations, compared with those with dural AVFs, have onset of symptoms at an earlier age (Fig. 8.2), a much higher incidence of haemorrhage (Table 8.3), a higher incidence of other vascular and axial bony anomalies, and are somewhat more balanced with respect to gender (Fig. 8.1) (Rosenblum *et al.* 1987). Intradural AVMs seem to be congenital lesions resulting from an inborn error of vascular embryogenesis.

Several mechanisms of cord injury have been proposed with the intradural types of AVMs. In contrast to patients with dural AVFs, an acute initial presentation occurs in over half of patients with intradural AVMs (Table 8.3); subarachnoid or intramedullary haemorrhage associated with the sudden onset of back pain, suboccipital pain and meningismus or sudden loss of consciousness is the initial symptom in 35–60% of them (Table 8.3). It is even higher in children. In 38 children less than 15 years old with intradural spinal AVMs reported by Riche *et al.* (1982), 84% had an acute initial onset of symptoms, 59% of which were associated with sudden impairment of motor function. The high incidence of associated arterial and venous aneurysms and the 13–37% incidence of associated vascular abnormalities of the CNS in patients with intradural spinal AVMs (Hurth *et al.* 1978; Riche *et al.* 1983a; Rosenblum *et al.* 1987) may, in part, explain the high incidence of haemorrhage.

On the other hand, many patients (40–65%) present initially with symptoms other than haemorrhage (Table 8.3) and in some series only about half have had a haemorrhage at diagnosis (Rosenblum *et al.* 1987), suggesting a different mechanism of cord injury. Mechanisms for the gradual progression in these patients include mechanical compression by aneurysm or varix, ischaemia secondary to vascular steal, and medullary venous congestion (Aminoff *et al.* 1974; Djindjian *et al.* 1978).

By the time the diagnosis of spinal AVM has been made or treatment performed haemorrhage has occurred in 40–55% of patients (Table 8.3) and about 75% are moderately or severely disabled (grades 3–5, Aminoff & Logue grading scale) and require a cane, two crutches, or are confined to a wheelchair or bed (Fig. 8.5b). In 54 patients with intradural AVMs at the NIH paresis (93%), sensory loss (74%) and disturbed bladder control (74%) were present in most patients at treatment (Rosenblum *et al.* 1987).

Natural history

The natural history of intradural AVMs is incompletely defined. Progression of symptoms and signs may be gradual or acute. Data on the long-term disability that occurs without therapy are unavailable. The limited information available suggests that most AVMs of the spinal cord cause recurrent haemorrhages and/or progressive neurological disability over the first few months or years after they are diagnosed. In the 90 patients with intradural AVMs of all types reported by Hurth *et al.* (1978), 69% had acute episodes of neurological progression ('stepwise progression'); 39% of the patients with previous haemorrhage had at least one additional haemorrhage (fatal in one patient). Similarly, in the 38 patients treated by Biondi *et al.* (1990) with repeated, yearly embolization with particles of polyvinyl alcohol, 31% relapsed with worsening between treatments (average of 6 years of treatment). In the 38 children treated by Riche *et al.* (1982) 71% had 'successive acute attacks' and 17% had a gradually progressing clinical evolution. Pregnancy, vigorous exertion and minor trauma may cause rapid progression of symptoms and seem to be associated with an increased risk of haemorrhage (Table 8.3). All authors characterize the prognosis of these patients as grave and have considered the condition sufficiently unpredictable and hazardous to justify the risks of treatment (Hurth *et al.* 1978; Riche *et al.* 1982; Cogen & Stein 1983; Yasargil *et al.* 1984; Gueguen *et al.* 1987; Rosenblum *et al.* 1987; Oldfield & Doppman 1988; Biondi *et al.* 1990).

However, it must be acknowledged that the natural history varies greatly among individual patients and that the course in some of them is not always grim. In Aminoff & Logue's series, in one half of the patients whose presentation was acute, a presentation more likely to be associated with intradural AVMs, there was no subsequent neurological progression (Aminoff & Logue 1974b). Similar observations were made by Tobin & Layton (1976) in their report on the natural history of patients with spinal AVMs, in which they report a progressive course leading to paraplegia over 2 to 3 years in patients with type I AVMs (dural AVFs), but 'such a relationship was not as clear' for the intradural types of AVMs. Hurth *et al.* (1978) noted that in 17 untreated patients with AVMs in the cervical segments of the spinal cord, 80% were independent and capable of carrying out their jobs at 5 years after diagnosis and five patients who were untreated or incompletely treated were unchanged 15 years after diagnosis, indicating the 'slow progression of disease that we have seen in a limited number of cases'. Further, 60% of

Table 8.4. *Intradural arteriovenous malformations*

Reference	Patients (n)	Level of nidus	Postoperative arteriography		Follow-up (mean)	Functional status after treatment		
			Immediate arteriography (persistent AVM)	Delayed arteriography (persistent AVM)		Improved	Unchanged	Worse
Surgery								
Rosenblum et al. 1987[a]	43	17% cervical, 83% thoracolumbar	32 (74%)	0	3 years	33%	51%	14%
Yasargil et al. 1984[b]	41	46% cervical, 54% thoracolumbar	0	0	3 years	48%	32%	20%
Embolization								
Biondi et al. 1990[b]	35	100% thoracic		35 (100%)	6 years	63%	26%	11%

[a] Includes patients with intradural AV fistulas.
[b] Includes only intramedullary AVMs.

their 17 untreated patients with thoracic AVMs at 5 years and 7 of 17 untreated or incompletely treated patients at 15 years were 'self-sufficient and relatively well' (Hurth *et al.* 1978). The dilemma in making decisions for individual patients is that we have no reliable guidelines that permit us to identify these patients prospectively.

Thus, although the neurological prognosis is guarded for untreated patients with the intradural types of AVMs, it may not be as dismal as it is in symptomatic, untreated patients with dural AVFs. This must be considered when undertaking treatment of patients with intradural AVMs, as treatment of some of them is associated with significant risks.

Effects of treatment

The ideal therapy for intradural vascular malformations should completely and permanently obliterate the AVM while preserving the blood supply to the cord. However, the feasibility of this goal, and how it can be best accomplished, with surgery alone, embolization, or surgery after embolization, depends on the type, size and location, and blood supply of the vascular malformation. In vascular malformations with certain adverse risk factors (large size, location in the thoracic or lumbar segments of the cord, involvement of the ventral half of the cord, a complex blood supply associated with extension anterior to the ventral cord surface, and multiple feeding vessels from the anterior spinal artery) preservation of neurological function and avoidance of iatrogenic disability may mandate less than definitive treatment regardless of the therapeutic approach.

The goal of surgery should be complete excision of the nidus of the AVM without injuring the spinal cord or interrupting the blood supply to it. The results are known only for up to 3 years after surgery (Table 8.4). Early postoperative arteriography reveals persistent AVM in as many as 40% of patients treated surgically during the 1960s and 1970s (Rosenblum *et al.* 1987). At an average of 3 years after surgery, about one-third to one-half of patients are improved, 30–50% remain unchanged, and 15–20% are worse. However, there are limited data on the incidence of persistent AVM, even as early as 3 years, and no long-term data exist on the incidence of clinical relapse or progression because of incomplete surgical excision. There are no studies of delayed arteriographic follow-up after surgical treatment of intradural AVMs. The short-term results (3 year follow-up) of surgery clearly indicate superior results in patients who receive treatment before serious neurological deficits arise (Fig. 8.5b).

Embolic occlusion of spinal AVMs developed as a natural extension of the introduction and refinement of selective spinal arteriography (Doppman *et al.* 1968, 1969, 1971; Djindjian 1975). With certain intradural AVMs embolization is used alone or, since the incidence of recanalization after embolic occlusion is quite high (Hall *et al.* 1989; Touho *et al.* 1992), antecedent to surgical excision in those lesions that can be excised with acceptable risk. Ideally embolization should permanently occlude all of the nidus of the AVM. However, this goal appears to be rarely achieved with the techniques now available. Use of the liquid embolizing materials, such as the polymerizing acrylics, may increase the likelihood of lasting obliteration of the AVM after embolization alone. However, since immediate arteriographic occlusion does not mean anatomical elimination of an AVM, and as lasting occlusion of the nidus does not occur in all patients (in fact, whether it occurs even in the minority of patients remains to be established, as there are no studies which evaluate, clinically or radiographically, embolized AVMs other than a few months after treatment), some clinicians who once advocated the use of glue for embolizing intradural spinal AVMs have abandoned it because of the incidence of complications associated with it (Riche et al. 1983a; Biondi et al. 1990).

The most commonly used particulate material for occlusion of spinal AVMs is polyvinal alcohol (PVA) sponge (Ivalon, Unipoint Industries, High Point, N.C.). Although embolization of spinal AVMs with PVA does not provide lasting elimination of flow through the AVM, it plays an important role in the current management of patients with intradural spinal AVMs. Presurgical embolization makes the surgery easier, as it reduces blood supply to the AVM and transiently reduces the size of the AVM. Treatment of completely paraplegic patients may eliminate an intractable pain syndrome, reduce the risk of subsequent haemorrhage (which could cause quadriplegia or death) and mollify the severity of spasticity in some patients. Furthermore, the recently reported results of Biondi et al. (1990) suggest efficacious serial, yearly endovascular embolization with PVA. Their long-term follow-up (mean of 6 years) showed that, although no patients had complete, permanent obliteration of the AVM (most patients had less than a 50% reduction in AVM size), nearly two-thirds of patients were clinically improved and only 11% were worse at the end of the study (Table 8.4). I have several patients with thoracic or lumbar ventral intramedullary AVMs which receive their blood supply from the anterior spinal artery whose neurological status has been stabilized repeatedly with repetitive embolic occlusion of the AVM when recurrent symptoms arise. On the other hand, since when further neurological disability occurs it may not be reversible, the approach of Biondi et al. (1990), who advocate routine yearly arteriography and embolization with PVA, regardless of symptoms, appears to be safe and eliminates neurological progression in most patients. However, these patients will presumably require repeated embolization indefinitely, with the cumulative risk of treatment increasing with each embolization. With surgical excision the risk may be greater, but with excision of the AVM treatment is completed and the risk occurs once.

As with surgery of intradural AVMs, the best results with embolization are obtained in patients without major neurological deficits before treatment (Doppman et al. 1968, 1971; Newton & Adams 1968; Djindjian 1975; Riche et al. 1983a; Horton et al. 1986; Theron et al. 1986; Biondi et al. 1990; Touho et al. 1992). Selective catheterization and embolization is associated with risks of occlusion of the anterior spinal artery and paraplegia or quadriplegia, perforation of an intradural vessel with the catheter and subarachnoid or intramedullary haemorrhage (Tuoho et al. 1992), and distal passage of the emboli through the AVM into the venous system causing haemorrhage or venous infarction

(Djindjian 1975), or into the distal vessels of the parent artery, such as the basilar artery when using the vertebral artery to reach the AVM, causing ischaemic infarction.

As a result of rapidly and simultaneously evolving classification schemes, diagnostic techniques, surgical instrumentation, catheter sophistication and other factors (listed below), the results of contemporary surgery, alone or after embolization, for intradural AVMs are unknown. The information on surgery is limited to series that began at least three decades ago. The two surgical and single embolization series included in Table 8.4 are the only two published series of over 10 patients that permit tabulation of the data included. Furthermore, there appear to be prominent selection biases for the use of surgery or embolization, or combined treatment, in individual patients in all series, surgical or embolization, large or small. For instance, although most intradural AVMs are in the thoracic or thoracolumbar segments of the cord, with few exceptions (Cogen & Stein 1983), the published reports emphasizing surgical success are greatly weighted towards patients with cervical lesions (Yasargil *et al.* 1975, 1984) – AVMs that arise in the segments of the cord known to have the greatest collateral blood supply. Further, there is an evident bias for surgery for the lesions in the dorsal half of the cord, exemplified by the tendency of surgical therapy for the 'long dorsal AVM' before it was recognized as the dural AVF. Dorsal intramedullary AVMs are less likely to receive their blood supply from the anterior spinal artery, and are associated with less surgical risk than are ventral ones. The tendency to avoid submitting a patient in good condition to a therapeutic procedure that risks leaving them paraplegic results in a longer delay from diagnosis to surgical treatment with the more difficult AVMs. In the NIH series the average duration from the onset of symptoms to treatment was 2.7 years for dural AVFs compared with 4.2 years for intradural AVMs (Rosenblum *et al.* 1987). Patients with intradural AVMs were more likely to be in the more severe functional grades at treatment than patients with the dural AVFs (Rosenblum *et al.* 1987). Some of the factors that underlie a bias in the selection of surgical or embolic therapy may act in opposite ways at different centres. Some centres reserve the use of surgery for patients who cannot be treated effectively with embolization, while others select the more accessible 'safer' lesions (smaller well-defined AVMs, direct AVFs, cervical AVMs, dorsal lesions) for surgery. Finally, there are nuances in the manner of reporting outcome that must be acknowledged. Patients who are treated when they are paraplegic or quadriplegic are rarely made worse as a result of therapy. Thus, those who treat patients earlier could easily have a greater fraction of patients who are worse after than before treatment, despite superior preservation of neurological function, than those who wait until later in the course of the disease.

Thus, the data from previous reports do not reflect significant advances in diagnostic techniques, current knowledge of the various subtypes of AVMs, the details of anatomy that can now be obtained before treatment with magnetic resonance imaging (MRI) and the rapid sequence imaging available with intra-arterial digital techniques, or the significant advances in the equipment and techniques of interventional radiology and surgery. Furthermore, certain lesions are treated more effectively with surgery and certain others are treated best with embolization. Others are more effectively treated by combining preoperative particulate embolization and surgery. Thus, direct comparisons of surgical and embolic therapy cannot be reliably made and, in the modern era of treatment, may not be very meaningful.

Summary

In most patients with intradural spinal AVMs treatment should be recommended when the diagnosis is established. When arteriography reveals that the anatomy of an in tradural AVM or AVF can be *completely excised with limited risk*, because of its permanence surgery alone, or surgery after embolization, should be considered. Many lesions can be identified, by arteriography or during surgery, as being associated with unacceptable risks for complete excision; for these lesions embolization should be recommended.

Cavernous angiomas

Cavernous angiomas, also known as cavernous malformations, cavernous haemangiomas and cavernomas, appear to be congenital vascular malfomations. They arise anywhere along the neuraxis, but represent only 5–12% of all spinal vascular abnormalities (Simard *et al.* 1986; Cosgrove *et al.* 1988). These mulberry-like lesions are typically small (5–15 mm), have low levels of blood flow, and are supplied by delicate thin-walled vessels. A well-demarcated rim of haemosiderin and gliosis typically surrounds them, suggesting previous small haemorrhages. Because they were rarely detected with myelography, arteriography and CT scanning, previously cavernous angiomas appeared to be exceptionally rare lesions. However, with the introduction of MRI and its use as the initial screening procedure in patients with myelopathy, it has become apparent that they are more common than was previously thought. They may occur at more than one level of the spinal cord, or may arise in association with intracranial cavernous angiomas when they are associated with familial multiple cavernous angiomatosis (Cosgrove *et al.* 1988; Rigamonti *et al.* 1988).

   Although they are low-flow lesions, the pathogenesis of myelopathy is usually via haematomyelia (Cosgrove *et al.* 1988; McCormick *et al.* 1988; Ogilvy *et al.* 1992). Small cavernous angiomas may remain clinically silent throughout life and become evident only at post-mortem examination. Symptomatic cavernous angiomas tend first to cause symptoms in early adulthood and middle age (third to sixth decades) (Voight & Yasargil 1976; Ogilvy *et al.* 1992). There are four common patterns of clinical presentation: discrete acute episodic progression over months or years, slowly progressive decline of neurological function over months or years, acute onset and rapid progression, and slowly progressive loss of function after an acute onset of mild neurological symptoms (Ogilvy *et al.* 1992). Although the natural history of spinal cavernous malformations has not been investigated, the available information on symptomatic lesions clearly indicates a tendency toward further neurological impairment associated with repeated small haemorrhages (Ogilvy *et al.* 1992).

Surgery is the only treatment available. The outcome after surgery, as with the dural and intradural spinal AVMs, depends greatly on the neurological function before surgery (Cosgrove *et al.* 1988; McCormick *et al.* 1988; Ogilvy *et al.* 1992; Anson & Spetzler 1993). The usual considerations for surgery of intraparenchymal cord lesions must be considered: lesions lying in the dorsal half of the cord, which are immediately access-ible with a limited myelotomy over the most superficial aspect of the lesion (frequently indicated by bluish-grey discoloration of the pia), require less manipulation of the spinal cord for exposure, and are associated with less risk of incurring additional neurological injury during surgery and a more favourable prognosis for improvement after removal than are the ventral lesions.

Unlike patients with neurological defects, whether asymptomatic spinal cord cav-ernous malformations should be excised is controversial, because their natural history is unknown. Some cavernous angiomas remain asymptomatic and undetected or are detected incidentally, for instance during spinal screening evaluations in a patient with a symptom-producing cavernous angioma of the brain. Recommendations for treat-ment must consider the patient's symptoms, evidence of progression, and the projec-ted risks of surgery. There are no data which support treatment of asymptomatic cavernous angiomas.

Summary

Modern methods of diagnosis and treatment permit early detection, exact anatomical definition and successful treatment of most patients with spinal AVMs. Dural AVFs are the most common type of spinal AVM, and the most amenable to treatment. Venous congestion, which underlies cord injury in these lesions, is effectively treated by interruption of the medullary vein between the dural nidus and the coronal venous plexus. Intradural AVMs impair cord function by haemorrhage or ischaemia due to vascular steal or venous congestion. Patients with ventral thoracic or lumbar intra-medullary AVMs are successfully managed with serial yearly endovascular emboliz-ation. Certain intradural AVMs are best treated surgically (with preoperative emboliz-ation, if it can be safely performed).

Although perfect understanding of the natural history of patients with spinal AVMs of all types is lacking, available information strongly indicates a natural history of pro-gression to severe disability in most untreated symptomatic patients. The outcome after treatment of spinal AVMs depends upon the type and location of the lesion, its blood supply, and the neurological function of the patient. Patients who are ambula-tory before treatment are usually ambulatory after treatment. Optimal outcome de-pends on early diagnosis and early intervention.

References

Aminoff, M. & Logue, V. (1974a). Clinical features of spinal vascular malformations. *Brain* 97, 197–210.

Aminoff, M. & Logue, V. (1974b). The prognosis of patients with spinal vascular malformations. *Brain* 97, 211–18.

Aminoff, M., Barnard, R. & Logue, V. (1974). The pathophysiology of spinal vascular malformations. *J. Neurol. Sci.* 23, 255–63.

Anson, J. & Spetzler, R. (1993). Surgical resection of intramedullary spinal cord cavernous malformations. *J. Neurosurg.* 78, 446–51.

Benhaiem, N., Poirier, J. & Hurth, M. (1983). Arteriovenous fistulae of the meninges draining into the spinal veins: a histological study of 28 cases. *Acta Neuropathol. (Berl.)* 62, 103–11.

Biondi, A., Merland, J. & Reizine, D. (1990). Embolization with particles in thoracic intramedullary arteriovenous malformations: long-term angiographic and clinical results. *Radiology* 177, 651–8.

Clavier, E., Tadie, M., Thiebot, J. *et al.* (1986). Common origin of the arterial blood flow for an arteriovenous medullar fistula and the anterior spinal artery: a case report. *Neurosurgery* 18, 660–3.

Cogen, P. & Stein, B. (1983). Spinal cord arteriovenous malformations with significant intramedullary components. *J. Neurosurg.* 59, 471–8.

Cosgrove, G., Bertrand, G., Fontaine, S. *et al.* (1988). Cavernous angiomas of the spinal cord. *J. Neurosurg.* 68, 31–4.

Criscuolo, G., Oldfield, E. & Doppman, J. (1989). Reversible acute and subacute myelopathy in patient with dural arteriovenous fistulas: Foix–Alajouanine syndrome reconsidered. *J. Neurosurg.* 70, 354.

Djindjian, R. (1975). Embolization of angiomas of the spinal cord. *Surg. Neurol.* 4, 411–20.

Djindjian, M., Djindjian, R., Rey, A. *et al.* (1977). Intradural extramedullary spinal arteriovenous malformations fed by the anterior spinal artery. *Surg. Neurol.* 8, 85–93.

Djindjian, M., Djindjian, R., Hurth, M. *et al.* (1978). Steal phenomenon in spinal arteriovenous malformations. *J. Neuroradiol.* 5, 187.

Doppman, J., DiChiro, G. & Ommaya, A. (1968). Obliteration of spinal-cord arteriovenous malformations by percutaneous embolisation. *Lancet* I, 477.

Doppman, J., DiChiro, G. & Ommaya, A. (1969). *Selective Arteriography of the Spinal Cord.* St Louis: Warren H. Green.

Doppman, J., DiChiro, G. & Ommaya, A. (1971). Percutaneous embolization of spinal cord arteriovenous malformations. *J. Neurosurg.* 34, 48–55.

Doppman, J., DiChiro, G. & Oldfield, E. (1985). Origin of spinal arteriovenous malformation and normal cord vasculature from a common segmental artery: angiographic and therapeutic considerations. *Radiology* 154, 687–9.

Foix, C. & Alajouanine, T. (1926). La myelite nécrotique subaique. *Rev. Neurol.* 2, 1.

Gueguen, B., Merland, J., Riche, M. *et al.* (1987). Vascular malformations of the spinal cord: intrathecal perimedullary arteriovenous fistulas fed by medullary arteries. *Neurology* 37, 969–79.

Hall, W., Oldfield, E. & Doppman, J. (1989). Recanalization of spinal cord arteriovenous malformations following embolization. *J. Neurosurg.* 79, 714.

Hassler, W., Thron, A. & Grote, E. (1989). Hemodynamics of spinal dural arteriovenous fistulas. An intraoperative study. *J. Neurosurg.* 70, 360.

Heros, R., Debrun, G., Ojemann, R. *et al.* (1986). Direct spinal arteriovenous fistula: A new type of spinal AVM: case report. *J. Neurosurg.* **64**, 134.

Horton, J., Latchaw, R. & Gold, L. (1986). Embolisation of intramedullary arteriovenous malformations of the spinal cord. *AJNR* **7**, 113–18.

Hurth, M., Houdart, R., Djindjian, R. *et al.* (1978). Arteriovenous malformations of the spinal cord: clinical, anatomical and therapeutic considerations-a series of 150 cases. *Prog. Neurol. Surg.* **9**, 238–66.

Kendall, B. & Logue, V. (1977). Spinal epidural angiomatous malformations draining into intrathecal veins. *Neuroradiology* **3**, 181–9.

Logue, V. (1979). Angiomas of the spinal cord: review of the pathogenesis, clinical features and results of surgery. *J. Neurol. Neurosurg. Psychiatry* **42**, 1–11.

McCormick, P., Michelsen, W., Post, K. *et al.* (1988). Cavernous malformations of the spinal cord. *Neurosurgery* **23**, 459–63.

Merland, J., Riche, M. & Chiras, J. (1980). Intraspinal extramedullary arteriovenous fistulae draining into the medullary veins. *J. Neuroradiol.* **7**, 271–320.

Merland, J., Assouline, E., Rufenacht, D. *et al.* (1985). *Dural Spinal Arteriovenous Fistulae Draining into Medullary Veins. Clinical And Radiological Results of Treatment (Embolization and Surgery) in 56 Cases.* Neuroradiology 1985/1986: Proceedings of the XIIIth Congress of the European Society of Neuroradiology. Amsterdam: Elsevier.

Morgan, M. & Marsh, W. (1989). Management of spinal dural arteriovenous malformations. *J. Neurosurg.* **70**, 832.

Muraszoko, K. & Oldfield, E. (1990). Vascular malformations of the spinal cord and dura. *Neurosurg. Clin. North Am.* **1**, 631–52.

Newton, T. & Adams, J. (1968). Angiographic demonstration and nonsurgical embolization of spinal cord angioma. *Radiology* **91**, 873.

Ogilvy, C., Louis, D. & Ojemann, R. (1992). Intramedullary cavernous angiomas of the spinal cord: clinical presentation, pathological features, and surgical management. *Neurosurgery* **31**, 219–30.

Oldfield, E. (1991). Spinal arteriovenous malformations. In *Neurosurgery Update II*, pp. 186–96. New York: McGraw-Hill.

Oldfield, E. & Doppman, J. (1988). Spinal arteriovenous malformations. *Clin. Neurosurg.* **34**, 161–83.

Oldfield, E., DiChiro, G., Quindlen, E. *et al.* (1983). Successful treatment of a group of spinal cord arteriovenous malformations by interruption of dural fistula. *J. Neurosurg.* **59**, 1019–30.

Riche, M., Modenesi-Freitas, J., Djindjian, M. *et al.* (1982). Arteriovenous malformations (AVM) of the spinal cord in children: a review of 38 cases. *Neuroradiology* **22**, 171–80.

Riche, M., Melki, J. & Merland, J. (1983a). Embolization of spinal cord vascular malformations via the anterior spinal artery. *AJNR* **4**, 378–81.

Riche, M., Scialfa, G., Gueguen, B. *et al.* (1983b). Giant extramedullary arteriovenous fistulas supplied by the anterior spinal artery: treatment by detachable balloons. *AJNR* **4**, 391–4.

Rigamonti, D., Hadley, M., Drayer, B. *et al.* (1988). Cerebral cavernous malformations: incidence and familial occurrence. *N. Eng. J. Med.* **319**, 343–7.

Rosenblum, B., Oldfield, E., Doppman, J. *et al.* (1987). Spinal arteriovenous malformations: a comparison of dural arteriovenous fistulas and intradural AVMs in 81 patients. *J. Neurosurg.* **67**, 795–802.

Simard, J., Garcia-Bengochea, F., Ballinger, W. *et al.* (1986). Cavernous angioma: a review of 126 collected and 12 new clinical cases. *Neurosurgery* **18**, 162.

Symon, L., Kuyama, H. & Kendall, B. (1984). Dural arteriovenous malformations of the spine: clinical features and surgical results in 55 cases. *J. Neurosurg.* **60**, 238–47.

Theron, J., Cosgrove, R., Melanson, D. *et al.* (1986). Spinal arteriovenous malformations: advances in therapeutic embolization. *Radiology* **158**, 163–9.

Tobin, W. & Layton, D. (1976). The diagnosis and natural history of spinal cord arteriovenous malformations. *Mayo Clin. Proc.* **51**, 637–46.

Touho, H., Karasawa, J., Ohnishi, H. *et al.* (1992). Superselective embolization of spinal arteriovenous malformations using the Tracker catheter. *Surg. Neurol.* **38**, 85–94.

Voight, K. & Yasargil, M. (1976). Cerebral cavernous hemangiomas or cavernomas: incidence, pathology, localization, diagnosis, clinical features and treatment. Review of the literature and report of an unusual case. *Neurochirurgia (Stuttg)* **19**, 59.

Yasargil, M., DeLong, W. & Guarnaschelli, J. (1975). Complete microsurgical excision of cervical extramedullary and intramedullary vascular malformations. *Surg. Neurol.* **4**, 211–24.

Yasargil, M., Symon, L. & Teddy, P. (1984). Arteriovenous malformations of the spinal cord. In *Advances and Technical Standards in Neurosurgery*, pp. 61–102. Berlin: Springer-Verlag.

9 Head injury

J. HSIANG AND L. F. MARSHALL

Treat a man as he is
And he will remain,
Treat him as he can become
And he will.

Anonymous (from San Diego Head Injury Foundation)

Introduction

Head injuries constitute a major health problem in industrialized countries. In the United States approximately 100 000 people die each year as a result of head injury (Department of Health and Human Services February, 1989). Many thousands are left with serious lifetime residual disabilities. However, reliable statistics of incidence are difficult to obtain because some of the fatal cases never reach the hospital, while many with milder injuries do not seek medical attention unless complications develop. Nevertheless, the overall estimate of incidence based on United States studies is approximately 200 per 100 000 population per year (Kraus 1993; Sorenson & Kraus 1991).

There are approximately 450 000 patients hospitalized in the United States for head injury each year. A great majority of these are mild head injuries where the period of unconsciousness can often be measured in seconds or minutes. Moderate and severe head injuries each contribute approximately 10% (Kraus *et al.* 1984). These figures imply that someone suffers a head injury in the United States every 15 seconds, and that every 5 minutes one of these individuals will die and another will become permanently disabled.

Transport-related events are the single largest cause of head injury. These events include motor vehicle accidents (50–60%), motorcycle accidents (20%), bicycle accidents (12%) and pedestrian injuries (Kraus *et al.* 1984). Falls are the second leading cause rated in most studies (Annegers *et al.* 1980b; Jagger *et al.* 1984; Klauber *et al.* 1981; Kraus *et al.* 1984). Brain injuries caused by assaults and firearms are increasing (Sosin *et al.* 1989). This trend is particularly prominent in high-density urban areas (Cooper *et al.* 1983; Whiteman *et al.* 1984).

Alcohol plays a significant role in many head injuries. The incidence of alcoholic intoxication or a crash involving one or more people who are either intoxicated or under the influence of alcohol is extremely high (Sparedo & Gill 1989). This problem is not unique to North America. Studies from Europe also showed a significant portion (32–51%) of brain-injured patients were intoxicated (Edna 1982; Vazquez-Barquero *et al.* 1991; Boyle *et al.* 1991).

The incidence of head trauma is highest among young adults, ages 15–24 years (Kraus 1993). A second peak incidence includes infants and children (Cooper *et al.* 1983; Whiteman *et al.* 1984). Head injury has become the leading cause of death and disability in children and young adults in the United States (Department of Health and Human Services, February 1989). Head injury also affects the elderly at higher rates than the general population, about 211 per 100 000 annually for those aged 75 years and over (Annegers *et al.* 1980b; Max *et al.* 1991). Most of the studies in the United States also indicate a higher rate of head injury in male (Kraus *et al.* 1984), nonwhite populations (Cooper *et al.* 1983; Jagger *et al.* 1984; Whiteman *et al.* 1984) and those of lower socioeconomic status (Kraus *et al.* 1984; Whiteman *et al.* 1984).

In industrialized countries, the financial impact of head injury is enormous. Survivors from head injury are often young, with long periods of social and physical disability. Furthermore, as most are male, and often the primary earner within their family unit, a whole generation is then subjected to brain-injury-induced poverty where the head injury results in the patient's permanent loss of the ability to earn a living. The long-term effects on these survivors not only place a tremendous emotional and financial burden on the patients' families, but also heavily drain the health care resources. The lifelong costs for care of a head injury survivor are estimated to be between $4.1 million and $9 million (Murer 1991). In the United States the total economic costs for all head injuries approaches $25 billion annually (Department of Health and Human Services, February 1989).

Outcome prediction

The outcome following traumatic brain injury is variable, with many factors contributing to the ultimate outcome. As we learn more about the heterogeneity of head injury, improvements in our ability to predict overall outcome have become more reliable. It is critically important for a disease which has such significant financial, social and societal implications to understand those factors which influence outcome. This is in part because society must plan to provide certain resources for these patients, but it is also important to be rational in application of our dwindling resources so that they are concentrated in those patients with some opportunity for significant improvement. As rehabilitation services have proliferated for the head injured it is becoming increasingly clear that a treatment plan must be based on a realistic view of what the patient's ultimate outcome is likely to be.

Classification of head injury

An ideal classification of head injury is one that can accurately predict the outcome of the injury. The commonly used classification currently is the one based on the Glasgow Coma Scale (GCS) (Jennett & Teasdale 1981). According to this scale, head injury is classified as mild (GCS scores 13–15), moderate (GCS scores 9–12) or severe (GCS scores 3–8). This arbitrary distinction, while helpful in subdividing head injury into three major groups, has significant limitations in terms of predicting the outcome of the injury. This is understandable if one recognizes that the GCS was not originally designed for classification of head injury, but for the assessment of the level of consciousness after brain injury.

The invention of computed tomography (CT) has revolutionized the management of head injury. The CT scan visually demonstrates varying patterns of macrostructural brain damage with high resolution. These include: contusion, haematoma, diffuse axonal injury (DAI), subarachnoid haemorrhage, as well as diffuse brain swelling. As we have become more sophisticated about the relationship between the pattern of structural brain injury and outcome, it has become obvious that a new classification of head injury, based on the varying CT findings, would be useful in predicting outcome in head injury (Marshall *et al.* 1991b). In addition to categorizing mass lesion as surgically or not surgically evacuated, this new classification also subdivides diffuse injury into four grades based on the volume status of the brain and the degree of midline shift (Table 9.1).

While this classification was initially developed within the Traumatic Coma Data Bank (TCDB) as a means of classifying severe head injury, it has gradually found its place in identifying those patients with less severe injuries based on the clinical examination. Often, the initial CT scan of these patients is interpreted as 'normal', but the recognition of the status of the mesencephalic cisterns, those subarachnoid spaces around the brain stem, which is well correlated with the presence or absence of intracranial hypertension, is a major change in the way we assess these patients. A classification based on GCS should not be abandoned, however, because a clinical examination is an extremely important guideline and should be used in concert with this new CT classification.

Factors affecting outcome of head injury

Head injury management can have a significant effect on the outcome of such patients. Most studies of the outcome of head injury have been done in developed nations. In these countries sophisticated systems of regional organization coupled with experienced trauma centres allow for the rapid evacuation and early treatment of these patients. Immediate access to a CT scanner and, thus, to the intracranial diagnosis can be rapidly obtained. With well-equipped intensive care units, ventilation to assure adequate gas exchange is now the rule rather than the exception. Intracranial pressure

Table 9.1. *Diagnostic categories of types of abnormalities visualized on CT scanning*

Category	Definition
Diffuse injury I	No visible intracranial pathology seen on CT scan
Diffuse injury II	Cisterns are present with midline shift 0–5 mm and/or: Lesion densities present No high- or mixed-density lesion $> 25\,cm^3$ May include bone fragments and foreign bodies
Diffuse injury III (swelling)	Cisterns compressed or absent with midline shift 0–5 mm, no high- or mixed-density lesion $> 25\,cm^3$
Diffuse injury IV (shift)	Midline shift $> 5\,mm$, no high- or mixed-density lesion $< 25\,cm^3$
Evacuated mass lesion	Any lesion surgically evacuated
Non-evacuated mass lesion	High- or mixed-density lesion $> 25\,cm^3$, not surgically evacuated

(ICP) monitoring is increasingly used as is rehabilitation for cognitive as well as physical and occupational disabilities.

One must not forget, however, that there are many nations and billions of people in regions prone to head injury where CT scanners and ventilators are items of luxury. ICP monitoring and rehabilitation are simply not available. One, therefore, should have differing expectations of outcome for head-injured patients depending on the locale in which they occur.

There are a number of well-identified risk factors that affect the outcome of head injury. Some of these, such as the age of the patient, post-resuscitation GCS/motor scores, abnormal pupils, admission hypotension, and intracranial diagnosis by CT scan, have been shown to be relatively independent and strong predictors of outcome. Others, such as disseminated intravascular coagulopathy (Crone *et al.* 1987; Kaufman & Mattson 1985; Miner *et al.* 1982), hyperglycaemia (Lam *et al.* 1991; Michaud *et al.* 1991; Young *et al.* 1989) and sepsis, although not shown to be independent predictors, can adversely affect the outcome of patients with traumatic brain injury.

Age

A recent report from the TCDB has shown that patients aged 45 years and older have a significantly higher rate of mortality (Table 9.2) (Vollmer *et al.* 1991). This study also shows that older patients are predisposed to intracranial mass lesions, particularly subdural haematoma (SDH), regardless of the mechanism of injury. The adverse effect of age on outcome after head injury is believed to be intrinsic to the aged brain in which pathophysiological response to injury is compromised.

Post-resuscitation GCS motor score

The GCS provides a great deal of information to assist in outcome prediction. It has

Table 9.2. *Outcome 6 months post-injury correlated with age[a]*

Outcome	Age (years)				
	16–25 (%)	26–35 (%)	36–45 (%)	46–55 (%)	≥56 (%)
Good recovery	33.4	27.8	16.9	11.1	0.0
Moderate disability	16.1	20.5	16.9	11.1	8.5
Severe disability	16.1	15.9	18.1	20.0	8.5
Vegetative survival	3.5	7.3	7.2	8.9	2.8
Death	30.9	28.5	41.0	48.9	80.3

[a] Outcome according to the Glasgow Outcome Scale.

very powerful predictive characteristics in severe head injury where it was initially applied. It was not designed, and therefore cannot be used, as a reliable predictor for outcome in mild and moderate head injury except to say that mortality is extremely unlikely (Marshall *et al.* 1991a). However, the motor score is a particularly important component in determining prognosis in patients with severe injuries (Braakman *et al.* 1980; Miller *et al.* 1981). A report by Butterworth *et al.* (1981) showed that a completely flaccid motor response (motor score = 1) after head injury was associated with a mortality rate of 76%.

Abnormal pupils

Pupillary size and reactivity have been linchpins of the neurological assessment of brain-injured patients. However, the loss of pupillary reactivity is an ominous finding and, therefore, while its predictive utility remains, every effort in the modern intensive care unit environment is directed at preventing brain stem compression which in turn produces the pupillary abnormalities. A detailed analysis done by the TCDB has demonstrated a close, very strong correlation between abnormal pupils and the outcome of head-injured patients (Marshall *et al.* 1991a). Among patients who had normal pupils throughout their hospital course, only 10% were dead or vegetative at discharge. This figure is compared with 61% mortality in those patients who had reactive pupils following resuscitation and then developed one pupillary abnormality, and with 82% mortality in those patients whose pupils were fixed and unreactive immediately following resuscitation. This study also revealed an interesting observation that patients with one abnormal pupil before and after the resuscitation fared better (47% dead or vegetative) than if one pupil became abnormal for at least one observation following resuscitation (61% dead or vegetative). Deterioration in the status of the pupils, a direct reflection of brain stem compression and clear evidence of herniation, has a strong and adverse affect on the outcome of such patients.

Table 9.3. *Outcome at discharge in relation to intracranial diagnosis[a]*

Outcome at discharge	Diffuse injury I (%)	Diffuse injury II (%)	Diffuse injury III (%)	Diffuse injury IV (%)	EVM (%)	NEVM (%)	Brain stem injury (%)
Good recovery	27.0	8.5	3.3	3.1	5.1	2.8	0
Moderate disability	34.6	26.0	13.1	3.1	17.7	8.3	0
Severe disability	19.2	40.7	26.8	18.8	26.1	19.4	33.3
Vegetative survival	9.6	11.3	22.9	18.8	12.3	16.7	0
Death	9.6	13.5	34.0	56.2	38.8	52.8	66.7

[a] Outcome classified by the Glasgow Outcome Scale.
EVM, evacuated mass; NEVM, nonevacuated mass.

Hypotension

Hypotension as a secondary brain insult is a major determinant of outcome from head injury. An association between arterial hypotension (systolic blood pressure < 90 mmHg) and poor outcome following head trauma was demonstrated by Miller and his colleagues (1981). This finding is reaffirmed by a recent analysis in TCDB, which showed that the presence of hypotension, in conjunction with a severe head injury, was associated with a doubling in the mortality rate (Chestnut *et al.* 1993).

Intracranial diagnosis by CT scan

A new classification of head injury based on CT findings was mentioned previously. This classification is shown in Table 9.1. An analysis of outcome in severely head-injured patients, in relation to the CT diagnostic categories utilized here, shows a strikingly direct correlation (Table 9.3) (Marshall *et al.* 1991b).

Diffuse axonal injury

Patients with diffuse injuries have varying degrees of shearing of the axons. This pattern of injury, originally described by Strich in 1956, is now recognized as a major pathophysiological process underlying almost all severe injuries. The mechanisms of injury usually involve rotational acceleration producing shear and tensile strains of high magnitude (Gennarelli *et al.* 1982b). Patients suffering from DAI show a spectrum of axonal injury. Radiologically, the CT scans of these patients can appear to be normal (as in Diffuse Injury I, Table 9.3) or to have multiple petechial haemorrhages. For the more severe type of DAI, petechial haemorrhage can usually be found in the corpus callosum and/or dorsolateral quadrants of the midbrain (Blumbergs & Jones 1989; Sahuquillo-Barris & Lamarca-Ciuro 1988). Over 90% of the patients who sustain severe DAI (as in Diffuse Injury IV, Table 9.3) are unconscious from the moment of injury, and remain unconscious, vegetative or at least severely disabled until death.

Intracranial mass lesions

Patients with acute SDH do much more poorly than those with extradural haematoma (EDH). This is because the SDH represents a more severe pattern of overall injury with high levels of brain shearing and other parenchymal lesions. In patients with EDH, the presence of other severe injuries, although not infrequent, is less common and usually direct pathology within the brain substance itself is less than in patients with acute SDH. A recent study by Haselsberger showed that the overall mortality for acute SDH is 57% versus 25% for EDH (Haselsberger *et al.* 1988). Another study of patients suffering from acute SDH showed a 66% mortality rate, and a 15% nonfunctional recovery (Wilberger *et al.* 1991). These findings suggest that the extent of primary underlying brain injury is more important than the SDH itself in dictating the outcome.

Traumatic basal ganglia haemorrhage is rarely seen in head injuries. A recent report showed that these injuries represent only 0.9% of all head injury patients undergoing CT scanning during a period of 5 years (Lee & Wang 1991). The haemorrhage is probably secondary to rupture of lenticulostriate or anterior choroidal arteries (Katz *et al.* 1989). In general, these patients have a favourable outcome, especially when the basal ganglia haemorrhage occurs in isolation (Katz *et al.* 1989; Lee & Wang 1991).

Pre-injury history affecting outcome

The pre-injury and social history have an enormous influence on the quality of outcome after mild to moderate head injury. As Sir Charles Symonds stated, 'The symptom picture depends not only upon the kind of injury, but upon the kind of brain' (Symonds 1937). For severe head injury, the extent of brain damage is so great that an individual's environment or intellectual endowment would not contribute much to the outcome. A report by Gronwall & Wrightson (1975) showed that a previous head injury lengthened the time of recovery from both mild and moderate head injuries. This notion is further supported by an independent study that showed reaction time was much slower and subjective sequelae were worse in individuals who had a history of multiple head injuries producing unconsciousness as compared with those with a single head injury (Carlsson *et al.* 1987).

Outcome of head injury

The outcome of head-injured patients often depends on the severity of the initial impact injury. This applies both to short-term survival as well as long-term functioning in society (Alexandre *et al.* 1983; Evans 1981; Jennett *et al.* 1976). Interestingly, the outcome for most patients with head injury is determined primarily by the intellectual and behavioural disabilities that remain, rather than by physical impairments which often improve materially over time.

Table 9.4. *The Glasgow Outcome Scale*

Score	Meaning
5	Good recovery: implies resumption of normal life even if there may be minor neurological and/or psychological deficits. This does not imply return to previous employment
4	Moderate disability: disabled but independent. Independent in so far as daily life is concerned. The disabilities include varying degrees of dysphasia, hemiparesis, ataxia, intellectual and memory deficits and personality change
3	Severe disability: conscious but disabled, dependent for daily support due to mental and/or physical disability. May be institutionalized, but this is not a criterion
2	Persistent vegetative state: unresponsive and speechless; after 2–3 weeks may open eyes and have sleep/awake cycles
1	Death

Assessment of outcome

In 1975, Jennett & Bond designed a system called the Glasgow Outcome Scale (GOS), which is widely used for measuring the quality of life after head injury. The GOS is a five-point scale which includes five categories (Table 9.4). When the outcome of brain injury is assessed by the GOS, the time of assessment should always be stated. This is important because of the prolonged time scale in head injury during which recovery appears to continue. The initial recovery from head injury can be characterized by a typical graphic relationship in which there is a steep upward slope during the first 1 to 3 months followed by a less steep continuing pattern of recovery and, ultimately, a plateauing of improvement. A study by Mandleberg & Brooks (1975) showed that a third of those who were severely disabled 3 months after head injury had improved to moderate disability by 1 year, but not one had made a good recovery. A third of those still moderately disabled at 3 months had made a good recovery by 12 months. The time scale of recovery may also be different for the various components of disability. Neurophysical features, such as spasticity and dysphasia, may continue to improve for years, while serial psychological testing indicates that most recovery in cognitive function occurs within 12 months (Mandleberg & Brooks 1975).

Outcome of mild head injury

The original design of GCS was not intended as a means of distinguishing between different types of milder head injury. With that in mind, it is generally accepted that GCS of 13–15 is considered as mild head injury (Kraus *et al.* 1984). Frequently, the patients present with a history of brief unconsciousness, with or without post-traumatic amnesia. Other acute and subacute symptoms following mild head injury include headache, nausea, dizziness and cognitive deficits, usually of short duration.

Some of these patients are hospitalized because of the risk, albeit low, of delayed complications such as a haematoma (Jennett 1976).

The mortality rate for mild head injury is virtually nil; however, the long-term sequelae of minor head injury are often underestimated. Although the head CT scan of mild injury patients may not reveal any neuroradiological abnormalities (Sabers *et al.* 1988), and the neurological examination can be completely normal, evidence of organic brain damage has been demonstrated by neuropsychological testing (Gronwall & Wrightson 1974; Rimel *et al.* 1981) and microscopic studies (Oppenheimer 1968; Povlishock *et al.* 1983). The loss of consciousness immediately after a blow to or rapid deceleration of the head is a result of the shearing forces on the brain stem. In an animal study of minor head injury, axonal degeneration was found scattered throughout the brain stem (Jane *et al.* 1985).

Although very few minor head injury patients exhibit objective focal neurological deficits, a significant portion of these patients complain of headache, dizziness, vertigo, irritability, inability to concentrate, impaired memory, and easy fatiguability. Sometimes, the organic brain damage can be so subtle that it is manifested only by difficulty processing information at a normal rate (Gronwall & Wrightson 1974). In some patients, these symptoms persist and, while this has been called the post-concussion syndrome, these patients can also be characterized as the 'miserable minority'. That is because for approximately 85% the residual disability is so mild that it can eventually be overcome by changes in areas such as work style or family interaction. But for this remaining small group no amount of physical, mental, cognitive or behavioural rehabilitation ever restores them to a completely functional role. These seemingly moderately disabling symptoms, when clustered in a constellation, often significantly affect the patient's ability to resume anything remotely resembling a normal life (Edna 1987; Khalek 1983; Rutherford *et al.* 1979).

The findings of Leininger *et al.* (1990) indicate that patients suffering minor head injury who report post-concussive symptoms often have measurable neuropsychological deficits. The severity of these deficits appears to be independent of the neurological status observed immediately after the injury. In Rimel's (1981) series of such patients, neuropsychological testing demonstrated some problems with attention, concentration, memory or judgement. Because of these symptoms, 34% of these patients, who were gainfully employed before the accident, became unemployed even 3 months after a seemingly insignificant head injury.

Levin *et al.* (1987), in a rather detailed report, showed that there was considerable improvement in patients with minor head injury in a pattern similar to that previously mentioned for more severe injuries. There was a steep recovery of function during the first month and then a slower, more gradual, recovery over the ensuing 2 months of the study. While many patients improved, and one might interpret the study as showing that the patients in many instances became normal, in fact a considerable number had significant residual problems in recent memory, abstract thinking and information processing, even at 3 months.

The results of all these studies are astonishing as they demonstrate that the long-term sequelae, particularly the psychosocial component, of mild head injury are much more significant than we have assumed in the past. These findings also suggest that a seemingly minor blow to the head can produce irreversible organic brain damage.

Outcome of moderate head injury

Moderate head injury has been rather poorly studied and these patients deserve more attention than they have received previously. Future attention from neurosurgeons, neuropsychologists and others interested in brain injury, such as physiatrists, should be directed to patients suffering moderate head injury, where the opportunities to improve are greater and where physical and cognitive rehabilitation may have an even more appreciable impact.

Head-injured patients with GCS scores between 9 and 12 following resuscitation are categorized as having suffered a moderate head injury. Virtually all the literature on head injury has focused on the sequelae of mild and severe injuries, and only a few studies have been dedicated to patients sustaining moderate head injuries (Rimel *et al.* 1982; Tabaddor *et al.* 1984).

In a more recent publication, Miller & Pentland (1989) studied the outcome of moderate head injury in older patients. This gives an even more dismal picture of outcome. This group demonstrates that when even a moderate-impact injury is sustained by an ageing brain the consequences can be truly devastating.

The largest study of moderate head injury to date is that of Rimel *et al.* (1982). Compared with those patients with minor head injury, the patients with moderate head injury were usually from a lower socioeconomic class, less educated, slightly older, had a higher incidence of alcohol abuse, and more often had a history of previous trauma. These factors, plus the greater severity of brain injury, suggest a less favourable outcome of patients with moderate head injury. Not surprisingly, the incidence of focal lesions was also higher in the moderate head injury group, and some of them required intracranial surgery. Those patients with a GCS score of 9 to 12 and harbouring a subdural haematoma had a very poor outcome. Sixty-five per cent died or were severely disabled and none made a good recovery as measured by the GOS. After following the moderate head injury patients for 3 months, only 38% made a good recovery – a significant decrease from the 75% of the minor head injury patients. Even within the good recovery category there was a higher rate of disability such as headache (93%), memory difficulties (90%) and difficulties with daily activities (87%). Only 7% of the patients were asymptomatic. Sixty-six per cent of the patients previously employed had not returned to work, compared with 33% of the minor head injury patients. Neuropsychological batteries performed in 32 moderately head-injured patients 3 months after the injury demonstrated significant deficits on all test measures.

These results are based on one study with a relatively small sample size (199 patients). It is appropriate to point out that information regarding the long-term sequelae of moderate head injury is scarce. Future attention from neurosurgeons and their colleagues in other medical disciplines should be directed to the patients suffering from moderate head injury, for whom the opportunities to improve the outcome are great, both in the acute phase of the injury and in physical and behavioural rehabilitation.

Outcome of severe head injury

Patients suffering head injury with GCS scores of 3–8 following resuscitation are classified as having suffered a severe head injury. These patients follow the trend of being less affluent, more poorly educated, and with a history of greater alcohol and substance abuse and of previous injury. In association with the higher degree of injury in these patients, the incidence of focal lesions is also significantly more frequent. Gennarelli et al. (1982a) reported that 56% of severely head-injured patients had focal lesions on CT scan. The severity of injury as indicated by the CT scan was also significant.

Outcome for the severely head-injured patient is dependent on many factors, some of which, such as the initial impact, are clearly beyond the control of the treating physician. In the care of these patients there is considerable evidence that early aggressive surgical treatment, successful control of intracranial hypertension, and careful attention to medical complications can improve the outcome (Marshall et al. 1979). However, regardless of the sophistication of the emergency medical services system and the advancement of intensive care therapies, the mortality rate of severe head injury patients remains high, ranging from 28% (Marshall et al. 1979) to 51% (Lyle et al. 1986).

A prospective analysis of 746 severe closed head injury patients was conducted using data from TCDB. It is important to mention that all these patients were admitted to state-of-the-art level I trauma centres with a commitment to head injury care and research. The results of this study demonstrated that 36% of these patients had died, 5% were vegetative, 16% were severely disabled, 16% were moderately disabled and 27% had made a good recovery. There was a strong correlation between the initial-resuscitation GCS score and outcome. This is demonstrated in Table 9.5. These outcome results are similar to those previously reported by Becker et al. (1977), Marshall et al. (1979), Bowers & Marshall (1980), and Miller et al. (1981).

Of 84 patients who were vegetative in the TCDB at the time of discharge, 41% were conscious at 6 months and 52% by 1 year. No strong predictor of recovery from a vegetative state could be identified, but the overall outcome, even with recovery of consciousness, was still poor (Levin et al. 1991).

Neuropsychological deficits are the most pervasive and permanent sequelae of severe head injury. Often they are rated as more disabling than physical limitations. Brooks and colleagues (1987) reported that sequelae involving memory, attention and emotional disturbances were the greatest impediment to the ability to return to work in survivors of severe closed head injury. Jennett et al. (1981) examined survivors from

Table 9.5. *Outcome at last contact with post-resuscitation Glasgow Coma Scale score[a]*

Outcome at last contact	Post-resuscitation Glasgow Coma Scale Score								
	Unknown (%)	3 (%)	3.3[b] (%)	4 (%)	5 (%)	6 (%)	7 (%)	8 (%)	≥ 9 (%)
Good recovery	0	4.1	25.4	6.3	12.2	29.2	46.6	54.8	40.3
Moderate disability	0	3.1	19.0	8.1	17.1	21.3	22.3	22.6	21.0
Severe disability	0	10.3	17.5	18.9	23.2	23.0	11.5	6.5	13.0
Vegetative survival	0	4.1	7.9	10.8	7.3	5.3	2.0	4.8	0
Death	100	78.4	30.2	55.9	40.2	21.2	17.6	11.3	25.8

[a] Outcome assessed by the Glasgow Outcome Scale.
[b] Patients who are untestable due to paralytic agents.

head injury whose outcomes were classified as good recoveries, moderate disabilities or severe disabilities. He noted that intellectual and memory deficits as well as personality changes were observed across a broad spectrum of outcomes.

Head injury in children

Paediatric head injury needs special consideration since the mechanism, pathophysiology and, therefore, the outcome of the injury are different from those in adults. Head injuries are the leading cause of death and disability in the paediatric age group. More than 1 million children in the United States sustain closed head injuries each year, and one-sixth of those cases require hospital admission (Eiben *et al.* 1984). About 80% of children who suffer multiple trauma also have significant head injuries, compared with 50% of adults (Walker *et al.* 1985). There are several factors contributing to children's greater susceptibility to head injury than adults. First, the younger the patient, the greater the head/body ratio. Second, the brain of the child, especially in early childhood, is less myelinated and hence more easily injured. Third, the cranial bones are thinner and afford less protection to the brain.

Mechanism of paediatric head injury

In order to assess outcome after head injury in children, it is important to take into account the various mechanisms of injury operating at different ages and their potential relationship to pathophysiology. Studies have shown that falls constitute a major source of closed head injury in children under 5 years (Annegers 1983; Kraus *et al.* 1984). In the 5- to 14-year-old range, recreational and sports-related injuries rise. Pedestrian–motor vehicle and bicycle accidents also predominate in this age group (Klauber *et al.* 1981). Motor vehicle injuries are more prevalent in the 15-years-old and older age group (Annegers *et al.* 1980b).

The difference in mechanisms plays an important role in the pathophysiology of closed head injury. Kalsbeek and colleagues (1980) have noted that coma caused by a motor vehicle accident is more often due to severe primary brain damage from acceleration/deceleration forces. On the other hand, coma after a head injury produced by a fall is likely to result in brain compression due to intracerebral haematoma. The experience of the TCDB revealed that the outcome of paediatric patients also depends on the age-defined subgroup to which they belong. The outcome was the poorest in those children younger than 4 years old. Five- to 10-years-olds have a more favourable outcome (Levin *et al.* 1992).

Pathophysiology of paediatric head injury

There are significant differences in the pathophysiology of brain injury between children and adults. In line with general research findings, children with severe head injury are more likely than adults to have intracranial hypertension: 80% and 40%, respectively (Walker *et al.* 1985). Intracranial haematomas from head injury are less frequent in the paediatric population than in adults: 26% versus 46% (Alberico *et al.* 1987; Bruce *et al.* 1978). Children are also more prone to develop 'malignant brain oedema' (Bruce *et al.* 1981), which is due to brain hyperaemia occurring shortly after the injury and is distinct from cytotoxic oedema, which may develop later.

An analysis from the TCDB revealed diffuse brain swelling occurred approximately twice as often in children as in adults. A high mortality rate (53%) was found in these children when compared with children without diffuse brain swelling (16%) (Aldrich *et al.* 1992). In one of their studies, Bruce and his associates noted that, while delayed deterioration in adults is most frequently associated with a focal intracranial mass lesion, delayed deterioration in children is associated with diffuse brain swelling (Bruce *et al.* 1981). The predisposition to cerebral hyperaemia and resulting intracranial hypertension makes children more vulnerable to secondary brain injury. Since a favourable outcome depends on the prevention of secondary brain injury, children with head injury do substantially better when therapy to decrease hyperaemia and brain oedema is started early (Bruce *et al.* 1978).

Outcome in paediatric head injury

The results of several studies on the outcome of paediatric head injury indicate that paediatric patients have a better outcome than their adult counterparts, except for children under 4 years of age (Levin *et al.* 1992; Walker *et al.* 1983). Mahoney *et al.* (1983) found that 61% of children with coma lasting more than 24 hours had a good survival. It was commonly believed that the immature brain responds to injury differently, allowing possibly for a better outcome in children due to the 'plasticity' of the nervous system. This belief is now in doubt, based on differences in the mechanism of injury, the effects of alcohol and drugs, and the increased frequency of mass lesions in the adult age group.

From a study with a large patient sample, Luerssen *et al.* (1988) concluded that paediatric patients exhibited a significantly lower mortality rate compared with adults, except for patients found to have SDH and for those who were profoundly hypotensive. Similarly, Alberico *et al.* (1987) found that although the overall mortality from head injury is lower in children than in adults, when those children with surgical mass lesions were compared with those of the adult population with mass lesions, the outcome in the two groups was similar.

Actually, the higher mortality rate in the 0- to 4-year age group revealed by Levin's study (Levin *et al.* 1992) can be explained by the correspondingly higher incidence of SDH, bilateral nonreactive pupils and hypotension in these patients. There is also evidence to suggest that infants and young children are as vulnerable as, or even more vulnerable than, adults to the effects of trauma on memory and cognition (Levin *et al.* 1983).

As in adults, deficits in neuropsychological functions are the major disabilities in paediatric head injury survivors. Even after mild head injury, parents often note behavioural changes such as increased crying or aggression, lowered frustration toler-ance, hypersensitivity, or timidity. While these symptoms may resolve in the first few weeks after injury, memory and attention deficits affecting school performance and behaviour may be more long-lasting. Unlike adults, whose recovery tends to plateau within 6 months or 1 year, children will often continue to show recovery of motor, speech and intellectual functions for several years after injury (Costeff *et al.* 1990; Mahoney *et al.* 1993). It has been noted that even after the most severe head injuries, most of the comatose children will regain consciousness (Costeff *et al.* 1985, 1990; Heiskanen & Kaste 1974). However, even though some of these patients may improve to a level consistent with employment and independent living, they continue to have significant neurobehavioural problems and poor social adjustment (Costeff *et al.* 1990; Filley *et al.* 1987; Kriel *et al.* 1988).

Non-accident head injury

Child abuse is a common cause of severe head injury in children particularly those under 1 or 2 years of age. It is often associated with a very high mortality and significant morbidity. Billmire and her colleagues found that 64% of all head injuries in children under 2 years of age, excluding uncomplicated skull fractures, and 95% of serious or life-threatening head injuries, were the result of child abuse (Billmire & Myers 1985). Paediatric head trauma resulting from non-accidental injury has become a more recognizable syndrome since the availability of CT scanning. The CT scan may reveal the presence of subdural haematoma, subarachnoid haemorrhage and a swollen brain. Close inspection may reveal areas of atrophic focal changes from old cerebral con-tusions, and the presence of some fresh subcortical–cortical bleeding and oedema (Zimmerman *et al.* 1979). Cerebral injuries and retinal haemorrhages without outward physical signs of trauma in an infant are suggestive of 'shaken baby syndrome' (Bruce &

Zimmerman 1989; Caffey 1974). The outcome in shaken babies is notably poor: 38% die, 30–50% show severe cognitive or neurological deficits, and only 30% have a chance of full recovery (Alexander *et al.* 1990).

In the presence of a comatose child, or severely obtunded infant who has a history that does not seem to concur with the clinical findings, child abuse should be a serious consideration. This is not only important because of the social implications and because of the patient's future management, but because it also suggests the possibility that this child has probably suffered another cerebral insult in the past and is being brought to the hospital usually after a considerable delay. It should be presumed, therefore, that seizures and/or hypoxic-ischaemic insults have been ongoing for an undetermined period, prior to the current emergency. All these explain the poor clinical outcome in many of these abused children.

Outcome of civilian craniocerebral gunshot wounds

Craniocerebral missile wounds are a major public health problem in the United States, where control of a wide variety of weapons is still rather rudimentary. Over 20 years ago, Raimondi & Samuelson (1970) reported that 1% of all trauma in inner city metropolitan hospitals involved gunshot wounds to the brain. This figure obviously underestimates the magnitude of the problem since the majority of patients die before hospital arrival (Freytag 1963; Kaufman *et al.* 1986). More recently, data from the Centers for Disease Control revealed that the mortality rate from firearm-related brain injuries was 2.4/100 000 annually. In 1991 more than 10 000 people died from craniocerebral gunshot wounds and it is the leading cause of death in black males in the United States under the age of 30 years. About 65% of these patients succumbed before hospital arrival and about 90% were dead within 24 hours (Clark *et al.* 1986; Freytag 1963; Graham *et al.* 1990).

In an autopsy series, homicides accounted for the majority of craniocerebral missile injuries in patients between 20 and 30 years of age, whereas in the age group in excess of 50 years these wounds are much more likely to be self-inflicted (Freytag 1963). The majority of injuries were caused by small-calibre (0.22–0.38) low-velocity (900–1300 feet/second) projectiles.

Unlike closed head injury, for which the mortality rate has been reduced by aggressive management, the mortality rate of civilian gunshot wounds of the brain remains high, ranging from 60% to 90% (Clark *et al.* 1986; Frahm *et al.* 1990; Nagib *et al.* 1986; Raimondi & Samuelson 1970). The high mortality rate is the result of the tremendous primary destruction as the bullet passes through the brain and the secondary effect of a highly resonating projectile which creates heat and shear stresses of almost unimaginable proportions.

There are few reliable predictors for the outcome of patients suffering from craniocerebral missile wounds. As with closed head injury, the outcome is closely correlated with the patient's level of consciousness at the time of admission. Patients who are alert upon admission have a low mortality ranging from 0 to 20% (Clark *et al.* 1986; Crockard 1974; Graham *et al.* 1990; Nagib *et al.* 1986). For patients who are decerebrate upon admission, the mortality rate is almost 96%. Of the few who survive, the majority will remain vegetative. The survival rate of patients who are flaccid upon admission is nil (Raimondi & Samuelson 1970; Rish *et al.* 1983). Similarly, patients with fixed dilated pupils upon admission rarely survive (Byrnes *et al.* 1974). The missile course also has a bearing on mortality. A missile course involving the ventricular system is associated with a poorer outcome than those with no ventricular involvement (Clark *et al.* 1986). Injuries that involve only a single lobe have a mortality of 35–45%, whereas those that involve multiple lobes or cross the midline are associated with a mortality as high as 51–90% (Kaufman *et al.* 1986; Nagib *et al.* 1986; Raimondi & Samuelson 1970).

Post-traumatic epilepsy

Post-traumatic epilepsy (PTE) is one of the sequelae for patients suffering head injury. It has not only a potential to affect the short-term outcome, but also is a major factor leading to social misadjustment and an inability to re-enter the work place. Seizures lead to secondary brain insults because of blood flow–metabolism mismatch, which creates local lactic acidosis and elevation of intracerebral pressure. Studies have shown that patients with PTE had poorer rehabilitation outcomes (Armstrong *et al.* 1990) and considerable difficulty obtaining or maintaining employment. About 20–25% of patients with moderate or severe head injuries experience at least one post-traumatic seizure (Jennett 1975).

PTE was classified by Jennett into two types: early and late (Jennett 1974, 1975). Early post-traumatic seizures are defined as those occurring within the first week after injury. This definition is clearly arbitrary and others have suggested that seizures might be better divided into those occurring within the first 24 hours, those occurring within the range of the first week, and those occurring more than 1 week after injury. Approximately one-third of early seizures occur within the first hour of injury, another one-third within the first day, and the rest during the remainder of the first week. A direct relationship exists between the incidence of early seizures and the severity of the head injury. About 33% of patients with subdural and intracerebral haematomas develop seizures. Epidural haematomas, depressed skull fractures and post-traumatic amnesia lasting longer than 24 hours result in approximately a 10% incidence of early seizures (Jennett 1974, 1975). About 25% of post-traumatic seizures, even when following a mild head injury, will progress to late post-traumatic seizures.

Late PTE is defined as seizures occurring after the first week of injury. Seventy per cent of the seizures develop within the first 2 years of injury (Jennett 1975). Like early PTE, the severity of the injury is a major determining factor in the incidence of late seizures. According to Jennett's series, almost 50% of patients with subdural or intracerebral haematomas or penetrating missile wounds develop late PTE, as compared with 20% of patients with epidural haematomas. Other factors, such as depressed skull fractures, focal brain injuries, post-traumatic amnesia for more than 24 hours, early seizures and dural laceration, have an additive effect on the rate of late PTE. A study by Weiss & Salazar (1986) showed that there is a 95% probability that epilepsy will not develop when the first 3 post-injury years are seizure-free.

Children of early age were found to be more susceptible to seizures. According to Jennett's series, individuals younger than age 5 years had a 9% epilepsy rate, whereas 5% of those older than age 5 years had early seizures (Jennett 1975). Similarly, Hahn *et al.* (1988) reported that 15.7% of patients aged under 2 years developed post-traumatic seizure, 11.6% in patients aged under 3 years, and 9.6% in the entire group of patients aged under 16 years of age. In children, early post-traumatic seizures often occur in the first hour or within 24 hours. Early seizures less often are followed by late seizures. Only 10–20% of children who develop early seizures subsequently develop late seizures (Annegers *et al.* 1980a; Jennett 1975).

Efficacy of prophylaxis

The most widely recognized study on prophylaxis is that of Temkin *et al.* (1990), which demonstrated that phenytoin reduced the risk of early seizures within the first week by 70% but had no efficacy in the prevention of late PTE. The previous study by Young *et al.* (1983a,b) was complicated by the fact that the patients in the active drug group occasionally had subtherapeutic levels during their early hospital stay which clearly might have influenced the overall result. Thus, their conclusion that the early adminis-tration of phenytoin is not prophylactically effective in reducing the occurrence of either early or late post-traumatic seizures must be viewed in that regard. Nevertheless, the studies of Young *et al.* (1983a,b) did show that early administration of phenytoin was not prophylactically effective in reducing the occurrence of either early or late post-traumatic seizures.

Today, prophylaxis of post-traumatic seizures remains a controversial topic. There are arguments for prophylaxis based on the relatively high incidence of post-traumatic seizures, especially if there are associated risk factors (Kuhl *et al.* 1990). Nevertheless, the adverse effects of phenytoin are well known (Rapp *et al.* 1983). There are also studies that phenytoin had a negative effect on neurobehavioural and cognitive function following head injury (Dikmen *et al.* 1991). In light of these findings, we advocate the use of prophylactic anticonvulsants after head injury only for the first week or so, unless an early post-traumatic seizure has occurred.

Post-acute brain injury rehabilitation

As we learn more and more about the outcome of head injury it becomes increasingly clear that higher-order executive functions, which include cognitive, affective, social and vocational activities, are the areas where disturbances are greatest in such patients. These form the main impediments for patients to attain a productive lifestyle, even after the physical disabilities have resolved. There has been an explosion in the development of rehabilitation programmes for patients suffering brain injury, in part in response to the increasing number of survivors and also because there is more general agreement that these programmes can have some effect in carefully selected patients on behavioural and cognitive disability.

In the early 1980s there were only a handful of rehabilitation programmes available. Towards the end of the 1980s there were more than 600 head injury rehabilitation programmes throughout the United States (Burke *et al.* 1988), and the number is increasing every year. These non-hospital-based programmes have developed cognitive, behavioural, social, educational and vocational strategies to address the higher-order traumatic brain injury deficits. Both outpatient and inpatient rehabilitation programmes are available, depending on the severity of the patient's post-traumatic injuries and the other services and support that are required. While this area is rapidly developing, it has been hampered by a lack of objective measures of outcome improvement. The problem in measuring outcome is complex because the natural history is one of improvement, particularly over the first several months when the patient is in the rehabilitation environment, and controlled trials have, in general, not been done, particularly in patients with severe injury. In trials of less severe injuries, the study by Ruff *et al.* (1991) demonstrated clear improvement in some cognitive functions, although in many patients the improvement was relatively small when patients undergoing an intense cognitive retraining programme were compared with a control group. Nevertheless, there is clear evidence that many of the social disabilities which affect cognitive function can be improved with rehabilitation in a structured environment, and as these programmes come under increasing cost pressure to produce measurable outcome results it is likely that strategies for rehabilitation in this area will improve.

While neurosurgeons and intensivists play a crucial role in the immediate mortality and morbidity of head injury patients, the post-acute phase of recovery is left in the hands of physiatrists and therapists. The major objective of a post-acute brain injury rehabilitation programme should be the achievement of increasingly independent function. A study by Kozloff (1987) has found that social support is an important outcome predictor of rehabilitation. Discharge to a group home with peer and professional support may provide a better social network than discharge to the family. Studies demonstrate substantial improvements in function during the post-acute rehabilitation of the patients and such improvements are unlikely to be the result of spontaneous improvement alone. Reported advantages to such rehabilitation approaches include increased patient motivation and acceptance of treatment, and an improvement of the patients' ability to integrate back into his or her community and home environment (Cope *et al.* 1991a,b).

Post-acute brain injury rehabilitation offers a potentially tremendous opportunity to return these patients to more useful roles in society if it can be shown that such interventions produce meaningful improvement in a cost-effective manner. It is important that neurosurgeons, intensivists and neuropsychologists, in addition to physiatrists, subject such programmes to a high level of intellectual scrutiny in order that they may improve. It is here, rather than in the intensive care unit and in the pre-hospital phase, that many of the gains that we are likely to see during the remainder of the 1990s can be made in more advanced societies. In areas where resources for pre-hospital and acute hospital care are not as great, better organization of pre-hospital care using limited or scarce resources and programmes of prevention are likely to be of tremendous importance.

References

Alberico, A. M., Ward, J. D. & Choi, S. C. (1987). Outcome after severe head injury: relationship to mass lesions, diffuse injury, and ICP course in pediatric and adult patients. *J. Neurosurg.* **67**, 648–56.

Aldrich, E. F., Eisenberg, H. M., Saydjari, C. & Luerssen, T. G. (1992). Diffuse brain swelling in severely head-injured children. A report from the NIH Traumatic Coma Data Bank. *J. Neurosurg.* **76**, 450–4.

Alexander, R., Sato, Y. & Smith, W. (1990). Incidence of impact trauma with cranial injuries abscribed to shaking. *AJDC* **144**, 724–6.

Alexandre, A., Colombo, F. & Nertempi, P. (1983). Cognitive outcome and early indices of severity of head injury. *J. Neurosurg.* **59**, 751–61.

Annegers, J. F. (1983). The epidemiology of head trauma in children. In *Pediatric Head Trauma*. New York: Futura.

Annegers, J. F., Grabow, J. D. & Groover, R. V. (1980a). Seizures after head trauma: a population study. *Neurology* **30**, 683–9.

Annegers, J. F., Grabow, J. D. & Kurland, L. T. (1980b). The incidence, causes, and secular trends in head injury in Olmsted County, Minnesota, 1934–1974. *Neurology* **30**, 912–19.

Armstrong, K. K., Sahgal, V. & Bloch, R. (1990). Rehabilitation outcomes in patients with posttraumatic epilepsy. *Arch. Phys. Med. Rehabil.* **71**, 156–60.

Becker, D. P., Miller, J. D. & Ward, J. D. (1977). The outcome from severe head injury with early diagnosis and intensive treatment. *J. Neurosurg.* **47**, 491–502.

Billmire, M. E. & Myers, P. A. (1985). Series head injury in infants: accident or abuse? *Pediatrics* **75**, 340–2.

Blumbergs, P. C. & Jones, N. R. (1989). Diffuse axonal injury in head trauma. *J. Neurol. Neurosurg. Psychiatry* **52**, 838–41.

Bowers, S. A. & Marshall, L. F. (1980). Outcome in 200 consecutive cases of severe head injury treated in San Diego County: a prospective analysis. *Neurosurgery* **6**, 237–42.

Boyle, M. J., Vella, L. & Moloney, E. (1991). Role of drugs and alcohol in patients with head injury. *J. R. Soc. Med.* **84**, 608–10.

Braakman, R., Gelpke, G. J. & Habbema, J. D. F. (1980). Systematic selection of prognostic features in patients with severe head injury. *Neurosurgery* **6**, 362–70.

Brooks, N., McKinlay, W. & Symington, C. (1987). Return to work within the first seven years of severe head injury. *Brain Injury* **1**, 5–19.

Bruce, D. A. & Zimmerman, R. A. (1989). Shaken impact syndrome. *Pediatr. Ann.* **18**, 482–94.

Bruce, D. A., Schut, L. & Bruno, L. A. (1978). Outcome following severe head injuries in children. *J. Neurosurg.* **48**, 679–88.

Bruce, D. A., Sutton, L. N. & Schut, L. (1981). Acute brain swelling and cerebral edema in children. In *Brain Edema*. New York: Wiley.

Burke, W. H., Wesolowski, M. D. & Guth, M. L. (1988). Comprehensive head injury rehabilitation: an outcome evaluation. *Brain Injury* **2**, 313–22.

Butterworth, J. F. I., Selhorst, J. B. & Greenberg, R. P. (1981). Flaccidity after head injury: diagnosis, management, and outcome. *Neurosurgery* **9**, 242–8.

Byrnes, D. P., Crockard, H. A., Gordon, P. S. & Gleadhill, C. A. (1974). Civilian penetrating craniocerebral missile injury in the civil disturbance in Northern Ireland. *Br. J. Surg.* **61**, 169–76.

Caffey, J. (1974). The whiplash infant syndrome: mannel shaking by the bleeding linked with residual permanent damage and mental retardation. *Pediatrics* **54**, 396.

Carlsson, G. S., Svardsudd, K. & Welin, L. (1987). Long-term effects of head injuries sustained during life in three male populations. *J. Neurosurg.* **67**, 197–205.

Chestnut, R. M., Marshall, L. F. & Klauber, M. R. (1993). The role of secondary brain injury in determining outcome from severe head injury. *J. Trauma* **34**, 216–22.

Clark, W. C., Muhlbauer, M. S. & Watridge, C. B. (1986). Analysis of 76 civilian craniocerebral gunshot wounds. *J. Neurosurg.* **65**, 9–14.

Cooper, J. D., Tabaddor, K. & Hauser, W. A. (1983). The epidemiology of head injury in the Bronx. *Neuroepidemiology* **2**, 70–88.

Cope, D. N., Cole, J. R. & Hall, K. M. (1991a). Brain injury: analysis of outcome in a post-acute rehabilitation system. 1. General analysis. *Brain Injury* **5**, 111–25.

Cope, D. N., Cole, J. R. & Hall, K. M. (1991b). Brain injury: analysis of outcome in a post-acute rehabilitation system. 2. Subanalysis. *Brain Injury* **5**, 127–39.

Costeff, H., Groswasser, Z. & Landman, Y. (1985). Survivors of severe traumatic brain injury in childhood, I, late residual disability. *Scand. J. Rehabil. Med.* (Suppl.) **12**, 10–15.

Costeff, H., Groswasser, Z. and Goldstein, R. (1990). Long-term follow-up review of 31 children with severe closed head trauma. *J. Neurosurg.* **73**, 684–7.

Crockard, H. A. (1974). Bullet injuries of the brain. *Ann. R. Coll. Surg. Engl.* **55**, 111–23.

Crone, K. R., Lee, K. S. & Kelly, D. L. (1987). Correlation of admission fibrin degradation products with outcome and respiratory failure in patients with severe head injury. *Neurosurgery* **21**, 532–6.

Department of Health and Human Services, P. H. S. (February 1989). *Interagency Head Injury Task Force Report*. Bethesda: National Institutes of Health, National Institute of Neurological Disorders and Stroke.

Dikmen, S. S., Temkin, N. R. & Miller, B. (1991). Neurobehavioral effects of phenytoin prophylaxis of posttraumatic seizures. *JAMA* **265**, 1271–7.

Edna, T. H. (1982). Alcohol influence and head injury. *Acta Chir. Scand.* **148**, 209–12.

Edna, T. H. (1987). Disability 3–5 years after minor head injury. *J. Oslo City Hosp.* **37**, 41–8.

Eiben, C., Anderson, T. P. & Lockman, L. (1984). Functional outcome of closed head injury in children and young adults. *Arch. Phys. Med. Rehabil.* **65**, 168–70.

Evans, C. D. (1981). *Future Developments in Rehabilitation after Severe Head Injury*. New York: Churchill Livingstone.

Filley, C. M., Cranbery, L. D. & Alexander, M. P. (1987). Neurobehavioral outcome after closed head injury in childhood and adolescence. *Arch. Neurol.* **44**, 194–8.

Freytag, E. (1963). Autopsy findings in head injuries from firearms. Statistical evaluation of 254 cases. *Arch. Pathol.* **76**, 215–25.

Gennarelli, T. A., Speilman, G. M. & Langfitt, T. W. (1982a). Influence of the type of intracranial lesion on outcome from severe head injury. *J. Neurosurg.* **56**, 26–33.

Gennarelli, T. A., Thibauly, L. E. & Adams, J. H. (1982). Diffuse axonal injury and traumatic coma in the primate. *Ann. Neurol.* **12**, 564–74.

Graham, T. W., Williams, F. C. & Harrington, T. (1990). Civilian gunshot wounds to the head: a prospective study. *Neurosurgery* **27**, 697–700.

Gronwall, D. & Wrightson, P. (1974). Delayed recovery of intellectual function after minor head injury. *Lancet* II, 605–9.

Gronwall, D. & Wrightson, P. (1975). Cumulative effect of concussion. *Lancet* II, 995–7.

Hahn, Y. S., Fuchs, S. & Flannery, A. M. (1988). Factors influencing posttraumatic seizures in children. *Neurosurgery* **22**, 864–7.

Haselsberger, K., Pucher, R. & Auer, L. M. (1988). Prognosis after acute subdural or epidural hemorrhage. *Acta Neurochir.* (Wien) **90**, 111–16.

Heiskanen, O. & Kaste, M. (1974). Late prognosis of severe brain injury in children. *Dev. Med. Child. Neurol.* **16**, 11–14.

Jagger, J., Levine, J. & Jane, J. (1984). Epidemiologic features of head injury in a predominantly rural population. *J. Trauma* **24**, 40–4.

Jane, J. A., Steward, O. & Gennarelli, T. (1985). Axonal degeneration induced by experimental noninvasive minor head injury. *J. Neurosurg.* **62**, 96–100.

Jennett, B. (1974). 'Early traumatic epilepsy: incidence and significance after nonmissile injuries.' *Arch. Neurol.* **30**, 394–8.

Jennett, B. (1975). *Epilepsy after Non-missile Head Injuries.* Chicago: Year Book Medical.

Jennett, B. (1976). Early complications after mild head injuries. *NZ Med. J.* **84**, 144–7.

Jennett, B. & Bond, M. (1975). Assessment of outcome after severe brain damage: a practical scale.' *Lancet* I, 480–4.

Jennett, B. & Teasdale, G. (1981). *Management of Head Injuries.* Philadelphia: F. A. Davis.

Jennett, B., Teasdale, G. & Braakman, R. (1976). Predicting outcome in individual patients after severe head injury. *Lancet* I, 1031–4.

Jennett, B., Snoek, J. & Bond, M. R. (1981). Disability after severe head injury observations on the use of the Glasgow Outcome Scale. *J. Neurol. Neurosurg. Psychiatry.* **44**, 285–93.

Kalsbeek, W. D., McLaurin, R. L. & Harris, B. S. H. (1980). The national head and spinal cord injury survey: major findings. *J. Neurosurg.* **53**(Suppl.), S19–S31.

Katz, D. I., Alexander, M. P. & Seliger, G. M. (1989). Traumatic basal ganglia hemorrhage: clinicopathologic features and outcome. *Neurology* **39**, 897–904.

Kaufman, H. H., Makela, M. E. & Lee, K. F. (1986). Gunshot wounds to the head: a perspective. *Neurosurgery* **18**, 689–95.

Kaufman, H. H. & Mattson, J. C. (1985). Coagulopathy in head injury. In *Central Nervous System Trauma Status Report 1985.* Bethesda: National Institute of Neurological and Communicative Disorders and Stroke.

Khalek, A. I. A. (1983). Head injuries persistent postconcussion symptoms. *Br. J. Clin. Pract.* [June], 209–11.

Klauber, M. R., Barrett-Connor, E. & Marshall, L. F. (1981). The epidemiology of head injury. A prospective study of an entire community: San Diego County, California, 1978. *Am. J. Epidemiol.* **113**, 500–9.

Kozloff, R. (1987). Networks of social support and the outcome from severe head injury. *J. Head Trauma Rehabil.* **2**, 14–23.

Kraus, J. F. (1993). Epidemiology of head injury. In *Head Injury.* Baltimore: Williams and Wilkins.

Kraus, J. F., Black, M. A. & Hessol, N. (1984). The incidence of acute brain injury and serious impairment in a defined population. *Am. J. Epidemiol.* **119**, 186–201.

Kriel, R. L., Krach, L. E. & Sheehan, M. (1988). Pediatric closed head injury: outcome following prolonged unconsciousness. *Arch. Phys. Med. Rehabil.* **69**, 678–81.

Kuhl, D. A., Boucher, B. A. & Muhlbauer, M. S. (1990). Prophylaxis of posttraumatic seizures. *DICP* **24**, 277–85.

Lam, A. M., Winn, H. R. & Cullen, B. F. (1991). Hyperglycemia and neurological outcome in patients with head injury. *J. Neurosurg.* **75**, 545–51.

Lee, J. P. & Wang, A. D.-J. (1991). Post-traumatic basal ganglia hemorrhages: analysis of 52 patients with emphasis on the final outcome. *J. Trauma* **31**, 376–80.

Leininger, B. E., Gramling, S. E. & Forrell, A. D. (1990). Neuropsychological deficits in symptomatic minor head injury patients after concussion and mild concussion. *J. Neurol. Neurosurg. Psychiatry* **33**, 293–6.

Levin, H. S., Eisenberg, H. M. & Miner, M. E. (1983). Neuropsychologic findings in head-injured children. In *Pediatric Head Trauma*. New York: Futura.

Levin, H. S., Mattis, S. & Ruff, R. M. (1987). Neurobehavioral outcome following minor head injury: a three-center study. *J. Neurosurg.* **66**, 234–43.

Levin, H. S., Saydjari, C. & Eisenberg, H. M. (1991). Vegetative state after closed-head injury. *Arch. Neurol.* **48**, 580–5.

Levin, H. S., Aldrich, E. F. & Eisenberg, H. M. (1992). Severe head injury in children: experience of the Traumatic Coma Data Bank. *Neurosurgery* **31**, 435–44.

Luerssen, T. G., Klauber, M. R. & Marshall, L. F. (1988). Outcome from head injury related to patients' age: a longitudinal prospective study of adult and pediatric head injury. *J. Neurosurg.* **68**, 409–16.

Lyle, D. M., Pierce, J. P. & Freeman, E. A. (1986). Clinical course and outcome of severe head injury in Australia. *J. Neurosurg.* **65**, 15–18.

Mahoney, W. J., D'Souza, B. J. & Haller, J. (1983). Long-term outcome of children with severe head trauma and prolonged coma. *Pediatrics* **71**, 756–62.

Mandleberg, I. A. & Brooks, D. N. (1975). Cognitive recovery after severe head injury, 1, serial testing on the Wechsler Adult Intelligence Scale. *J. Neurol. Neurosurg. Psychiatry* **38**, 1121–6.

Marshall, L. F., Smith, R. W. & Shapiro, H. M. (1979). The outcome with aggressive treatment in severe head injuries, part 1. The significance of intracranial pressure monitoring. *J. Neurosurg.* **50**, 20–5.

Marshall, L. F., Gautille, T. & Klauber, M. R. (1991). The outcome of severe closed head injury. *J. Neurosurg.* **75**(Suppl.), S28–S36.

Marshall, L. F., Marshall, S. B. & Klauber, M. R. (1991). A new classification of head injury based on computed tomography. *J. Neurosurg.* **75**(Suppl.), S14–S20.

Max, W., MacKenzie, E. J. & Rice, D. P. (1991). Head injuries: costs and consequences. *J. Head Trauma Rehabil.* **6**, 76–87.

Michaud, L. J., Rivara, F. P. & Longstreth, W. T. J. (1991). Elevated initial blood glucose levels and poor outcome following severe brain injuries in children. *J. Trauma* **31**, 1356–62.

Miller, J. D. & Pentland, B. (1989). The factors of age, alcohol, and multiple injury in patients with mild and moderate head injury. In *Mild to Moderate Head Injury*. Boston: Blackwell Scientific.

Miller, J. D., Butterworth, J. F. & Gudeman, S. K. (1981). Further experience in the management of severe head injury. *J. Neurosurg.* **54**, 289–99.

Miner, M. E., Kaufman, H. H. & Graham, S. H. (1982). Disseminated intravascular coagulation and fibrinolytic syndrome following head injury in children: frequency and prognostic implications. *J. Pediatr.* **100**, 687–91.

Murer, C. G. (1991). Coma to community. *Contin. Care* **10**(7), 26–7.

Nagib, M. G., Rockswold, G. L. & Sherman, R. S. (1986). Civilian gunshot wounds to the brain: prognosis and management. *Neurosurgery* **18**, 533–7.

Oppenheimer, D. R. (1968). Microscopic lesions in the brain following head injury. *J. Neurol. Neurosurg. Psychiatry* **31**, 299–306.

Povlishock, J. T., Becker, D. P. & Cheng, C. L. Y. (1983). Axonal change in minor head injury. *J. Neuropathol. Exp. Neurol.* **42**, 225–42.

Raimondi, A. J. & Samuelson, G. H. (1970). Craniocerebral gunshot wounds in civilian practice. *J. Neurosurg.* **32**, 647–53.

Rapp, R. P., Norton, J. A. & Young, B. Y. (1983). Cutaneous reactions in head-injured patients receiving phenytoin for seizure prophylaxis. *Neurosurgery* **13**, 272–5.

Rimel, R. W., Giordani, B. & Barth J. R. (1981), Disability caused by minor head injury. *Neurosurgery* **9**, 221–8.

Rimel, R. W., Giodani, B. & Barth, J. T. (1982). Moderate head injury: Completing the clinical spectrum of brain trauma. *Neurosurgery* **11**, 344–51.

Rish, B. L., Dillon, J. D. & Weiss, G. H. (1983). Mortality following penetrating craniocerebral injuries: an analysis of the deaths in the Vietnam Head Injury Registry population. *J. Neurosurg.* **59**, 775–80.

Ruff, R. M., Young, D. & Gautille, T. (1991). Verbal learning deficits following severe head injury: heterogeneity in recovery over 1 year. *J. Neurosurg.* **75**(Suppl.), S50–8.

Rutherford, W. H., Merrett, J. D. & McDonald, J. R. (1979). Symptoms at one year following concussion from minor head injuries. *Injury* **10**, 225–30.

Sabers, A., Heyn, J. & Karle, A. (1988). Computed tomography in brain concussion. *Ugeskr. Læg.* **150**, 1161–3.

Sahuquillo-Barris & Lamarca-Ciuro, J. (1988). Acute subdural hematoma and diffuse axonal injury after severe head injury. *J. Neurosurg.* **68**, 894–900.

Sorenson, S. & Kraus, J. F. (1991). Occurrence, severity, and outcomes of brain injury. *J. Head Trauma Rehabil.* **6**, 1–10.

Sosin, D. M., Sackes, J. J. & Smith, S. M. (1989). Head injury-associated deaths in the United States from 1979 to 1986. *JAMA* **262**, 2251–5.

Sparedo & Gill (1989). Effects of prior alcohol use on head injury recovery. *J. Head Trauma Rehabil.* **4**, 75–82.

Strich, S. J. (1956). Diffuse degeneration of the cerebral white matter in severe dementia following head injury. *J. Neurol. Neurosurg. Psychiatry* **19**, 163–85.

Symonds, C. (1937). The assessment of symptoms following head injury. *Guys Hosp. Gazette* **51**, 461–8.

Tabaddor, K., Mattis, S. & Iazula, T. (1984). Cognitive sequelae and recovery course after moderate and severe head injury. *Neurosurgery* **14**, 701–8.

Temkin, N. R., Dikman, S. S. & Wilensky, A. J. (1990). A randomized, double-blind study of phenytoin for the prevention of posttraumatic seizures. *N. Engl. J. Med.* **323**, 497–502.

Vazquez-Barquero, J. L., Gaite, L. & Diez-Manrique, J. F. (1991). The contribution of alcohol intoxication to head injuries. *Eur. J. Psychiatry* **5**, 216–23.

Vollmer, D. G., Torner, J. C. & Jane, J. A. (1991). Age and outcome following traumatic coma: why do older patients fare worse? *J. Neurosurg.* **75**(Suppl.), S37–S49.

Walker, M. C., Storrs, B. B. & Meyer, T. (1983). Factors affecting outcome in the pediatric patients with multiple trauma. *Concepts Pediatr. Neurosurg.* **4**, 243–52.

Walker, M. L., Mayer, T. A., Storrs, B. B. & Hylton, P. D. (1985). Pediatric head injury: factors which influence outcome. In *Concepts in Pediatric Neurosurgery*. Basel: Karger.

Weiss, G. H. & Salazar, A. M. (1986). Predicting posttraumatic epilepsy in penetrating head injury. *Arch. Neurol.* **43**, 771–3.

Whiteman, S., Coonley-Hoganson, R. & Desai, B. T. (1984). Comparative head trauma experiences in two socioeconomically different Chicago-area communities. A population study. *Am. J. Epidemiol.* **119**, 570–80.

Wilberger, J. E., Harris, M. & Diamond, D. C. (1991). Acute subdural hematoma: morbidity, mortality, and operative timing. *J. Neurosurg.* **74**, 212–18.

Young, B. Y., Rapp, R. P. & Norton, J. A. (1983a). Failure of prophylactically administered phenytoin to prevent early posttraumatic seizures. *J. Neurosurg.* **58**, 231–5.

Young, B. Y., Rapp, R. P. & Norton, J. A. (1983b). Failure of prophylactically administered phenytoin to prevent late posttraumatic seizures. *J. Neurosurg.* **58**, 236–41.

Young, B., Ott, L. & Dempsey, R. (1989). Relationship between admission hyperglycemia and neurologic outcome of severely brain-injured patients. *Ann. Surg.* **210**, 466–73.

Zimmerman, R. A., Bilamick, L. T., Bruce, D., Schut, L. & Uzzell, B. (1979). Computed tomography of craniocerebral injury in the abused child. *Radiology.* **130**, 687–90.

10 Outcomes in spinal cord injuries

H. L. FRANKEL

This chapter is confined to consideration of closed spinal cord injuries. The term paraplegia indicates paralysis of the lower limbs with sensory loss and involvement of bladder, bowel and autonomic functions. The term will be used for any clinically complete spinal cord lesion below the cervical cord. The term tetraplegia (quadraplegia) indicates a higher lesion causing, in addition, total or partial paralysis and sensory loss in the upper limbs. The terms paraplegia and tetraplegia, unless further defined, describe a clinically complete lesion. The terms paraparesis and quadraparesis are not used in this chapter but are widely used to describe incomplete lesions. The term 'paraplegia' has also been widely used to encompass both tetraplegia and paraplegia.

Descriptions and scales used to quantify initial severity of spinal cord lesion and outcomes

Until the late 1960s, descriptive terms were usually employed to describe initial severity such as 'complete', 'virtually complete' and 'incomplete'. Outcomes were described as 'unchanged', 'improved' and 'worse'. These descriptions enabled various authors to claim success for their chosen methods of treatment!

In 1969 Frankel *et al.* in a retrospective analysis of the outcome of non-surgical postural reduction of spinal injuries introduced a simple classification which was subsequently called the Frankel classification. This classification remained the standard for almost 20 years. The Frankel classification consists of the letters A–E as follows:

A *Complete*: the lesion is found to be complete, both motor and sensory, below the segmental level named.

B *Sensory incompleteness only*: implies that there is some sensation present below the level of the lesion but that the motor paralysis is complete below that level. This does not apply when there is slight discrepancy between motor and sensory levels but does apply to 'sacral sparing'.

C *Motor useless*: implies that there is some motor power present below the lesion but it is of no practical use to the patient.

D *Motor useful*: implies that there is useful motor power below the level of the lesion. Patients in this group can move the lower limbs and many can walk with or without aids.

E *Recovery*: implies that the patient is free of neurological symptoms, i.e. no weakness, no sensory loss, and no sphincter disturbance. Abnormal reflexes may be present.

Figures 10.1 and 10.2 show examples of the use of the Frankel classification.

A somewhat similar system with more emphasis on sensory functions was introduced by Bohlman in 1979 and modified by Bohlman *et al.* (1985). For prospective studies more sophisticated classifications were introduced such as the Yale Index (Bracken *et al.* 1978; Chehrazi *et al.* 1981). These methods require disciplined and uniform note keeping and were modified by the American Spinal Injuries Association (ASIA) into their standards for neurological classification for spinal cord injury in 1982.

The ASIA standards were revised in 1992 (Ditunno 1992). The American Spinal Injuries Association and the International Medical Society of Paraplegia (IMSOP) have now agreed to a very slight modification of the previous ASIA standards as the International Standards for Neurological and Functional Classification of Spinal Cord Injury (Ditunno 1994). The International Standard consists of routine 0–5 muscle testing of ten key muscles (Fig 10.3). Sensory testing for pin-prick and light touch is performed at key sensory points within 28 dermatomes on each side (both motor and sensory testing have been stereotyped so that testing can be performed by specially trained nurses and therapists). The ASIA/IMSOP Standards booklet also contains an outcome measure – the ASIA Impairment scale, which is graded A to E and is very similar to the Frankel scale.

The booklet also contains the functional independence measure (FIM) which enables independence of a patient admitted for rehabilitation to be assessed on admission and discharged (Centre for Functional Assessment Research 1990). The interinstitutional agreement of FIM has been demonstrated by Segal *et al.* (1993). FIM is an attempt to assess the outcome of the rehabilitation process. Research into the efficacy of individual components of a rehabilitation process is difficult and rarely shows a clear-cut benefit relative to other treatments or no treatment at all. There are, however, many methods of evaluating the outcome of the entire rehabilitation process. Whiteneck (1992) identifies six primary outcomes of spinal cord injury; impairment, disability, handicap, health, life satisfaction and cost. It is obvious that bulk purchasers of health care will show an increasing interest in this type of outcome measure.

Li, Houlden & Rowed (Li *et al.* 1990) performed an analysis of motor index score, pin-prick sensory score, joint sensation score, somatosensory evoked potential grade in the ulnar and posterior tibial regions and the overall somatosensory evoked potential grade from 36 patients with cervical cord injuries to determine the relationship of these scores, both individually and in combination, to functional outcomes (as determined in using the Barthel Index at 6 months after injury). The authors concluded that their

Cervical Injuries

SKELETAL INJURY			CORD INJURY									
			On admission					On discharge				
Type		Degree of reduction	A	B	C	D	E	A	B	C	D	E
Compression		Anatomical 13	5	1	1	6	–	–	2	1	7	3
Fractures	36	Residual wedge 20	9	5	4	2	–	4	4	2	9	1
		Partial 3	1	–	–	?	–	1	–	–	?	–
		Failed –	–	–	–	–	–	–	–	–	–	–
Burst		Anatomical 9	2	5	–	2	–	1	5	–	2	1
Fractures	12	Residual wedge 2	2	–	–	–	–	2	–	–	–	–
		Partial 1	–	1	–	–	–	–	1	–	–	–
		Failed –	–	–	–	–	–	–	–	–	–	–
Fracture–		Anatomical 37	16	5	4	12	–	9	3	4	14	7
Dislocations	129	Residual wedge 34	25	4	4	1	–	17	6	1	8	2
Displaced $<\frac{1}{2}$		Partial 50	32	8	5	5	–	28	4	6	9	3
		Failed 8	6	1	–	1	–	4	1	1	–	2
Fracture–		Anatomical 7	5	2	–	–	–	2	3	1	1	–
Dislocations	25	Residual wedge 4	3	–	1	–	–	3	–	–	1	–
Displaced $<\frac{1}{2}$		Partial 11	10	–	–	1	–	8	1	–	2	–
		Failed 3	2	–	–	1	–	2	–	–	–	1
No bony injury	16		5	1	2	8	–	3	1	–	11	1
Total	218		123	33	21	41	–	84	31	16	66	21

Fig. 10.1. Frankel Classification of cervical injuries. Reproduced from Frankel *et al.* (1969) with permission.

Cervical Injuries

AA 81	AB 21	AC 10	AD 11	AE 0
BA 3	BB 9	BC 2	BD 14	BE 5
CA 0	CB 1	CC 4	CD 11	CE 5
DA 0	DB 0	DC 0	DD 30	DE 11
EA 0	EB 0	EC 0	ED 0	EE 0

Fig. 10.2. Frankel Classification of cervical injuries. In each square of the grid are two letters of the alphabet, the first related to the neurological lesions on admission and the second to the neurological lesions on discharge. Reproduced from Frankel *et al.* (1969) with permission.

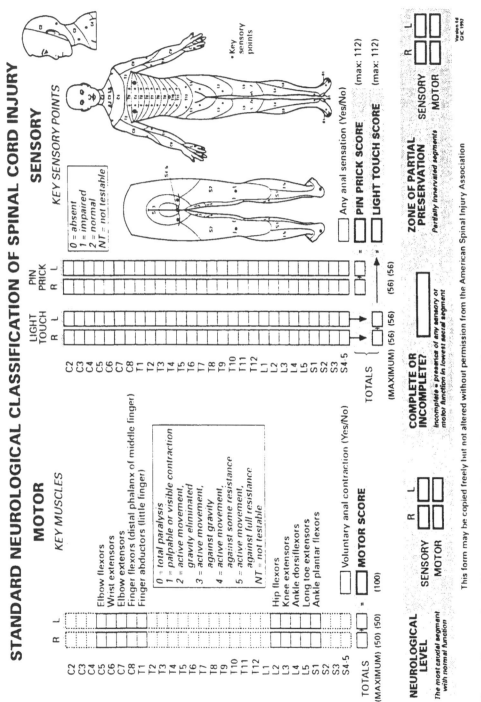

Fig. 10.3. Key muscles and key sensory points for the ASIA/IMSOP standards.

study confirmed the prognostic value of quantitative somatosensory evoked potential analysis for patients with acute spinal cord injuries.

Prognostic value of MRI

Kulkarni *et al.* (1987) described three types of magnetic resonance imaging (MRI) signal pattern in the acute phase of spinal cord injury. Pattern I was where the T1 weighted image was inhomogenous and the T2 weighted image showed a large central area of hypointensity and a thin rim of hyperintensity. The authors concluded that this pattern was due to intra-spinal haemorrhage and the patients had severe or complete neurological lesions and did not recover. Pattern II showed normal T1 weighted images and in the T2 weighted images there was central and peripheral hyperintensity and this was deduced to be due to cord oedema and contusion. These patients had predominantly incomplete spinal lesions with subsequent improvement. Type III had normal T1 weighted images and in the T2 weighted images a small central area of hypointensity and a thick rim of hyperintensity at the periphery. This method of classification was also used by Bondurante *et al.* (1990) in a larger series, which possibly included some from Kulkarni *et al.* (1987). Ten patients with Type I images had complete lesions that remained complete. In Type II, four patients with initially complete lesions recoverd partially. Six patients with incomplete lesions improved and one remained unchanged, five patients had no neurological lesion either at onset or at follow-up. There were only three patients with Type III injury, all of whom improved. These authors also found three patients with normal MRI images who had clinical cord lesions, all of them improved.

Schaefer *et al.* (1992) used a similar classification, but based on T2 images only. They based their findings on the median recovery of motor scores (ASIA). In Group 1 in 21 patients they found a 9% median motor recovery. In group 2 in 17 patients, a 41% median motor recovery and in group 3 in 19 patients, a 72% median motor recovery.

Sato *et al.* (1994) also found that patients with slightly low intensity on T1 weighted images and low intensity on T2 weighted images in the acute MRI had complete or severe lesions and did not recover. They also described patterns of development of the MRI signals over time; these later changes, although of interest, add little to the prognosis.

It seems that most of the prognostic value of MRI in the acute stage is related to the density of the clinical lesion. However, MRI might predict those patients with initially complete lesions who have a potential for partial recovery.

Outcome

Survival

The natural history of complete tetraplegia is for the patient to die of respiratory complications within the first week or two after injury. Inability to cough leads to retained secretions and, in the absence of any intervention, to the early death of the patient. The natural history of complete traumatic paraplegia is for the patient to develop severe pressure sores and urinary tract complications and to die of one or other or a combination of these within 1 year of injury (Thomson-Walker 1937).

This natural history is of course never seen today. Since the development of spinal injuries centres during the Second World War simple methods of preventing life-threatening complications have been evolved. It is not possible to give a meaningful figure of early survival for spinal cord injuries as the result depends largely on the level of the injury, presence of associated injuries and whether the first hours after injury are included in the figures. Gerhart (1991) reported a fatality rate during hospitalization of less than 4%. Devivo *et al*. 1990 compared patients aged at least 61 years at injury with those aged 16–30 years. They found a greatly increased incidence of complications in the older age group. The 2 year survival rate was 59% for patients aged 61–86 years and 95% for patients aged 16–30 years.

Long-term survival

Geisler *et al*. (1983) calculated the life expectancy of complete and incomplete tetra-plegics and complete and incomplete paraplegics who had survived the first year after injury; the patients had all been treated in the same centre in Toronto. They calculated the relative mortality of each group of patients against the general population and found that for complete tetraplegics it was 7.67, incomplete tetraplegics 2.09, for complete paraplegics 3.18 and for incomplete paraplegics 1.86. This study remains the most comprehensive study published so far. Whiteneck *et al*. (1992) in a study that concentrated on morbidity found that in England survival was somewhat better.

Progression of traumatic spinal cord lesions

From the clinical standpoint, in the majority of cases, the neurological deficit is maximal immediately after the injury. The ascent of the lesion by one or at the most two spinal cord segments within the first 3 or 4 days is by no means unusual and is almost always followed by recovery to the original level and often to a level one segment lower than that. Occasionally a more serious form of ascending lesion occurs (Frankel 1969). In those cases the level of the lesion can ascend by many segments. The onset of this phenomenon is usually between the second and eleventh days and the lesion ascends segment by segment over a number of days. The phenomenon is usually associated with pyrexia and sometimes with severe pain in the segments which are about to be lost. These ascending lesions are most common in patients with dorso-lumbar lesions and in one personal case the lesion rose from L4 to C8. The incidence of the phenomenon with dorsolumbar lesions is probably between 1.5% and 2%. The pathology in these cases is uncertain. It is also unlikely that the pathology is the same in all cases. The most obvious aetiologies are ascending thrombosis and ascending haematomyelia. The possibility of extrinsic compression by extending haematoma has to be excluded. In my opinion the majority of cases are due to an inflammatory or necrotizing lesion which, for lack of a better term I would call 'ascending myelitis'. For this reason, I treat such patients with systemic corticosteroids once the lesion has ascended more than two segments. It is also reasonable to treat patients whose lesions go up one or two segments with corticosteroids, even though this rise is usually temporary. The aetiology in these cases is probably post-traumatic oedema. In a patient who already has a lesion below C4 or C5, ascent of the lesion is life-threatening.

Neurological outcome

The prognosis of groups of patients treated at Stoke Mandeville Hospital by conservative means (without open surgery, usually by postural reduction and in cervical cases, with the use of skull traction) is shown in Figure 10.1 and 10.2. From these figures it will be seen that there was a correlation between severity of spinal dislocation and the initial and final neurological result. There is, however, no correlation between the degree of reduction achieved and the improvement in neurological status. There are individual cases where gross dislocations are associated with slight neurological lesions.

In the cervical region in spite of having an initially clinically complete lesion, 17% of patients improve from group A to group C or D. Patients who had initially incomplete lesions fared very much better. This is in keeping with the statement of Stauffer (1984) that 'partial lesions recover partially' and 'the less the injury the greater the recovery'. I cannot agree with Stauffer's statement that 'complete cord lesions do not recover cord functional motor control'. Our Stoke Mandeville results shown in Figures 10.1 and 10.2 have been confirmed by Maynard *et al.* (1979) and Young & Dexter (1978).

For patients with thoracic injuries Frankel *et al.* (1969) found fewer incomplete cases than in the cervical region and even in this group 7.4% improved from Grade A to C, D or E. This finding is at variance with that of Bohlman *et al.* (1985).

Surgical interventions

There have been no prospective controlled trials of surgery against conservative management of spinal cord injuries and it would be extremely difficult to organize such trials. Using retrospective analysis on groups of patients it has not been possible to demonstrate any improvement in neurological function as a result of early surgery (Young & Dexter 1978; Bohlman, Freehaffer & Dejak 1985; Hardy 1965). In a study of cervical injuries, Donovan, Cifu & Schotte (1992) found that the neurological recovery did not depend on surgical versus non-surgical treatment; they demonstrated significantly less vertebral angulation, more rapid stabilization and less anterior callus formation amongst the patients in the surgical group. In addition, the surgical patients had

Table 10.1. *Physical rehabilitation after C3-level lesion. Lowest muscles; sternomastoid; trapezius part; diaphragm – part*

Independent	Assisted		Dependent
Talking	Breathing – **ventilator**, part or full time		Drinking
Swallowing	Coughing		Feeding
	Writing	⎫	Turning
	Typing	**mouthstick** or **Possum** or	Lifting
	Computer operation ⎬	**other environmental**	
		controls	Washing
	Telephoning		Shaving
	Environmental controls – **Possum**		Dressing
	Electric wheelchair		Bowels
			Urinal
			Transfers – sometimes
			hoist
			Car – **special safety belt**

From Frankel (1990)

marginally shorter lengths of hospitalization. Murphy *et al.* (1990) found that patients with cervical cord injuries treated with early surgical stabilization of the cervical column were hospitalized a mean of 21 days fewer than their non-surgical counterparts; at final follow-up however, no appreciable differences in achievement in activities of daily living and mobility were noted between patients treated with surgical stabilization of the cervical spinal column and those treated non-surgically. There was some evidence that laminectomy may worsen the neurological prognosis (Holdsworth & Hardy 1953; Holdsworth 1970; Morgan, Wharton & Austin 1971).

Piepmeier & Collins (1992), in a comprehensive review of the literature, confirmed the positive correlation between the status on admission and outcome regardless of the method of management. The percentage in each functional group that improved or deteriorated was generally similar.

Pharmacological interventions

The NASCIS1 trial (Bracken 1984) showed no difference in neurological outcome between 1000 mg of methylprednisolone daily for 10 days and 100 mg of methylprednisolone daily for 10 days. The NASCIS2 trial (Bracken *et al.* 1990, 1993) was a double-blind prospective trial of methylprednisolone, naloxone and placebo. Methylprednisolone was given to 162 patients as a bolus of 30 mg/kg body weight followed by an infusion of 5.4 mg/kg per hour for 23 hours. Naloxone was given to 154 patients as a bolus of 5.4 mg/kg followed by infusion at 4.0 mg/kg per hour for 23 hours. Placebo was given to 171 patients by bolus infusion. The neurological assessments were performed on admission, 6 weeks and 6 months after injury, the method of examination was that of Bracken *et al.* (1978). After 6 months the patients who were treated with methylpred

Table 10.2. *Physical rehabilitation after C4-level lesion. Lowest muscles: trapezius; rhomboid; diaphragm – part*

Independent	Assisted	Dependent
Talking	Coughing	Feeding
Swallowing	Writing – **mouthstick**	Turning
Breathing	Typing – **electric continuous paper**	**Lifting**
	Computer operation	**Washing**
	Telephoning – possum and other adaption	Dressing
	Environmental controls – **Possum**	Bowels
	Shaving – **electric razor on stand**	Urinal
	Electric wheelchair	Transfers – sometimes **hoist**
	Drinking	Car – **special safety belt**

From Frankel (1990)

Table 10.3 *Physical rehabilitation after C5-level lesion. Lowest muscles: deltoids; biceps; diaphragm*

Independent	Assisted	Dependent
Talking	Coughing	Bowels
Swallowing	Feeding – help with cutting	Urinal
Breathing		
Drinking – **Thermos mug**		
Teeth cleaning – **strap to hold brush**		
Hair brushing – **strap to hold brush**	Transfers – sometimes **hoist**	Car
Make-up (some)	Turning	
Push self-propelled **wheelchair** on flat surface	Lifting	
Writing – **pen holder**	Washing	
Typing – **electric typewriter**	Dressing	
Telephoning – **Possum** or **adaptation**		
Feeding (easy food)		
Shaving – **electric shaver**		

From Frankel (1990)

nisilone within 8 hours of their injury had significant improvement, as compared with those given placebo, in motor function and sensation. Following publication of these results this method of treatment has been widely adopted in the USA. The method did not gain immediate acceptance in the United Kingdom, partly because of premature disclosure of the results and due to the lack of information about the effects of therapy on the level of the lesion relative to the density of the lesion. This information was eventually released (Bracken & Holford 1993). The authors conclude that the greatest proportion of all neurological recovery attributed to methylprednisolone treatment administered early after injury occurred below the lesion although there was a relatively small improvement in the injury level. This method of treatment is still only used sporadically in the United Kingdom, where clinicians still fear the side effects of the

Table 10.4 *Physical rehabilitation after C6-level lesion. Lowest muscles: brachioradialis; extensor carpi radialis longus; triceps – sometimes*

Independent	Assisted	Dependent
As C5 plus:		
Typing – **standard typewriter**	Coughing	Bowels
Feeding	Turning	Urinal
Teeth cleaning		
Hair brushing		
Hair washing		
Lifting (most)		Car (some)
Dressing (some)	Dressing (some)	
Cooking (easy)		
Kitchen work	Cooking (difficult)	
Writing (some) – no aid		
Transfers (some) using **sliding board**	Transfers – (some) **hoist** or manual	
Push **wheelchair** up incline 1 in 15	Standing – in **standing frame**	
Car (some) – **hand-controlled car, automatic gearbox**	Family shopping	

From Frankel (1990)

Table 10.5 *Physical rehabilitation after C7-level lesion. Lowest muscles: triceps; wrist flexors*

Independent	Assisted	Dependent
As C6 plus:		
Turning (most)	Coughing	Bowels (some)
Washing (most)	Turning (few)	Urinal (some)
Dressing (most)	Washing (some)	Car (some)
Wheelchair – 'back wheel balance' (some)	Dressing (few)	
Bowels (few) – **suppository insertor**	Transfers (few) – **hoist** or manual	
Urinal (some) apply and empty	Standing in **standing frame**	
Transfers (most) – some using **sliding board**		
Family shopping (some)	Family shopping (most)	
Car (some) – **hand-controlled, automatic gearbox**		
Chair into car (some)		

From Frankel (1990)

treatment. Since the first publication of the NASCIS2 trial it has become ethically very difficult to mount any further prospective trials that do not include methylprednisolone in this exact dosage. The NASCIS2 trial represents a serious attempt to evaluate pharmacological treatment and it is extremely difficult to mount prospective trials of any therapy for closed spinal cord injuries as the outcome is so variable. When the full data from the NASCIS2 trial is eventually thrown open for inspection, the placebo data is likely to be an invaluable database for other workers.

Table 10.6 *Physical rehabilitation after C8-level lesion. Lowest muscles: finger extensors, finger flexors*

Independent	Assisted	Dependent
As C7 plus: Turning	Coughing with respiratory infection	
Washing		
Dressing	Ambulate with **calipers** in parallel	
Transfers	bars (not usually attempted)	
Full control of **wheelchair** – can mount 15 cm kerb		
Car – **hand controls, automatic gearbox**		
Chair into car (most)		
Bowels		
Urinals		
Standing – in **standing frame**		

From Frankel (1990)

Geisler *et al.* (1991) reported a double-blind controlled trial of a ganglioside, GM-1. Dosage of 100 mg per day for 18–32 days was started at 48–72 hours after injury. The 18 treated patients were compared with placebo treatment at one year following injury and found to have a greater return of motor function and a greater chance of improvement of 2 Frankel Grades. If these results are confirmed it would indicate that pharmacological agents administered 48 hours after injury may still affect the neurological outcome (in this trial patients were also given methylprednisolone 250 mg intravenously followed by 125 mg intravenously 6-hourly for 72 hours).

Other medical management, nursing and therapy

There are no clearly defined outcomes of various medical interventions in the management of the paralysed patient. The development of pressure sores is unfortunately still quite common but can be almost completely avoided if patients are transferred to a spinal injuries centre within the first few hours of the injury. Likewise therapy is very effective in preventing complications such as contractures but there is no statistical proof that any particular component of the therapy is superior to other methods of performing the same task. Useful accounts of therapy techniques are given by Bromley (1991) and Bergstrom & Rose (1992).

The final functional capacity of patients with spinal cord lesions is infinitely varied in those with incomplete lesions. For those with complete lesions the best expected outcome can be documented (Frankel 1990). The best expected outcome at every segmental level from C3 to C8 is shown in Tables 10.1 to 10.6. It can be seen that with every additional segment independence increases markedly.

Motivation and age greatly influence the outcome in individual cases. Bergstrom *et al.* (1985) studied the physical ability, in particular the ability to do independent transfers, in patients with complete lesions below the C6 segment. They demonstrated influence of anthroprometic measurements in the achievment of this particular function.

References

Bergstrom, E. M. K., Frankel, H. L., Galer, I. A. R., Haycock, E. L., Jones, P. R. M. & Rose, L. S. (1985). Physical ability in relation to anthropometric measurments in persons with complete spinal cord lesion below the sixth cervical segment. *Int. Rehabil. Med.* **7**, 51–5.

Bergstrom, E. M. K. & Rose, L. S. (1992). Physical rehabilitation: principles and outcome. (1992) In *Handbook of Clinical Neurology: Spinal Cord Trauma*, rev. edn., ed. P. J. Vinken, G. W. Bruyn, H. L. Klawans & H. L. Frankel. Amsterdam, Elsevier Science Publishers, pp. 457–78.

Bohlman, H. H. (1979). Acute fractures and dislocations of the cervical spine. *J. Bone Joint Surg.* **61A**, 1119–42.

Bohlman, H. H., Freehaffer, A. & Dejak, J. (1985). The results of treatment of acute injuries of the upper thoracic spine with paralysis. *J. Bone Joint Surg.* **67A**, 360–9.

Bondurante, F. J., Cotler, H. B., Kulkarni, M. V., McArdle, C. B. & Harris, J. H. (1990). Acute spinal cord injury: a study using physical examination and magnetic resonance imaging. *Spine,* **15**, 161–8.

Bracken, M. B. & Holford, T. R. (1993). Effects of timing of methylprednisolone or naloxone administration on recovery of segmental and long-tract neurological function in NACSIS2. *J. Neurosurg.* **79**, 500–7.

Bracken, M. B., Webb, S. B. & Wagner, F. C. (1978). Classification of the severity of acute spinal cord injury: implications for management. *Paraplegia,* **15**, 319–26.

Bracken, M. B. *et al.* (1984). Efficacy of Methyl Prednisolone in acute SCI. *J. Amer. Med. Assoc.,* **251**, 45–52.

Bracken, M. B. *et al.* (1990). A randomized, controlled trial of methylprednisolone or naloxone in the treatment of acute spinal cord injury. *N. Engl. J. Med.,* **322**(20), 1405–11

Bromley, I. (1991). *Tetraplegia and Paraplegia. A Guide for Physiotherapists*, 4th edn. London: Churchill Livingstone.

Chehrazi, B., Wagner, F. C. Jr, Collins, W. F. Jr, & Freeman, D. H. Jr, (1981). A scale for evaluation of spinal cord injury. *J. Neurosurg.* **54**, 310–15.

DeVivo, M. J., Kartus, P. L., Rutt, R. D., Stover, S. L. & Fine, P. R. (1990). The influence of age at time of spinal cord injury on rehabilitation outcome. *Arch. Neurol.* **47**, 687–91.

Ditunno, J. F. Jr. (1992). Functional assessment measures in CNS trauma. *J. Neurotrauma,* **9** (Suppl. 1), S301–5.

Ditunno, J. F. Jr. (1994). The International Standards Booklet for Neurological and Functional Classification of Spinal Cord Injury. *Paraplegia,* **32**, 70–80.

Donovan, W. H., Cifu, D. X. & Schotte, D. E. (1992). Neurological and skeletal outcomes in 113 patients with closed injuries to the cervical spinal cord. *Paraplegia* **30**(8), 533–42.

Frankel, H. L. (1969). Ascending cord lesion in the early stages following spinal cord injury. *Paraplegia* **7**, 111–18.

Frankel, H. L. (1990). Spinal trauma – neurological assessment and rehabilitation. In *Spinal Surgery: Science and Practice*, ed. R. A. Dickson. Butterworths, London, pp. 324–36.

Frankel, H. L., Hancock, D. O. & Hyslop, G., Melzak, J., Michaelis, L. S., Ungar, G. H., Vernon, J. D. S. & Walsh, J. J. (1969). The value of postural reduction in the initial management of closed injuries of the spine with paraplegia and tetraplegia. *Paraplegia* 7, 179–92.

Geisler, W. O., Jousse, A. T., Wynne-Jones, M. & Breithaupt, D. (1983). Survival in traumatic spinal cord injury. *Paraplegia* 21, 364–73.

Geisler, F. H., Dorsey, F. C. & Coleman, W. P. (1991). Recovery of motor function after spinal cord injury – a randomized placebo-controlled trial with GM-1 Ganglioside. *N. Engl. J. Med.*, 324(26), 1829–38

Gerhart, K. A., (1991). Spinal cord injury outcomes in a population based sample. *J. Trauma*, 31(11), 1529–35.

Hardy, A. G. (1965). The treatment of paraplegia due to fracture dislocations of the dorso-lumber spine. *Paraplegia* 3, 112.

Holdsworth, F. (1970). Fractures, dislocations and fracture-dislocations of the spine. *J. Bone Joint Surg.* 52A, 1534–51.

Holdsworth, F. W. & Hardy, A. G. (1953). Early treatment of paraplegia from fractures of the thoraco-lumbar spine. *J. Bone Joint Surg.* 35B, 540–50.

Kulkarni, M. V., McArdle, C. B., Kopanicky, D., Miner, M., Cotler, H. B., Lee, K. F. & Harris, J. H. (1987). Acute spinal cord injury: MR imaging at 1.5 T¹. *Neuroradiology*, 164(3), 837–43.

Li-C., Houlden, D. A. & Rowed, D. W. (1990). Somatosensory evoked potentials and neurological grades and predictors of outcome in acute spinal cord injury. *J. Neurosurg.* 72, 600–9.

Maynard, F. M., Reynolds, G. G., Fountain, S., Wilmot, C. & Hamilton, R. (1979). Neurological prognosis after traumatic quadraplegia. Three year experience of California Regional Spinal Cord Injury Care System. *J. Neurosurg.*, 50, 611–16.

Morgan, T. H., Wharton, G. W. & Austin, G. M. (1971). The results of laminectomy in patients with incomplete spinal cord injuries. *Paraplegia* 9, 14–23.

Murphy, K. P., Opitz, J. L., Cabanela, M. E. & Ebersold, M. J. (1990). Cervical fractures and spinal cord injury: outcome of surgical and nonsurgical management. *Mayo Clin. Proc.* 65, 949–59.

Piepmeier, J. M. & Collins, W. F. (1992). Recovery of function following spinal cord injury. In *Handbook of Clinical Neurology: Spinal Cord Trauma*, rev. edn., ed. P. J. Vinken, G. W. Bruyn, H. L. Klawans & H. L. Frankel. Amsterdam, Elsevier Science Publishers, pp. 421–33.

Sato, T., Kokubun, S. Rijal, K. P., Ojima, T., Moriai, N., Hashimoto, M., Hyodo, H. & Oonuma, H. (1994). Prognosis of cervical spinal cord injury in correlation with magnetic resonance imaging. *Paraplegia*, 32, 81–5.

Schaefer, D. M., Flanders, A. E., Osterholm, J. L. & Northrup, B. E. (1992). Prognostic significance of magnetic resonance imaging in the acute phase of cervical spine injury. *J. Neurosurg.*, 76, 218–23.

Segal, M. E., Ditunno, J. F. & Staas, W. E. (1993). Interinstitutional agreement of individual functional independence measure (FIM) items measured at two sites on one sample of SCI patients. *Paraplegia*, 31, 622–31.

Stauffer, E. S. (1984). Neurologic recovery following injuries to the cervical spinal cord and nerve roots. *Spine* 9, 532–4.

Thomson-Walker, Sir J. (1937). The treatment of the bladder in spinal injuries in war. *Br. J. Urol.*, 9, 217–30.

Whiteneck, G. G. (1992). Outcome evaluation and spinal cord injury. *Neurorehabilitation*, 2(4), 31–41.

Whiteneck, G. G., Charlifue, M. A., Frankel, H. L., Fraser, M. H., Gardner, B. P., Gerhart, K. A., Krishnan, K. R., Menter, R. R., Nuseibeh, I., Short, D. J. & Silver, J. R. (1992). Mortality, morbidity, and psychosocial outcomes of persons spinal cord injured more than 20 years ago. *Paraplegia*, **30**(9), 617–30.

Young, J. S. & Dexter, W. R. (1978). Neurological recovery distal to the zone of injury in 172 cases of closed, traumatic spinal cord injury. *Paraplegia* **16**, 39–49.

11 Extrinsic lesions of the CNS

H. I. SABIN

In this chapter the focus will be restricted to the following:

> Tumours of the meninges
> Tumours of the nerve sheaths
>> Acoustic neuroma
>> Trigeminal neuroma
>> Jugular neuroma
> Tumours of developmental origin
>> Dermoid and epidermoid cysts
>> Craniopharyngiomas
>> Colloid cysts
> Tumours involving the nervous system secondarily
>> Chemodectomas (glomus tumours)
>> Chordomas and chondrosarcomas

Pituitary tumours and vascular developmental abnormality are covered elsewhere in this book (Chapters 7 and 12).

Neurosurgery has evolved rapidly, helped by development of reliable anaesthesia, excellent preoperative imaging, improved microscopes, specialist microinstruments and a better understanding of the pathophysiology of the nervous system. Large strides are being made in the subspecialties of paediatric, spinal, oncologic, neurovascular and skull base surgery, with surgeons now tackling problems which would have been considered inoperable only a decade ago. Such major changes in surgical practice make it difficult to include the older series in this chapter for as the techniques change so do the outcomes. Even the risks of general complications such as deep venous thrombosis and pneumonia have been modified by early postoperative mobilization, aggressive physiotherapy and the use of perioperative prophylaxis such as subcutaneous heparin. Wherever possible, large, recent series have been consulted in an attempt to establish the current mortality and morbidity for each of the lesions covered. However, it is disappointing to note that although many of the publications list the complications of surgery for these diseases, most do not objectively assess the overall outcome in terms of postoperative functional state, quality of life and patient satisfaction with treatment. Most rely on relatively subjective grading using terms such

Table 11.1. *The grading of meningioma excision related to the risk of symptomatic recurrence (Simpson 1957)*

Grade	Description	Recurrence (%)
I	Complete macroscopic resection of tumour, dural attachment and abnormal bone	9
II	Complete macroscopic resection of tumour and visible extensions with diathermy of dural origin	19
III	Complete macroscopic resection of tumour without resection or diathermy of attachment	29
IV	Partial resection, leaving obvious tumour behind	44
V	Simple decompression	N/A

as 'excellent outcome' or 'good result' within arbitrary scales devised by the authors of each paper.

Tumours of the meninges

Meningiomas form approximately 15% of the total number of intracranial tumours. They can occur anywhere that arachnoidal cell rests exist; from skull base to convexity as well as intraventricular sites. Although benign histologically, they do not always run a benign clinical course and their location can make resection particularly hazardous. In addition to the risks of surgery there is the additional risk of recurrence if excision is not complete.

Recurrence

Meningiomas are generally regarded as having a favourable outcome after resection, and indeed many can be resected with permanent cure. Some, however, will recur even when removal appears total. The reasons for recurrences were thoughtfully presented by Donald Simpson in 1957 in a series of 242 tumours treated in Oxford between 1938 and 1954, and in a further 97 tumours treated at the London Hospital by Sir Hugh Cairns. He found that 55 patients had developed symptomatic recurrences, 44 in the Oxford series and 11 in the London series (combined incidence of 21%). This must have been an underestimate as imaging techniques were crude and the length of follow-up in the Oxford series was no longer than 17 years. His conclusions were that the incidence of recurrence varied according to the experience of the surgeon and the adequacy of surgery (Table 11.1).

The possibility of achieving a 'grade I' resection varies according to the site of origin with convexity tumours being easier to remove completely than the basal meningiomas. The same remains true even with modern methods and recurrence remains a source of considerable concern. It is, however, difficult to estimate the incidence of recurrence in many of the recent series owing to the small patient numbers, often presented with a relatively short follow-up, usually in relation to a new surgical approach. Clearly, the treatment of meningioma is evolving.

For the assessment of recurrence to be accurate, follow-up has to be prolonged. If the tumour doubling rate is 1000 days, it will take many years for the recurrence to be visible on a CT scan. Meningioma doubling times are very variable, ranging from 50 to 500 days (Phillippou & Cornu 1991). Table 11.2 records the estimated risk of incomplete resection and/or recurrence by region. It must be emphasized that the relatively high risk quoted for some regions does not in itself argue against an attempt at complete removal – the concept that radical resection carries the best chance of cure still applies. Most of the operations that were not curative, however, were halted in an attempt to reduce the morbidity associated with the stripping of tumours from vital structures. It must also be appreciated that these figures do not imply symptomatic recurrence –

Table 11.2. Risk of recurrence or incomplete resection related to meningioma origin

Origin	Surgical approach	Recurrence/incomplete resection	Reference
Foramen magnum	Far lateral	0.5%	Meyer et al. 1984
	Postero-lateral		Guidetti & Spallone 1988
	Transoral (rare, selected)		Hakuba & Tsujimoto 1993
Clivus	Mid third: Retrosigmoid (small tumours)		Mayberg & Symon 1986
	Lower third: Far lateral		Samii et al. 1989
	Upper third: Cranio-orbito-zygomatic transylvian		
	Complex: Lateral infratemporal fossa	30–60%	Sekhar et al. 1993
	Combined supra-infratentorial		Couldwell et al. 1996
	Petrosectomy/transcochlear		
Sphenoid wing/clinoidal	Pterional ± zygomatic osteotomy		Al-Mefty 1991
Cavernous sinus	Cranio-orbital	16–38%	Sekhar et al. 1993
			DeMonte et al. 1994
			Cusimano et al. 1995
			Knosp et al. 1996
Convexity	Standard craniotomy flap over		Simpson 1957
Parasagittal	the tumour origin	9–25%	Baird & Gallagher 1989
			Phillipou & Cornu 1991
			Samii et al. 1996
Tentorial	Supracerebellar/infratentorial	Approx. 20%	
	Suboccipital		
	Combined supra/infratentorial		
Intraventricular	Transcortical	0–10%	Crisculo & Symon 1986
	Transcallosal		Guidetti & Delfini 1991
Olfactory groove	Subfrontal		Kadis et al. 1979
Suprasellar	Pterional	0–60%	Symon & Rosenstein 1984
			Ojemann 1991
			Al-Mefty & Smith 1991

generally these rates are much lower, but will probably increase as the length of follow-up increases.

Morbidity/mortality

As surgeons develop new techniques for the resection of tumours previously considered 'inoperable' the complications from surgery inevitably increase. This is balanced to a certain extent by developments in surgical equipment, imaging, neurophysiological monitoring and anaesthesia. The morbidity following meningioma resection is shown in Table 11.3. The question of how radical an attempt at resection should be in areas such as the cavernous sinus is still being debated. The microanatomy of the region has now been well described and radical removal is tempting as theoretically it allows the patient the chance of cure. The principal morbidity is secondary to injury to the carotid artery or the cranial nerves leading to stroke, ophthalmoplegia and facial sensory loss. Diplopia is particularly disabling and should be avoided wherever possible. It has been stated that in 90% of cases the diplopia resulting from cavernous sinus surgery is transient and will recover with time but extension of the resection of a clinoid meningioma into the cavernous sinus may lead to an unacceptable deficit. Removal of the tumour to a point flush with the lateral wall of the sinus and stereotactic radiotherapy in the event of disease progression may be a better option.

The carotid artery is often intimately involved with the tumour and there is a grave risk of injury if attempts are made to strip the tumour free of the arterial wall. There is general agreement that the artery should not be resected in an attempt to achieve cure as there is likely to be microscopic disease remaining around the cranial nerves in the cavernous sinus which may well lead to recurrence in the future. The risk of stroke is also a concern. A bypass graft can be used between the petrous carotid and the supraclinoid carotid but generally requires 120 minutes to perform and if the patient can tolerate this period of arterial occlusion he or she is likely to have sufficient collateral circulation not to require the bypass.

Petroclival tumours are also particularly difficult to resect without significant morbidity. It has been said that there are two types of petroclival tumour: those that are too large to resect and those that are too small. It is difficult, however, to allow a patient to become progressively disabled as a result of neuraxis compression without at least attempting to relieve that compression. Unfortunately non-surgical methods of treatment are not yet effective: neither radiotherapy nor hormonal manipulation seem to influence their progression.

Tumours of the nerve sheaths

Acoustic neuromas

The outcome information on acoustic neuromas presented here relates to those individuals with sporadic tumours, not associated with neurofibromatosis 2 (NF2). Presen-

Table 11.3. *Mortality and principal morbidity following meningioma resection*

Site	Morbidity		Mortality	Reference
Foramen magnum	Respiratory failure			George *et al.* 1988
	Vertebral artery injury			Hakuba & Tsujimoto 1993
	CSF leak		10–21%	Sen & Sekhar 1993
	Lower cranial nerve deficit			
	Craniovertebral instability			
Petroclival	Vascular injury	7%		Mayberg & Symon 1986
	Cranial nerve deficits	10–50%		Al-Mefty *et al.* 1988
	Pneumonia	12%	0–9%	Samii *et al.* 1989
	CSF leak	22%		Sekhar *et al.* 1990
	Epilepsy	7%		Sekhar *et al.* 1993
Sphenoid wing/clinoidal	Eye movement disorder	13–50%		Al-Mefty & Smith 1988
Cavernous sinus	Trigeminal disturbance	6–30%		Sekhar *et al.* 1989
	Vascular injury	3–10%	0–6%	DeMonte *et al.* 1994
	CSF leak	5–28%		Rigi *et al.* 1994
	Visual loss	2–18%		Cusimano *et al.* 1995
				Knosp *et al.* 1996
Olfactory groove	Visual deterioration	3–25%		Symon & Rosenstein 1984
Parasellar	Early epilepsy	6%		Al-Mefty & Smith 1991
	Late epilepsy	11%		Ojemann 1991
	Permanent diabetes insipidus	5%	4–8%	Kinjo *et al.* 1995
	Hypopituitarism	4%		
	CSF leak	4–6%		
	Vascular injury	1%		
Convexity	Epilepsy	17–50%		Foy *et al.* 1981
Parasagittal	Cerebral swelling		3–7%	Chan & Thompson 1984
	Haematoma			Giombini *et al.* 1984
				Giombini & Fornari 1991

ting symptoms and signs of these tumours include deafness, ataxia and tinnitus. Postoperatively these are likely to be unchanged or worse, but all too often there are, in addition, signs of trigeminal, facial and lower cranial nerve damage. The treatment of acoustic neuromas has changed within the last decade with the introduction of MRI, radiosurgery, intraoperative monitoring of cranial nerve function and the evolution of surgical techniques. It has become clear that many of the tumours grow only very slowly and when found in an elderly patient may well not require treatment. Serial MRI scans allow these to be followed non-invasively.

Table 11.4. *Operative approaches: acoustic neuroma*

Approach	Indication	Disadvantage
1 Suboccipital retromastoid	Attempted hearing preservation	More risk to the facial nerve compared with translabyrinthine approach
	Tumour $<$ 2.5 cm diameter	
	Good preoperative hearing	Scar pain/headaches
	Distal porus free of tumour	
2 Translabyrinthine	Large tumours or all tumours if preoperative hearing poor, or tumour extends to the labyrinth/cochlea	Inevitable hearing loss Large bone defect
3 Middle fossa	Hearing preservation	Slight increase in risk of injury to facial nerve
	Tumour not extending to labyrinthe	Limited access
	Not projecting into the CP angle $>$ 1.5 cm	

Table 11.5. *Outcome of acoustic neuroma treatment*

	Surgery		Radiosurgery
	Translabyrinthine	Retromastoid	
Hearing preservation	0	25–43%	25–62%
Facial nerve function (Grade I & II House & Brackmann 1985)			
Small tumours (< 1.5 cm)	95%	90%	70–80%
Large tumours (> 3.0 cm)	42%	12–56%	(All sizes, generally only treated when < 3.0 cm)
Trigeminal nerve dysfunction	Unknown	Unknown	28%
Recurrence/regrowth	Unknown (probably very low)	5–10%	10–20%
Mortality	0–4%	0–2%	0
Miscellaneous morbidity			
Haematoma	2%	1%	0
CSF leak	10%	7–15%	0
Meningitis	7%	6%	0
Hydrocephalus	2%	2%	10%
Brainstem infarcts	2%	1%	0
References	Tos & Thomsen 1982 Hardy et al. 1989 Briggs et al. 1994	Tator & Nedzelski 1985 Frerebeau et al. 1987 Bentivoglio et al. 1988a,b Symon et al. 1989 Ojemann et al. 1992 Comey et al. 1995 Mazzoni et al. 1996	Leksell 1987 Flickinger et al. 1991 Forster et al. 1996

Radiosurgery has been increasingly employed as a treatment, initially for small tumours in those patients considered medically unfit for the major surgery, but more recently for anyone not wishing an operation (Flickinger *et al.* 1991; Pollock *et al.* 1995; Forster *et al.* 1996). Long-term follow-up is awaited with interest but although this treatment may well have a place, warnings have been sounded about the risks of facial nerve injury, trigeminal nerve damage, progressive decline of hearing and failure to control tumour growth. In addition, in those who subsequently require surgery the chances of preserving the facial nerve may well be reduced by the radiotherapy given. Of even more concern are the reports, as yet unpublished, of malignant change in two tumours after radiotherapy. The surgical treatment options are listed in Table 11.4, with outcomes for all forms of treatment in Table 11.5. There has been much debate about the value of hearing preservation with these tumours. Interestingly the neurosurgeons are often the advocates of hearing with the otologists pleading the case for the facial nerve (Tos & Thomsen 1982; Samii & Matthies 1996).

In an attempt to reduce the risk of facial nerve injury and increase the chance of hearing preservation electrophysiological monitoring has been promoted, although its role has yet to be fully evaluated. Certainly facial nerve monitoring appears to have considerable value both in locating the nerve and in protecting it from vigorous manipulation during the removal of the tumour. Brainstem auditory evoked potentials, electrocochleography and direct recording from the cochlear nerve during surgery have all been employed in the search for aids to the preservation of hearing. Of these, direct recording of the nerve action potential seems to hold most promise as the waveform is large and requires only a few repetitions to be visible on the evoked potential averager.

The whole issue of hearing preservation in acoustic neuroma surgery remains somewhat controversial. It appears reasonable to attempt to retain good hearing in a patient with a small tumour arising from the vestibular nerve which is causing hearing loss by compression of the cochlear nerve but in the light of recent reports of recurrence rates up to 10% it may be preferable to sacrifice hearing by performing a translabyrinthine operation, so ensuring that the distal porus is clear of tumour.

Particular difficulties are encountered in patients with a single hearing ear. Generally these individuals will be offered a confusing choice of therapy: immediate microsurgical resection employing a hearing-saving approach, delayed microsurgical resection if the tumour shows growth on serial scans and the hearing is noted to be decreasing, or stereotactic radiotherapy or observation until the hearing is lost. The choice cannot be made on the basis of published series comparing the options as the data do not exist. Even in the best hands the chance of hearing being present after surgery is in the region of 40–60%. What happens to this hearing with time is still not known but there are indications that it decreases more rapidly than would be expected through ageing alone. Radiotherapy also may result in delayed hearing loss, possibly due to continued tumour growth or possibly due to direct effects on the nerves or blood supply to the

Table 11.6. *Complications of trigeminal neuroma resection*

	Pollock & Sekhar 1993	McCormick *et al.* 1988
Incomplete resection	4/22 (18%) (All had symptomatic recurrences within 3 years of surgery)	8/14 (57%) (Four had symptomatic recurrences within 5 years and one 20 years after surgery)
Deterioration of trigeminal nerve function	10/22 (45%) (Some of the remaining twelve had improvement of function)	9/14 (64%) (All new deficits tended to be permanent)
Other cranial nerve deficits		
Diplopia		
Facial weakness	10/22 transient (45%) 3/22 permanent (14%)	1/14 permanent (7%)
Hearing loss		
CSF leak	2/22 (9%)	1/14 (7%)

cochlea. The choice is probably best left to the patient after a frank explanation of the risks, with some guidance from an experienced clinician.

Trigeminal neuroma

Trigeminal neuromas are rare tumours and published series are small. They may be entirely infratentorial (20%) or be within the ganglion and extend in a dumbbell fashion below the tentorium (25%). The principal complications of surgery are due to injury to tho trigominal and adjacent cranial nerves (Table 11.6).

Jugular neuroma

Jugular neuromas are even less common than trigeminal neuromas; in 1979 a literature review reported only 56 cases (Maniglia *et al.* 1979) and it would be unusual for even a busy skull base centre to treat more than one or two cases each year. They generally present with palsies of the lower cranial nerves which will influence the eventual outcome, as these often do not recover after resection of the tumour. They may be predominantly intracranial (type A), confined to the skull base (type B) or extend inferiorly into the neck from the jugular foramen (type C) (Kaye *et al.* 1984). Should surgery be contemplated the aim is complete resection with preservation of existing cranial nerve function. The size of the tumour and any pre-existing deficit will heavily influence the outcome. In a series of 14 patients operated between 1976 and 1993 all experienced postoperative swallowing problems and six required vocal cord injection. Four patients had transient facial nerve weakness but all were able to return to their presurgery lifestyle (Kinney 1993).

Tumours of developmental origin

Dermoid and epidermoid cysts

Dermoid and epidermoid cysts have characteristic CT and MRI appearances and within the cranium tend to be distributed in the parasellar region, the cerebello-pontine angle and within the ventricular system (Tytus & Pennybacker 1956; Ulrich 1964). The natural history of these slowly expanding lesions is to cause focal deficit and symptoms of raised intracranial pressure until the death of the patient. The early appalling results of surgery were recorded by Critchley & Ferguson in 1928. Recent surgical results have been a little more favourable (Table 11.7).

Problems persist with recurrence of the lesions as the capsule of an epidermoid cyst usually insinuates itself around adjacent nerves and vessels. Vigorous attempts to resect all the capsular fragments may well cause significant morbidity and are probably best avoided. If a radical resection of the cyst contents is completed with resection of part of the capsule the lesion will probably become symptomatic again only after many

Table 11.7. *Results of surgical treatment for intracranial dermoid and epidermoid cysts*

	Risk
Mortality	0–20%
Morbidity	
New or worse cranial nerve deficits	10–67%
Epilepsy	Approx. 10%
Chemical meningitis	2.5%–25%
Vascular injury/stroke	11–15%
CSF leak	Approx. 5%
Hydrocephalus needing shunt	2.5–15%
Recurrence	0–30%[a]

References: Guidetti & Gagliardi (1977); Sabin *et al.* (1987); Vinchon *et al.* (1995); Samii *et al.* (1996); Doyle & Cruz (1996).
[a] Follow-up periods generally too short for meaningful data about recurrence.

years and then may be suitable for another resection. Chemical meningitis from release of cyst contents into the CSF space has been largely avoided by the routine use of perioperative steroids. Those who do develop this complication often require delayed ventriculoperitoneal (VP) shunting to treat the resulting hydrocephalus.

Craniopharyngiomas

Craniopharyngiomas account for approximately 3% of all intracranial tumours, with 50% being diagnosed in childhood. There is continued debate about management (Sandford *et al.* 1996) with support for aggressive and/or conservative surgery. Considerable morbidity can be anticipated with either approach (Table 11.8). Given that the tumours are histologically benign it is logical that complete resection should be curative but the difficulty is the location of the mass around the optic nerves, carotid arteries and hypothalamus. Supporters of radical excision point out that there is a layer of gliotic brain around the tumours allowing robust dissection of solid tumours from the hypothalamus but the majority of series show that the most severely disabled individuals with regard to hypothalamic damage (morbid obesity and chronic hyperosmolar states) have undergone radical resection.

There is no doubt that simple decompression or subtotal resection alone carries a very high risk of recurrence. When adjuvant radiotherapy and/or intracyst chemotherapy is added this risk appears to fall to match that after radical resection. Opponents of radiotherapy, especially in children, point to the reduction in IQ seen after standard external beam treatment and worry about the risk of radiation-induced second tumours. Stereotactic radiotherapy and/or intracyst instillation of radioactive phosphorus or yttrium may avoid these complications while achieving similar rates of disease control. The goal of treatment should be the control of tumour growth with

Table 11.8. *Radical versus conservative therapy of craniopharyngiomas*

	Radical surgery	Conservative surgery and radiotherapy ± intracyst chemotherapy/radiotherapy
Recurrence	20–25%	20–25%
Endocrinopathy	95%	95%
Diabetes insipidus	up to 80%	6%
Mortality	2–4%	0–1%
References	Yasargil *et al.* 1990	Takahashi *et al.* 1985
	Symon *et al.* 1991	Weiner *et al.* 1994
	Epstein & Handler 1994	Cavalheiro *et al.* 1996
	De Vile *et al.* 1996	Sandford *et al.* 1996

preservation of the patient's cognitive, visual and endocrine function. Table 11.9 gives a suggested protocol taken from the monograph of Epstein & Handler (1994).

Colloid cysts

Colloid cysts are thought to comprise 1–2% of all intracranial tumours and are of uncertain histogenesis, with most workers favouring a neuroepithelial origin. Their clinical significance is the risk of significant morbidity and mortality when they enlarge sufficiently to obstruct the foramen of Monro with the development of hydrocephalus. Nitta & Symon (1985) found three patterns of clinical presentation:

> Group 1: Headache, papilloedema but no neurological deficit (47%)
> Group 2: Fluctuating or progressive dementia (17%)
> Group 3: 'Classical' features of epilepsy, headache and drop attacks (33%)
> Unclassified (3%)

As with most other CNS lesions, colloid cysts are increasingly being discovered incidentally, often in patients complaining of headache in whom the cyst is not obviously causing hydrocephalus. There are a number of management options including the conservative approach of clinical observation, CSF shunting, stereotactic aspiration or microsurgical resection. The advantages and disadvantages of each are shown in Table 11.10.

Simple observation has been described in a series of 24 patients with a mean follow-up of 19 months (range 1–89 months). Of these 70% had normal ventricular size but the reasons for not operating on the 30% with hydrocephalus were not given. There were no deaths in this group (Camacho *et al.* 1989). In the same paper, four of a group of five patients treated initially with VP shunting required subsequent resection of the cyst after shunt malfunction, the fifth required shunt revision. Primary treatment of hydrocephalus by VP shunting is still described but it would appear to be increasingly difficult to justify in view of the potential risks of shunt occlusion and infection.

Stereotactic surgery has its advocates (Mohadjer *et al.* 1987; Rivas & Hobato 1985).

Table 11.9. *Craniopharyngioma: suggested treatment*

Microsurgical resection	Intracyst therapy	Radiotherapy
Rapid visual deterioration	Primarily cystic tumours with little solid component (choice of bleomycin, ^{32}P, ^{90}Y)	Incomplete resection at first operation by skilled surgeon because of adherence to vital structures if signs of progression on serial CT scans
Hydrocephalus		
Child under 5 years of age (to avoid deleterious effects of radiation to developing brain)		Stereotactic radiotherapy: reserved for solid components that are small (< 20 mm) and separated from the optic apparatus (> 5 mm)
Large solid component to tumour		
Location within sella turcica (transsphenoidal operation)		
Ready access to appropriate endocrine follow-up, hormone therapy		
Solid or mixed tumour recurrence after initial 'total resection' (50% can be cured by further operation)		

Table 11.10. *Colloid cysts: treatment options*

Treatment	Advantage	Disadvantage
Clinical observation	No risks from surgical intervention but only suitable for those without hydrocephalus. Ventriculomegaly is an indication for operation	May rapidly become symptomatic: risk of acute hydrocephalic attack and death
CSF shunting	Relatively low-risk procedure	Does not treat cause of hydrocephalus. Sudden obstruction of shunts may lead to acute hydrocephalic attack and death Bilateral shunts usually required
Stereotactic aspiration	Relatively low-risk procedure. Minimally invasive	Cyst walls are often difficult to puncture. Cyst contents are often too thick to aspirate. Risk of haemorrhage. Risk of recurrence
Endoscopic craniotomy	Minimally invasive	Insrumentation still being developed. Haemostasis can be difficult. Often resection incomplete: risk of recurrence
Microsurgery	Good view of lesion Complete resection possible Low risk of recurrence	Risk of epilepsy. Risk of neuropsychological injury

Table 11.11. *Microsurgical approaches to colloid cysts (Rhoton* et al. *1981; Carmel 1985)*

	Advantages	Disadvantages
Transcortical	Wide operative exposure. Easy landmark identification. Good view of anatomy of ipsilateral foramen of Monro and contralateral wall of III	Division of frontal cortex. Requires hydrocephalus
Transcallosal	Does not require hydrocephalus. Largely extra-axial. Good view of both walls of III	Divides anterior corpus callosum. Risk of bilateral forniceal injury. Difficult landmarks. Risk of injury to cortical bridging veins

One recent report details the results of stereotactic aspiration of colloid cysts in 37 patients (Ostertag & Kreth 1996). In 18, the cyst was 'completely evacuated', in 12 a reduction in volume of 75% was obtained and in seven there was no change seen on postoperative imaging. Ten patients already had biventricular shunts *in situ*. In two patients recurrence was demonstrated at 4 and 5 years after an incomplete evacuation of the contents. The mean follow-up period was 5.2 years (range 1–14 years).

Microsurgical resection remains the favored treatment of many neurosurgeons. A number of approaches have been described but the most commonly used routes to the third ventricle are the transcallosal and the transcortical. The advantages and disadvantages of each are listed in Table 11.11. Much has been made of the risk of cognitive impairment after craniotomy, but in at least one series of patients, studied with formal psychometric evaluation before and after surgery this deficit was not observed (Petrucci *et al.* 1987).

Finally, neuroendoscopy deserves mention. One early paper (Powell *et al.* 1983) described the endoscopic appearance of colloid cysts as an aid to diagnosis; attempts were made to aspirate six of nine cysts examined and were successful in five. More recently a further five cases treated endoscopically using stereotactic placement of the endoscope have been reported (Caemaert & Abdullah 1996). The authors state that their technique was in evolution during the treatment period. They achieved complete resection in only three of the five patients treated and one required two procedures before the cyst wall was removed. With continued development of the endoscopic equipment, this method may supersede microsurgery as the treatment of choice in the future.

Tumours involving the nervous system secondarily

Chemodectomas (glomus tumours)

Glomus tumours form part of a family of tumours arising from paraganglionic structures including the carotid body, glomus jugulare and glomus tympanicum. They tend to arise in middle age and are commoner in women, presenting with hearing loss,

Table 11.12. *Classification of glomus tumours (Oldring & Fisch 1979)*

Type A	Middle ear cleft and tympanic area
Type B	Tympanomastoid area, no destruction of bone in the infralabyrinthine temporal bone
Type C (C_1–C_3)	Infralabyrinthine and apical compartment tumours causing temporal bone destruction
Type D (D_1–D_3)	Intracranial extension

Table 11.13. *Complications of resection of glomus jugulare tumours*

Mortality	0–6%
Morbity (new deficits)	
Lower cranial nerve palsies	30–75%
Facial nerve palsy	11–28%
CSF	8–15%
Meningitis	2–6%

References: Bordi *et al.* (1989); Robertson *et al.* (1990); Jackson *et al.* (1993).

tinnitus, ataxia and lower cranial nerve palsies depending on their site of origin and direction of growth. There has been debate about the preferred management for many years but surgical resection seems to offer the best chance of cure. They are, however, relatively slow in their growth and may not cause significant problems to an elderly individual during the remainder of their lifetime. The question that has to be addressed having decided that surgery offers the best chance of cure is: Who should not be operated on? The consensus view is that individuals aged over 60–65 years are unlikely to benefit from surgery. This is based on the consideration that the growth of these tumours is slow and also on the balance of benefit against surgical mortality. It is possible that radiotherapy with or without subtotal tumour resection would provide sufficient palliation.

If surgery is felt to be advisable the aim of operation has to be the complete resection of the tumour in a single stage preserving as much normal anatomy and function as possible. Preoperative investigations have to show exactly the extent and size of the tumour, the presence of associated lesions and the relationship to major vessels, particularly the carotid artery. Endocrine-active tumours are not unusual and must be screened for before surgery (Bordi *et al.* 1989). In a series of 84 patients treated for glomus jugulare tumours between 1970 and 1989, 20% had multiple tumours and 5% were 'secretor' tumours (Jackson *et al.* 1993).

Fisch has a very large experience with the management of these tumours and has classified them according to their extent (Table 11.12). The majority of neurosurgical cases have intracranial extensions (type D) and present a formidable surgical challenge. The smaller lesions restricted to the jugular foramen can be resected without destruction of the ear anatomy (Jackson *et al.* 1993) but those which destroy more of the temporal bone will require extensive surgery leading to damage of cranial nerve function (if not already destroyed by the tumour) (Fisch 1982; Bordi *et al.* 1989) Pre-operative embolization is often employed in an attempt to reduce surgical blood loss from these extremely vascular tumours.

Postoperative complications are related mainly to cranial nerve deficits but may also be secondary to uncontrolled hypertensive episodes in patients not adequately treated or investigated before surgery (Table 11.13).

Chordomas and chondrosarcomas

Chordomas and chondrosarcomas are considered together owing to their biological and histological similarities. Indeed it is only with the advent of immunohistochemical techniques that it has been possible to reclassify 'chondroid chordomas' as low-grade chondrosarcomas. Chondrosarcomas within the cranium tend to arise within the skull base from those bones preformed in cartilage. They often cause extensive bone destruction and invade the middle and posterior fossae. Chordomas arise from notochord remnants and tend to occur at either end of the vertebral column. These intracranial tumours usually cause extensive destruction of the skull base, compressing the neuraxis and local cranial nerves. Histologically benign, they generally have a poor prognosis due to the difficulty achieving a complete resection given their location. In addition, metastases from chordomas are seen in 10–40% of affected individuals, but usually only many years after onset.

Treatment for these tumours over the years has included biopsy, subtotal resection or radical resection. Standard external beam radiotherapy has often been added to the surgery but appears to have little effect with regard to tumour control. Proton beam radiation and stereotactic radiotherapy to residual tumour are still under evaluation. Untreated the mean survival of 11 Swedish patients was under 1 year (Eriksson *et al.* 1981). Five-year recurrence-free survival of 90% for chondrosarcoma and 65% for chordomas is now being reported (Gay *et al.* 1995).

Current surgical opinion favours radical primary surgery in those fit enough to withstand it. The approaches used vary according to the tumour location but are all essentially extradural and include: subtemporal, preauricular infratemporal, extreme lateral transcondylar and transoral with extended maxillolotomy (Sen *et al.* 1989; Lanzino *et al.* 1993; Watkins *et al.* 1993; Borba *et al.* 1996). Multiple procedures have often been required to deal with the tumour and many patients needed additional surgery to deal with recurrence. Although rare in children, the clinical behaviour of chordomas seems to depend on the age at presentation and the histological pattern. Children under 5 years of age tend to present with raised intracranial pressure and their tumours show atypical histology and more aggressive behaviour. The incidence of metastases also appears to be much higher in this age group (Borba *et al.* 1996). For adults with

Table 11.14. *Mortality and morbidity after resection of chordomas/chondrosarcomas*

Mortality	0–5%
Morbidity	
CSF leak	11–25%
Hydrocephalus	16%
SIADH	13%
Hemiparesis	3–6%
Diabetes insipidus	6%
Hypopituitarism	3–6%
New cranial nerve deficit[a]	10–80%

[a] Many may be transient and recoverable.
References: Sen *et al.* (1989); Larzino *et al.* (1993); Watkins *et al.* (1993); Gay *et al.* (1995); Bordi *et al.* (1966).

chordomas, it appears that there are two distinct groups with regard to tumour behaviour plus overall prognosis. Morbidity is highest in the first 5 years after presentation but thereafter the prognosis appears to impove and is excellent for those surviving more than 5 years (Watkins *et al.* 1993). Previously this finding was thought to represent inclusion of chondrosarcomas, but it appears true even when immunohistochemistry has excluded these latter tumours.

The morbidity and mortality of surgery is shown in Table 11.14. Risks generally were much higher in those who had undergone previous surgery and in those who had received prior radiotherapy, as might be expected.

Very few studies have reported thorough assessments of overall outcome of treatment. Karnofsky scores have been assessed (Gay *et al.* 1995) and a transient reduction found in 60% immediately after surgery. In 40% a permanent functional deterioration was found, usually by 10 points on the scale; however, 20% experienced an improvement, usually by 10 points. Of the 60 patients treated, 50 had preoperative Karnofsky scores between 80 and 100 (normal or minimal symptoms and working) with 46 having that score between 6 and 12 months postoperatively.

References

Al-Mefty, O. (1991). Clinoidal meningiomas. In *Meningiomas*, ed. O. Al-Mefty, pp. 427–43. New York: Raven Press.

Al-Mefty, O. & Smith, R. R. (1988). Surgery of tumours invading the cavernous sinus. *Surg. Neurol.* **30**, 370–81.

Al-Mefty, O. & Smith, R. R. (1991). Tuberculum sellae meningiomas. In *Meningiomas*, ed. O. Al-Mefty, pp. 395–411. New York: Raven Press.

Al-Mefty, O., Fox, J. L. & Smith, R. R. (1988). Petrosal approach for petroclial meningiomas. *Neurosurgery* **22**, 510–17.

Baird, M. & Gallagher, P. J. (1989). Recurrent intracranial and spinal meningiomas: clinical and histological features. *Clin. Neuropathol.* **8**, 41–4.

Bentivoglio, P., Cheesman, A. D. & Symon, L. (1988*a*). Surgical management of acoustic neuromas during the last five years: part 1. *Surg. Neurol.* **29**, 197–204.

Bentivoglio, P., Cheesman, A. D. & Symon, L. (1988*b*). Surgical management of acoustic neuromas during the last five years. II. Results for facial and cochlear nerve function. *Surg. Neurol.* **29**, 205–9.

Borba, L. A. B., Al-Mefty, O., Mrak, R. E. *et al.* (1996). Cranial chordomas in children and adolescents. *J. Neurosurg.* **84**, 584–91.

Bordi, L., Cheesman, A. D. & Symon, L. (1989). The surgical management of glomus jugulare tumours – description of a single-staged postero-lateral combined otoneurological approach. *Br. J. Neurosurg.* **3**, 21–30.

Briggs, R. J. S., Luxford, W. M., Atkins, J. S. (1994). Translabyrinthine removal of large acoustic neuromas. *Neurosurgery* **34**, 785–92.

Caemaert, J. & Abdullah, J. (1996). Endoscopic management of colloid cysts. *Techn. Neurosurg.* **1**, 185–200.

Camacho, A., Abernathy, C. D., Kelly, P. *et al.* (1989). Colloid cysts: experience with the management of 84 cases since the introduction of computed tomography. *Neurosurgery* **24**, 693–700.

Carmel, P. W. (1985). Tumours of the third ventricle. *Acta Neurochir.* **75**, 136–46.

Cavalheiro, S., de Castro Sparapani, F. V., Franco, J. O. B. *et al.* (1996). Use of bleomycin in intratumoral chemotherapy for cystic craniopharyngioma. *J. Neurosurg.* **84**, 124–6.

Chan, R. C. & Thompson, G. B. (1984). Morbidity, mortality and quality of life following surgery for intracranial meningiomas. A retrospective study in 257 cases. *J. Neurosurg.* **60**, 52–60.

Comey, C. H., Jannetta, P. J., Sheptak, P. E. *et al.* (1995). Staged removal of acoustic tumours: techniques and lesions learned from a series of 83 patients. *Neurosurgery* **37**, 915–21.

Couldwell, W. T., Fukushima, T., Gianotta, S. L. *et al.* (1996). Petroclival meningiomas: surgical experience in 109 cases. *J. Neurosurg.* **84**, 20–8.

Criscuolo, G. R. & Symon, L. (1986). Intraventricular meningioma: a review of 10 cases. *Acta Neurochir.* (Wien) **83**, 83–91.

Critchley, M. & Ferguson, F. R. (1928). The cerebrospinal epidermoids (cholesteatomata). *Brain* **51**, 334–85.

Cusimano, M. D., Sekhar, L. N., Sen, C. *et al.* (1995). The results of surgery for benign tumours of the cavernous sinus. *Neurosurgery* **37**, 1–10.

DeMonte, F., Smith, H. K., Al-Mefty, O. (1994). Outcome of aggressive removal of cavernous sinus meningiomas. *J. Neurosurg.* **81**, 245–51.

De Vile, C. J., Grant, D. B., Kendall, B. E. *et al.* (1996). Management of childhood craniopharyngioma: can the morbidity of radical surgery be predicted. *J. Neurosurg.* **85**, 73–81.

Doyle, K. J. & De la Cruz, A. (1996). Cerebellopontine angle epidermoids: results of surgical treatment. *Skull Base Surg.* **6**, 27–33.

Epstein, F. J. & Handler, M. H. (eds.) (1994). *Craniopharyngioma: the Answer.* Paediatric Neurosurgery, vol. 21 (Suppl. 1). Philadelphia: Saunders.

Eriksson, B., Gunterberg, B. & Kindblom, L. G. (1981). Chordoma: a clinicopathological and prognostic study of a Swedish national series. *Acta Orthop. Scand.* **52**, 49–58.

Fisch, U. (1982). Infratemporal approach for glomus tumours of the temporal bone. *Ann. Otol. Rhinol. Laryngol.* **91**, 474–9.

Flickinger, J. C., Lunsford, L. D., Coffey, R. J. *et al.* (1991). Radiosurgery of acoustic neuromas. *Cancer* **67**, 345–53.

Forster, D. M. C., Kemeny, A. A., Pathak, A. *et al.* (1996). Radiosurgery: a minimally interventional alternative to microsurgery in management of acoustic neuroma. *Br. J. Neurosurg.* **10**, 169–74.

Foy, P. M., Copeland, G. P. & Shaw, M. D. M. (1981). The incidence of post-operative seizures. *Acta Neurochir.* (Wien) **55**, 253–64.

Frerebeau, P., Benezech, J. & Uziel, A. (1987). Hearing preservation after acoustic neurinoma operation. *Neurosurgery* **21**, 197–200.

Gay, E., Sekhar, L. N., Rubinstein, E. *et al.* (1995). Chordomas and chondrosarcoma of the cranial base: results and follow-up of 60 patients. *Neurosurgery* **36**, 887–97

George, B., Dematous, C. & Cophignon, J. (1988). Lateral approach to the anterior portion of the foramen magnum. Application to surgical removal of 14 benign tumours: technical note. *Surg. Neurol.* **29**, 484–90.

Giombini, S. & Fornari, M. (1991). Convexity meningiomas. In *Meningiomas*, ed. O. Al-Mefty, pp. 321–8. New York: Raven Press.

Giombini, S., Solero, C. L., Lasio, G. *et al.* (1984). Immediate and late outcome of operations for parasagittal and falx meningiomas: report of 342 cases. *Surg. Neurol.* **21**, 427–35.

Guidetti, B. & Delfini, R. (1991). Lateral and fourth ventricle meningiomas. In *Meningiomas*, ed. O. Al-Mefty, pp. 569–81. New York: Raven Press.

Guidetti, B. & Gagliardi, F. M. (1977). Epidermoid and dermoid cysts. Clinical evaluation and late surgical results. *J. Neurosurg.* **47**, 12–18.

Guidetti, B. & Spallone, A. (1988). Benign extramedullary tumours of the foramen magnum. In *Advances and Technical Standards in Neurosurgery*, vol. 16, ed. L. Symon, pp. 83–120. Vienna: Springer-Verlag.

Hakuda, A. & Tsujimoto, T. (1993). Transcondyle approach for foramen magnum meningiomas. In *Surgery of Cranial Base Tumors*, ed. L. N. Sekhar & I. P. Janecka, pp. 671–8. New York: Raven Press.

Hardy, D. G., MacFarlane, R., Baguley, D. *et al.* (1989). Surgery of acoustic neuroma: An analysis of 100 translabyrinthine operations. *Neurosurgery* **71**, 799–804.

House, J. W. & Brackmann, D. E. (1985). Facial nerve grading system. *Otolaryngol. Head Neck Surg.* **93**, 146–7.

Jackson, C. G., Woods, C. I. & Chironis, P. N. (1993). Glomus jugulare tumours. In *Surgery of Cranial Base Tumours*, ed. L. N. Sekhar & I. P. Janecka, pp. 747–62. New York: Raven Press.

Kadis, G. N., Mount, L. A. & Ganti, S. R. (1979). The importance of early diagnosis and treatment of the meningiomas of the planum sphenoidale and tuberculum sellae. A retrospective study of 105 cases. *Surg. Neurol.* **12**, 367–71.

Kaye, A., Hahn, J., Kinney, S. *et al.* (1984). Jugular foramen schwannomas. *J. Neurosurg.* **60**, 1045–53.

Kinjo, T., Al-Mefty, O. & Ciric, I. (1995). Diaphragma sellae meningiomas. *Neurosurgery* **36**, 1082–92.

Kinney, S. E. (1993). Jugular foramen neurilemoma. In *Surgery of Cranial Base Tumours*, ed. L. N. Sekhar & I. P. Janecka, pp. 731–5. New York: Raven Press.

Knosp, E., Perneczky, A., Koos, W. T. *et al.* (1996). Meningiomas of the space of the cavernous sinus. *Neurosurgery* **38**, 434–44.

Lanzino, G., Sekhar, L. N., Hirsch, W. L. *et al.* (1993). Chordomas and chondrosarcomas involving the cavernous sinus: review of surgical treatment and outcome in 31 patients. *Surg. Neurol.* **40**, 359–71.

Leksell, D. G. (1987). Stereotactic radiosurgery: present status and future trends. *Neurol. Res.* **9**, 60–8.

Maniglia, A., Chandler, J., Goodwin, W. *et al.* (1979). Schwannomas of the parapharyngeal space and jugular foramen. *Laryngoscope* **89**, 1405–14.

Mayberg, M. R. & Symon, L. (1986). Meningiomas of the clivus and apical petrous bone. Report of 35 cases. *J. Neurosurg.* **65**, 160–7.

Mazzoni, A., Calabrese, V. & Moschini (1996). Residual and recurrent acoustic neuromas in hearing preservation procedures. Neuroradiologic and surgical findings. *Skull Base Surg.* **6**, 105–12.

McCormick, P. C., Bello, J. A. & Post, K. D. (1988). Trigeminal schwannoma. Surgical series of 14 cases with review of the literature. *Neurosurgery* **69**, 850–60.

Meyer, F. B., Ebersold, M. J. & Reese, D. F. (1984). Benign tumours of the foramen magnum. *J. Neurosurg.* **61**, 136–42.

Mohadjer, M., Teshmar, E. & Mundinger, F. (1987). CT – stereotaxic drainage of colloid cysts in the foramen of Munro and the third ventricle. *J. Neurosurg.* **67**, 220–3.

Nitta, M. & Symon, L. (1985). Colloid cysts of the third ventricle: a review of 36 cases. *Acta Neurochir.* **76**, 99–104.

Ojemann, R. G. (1991). Olfactory groove meningiomas. In *Meningiomas*, ed. O. Al-Mefty, pp. 383–93. New York: Raven Press.

Ojemann, R. G. (1992). Management of acoustic neuromas (vestibular schwannomas). *Clin. Neurosurg.* **40**, 498–535.

Oldring, D. & Fisch, U. (1979). Glomus tumours of the temporal region: surgical therapy. *Am. J. Otolaryngol.* **1**, 7–18.

Ostertag, C. B. & Kreth, F. W. (1996). The stereotactic approach to colloid cysts. In *Controversies in Neurosurgery*, ed. O. Al-Mefty *et al.*, pp. 32–54. New York: Thieme.

Petrucci, R. J., Bucheit, W. A., Woodruff, G. C. *et al.* (1987). Transcallosal parafornicial approach for third ventricle tumours. Neuropsychological consequences. *Neurosurgery* **20**, 457–64.

Phillippou, J. & Cornu, P. (1991). The recurrence of meningiomas. In *Meningiomas*, ed. O. Al-Mefty, p. 89. New York: Raven Press.

Pollack, I. F. & Sekhar, L. N. (1993). Trigeminal neurilemoma. In *Surgery of Cranial Base Tumors*, ed. L. N. Sekhar & I. P. Janecka, pp. 737–46. New York: Raven Press.

Pollock, B. E., Lunsford, L. D., Kondziolke, D. *et al.* (1995). Outcome analysis of acoustic neuroma management: a comparison of microsurgery and stereotactic radiosurgery. *Neurosurgery* **36**, 215–29.

Powell, M. P., Torrens, M. J., Thomson, J. L. G. *et al.* (1983). Isodense colloid cysts of the third ventricle: a diagnostic and therapeutic problem resolved by ventriculoscopy. *Neurosurgery* **13**, 234–7.

Rhoton, A. L., Yamamoto, I. & Peace, D. A. (1981). Microsurgery of the third ventricle. 2. Operative approaches. *Neurosurgery* **8**, 357–73.

Risi, P., Uske, A. & DeTribolet, N. (1994). Meningiomas involving the anterior clinoid process. *Br. J. Neurosurg.* **8**, 295–305.

Rivas, J. J. & Lobato, R. D. (1985). CT-assisted stereotaxic aspiration of colloid cysts of the third ventricle. *J. Neurosurg.* **62**, 238–42.

Robertson, J. T., Clark, W. C., Robertson, J. H. *et al.* (1990). Glomus jugulare tumours. In *Neurological Surgery*, ed. J. R. Youmans, pp. 3654–66. Philadelphia: Saunders.

Sabin, H. I., Bordi, L. T. & Symon, L. (1987). Epidermoid cysts and cholesterol granulomas centered on the posterior fossa. Twenty years of diagnosis and management. *Neurosurgery* **21**, 798–805.

Samii, M. & Matthies, C. (1996). Hearing preservation in acoustic tumour surgery. In *Current Techniques in Neurosurgery*, ed. M. Salcman, pp. 93–108.

Samii, M., Ammirati, M., Mahran, A. *et al.* (1989). Surgery of petroclival meningiomas. Report of 24 cases. *Neurosurgery* **24**, 12–17.

Samii, M., Carvalho, G. A., Tatagiba, M. *et al.* (1996*a*). Meningiomas of the tentorial notch: surgical anatomy and management. *J. Neurosurg.* **84**, 375–81.

Samii, M., Tatgiba, M., Piquer, J. *et al.* (1996*b*). Surgical treatment of epidermoid cysts of the cerebellopontine angle. *J. Neurosurg.* **84**, 14–19,

Sandford, R. A., Hoffman, H. J. & Boop, F. A. (1996). Conservative vs aggressive treatment of craniopharyngiomas. In *Controversies in Neurosurgery*, ed. O. Al-Mefty *et al.*, pp. 23–9. New York: Thieme.

Sekhar, L. N., Sen, C. N., Jho, H. D. *et al.* (1989). Surgical treatment of intracavernous neoplasms: a four-year experience. *Neurosurgery* **24**, 18–30.

Sekhar, L. N., Jannetta, P. J., Burkhart, L. E. *et al.* (1990). Meningiomas involving the clivus: a six-year experience with 41 patients. *Neurosurgery* **27**, 764–81.

Sekhar, L. N., Javed, T. & Jannetta, P. (1993*a*). Petroclival meningiomas. In *Surgery of Cranial Base Tumours*, ed. L. N. Sekhar, & I. P. Janecka, pp. 605–59. New York: Raven Press.

Sekhar, L. N., Ross, D. A. & Sen, C. (1993*b*). Cavernous sinus and sphenocavernous neoplasm. In *Surgery of Cranial Base Tumours*, ed. L. N. Sekhar & I. P. Janecka, pp. 521–604. New York: Raven Press.

Sen, C. & Sekhar, L. N. (1993). Extreme lateral transcondylar and transjugular approaches. In *Surgery of Cranial Base Tumours*, ed. L. N. Sekhar & I. P. Janecka, pp. 389–411. New York: Raven Press.

Sen, C. N., Sekhar, L. N., Schramm, V. L. *et al.* (1989). Chordoma and chondrosarcoma of the cranial base: an 8-year experience. *Neurosurgery* **25**, 931–41.

Simpson, D. (1957). The recurrence of intracranial meningiomas after surgical treatment. *J. Neurol. Neurosurg. Psychiatry* **20**, 22–9.

Symon, L., Bordi, L. T., Compton, J. S. *et al.* (1989). Acoustic neuroma: a review of 392 cases. *Br. J. Neurosurg.* **3**, 343–8.

Symon, L., Pell, M. F. & Habib, H. A. (1991). Radical excision of craniopharyngiomas by the temporal route: a review of 50 patients. *Br. J. Neurosurg.* **5**, 539–49.

Symon, L. & Rosenstein, J. (1984). Surgical management of suprasellar meningioma. *J. Neurosurg.* **61**, 633–41.

Takahaski, H., Nakazawa, S. & Shimura, T. (1985). Evaluation of postoperative intratumoural injection of bleomycin for craniopharyngioma in children. *J. Neurosurg.* **62**, 120–7.

Tator, C. H. & Nedzelski, J. M. (1985). Preservation of hearing in patients undergoing excision of acoustic neuromas and other cerebello-pontine angle tumours. *J. Neurosurg.* **63**, 168–74.

Tos, M. & Thomsen, J. (1982). The price of preservation of hearing in acoustic neuroma surgery. *Ann. Otol. Rhinol. Laryngol.* **91**, 240–5.

Tytus, J. S. & Pennybacker, J. (1956). Pearly tumours in relation to the central nervous system. *J. Neurol. Neurosurg. Psychiatry.* **19**, 241–59.

Ulrich, J. (1964). Intracranial epidermoids. A study on their distribution and spread. *J. Neurosurg.* **21**, 1051–8.

Vinchon, M., Pertuzon, B., Lejeune, J. P. *et al.* (1995). Intradural epidermoid cysts of the cerebellopontine angle: diagnosis and surgery. *Neurosurgery* **36**, 52–7.

Watkins, L., Khudados, E. S., Kaleoglu, M. *et al.* (1993). Skull base chordomas: a review of 38 patients 1958–88. *Br. J. Neurosurg.* **7**, 241–8.

Weiner, H. L., Wisoff, J. H. & Rosenberg, M. E. (1994). Craniopharyngiomas: a clinicopathological analysis of factors predictive of recurrence and functional outcome. *Neurosurgery* **35**, 1001–11.

Yasargil, M. G., Circic, M., Kis, M. *et al.* (1990). Total removal of craniopharyngiomas. Approaches and long-term results in 144 patients. *J. Neurosurg.* **62**, 174–81.

12 Outcome measurements for intrinsic brain and pituitary tumours

EDWARD R. LAWS, JR

Introduction

There is increasing interest in outcome measurement associated with the management of patients with tumours affecting the central nervous system. This interest is largely the result of the significant costs of diagnosis and therapy, and also relates to the nature and extent of neurological disabilities which have a tremendous impact on both public health and economic productivity.

Brain tumours rank second in relative incidence of tumours of childhood and from sixth to eighth among tumours of adults, depending upon whether pituitary tumours and tumours metastic to the brain are included (Berens *et al.* 1990, Black 1990, Walker *et al.* 1985). The most common primary brain tumours are the gliomas. These include the astrocytoma which appears in benign and malignant forms, the glioblastoma which is a highly malignant astrocytoma and the oligodendroglioma. The gliomas comprise approximately 40–60% of primary brain tumours, and of these about half fall into a relatively benign category and half into a rapidly progressive, more malignant, classification. Other tissues within the brain also give rise to tumours and these include the ependyma and the choroid plexus. Primitive developmental tumours such as the primitive neuroectodermal tumour (PNET), medulloblastoma, ependymoblastoma and the pineoblastoma may occur, usually appearing in infancy and childhood.

The second most common type of intracranial tumour is the meningioma (Barbaro *et al.* 1987) that arises from the lining of the skull and produces symptoms by external pressure on the brain. These tumours are considered 'extra-axial' lesions and occur more commonly in women and in older patients.

Benign nerve sheath tumours occur in relationship to the cranial nerves and the most common of these is the acoustic neurinoma or vestibular schwannoma. This also is a tumour generally related to the elderly population, but it can occur in association with neurofibromatosis. Neurofibromatosis (NF) has now been classified on a genetic basis as well as a clinical basis and patients with both NF type 1 and NF type 2 are subject to a variety of different intracranial tumours, with the hallmark of NF2 being bilateral acoustic neurinomas.

Pituitary tumours, most of which are quite benign, make up approximately 10% of intracranial tumours in some series. They are a common cause of both neurological and endocrinological disability, and modern methods of diagnosis and treatment have been responsible for increasing success in the long-term management of these tumours.

Tumours of the pineal region are uncommon and include both intrinsic tumours of the brain and germ cell tumours that are of primitive or embryonic origin. The germ cell tumours tend to occur more commonly in adolescent males. Modern methods of diagnosis and therapy have become increasingly successful in the long-term management of these tumours as well.

Age as a prognostic factor

Age has a striking influence on the outcome and prognosis for patients with gliomas and, except for the very primitive tumours, there is an age-specific increasing incidence in malignancy that is quite striking and is yet not fully explained. The prognosis of the primitive primary brain tumours affecting infants and children under 2 years of age is also characteristic, and the outcome for this population is almost uniformly poor. Tumours occurring later in childhood tend to have a much better prognosis, and this is particularly true of the gliomas, with the characteristic 'juvenile' pilocytic cystic astrocytoma of the cerebellum being one of the potentially curable astrocytomas of the central nervous system. Among the elderly population, there is an increasing incidence in frequency of meningiomas and also of acoustic tumours and to a lesser extent other schwannomas affecting the cranial nerves.

Outcome with regard to surgical management is affected to some degree by the age of the patient; however, numerous studies of neurosurgical procedures in the elderly tend to support the concept of surgical resection for benign tumours in these patients as a reasonable recommendation with quite satisfactory outcomes in most cases.

Criteria for outcomes analysis

In considering criteria for the outcome of strategies used for the treatment of brain tumours, a number of different endpoints have been utilized in retrospective studies and attempts have been made to improve upon these both in retrospective and in prospective studies of brain tumour treatment.

Survival alone has tended to be the most commonly used endpoint and clearly is a very crude measure of the efficacy of therapy (Table 12.1).

Quality of life has become probably the most important outcome measure for patients with neurological disease and disability. It is, however, very difficult to measure in a precise fashion, particularly as it may differ from one patient to another or one cultural setting to another.

Attempts have been made to measure *neurological status* of patients in a systematic

Table 12.1. *Outcome results for malignant glioma (malignant astrocytoma and glioblastoma multiforme)*

Treatment modality	Median survival	Survival (%) 2 years	Survival (%) 5 years
Surgery alone	17 weeks	0	0
Surgery and radiotherapy	37.5 months	1	0
Surgery and radiotherapy and BCNU	40.5–50 months	5	0

Quality of life not measured
Other forms of chemotherapy have not provided improved survival.

fashion in order to determine outcomes related to therapeutic intervention; however, this also tends to be quite difficult as there is a considerable disagreement about standard measurements of neurological function. Standard measurement criteria have been developed for injuries of the head and of the spinal cord, but there is no current consensus with regard to methods of measurement for patients with brain tumours.

Performance status has been the most widely utilized outcome measurement for patients with tumours who are treated by surgery, radiation therapy, chemotherapy or combinations of these modalities. The most generally accepted and utilized measure of performance is the *Karnofsky Index*, which has proved relatively simple, fairly standard in its application and reasonably reproducible. Outcomes as measured by this index tend to reflect both quality of life and ability for a patient to remain productive at work.

Disease-specific outcomes

Outcome can be measured with respect to specific symptoms related to brain tumours as well. These symptoms include non-specific signs of *increased intracranial pressure* including headache, nausea and vomiting, and visual distortions. Obviously, the relief of these symptoms by measures designed to decrease intracranial pressure produced by a given brain tumour can be utilized as an outcome measure, though there is no agreed systematic way to do this. Many brain tumours, both intrinsic and extrinsic, present with *epileptic seizures* as a manifestation of the tumour, and outcomes can be measured with regard to reduction in seizure frequency or severity or elimination of seizures. This, however, is a complex issue as even with perfect removal of a benign tumour, seizure disorders may persist. Other forms of *progressive neurological difficulties* associated with brain tumours include paralysis, loss of sensation and loss of visual function. The stabilization of progressive symptoms or reversal of a neurological or visual deficit can also be used as effective outcome measures depending upon the type of tumour and the patient population studied.

In those situations where improvement in neurological or performance functions occurs, the *time to recovery* can be measured and utilized as an outcome measure. In general, the pace of neurological loss reflects the reversibility of many symptoms and

Table 12.2. *Outcome results for low-grade astrocytomas (excluding pilocytic astrocytomas)*

Treatment modality	Median survival	Survival (%)		
		3 years	5 years	10 years
Surgery alone	28 months	35–58	30–37	10–11
Surgery and radiotherapy	8 years	59–64	36–55	17–36

Quality of life not addressed in these studies.
Selection bias for radiotherapy makes rigid comparisons unreliable.
Chemotherapy has not been demonstrated to be of benefit.
Age of the patient is a major prognostic factor.

7Table 12.3. *Outcome results for oligodendroglioma*

Treatment modality	Median survival	Survival (%)		
		3 years	5 years	10 years
Surgery alone	26.5 months	35	27	12
Surgery and radiotherapy	38 months	53	36	8

Quality of life not addressed.
Selection bias for radiotherapy should be considered.
Chemotherapy may be of benefit in some cases.

signs. Those patients with longstanding neurological disability have a poorer chance of regaining normal function than those who have had a relatively shorter period of symptomatology. *Higher cortical functions* consisting of memory, language, judgement and orientation can all be evaluated and potentially can be used as outcome measures. There are a number of well-standardized psychometric tests which can be utilized for evaluation of memory function, both written and verbal, and specific tests are available with regard to orientation and various aspects of language function. Alterations in *emotions*, *judgement* and *personality* which may occur as a result of brain tumours are much more difficult to measure and, therefore, much more difficult to use as outcome criteria.

Levels of intervention for the treatment of brain tumours

The most commonly utilized modality for the diagnosis and treatment of brain tumours is surgery. Neurosurgical procedures include craniotomy and various types of biopsy ranging from open biopsy to computer-guided stereotactic methods. Surgical procedures are generally graded by the extent of removal of the tumour involved, from complete to subtotal to incomplete or biopsy only, and for many tumours the extent of resection is directly related to the outcome with regard to survival and occasionally to other measures such as performance status. Obviously one of the major criteria for a successful surgical intervention is getting reliable histological diagnosis of the tumour

Table 12.4. *Outcome results for meningioma*

Treatment modality	Survival (%)	
	5 years	10 years
Gross total resection	93	80
Subtotal resection	63	45
All surgically treated	83	77

Quality of life is not addressed.
Radiation therapy and chemotherapy are reserved for
aggressive variants and are of limited efficacy.
Recurrence rates and survival highly correlated with location
of tumour.

involved, and this is possible at present approximately 98% of the time. Depending upon the type of tumour involved, surgical intervention can provide excellent outcomes with regard to longevity and reversal of neurological symptoms in approximately 70% of patients. For gliomas the nature and extent of involvement of the brain tends to play a major role in determining outcome and some patients with intrinsic tumours will have a decrease in performance status directly related to the surgical intervention, particularly if major resection is carried out (Salcman 1990).

Radiation therapy is commonly used following surgery for brain tumours, particularly for malignant lesions (Leibel & Sheline 1987). A number of advances in the delivery of radiation therapy have improved both the safety and efficacy of this modality of brain tumour treatment (Larson *et al.* 1990). It is clear that appropriately administered external radiation therapy increases the survival of patients with gliomas of the brain, though radiation therapy is rarely, if ever, curative for these tumours. Stereotactically delivered focused radiation therapy or radiosurgery has been applied to a number of brain tumours, both benign and malignant, and is currently under evaluation. There is some prospect that considerable advantages in outcome will be achieved using these newer computer-based techniques.

Pituitary tumours

Clinical features of pituitary tumours reflect both the size of the lesion and its potential for producing endocrinological abnormalities. Larger tumours greater than 10 mm in diameter are classified as macroadenomas, and smaller tumours are known as microadenomas. The ability of some pituitary tumours to secrete abnormally high levels of normal pituitary hormones leads to characteristic syndromes of endocrine-active tumours. These are acromegaly, related to excess growth hormone (GH), Forbes–Albright syndrome (amenorrhoea–galactorrhoea) related to prolactin (PRL), Cushing's disease and Nelson's syndrome related to corticotropin (ACTH) and, much less commonly, hyperthyroidism related to thyrotropin (TSH). Gonadotropic tumours (FSH/LH) exist, but rarely present with clinical syndromes related to hypersecretion.

Table 12.5. *Outcome results for pituitary adenoma treated by surgery*

Type of pituitary tumour	Remission of hormonal hypersecretion (%)	Recovery of visual loss (%)	Recurrence-free survival (%)
GH adenoma (acromegaly)	60–80	95	92
Prolactinoma	50–80	90	75
ACTH adenoma (Cushing's disease)	80–90	95	90
Non-functioning adenoma	N.A.	92	84

Clinically non-functioning pituitary tumours are common and they ordinarily are associated with hypopituitarism and symptoms related to mass effect, as most of these are macroadenomas. Typical symptoms include headache and visual loss, usually a bitemporal hemianopsia. Pituitary tumours may extend laterally to involve the cranial nerves within the cavernous sinus, producing diplopia, craniofacial pain or facial numbness.

Assessments of hormonal activity, or lack thereof, can be made by laboratory tests of pituitary hormones in serum. These tests can be done in basal and provoked (stimulated) settings, and excellent characterization of pituitary physiology can be accomplished. For pituitary tumours associated with hyperfunctioning syndromes, these laboratory tests provide a rigorous measure of outcome, and they are used for purposes of longitudinal follow-up.

Another endocrinologically based outcome measurement is recovery from hypopituitarism associated with macroadenomas. This does not occur frequently, but also can be accurately measured by laboratory tests of pituitary hormone levels.

Clinical measures of outcome in pituitary tumours include reversal of symptoms of endocrine active syndromes, restoration of energy, stamina, libido and potency, and improvement in visual function. Most of these are difficult to quantify in a reproducible fashion. Visual function, however, can be tested accurately, and restoration of vision is an excellent outcome in those patients with visual loss as a presenting symptom. In conjunction with our colleagues in neuro-ophthalmology, accurate measures of visual acuity and visual fields can be made, both of which may be impaired by a pituitary tumour. The optic atrophy seen on funduscopic examination may be graded or even photographed, but does not serve as a useful outcome measure, as the colour of the optic disc rarely recovers to normal, even when visual function improves.

Because pituitary tumours so rarely are malignant, survival alone is not a useful outcome measurement. Performance or work status evaluations are useful in some situations, but generally tend to be irrelevant. Sexual activity and reproductive capacity are often affected by pituitary tumours and outcome measurements in this area can be important. Recovery from sexual dysfunction, resumption of spermatogenesis in the male and ovulation, conception and pregnancy in the female can all be effectively used as measures of outcome. For prolactin-secreting tumours, resolution of galactorrhoea can be an effective outcome measure.

Although benign, many pituitary tumours have the capability of involving the dura and bone of the sella turcica. These invasive tumours have a tendency toward recurrence, but tumour recurrence can be seen with all types of pituitary tumours, varying in incidence from 7% to 20% depending upon the type of tumour and the length of follow-up. Thus recurrence and time to recurrence are both important outcome measures for pituitary tumours.

The majority of pituitary tumours are detectable on modern imaging studies. Outcomes of various types of therapy can be assessed by evaluation of post-therapeutic imaging studies. These can detect resolution of mass, persistence of tumour, restoration of normal anatomy and occasionally they even show correlates of pituitary physiology. The best current method for such assessment is MRI with gadolinium contrast.

Levels of intervention for the treatment of pituitary tumours

For some patients with small tumours that are not producing endocrine abnormalities that interfere with day-to-day life and activity, observation alone may suffice. These patients are usually followed with periodic endocrine laboratory and imaging tests.

Pharmacotherapy is effective in some pituitary tumours. Prolactin-secreting adenomas often respond well to dopamine agonist therapy. The most common agent used is bromocriptine (Parlodel). Responses may be assessed both by lowering the serum prolactin levels and by shrinkage of tumour mass on MRI. Growth-hormone-secreting tumours can also have a favourable response to dopamine agonist therapy, but tumours rarely shrink and excess levels of growth hormone are almost never normalized. Much more effective in acromegaly, is the somatostatin analogue octreotide (Sandostatin), which can provide effective control of excess growth hormone and can occasionally produce shrinkage of tumour mass. In Cushing's disease, treatment with ketaconazole can lower circulating levels of cortisol, but this drug has no effect on the pituitary tumour.

Surgical therapy currently is the most effective and rapid method for dealing with tumours other than prolactinomas. The trans-sphenoidal microsurgical approach has evolved into a safe and effective means of dealing with most pituitary tumours, and currently craniotomy is utilized in only 4–6% of surgically treated cases. Clinical response, laboratory tests and MRI provide excellent measures of surgical outcome. Incomplete removal and tumour recurrence remain a problem and often prompt the use of adjunctive pharmacological or radiation therapy.

Radiation therapy is effective in the management of some pituitary tumours, and newer methods of focused radiation therapy promise to improve both the safety and the efficacy of this modality. Major disadvantages have been delayed responses to therapy, potential damage to adjacent structures (optic nerves and chiasm, hypothalamus, carotid arteries), and ultimate development of hypopituitarism. These disadvantages are being addressed by new techniques and concepts.

The best outcome for patients with brain tumours and pituitary tumours alike depends upon a carefully considered programme of diagnosis and management, which usually involves a multispecialty collaborative approach, multimodality therapy, rigorous assessment of results of therapies, and consistent, rigorous follow-up studies. The application of these principles will ensure continuing improvement in outcome for our patients.

References

Barbaro, N. M., Gutin, P. H., Wilson, C. B., Sheline, G. E., Boldrey, E. B. & Wara, W. M. (1987). Radiation therapy in the treatment of partially resected meningiomas. *Neurosurgery* **20**, 525–8.

Berens, M. E., Rutka, J. T. & Rosenblum, M. L. (1990). Brain tumor epidemiology, growth and invasion. *Neurosurg. Clin. North Am.* **1**, 1–18.

Black, P. M. (1990). Brain tumors. *N. Engl. J. Med.* **324**, 1555–64.

Larson, D. A., Gutin, P. H., Leibel, S. A. *et al.* (1990). Stereotaxic irradiation of brain tumors. *Cancer* **65**, 792–9.

Leibel, S. A. & Sheline, G. E. (1987). Radiation therapy for neoplasms of the brain. *J. Neurosurg.* **66**, 1–22.

Salcman, M. (1990). Malignant gliomas: management. *Neurosurg. Clin. North Am.* **1**, 49–63.

Walker, A. E., Robins, M. & Weinfeld, F. D. (1985). Epidemiology of brain tumors: the national survey of intracranial neoplasms. *Neurology* **35**, 219–26.

13 Spinal tumours

JACQUES BROTCHI

Introduction

Spinal tumours may be classified as extradural or intradural. Intradural may be divided into extramedullary and intramedullary. The true incidence of spinal cord tumours is unknown and should be reviewed in the light of modern neuroradiological diagnosis. Estimates based on population studies vary from 1 to 13 per 100 000 population (Connolly 1982). In this chapter, intradural tumours are described first. Clinical signs, diagnosis and treatment are reviewed according to the modern literature.

Intradural tumours

Extramedullary tumours

Incidence and clinical signs
About 70% of intradural tumours are extramedullary, the majority being meningiomas or schwannomas (Foy 1992). Pain of spinal root origin is the commonest initial symptom, occurring mostly at night; it may precede by months or years the signs of spinal cord compression. Motor disturbances are often the second symptom to be noticed involving the legs first, with spasticity and increased reflexes. Sensory deficits nearly always appear after the motor disturbances. At the beginning, a sensory level due to cord compression will not correspond with the true site of the tumour. Sphincter disturbances always occur at a late stage.

Meningiomas Cushing & Eisenhardt (1938) gave an informative description of these tumours, which account for approximately 25% of spinal cord tumours. They occur predominantly in women. They are encountered most frequently in patients between the ages of 40 and 70 years. Meningiomas may develop in any part of the spinal canal but arise most frequently in the thoracic region, then the cervical area and rarely in the lumbosacral canal (Nittner 1976). As opposed to intracranial meningiomas, spinal meningiomas do not involve bone. This is probably due to the space existing between dura and bone, filled with fat, venous plexuses and nerve roots. Extradural spread is uncommon.

Schwannomas This tumour, as well as neurofibroma, is derived from the sheath of Schwann (Russell & Rubinstein 1989). Schwannomas arise indiscriminately from any of the spinal nerves and almost invariably from the sensory roots (Russell & Rubinstein 1989). This explains why radicular pain is so frequent during the months and years before diagnosis in spinal schwannomas. The clinical signs are similar to those encountered in meningiomas and the incidence is equal in males and females. They may be found anywhere in the spine, even in the lumbosacral area where they may mimic common sciatica. They may grow out of the canal, in an hourglass shape, mostly in the cervical and thoracic regions, through the intervertebral foramina. Sometimes, they may be multiple or associated with meningiomas, as in Von Recklinghausen's disease.

Other lesions Most of these are cysts, either arachnoidal or enterogenous. They are very rare, as are teratomas, as reported by Sloof *et al.* (1964), and Agnoli *et al.* (1984) where reviews may be found.

Diagnostic imaging

When the site of the tumour can be determined on clinical grounds, CT scan with intravenous contrast and MRI with paramagnetic agents are the best investigations (Balériaux *et al.* 1989) (Fig. 13.1*a*). However, when the clinical level is indefinite, myelography with water-soluble contrast associated with CSF analysis may still be very useful. In the thoracic area, CT scan may be disappointing. MRI remains the gold standard anywhere in the spine as it demonstrates schwannomas and meningiomas very well. But in case of arachnoidal cyst, myelography may be useful because it fills the cavity with the dye. Again, MRI should image these lesions adequately. Finally, plain radiographs have no current interest, except in hourglass schwannoma when they may demonstrate an enlargement of an intervertebral foramen.

Treatment

Most schwannomas and meningiomas may be approached through a laminectomy. However, one should always have in mind the need to avoid any damage to the spinal cord. It is very important to ask the neuroradiologist on which side the lesion is located. Therefore, knowing that the tumour is laterally situated, the exposure can be more generous over that side in order to avoid retraction of the spinal cord (Balériaux & Brotchi 1992). This allows the dura to be opened over the tumour rather than over the spinal cord, giving better visualization of the operative field and diminishing the risks of spinal cord injury during surgery. We like to put a 6–0 atraumatic suture through the dentate ligament after cutting its attachment and to hold it up which gives space in the anterior part of the spinal canal, particularly in meningiomas (Fig. 13.1*b*). Tumours must be debulked by piecemeal intracapsular removal in order to avoid any traction on the spinal cord. Ultrasonic aspiration may be useful but care should be taken not to damage the spinal cord. Most schwannomas can be totally cured only by sacrificing

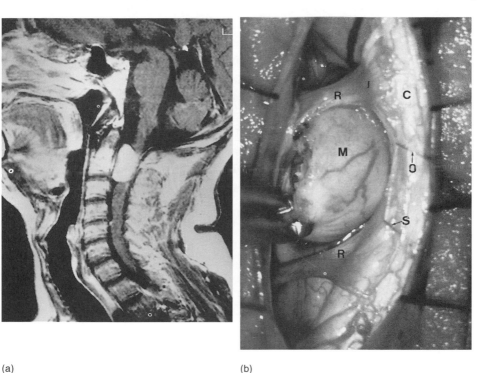

(a)   (b)

Fig. 13.1. Cervical meningioma. *a* MRI (T1-weighted with gadolinium) showing the tumor. *b* Operative view: M, meningioma; R, posterior roots; C, cord; S, sutures on dentate ligament.

sensory and motor roots. A conservative approach has been advocated in the past with partial excision of the tumour at spinal levels concerned for arm or leg functions (Stein 1985), but we favour an aggressive treatment with total removal, and nerve root sacrifice. Our experience has shown that patients may have minor or no deficit with such a policy, in agreement with the results of Kim *et al.* (1989). Surgical results are gratifying (Levy *et al.* 1986).

In hourglass tumours, it is often necessary to undertake an extraspinal approach to complete the intraspinal removal and achieve a total excision. However, this can seldom be made in Von Recklinghausen's disease where it is usually impossible to remove all the multiple spinal neurofibromas. The removal of spinal meningiomas differs from that of a schwannoma, which is a mobile tumour. Meningiomas are fixed to the dura and gradual tumour exenteration is essential except in posteriorly situated tumours. Caution should be taken with adherent blood vessels which must be preserved. Most spinal meningiomas are extra-pial lesions, not adherent to the spinal cord, and they may be removed without neurological deficit.

Operative mortality is low (less than 1%) (Solero *et al.* 1989) and neurological recovery good, even in those patients who had severe preoperative neurological deficits (Levy *et al.* 1982). Opinions differ on the necessity for dural excision. However, Levy *et al.* (1982) and Solero *et al.* (1989) had fewer recurrences when the dura was coagulated than when the dural attachment was excised. In our opinion, dural excision is seldom necessary as spinal meningiomas never invade bone, and very rarely invade the extradural space. We coagulate the attachment and peel the dura sheet by sheet until we get a normal white aspect. With such a policy we have had no recurrence so far, but we know that it may develop after a long delay as described by Philippon *et al.* (1986). To succeed, it is necessary to have control of the dural attachment which is sometimes very difficult in ventral tumours. In that case, an extreme lateral approach as described by Shucart & Kleriga (1980) or by Sen & Sekhar (1990) may be of great interest, as is the anterior approach using a transoral route as reported by Crockard & Sen (1991) in ventral tumours of the foramen magnum.

Intramedullary tumours

Incidence and clinical signs

Intramedullary tumours are relatively uncommon and they represent approximately 15% of all primary intradural tumours (Cooper & Epstein 1992). They are less frequent in adults than in children, in whom astrocytomas predominate (Reimer & Onofrio 1985). Over 50% are located in the cervical or cervicodorsal regions (Cooper & Epstein 1985; Cooper 1989). The most common initial symptom is spinal pain, particularly in children.

A number of patients will be noted to have a scoliosis, meaning that non-malignant tumours of the spinal cord, which are the majority, develop over a period of years. Later, weakness of limbs may develop, with sphincter disturbances in conus medullaris tumours. It is sometimes very difficult to assess on clinical signs the differential diagnosis between intra- and extramedullary tumours.

Diagnostic imaging

Since the advent of MRI, the diagnosis of intramedullary tumours has been much easier. However, MR study must be based on T1- and T2-weighted images as well as gadolinium-enhanced T1-weighted images (Fig. 13.2). Ideally, it should include sequences acquired in the sagittal, coronal and axial planes. In the case of scoliosis, three-dimensional acquisitions which allow reconstructions in all planes including the oblique and curved planes, are very useful (Balériaux & Brotchi 1992). In intramedullary tumours, a perfect MRI study is essential, with a close relationship between neuroradiologists and neurosurgeons. We need to know if the tumour is intra- or extra-axial, solid or cystic, the limits of the tumour versus the cyst, and its histology, whenever possible. Several tumours have a typical MRI pattern, e.g. lipomas, epidermoid cysts and haemangioblastomas. The last may sometimes be solid and accompanied by an

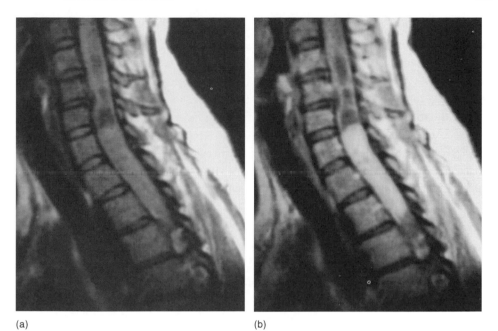

(a)   (b)

Fig. 13.2. Cervical ependymoma. *a* T1-weighted image showing a widened cord with cystic cavities. *b* Only the tumour is enhanced by gadolinium.

extensive secondary oedematous enlargement of the cord, but most of the time these gadolinium-enhancing tumours have an extensive cystic component.

The most frequent tumours, ependymomas and astrocytomas, are very difficult to distinguish one from the other. Many ependymomas resemble astrocytomas (Parizel *et al.* 1989). Both histological types may be either strictly solid or partially cystic. Contrast enhancement is usually more rapid and homogeneous in ependymomas while it appears to be slowly progressive and heterogeneous in astrocytomas (Balériaux & Brotchi 1992). In a series of 65 intramedullary tumours (Brotchi *et al.* 1991) the pre-operative histological diagnosis predicted by MRI was correct in approximately 70% of cases.

In the absence of a known primary cancer, it is often impossible to suspect a metastatic origin to a solitary intramedullary tumour. It has been encountered six times in our series of 65 cases (Brotchi *et al.* 1991). The differential diagnoses of intramedullary tumour also include multiple sclerosis, transverse myelitis, abscesses, syringomyelia and sarcoidosis (Levivier *et al.* 1991*a*,*b*). A brain MRI must be performed whenever a diffuse intramedullary lesion is discovered in order to eliminate multiple sclerosis. Plain films of the spine may have some value in showing a widening of the pedicles on frontal views or scalloping of the vertebral bodies in the sagittal plane, suggesting an intraspinal mass. Angiography is not indicated except in large haemangioblastomas, for which preoperative embolization may be useful and is mandatory in vascular malformations. With rare exceptions, MRI is the only modality necessary for the diagnosis of intramedullary tumours.

Treatment

We shall focus on the most frequent tumours. Surgical strategy will depend on the solid or cystic aspect of the tumour. It is well known that in haemangioblastomas, the elective removal of the tumoral nodule induces a progressive reduction of the cyst, even in the case of a cystic cavity apparently involving the whole cord.

Only the tumour should be removed and the satellite cysts opened. It is unnecessary to actively drain the cyst itself (Balériaux & Brotchi 1992). This is also true for cystic ependymomas and astrocytomas. It is mandatory to realize that the satellite cysts are non-tumorous. They are lined merely by glia and the fluid they contain is produced by the tumour itself (Cooper & Epstein 1992). That is why it is so important to know before surgery the exact relationship between the tumour and the cyst. As the cyst walls are non-tumorous, it is possible to limit exposure to the solid portion of the tumour and to avoid laminectomy. Of course, when cystic cavities are into the tumour, they should be treated and removed as the tumour itself. In children, however, laminotomy is necessary. The use of ultrasonography prior to opening the dura permits accurate localization of the solid portion of the tumour. It may help in tumoral diagnosis as astrocytomas have different echo features from ependymomas (Rubin & Chandler 1990).

Except in lipomas, where a decompressive procedure with a moderate reduction of the mass should be done, and in haemangioblastomas, which may be dissected from normal spinal cord, the surgical procedure begins with an approach strictly in the midline over the solid portion of the tumour (Brotchi *et al.* 1992). We like to use 6–0 atraumatic sutures through the pia at intervals of 2 cm on either side of the midline to maintain the spinal cord open. This enables one to do intramedullary surgery without manipulation of the spinal cord. We search for the poles and open there the frequently associated cystic cavities. Some authors like to use the CO_2 laser (Epstein & Epstein 1982; Roux *et al.* 1984; Cooper & Epstein 1985). As the only intramedullary landmark between the tumour and the normal tissue is a difference of colour, we are not in favour of the CO_2 laser, which may char the tissue. We prefer to use ultrasonic aspiration for debulking the tumour, working inside the lesion and stopping when the colour changes. This was of great help in our hands to remove most ependymomas and many astrocytomas (Brotchi *et al.* 1991). We like to close the spinal cord opening with separate atraumatic 8–0 non-watertight sutures and to try to close the arachnoid layer whenever possible. A watertight dural closure is then performed.

As shown by Cooper (1989) and by Cooper & Epstein (1985), the postoperative results depend on the preoperative status. No paraplegic patient was able to walk after surgery. In our recent publications (Brotchi *et al.* 1991, 1992), all our patients were evaluated 3 months after surgery. We observed 53% improvement, 37% stabilization and 10% postoperative deterioration whatever the surgical technique used (partial or total resection). That means that intramedullary tumours should be operated when the patient is still able to walk. There is no benefit in stabilizing somebody in a wheelchair!

Modern literature is in favour of aggressive surgical treatment of ependymomas and astrocytomas (Fischer & Mansuy 1980; Cooper 1989; Guidetti *et al.* 1981; Stein 1985;

Epstein & Wisoff 1987; McCormick *et al*. 1990). Some authors are in favour of adjunctive radiotherapy (Stein 1979; Kopelson *et al*. 1980, Cooper & Epstein 1992) in astrocytomas and incomplete ependymoma removal. Others find no benefit from radiotherapy (Fischer & Mansuy 1980; Guidetti *et al*. 1981; Brotchi *et al*. 1991, 1992) except in malignant gliomas, which are very rare in the spinal cord. The use of intraoperative spinal cord monitoring may be useful but long-term survival and neurological function are related to tumour histology, the patient's preoperative neurological status and extent of tumour resection. All these concepts have been recently detailed in a cooperative work between the Universities of Lyons and Brussels (Fischer & Brotchi 1994, 1996).

Extradural tumours

The commonest neoplastic disease affecting the spine is undoubtedly metastatic disease. Some primary malignant disease may also appear: chordoma, chondrosarcoma, Ewing's sarcoma, osteosarcoma and myeloma, and also benign processes such as aneurysmal bone cyst or osteoid osteoma. All these illnesses have a common symptom: midline pain local to the level of spinal involvement. In malignant tumours, neurological deficit will rapidly develop, with motor and sensory disturbances and sphincteric dysfunction, either acute or chronic, even in metastases as reported by Shapiro & Posner (1983).

Diagnosis

Differential diagnosis of spinal cord compression is mandatory, for example between primary neoplasia of bone and cartilage of the spinal column, and metastasis. One should not forget that thoracic disc protrusion may present in a very similar manner to metastatic disease.

If chest radiography is mandatory, there is no place for the practice of attempting to discover the presumed underlying primary lesion by additional investigation when there is a cord compression (Findlay 1992). Plain radiography of the spine shows evidence of metastatic disease in approximately 60% of patients with cord or root compression (Black 1979), the most common features being pedicular loss or vertebral collapse. However, one should have in mind that lymphomas do not induce any plain radiographic abnormality. Isotope bone scanning can be useful in assessment as it is more sensitive than plain radiography, although it may be positive in benign disease, e.g. arthritis, and both false-positive and false-negative results are not uncommon! Water-soluble myelography remains the most popular test, completed by a CT scan following the myelogram, although MRI is preferable as the primary investigation.

The usefulness of MRI in metastatic spinal compression has been defined (Sarpel *et al*. 1987) but the main problem remains difficulty in obtaining an MR scan in an emergency.

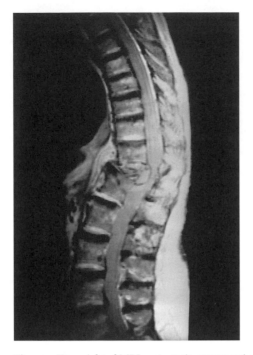

Fig. 13.3. T2-weighted MRI metastatic compression. In this case, a laminectomy would be wrong. An anterior approach combined with pedicle screws and fixation is the ideal surgery.

Treatment

Several studies have shown that radiotherapy alone may give the same good results as surgery followed by radiotherapy (Gilbert *et al.* 1978; Dunn *et al.* 1980; Young *et al.* 1980). Obviously this reinforces the need for a histological diagnosis. The strategy will be adapted according to the radiosensitivity of the lesion and to its location in the spinal canal. Benign lesions will be cured either by surgery or, for example, by embolization or methylmethacrylate injection in aneurysmal bone cyst (Galibert *et al.* 1987). Malignant radio-resistant tumours like sacral chordomas must be treated by extensive surgery. The same policy should be applied to primary malignant diseases which are seldom radiosensitive, even if radiotherapy is given after surgery. In metastatic disease, although neoplasms of the bronchus and the breast account for the vast majority (Constans *et al.* 1983), some other origin such as prostate, haematopoietic system or renal neoplasm may occur (Sundaresan *et al.* 1985). That is why a formal histological confirmation is sought in all cases when no primary is known, either through a surgical approach or by a percutaneous needle biopsy as described by Fyfe *et al.* (1983). CT study shows the tumoral invasion which, in most cases, involves vertebral pedicles and bodies. Nowadays, it has become clear that laminectomy carries a very significant incidence of adverse effects (Findlay 1984, 1987). Except in biopsy or in very rare posterior tumoral locations, it has little relevance.

Several reports describe the use of posterior spinal stabilization at the time of laminectomy, the most popular being Harrington distraction rods with or without segmental wiring (Sundaresan *et al*. 1984) and pedicle screw fixation combined with the Cottrel–Dubousset instrumentation (Aprin 1988). However, laminectomy even with instrumentation fails to decompress the cord adequately when severely compressed by an anterior mass (Fig. 13.3). This has led many neurosurgeons to perform anterior approaches. This is well established in the cervical spine and was first reported by Scoville *et al*. (1967) who resected a cervical vertebral body followed by an acrylic stabilization.

The use of the anterior approach allows maximum tumour removal but is quite difficult to perform in thoracic and lumbar areas. Sundaresan *et al*. (1985) have reported a series of 101 consecutive patients treated by vertebral body resection and stabilization, 13 in the cervical region, 68 in the thoracic and 20 in the lumbar area. Using an anterolateral surgical exposure, the vertebral body was resected along with all epidural tumour. Immediate stabilization was achieved with methylmethacrylate and Steimmann pins with a 78% overall ambulatory rate and 85% pain relief. However, these techniques require considerable surgical experience and expertise and should be restricted to patients who are not in the terminal phase of their disease.

These treatments should be offered to patients who may hope for some preservation or restoration of neurological functions, e.g. ambulation and control of bowel and bladder, which are the criteria of successful therapy in metastatic disease as defined by Siegal & Siegal (1985). Patients in poor condition should have radiotherapy alone. Surgery should be restricted to those who demonstrate neurological progression during the course of radiotherapy and to those patients who have recurrent symptoms referable to a previously irradiated metastasis (Dunn *et al*. 1980).

References

Agnoli, A. L., Laun, A. & Schönmayr, R. (1984). Enterogenous intraspinal cysts. *J. Neurosurg.* **61**, 834–40.

Aprin, H. (1988). Metastatic tumours of the spine. In *Spinal Tumours*, ed. B. Akbarnia, pp. 301–313. Philadelphia: Hanley & Belfus.

Balériaux, D. & Brotchi, J. (1992). Spinal cord tumors. Neuroradiological and surgical considerations. *Riv. Neuroradiol.* **5**, 29–41.

Balériaux, D., Parizel, P. & Segebarth, C. (1989). Pathologie intrarachidienne et médullaire. In *Imagerie du rachis et de la moelle*, ed. C. Manelfe, pp. 499–545, Paris: Vigot.

Black, P. (1979). Spinal metastasis: current status and recommended guidelines for management. *Neurosurgery* **5**, 726–46.

Brotchi, J., Dewitte, O., Levivier, M., Balériaux, D., Vandesteene, A., Raftopoulos, C., Flament-Durand, J. & Noterman, J. (1991). A survey of 65 tumors within the spinal cord: surgical results and the importance of preoperative magnetic resonance imaging. *Neurosurgery* **29**, 651–7.

Brotchi, J., Noterman, J. & Balériaux, D. (1992). Surgery of intramedullary spinal cord tumours. *Acta Neurochir.* **116**, 176–178.

Connolly, E. S. (1982). Spinal cord tumours in adults. In *Neurological Surgery*, 2nd edn, vol. 5, ed. J. R. Youmans, pp. 3196–214, Philadelphia: Saunders.

Constans, J., de Divitiis, E., Donzelli, R., Spazianti, R., Meder, J. & Haye, C. (1983). Spinal metastases with neurological manifestations: review of 600 cases. *J. Neurosurg.* **59**, 111–18.

Cooper, P. R. (1989). Outcome after operative treatment of intramedullary spinal cord tumours in adults. Intermediate and long-term results in 51 patients. *Neurosurgery* **25**, 855–9.

Cooper, P. R. & Epstein, F. (1985). Radical resection of intramedullary spinal cord tumours in adults. Recent experience in 29 patients. *J. Neurosurg.* **63**, 492–9.

Cooper, P. R. & Epstein, F. J. (1992). Intramedullary tumours. In *Surgery of the Spine*, ed. G. Findlay & R. Owen, pp. 587–600. Oxford: Blackwell Scientific.

Crockard, H. A. & Sen, C. N. (1991). The transoral approach for the management of intradural lesions at the craniovertebral junction: review of 7 cases. *Neurosurgery* **28**, 88–9.

Cushing, H. & Eisenhardt, L. (1938). *The Meningiomas.* Springfield: C. C. Thomas.

Dunn, R. C., Kelly, W. A., Wohns, R. N. W. & Howe, J. F. (1980). Spinal epidural neoplasia. A 15-year review of the results of surgical therapy. *J. Neurosurg.* **52**, 47–51.

Epstein, F. & Epstein, N. (1982). Surgical treatment of spinal cord astrocytomas of childhood. A series of 19 patients. *J. Neurosurg.* **57**, 685–9.

Epstein, F. & Wisoff, J. (1987). Intra-axial tumors of the cervicomedullary junction. *J. Neurosurg.* **67**, 483–7.

Findlay, G. (1984). Adverse effects of the management of malignant spinal cord compression. *J. Neurol. Neurosurg. Psychiatry* **47**, 761–8.

Findlay, G. (1987). The role of vertebral body collapse in the management of malignant spinal cord compression. *J. Neurol. Neurosurg. Psychiatry* **50**, 151–4.

Findlay, G. F. G. (1992). Metastatic spinal disease. In *Surgery of the Spine*, ed. G. Findlay & R. Owen, pp. 557–572. Oxford: Blackwell Scientific.

Fischer, G. & Brotchi, J. (1994). Les tumeurs intramédullaires. *Neurochirurgie* **40** (Suppl. 1), 1–108.

Fischer, G. & Brotchi, J. (1996). *Intramedullary spinal cord tumors*, pp. 1–115. New York: Thieme.

Fischer, G. & Mansuy, L. (1980). Total removal of intramedullary ependymomas: follow-up study of 16 cases. *Surg. Neurol.* **14**, 243–9.

Foy, P. M. (1992). Intradural extramedullary tumours. In *Surgery of the Spine*, ed. G. Findlay & R. Owen, pp. 573–86. Oxford: Blackwell Scientific.

Fyfe, I., Henry, A. & Mulholland, R. (1983). Closed vertebral biopsy. *J. Bone Joint Surg. Br.* **65**, 140–3.

Galibert, P., Deramond, H., Rosat, P. & Le Gars, D. (1987). Note préliminaire sur le traitement des angiomes vertébraux par vertébroplastie acrylique percutanée. *Neurochirurgie* **33**, 166–8.

Gilbert, R., Kim, J. & Posner, J. (1978). Epidural spinal cord compression from metastatic tumour: diagnosis and treatment. *Ann. Neurol.* **3**, 40–51.

Guidetti, B., Mercuri, S. & Vagnozzo, R. (1981). Long-term results of the surgical treatment of 129 intramedullary spinal gliomas. *J. Neurosurg.* **54**, 323–30.

Kim, P., Ebersold, M. J., Onofrio, B. M. & Quast, L. M. (1989). Surgery of spinal nerve schwannoma. Risk of neurological deficit after resection of involved root. *J. Neurosurg.* **71**, 810–14.

Kopelson, G., Linggood, R. M., Kleinman, G. M., Doucette, J. & Wang, C. C. (1980). Management of intramedullary spinal cord tumours. *Radiology* **135**, 473–9.

Levivier, M., Balériaux, D., Matos, C., Pirotte, B. & Brotchi, J. (1991*a*). Sarcoid myelopathy. *Neurology* **41**, 1539–40.

Levivier, M., Brotchi, J. Balériaux, D., Pirotte, B. & Flament-Durand, J. (1991*b*). Sarcoidosis presenting as and isolated intramedullary tumour. *Neurosurgery* **29**, 271–6.

Levy, W., Bay, J. & Dohn, D. (1982). Spinal cord meningioma. *J. Neurosurg.* **57**, 804–12.

Levy, W. J., Latchaw, J., Hahn, J. F., Sawhny, B., Bay, J. & Dohn, D. F. (1986). Spinal neurofibromas: a report of 66 cases and a comparison with meningiomas. *Neurosurgery* **18**, 331–4.

McCormick, P. C., Torres, R., Post, K. D. & Stein, B. M. (1990). Intramedullary ependymoma of the spinal cord. *J. Neurosurg.* **72**, 523–32.

Nittner, K. (1976). Spinal meningiomas, neurinomas and neurofibromas, and hourglass tumours. In *Handbook of Clinical Neurology*, vol. 20, part II, *Tumours of the Spine and Spinal Cord*, ed. P. J. Vinken & G. W. Bruyn, pp. 177–322, Amsterdam: North-Holland.

Parizel, P. M., Balériaux, D., Rodesch, G., Segebarth, C., Lalmand, B., Christophe, C., Lemort, M., Haesendonck, P., Niendorf, H. P., Flament-Durand, J. & Brotchi, J. (1989). Gd-DTPA-Enhanced MR imaging of spinal tumours. *Am. J. Neuroradiol.* **10**, 249–58.

Philippon, J., Cornu, P. R., Grob, R. & Rivierez, M. (1986). Les méningiomes récidivants. *Neurochirurgie* **32** (Suppl. 1), 54–62.

Reimer, R. & Onofrio, B. M. (1985). Astrocytomas of the spinal cord in children and adolescents. *J. Neurosurg.* **63**, 669–75.

Roux, F. X., Rey, A., Lecoz, P., George, B., Thurel, C., Cophignon, J. & Mikol, J. (1984). Astrocytomes et épendymomes intramédullaires de l'adulte. La tactique thérapeutique influe-t-elle sur les résultats à long terme? Bilan de 23 cas opérés et discussion de la littérature. *Neurochirurgie* **30**, 99–105.

Rubin, J. M. & Chandler, W. F. (1990). *Ultrasound in Neurosurgery*. New York: Raven Press.

Russell, D. S. & Rubinstein, L. J. (1989). *Pathology of Tumours of the Nervous System*, 5th edn. London: Edward Arnold.

Sarpel, S., Sarpel, G., Yu, E., Hyder, S., Kaufman, B. & Hindo, W. (1987). Early diagnosis of spinal-epidural metastasis by magnetic resonance imaging. *Cancer* **59**, 1112–16.

Sen, C. N. & Sekhar, L. N. (1990). An extreme lateral approach to intradural lesions of the cervical spine and foramen magnum. *Neurosurgery* **27**, 197–204.

Shucart, W. A. & Kleriga, E. (1980). Lateral approach to the upper cervical spine. *Neurosurgery* **6**, 278–81.

Scoville, W., Palmer, A., Samra, K. & Chong, G. (1967). The use of acrylic plastic for vertebral replacement of fixation in metastatic disease of the spine. *J. Neurosurg.* **27**, 274–9.

Shapiro, W. & Posner, J. (1983). Medical versus surgical treatment of metastatic spinal cord tumours. In *Controversies in Neurology*, ed. R. Thompson & J. Green, pp. 57–65. New York: Raven Press.

Siegal, T. & Siegal, T. (1985). Surgical decompression of anterior and posterior malignant epidural tumours compression of the spinal cord: a prospective study. *Neurosurgery* **17**, 424–32.

Sloof, J. L., Kernohan, J. W. & MacCarty, C. S. (1964). *Primary Intramedullary Tumours of the Spinal Cord and Filum Terminale*. Philadelphia: Saunders.

Solero, C. L., Fornari, M., Giobini, S., Lasio, G., Oliveri, G., Cimino, C. & Pluchino, F. (1989). Spinal meningiomas: review of 174 operated cases. *Neurosurgery* **25**, 153–60.

Stein, B. M. (1979). Surgery of intramedullary spinal cord tumours. *Clin. Neurosurg.* **26**, 529–42.

Stein, B. M. (1985). Spinal intradural tumours. In *Neurosurgery*, vol. 1, ed. R. H. Wikins & S. S. Rengachary, pp. 1048–61, New York: McGraw-Hill.

Sundaresan, N., Galicich, J. & Lane, J. (1984). Harrington rod stabilisation for pathological fractures of the spine. *J. Neurosurg.* **60**, 282–6.

Sundaresan, N., Galicich, J., Lane, J., Bavis, M. & McCormack, P. (1985). Treatment of neoplastic epidural cord compression by vertebral body resection and stabilisation. *J. Neurosurg.* **63**, 676–84.

Young, R., Post, E. & King, G. (1980). Treatment of spinal epidural metastases. Randomised prospective comparison of laminectomy and radiotherapy. *J. Neurosurg.* **53**, 741–8.

14 Multiple sclerosis

ALAN J. THOMPSON

Introduction

Multiple sclerosis (MS) is an inflammatory, demyelinating disorder. Its prevalence varies greatly throughout the world and appears to be influenced by a complex combination of geographical location and genetic background (Skegg 1991). In the temperate zones of northern Europe, North America and Australasia prevalence rates in the region of 100/100 000 are frequently recorded, reaching 300/100 000 in the Orkney and Shetland Islands. By contrast, most of Asia and Africa have a very low prevalence in the order of 5/100 000. There is a female preponderance with a male/female ratio of approximately 1–1.5. Mean age at onset is 30 years, but there is bimodal distribution with a major peak between 21 and 25 years and a lesser one at 41–45 years of age (Confavreux *et al.* 1980; Thompson *et al.* 1986). Childhood onset, although rare, is well recognized, and diagnosis has also been made in patients over 70 years of age (Noseworthy *et al.* 1983).

One of the hallmarks of MS is its inherent variation, which is seen within the individual patient, between patients and between groups of patients. This feature, together with an inability to predict the outcome of individual patients in terms of disability, is one of the most difficult aspects of the condition for the patient and for the development of a management plan. As MS frequently affects young adults the disability which results has a major impact on the areas of employment, family role and society, all of which have major implications in terms of resourcing and support (Inman 1984). A recent study has suggested that the 87 000 people with MS in the UK result in an annual financial loss of £1.2 billion sterling, the majority of which is made up of lost earnings for both patient and carer, and subsequent support from the state (Holmes *et al.* 1995).

Other demyelinating disorders

This small group of rare conditions may be usefully divided into those in which the demyelinating disorder is the sole disease process and those in which demyelination occurs in the context of systemic disease (Allen & Kirk 1992). The former group includes genetic disorders of myelin formation such as the lipid storage diseases and metabolic disorders such as phenylketonuria (Thompson *et al.* 1993). A number of rare conditions, many of which are probably variants of MS, have been described. They are usually of acute onset, fulminant course and poor prognosis (Marburg type, Balo's concentric sclerosis, Schilder's cerebro-sclerosis) or may involve specific parts of the central nervous system (Devic's syndrome or neuromyelitis optica). Devic's syndrome is the most common of the four conditions and is ascribed to patients in whom the optic nerve and spinal cord are involved in the early stage of the disease, usually in quick succession and frequently with limited recovery (O'Riordan *et al.* 1996*a*).

The most common demyelinating condition associated with systemic disease is central pontine myelinolysis, which predominantly involves the pons but also affects the tegmentum and cerebrum. It is usually seen in the setting of either chronic alcoholism or malnutrition and is thought to be precipitated by a rapid change in plasma sodium.

Clinical course

While MS may involve any area of the central white matter there are certain areas of predilection notably the optic nerve, periventricular area and cervical cord. Clinically the most common initial presentations are optic neuritis and sensory disturbance, though motor dysfunction and symptoms attributable to the brain stem, such as diplopia and ataxia, also occur frequently (Weinshenker *et al.* 1989*a*). Classically patients begin with a *relapsing and remitting course*; however, with time, remissions tend to be less than complete and residual deficit may accrue. Approximately two-thirds of patients pass into a progressive phase of the disease (*secondary progressive MS*) with gradual accumulation of irreversible disability, and not infrequently superimposed relapses. The remaining one-third of patients do not develop progressive disability and remain relatively unimpaired for many years (*benign MS*). A smaller proportion of patients (less than 10%) develop progressive disability from onset without relapses and remission (*primary progressive MS*) (Weinshenker *et al.* 1989*b*; Thompson et al 1997). These terms have been endorsed by a recent international survey which was carried out to review the nomenclature used to describe disease course (Lublin & Reingold 1996).

Establishing the diagnosis

The diagnosis of MS remains essentially clinical and requires the involvement of two areas of the CNS, affected at two separate times, i.e. dissemination in time and place. The third essential component of the diagnosis is the exclusion of other conditions which may produce a similar clinical picture. This is clearly laid out in Poser's criteria (Poser *et al.* 1983). The investigations that may be carried out in establishing the diagnosis include: (1) those which demonstrate an underlying immunological disturbance, i.e. the presence of IgG oligoclonal bands in the CSF; (2) those which provide

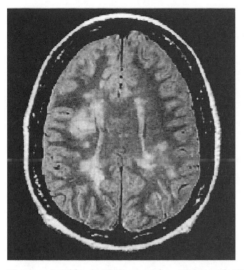

Fig. 14.1. Axial brain MRI scan of a patient with MS (fast spin echo with TE$_{eff}$ 100 ms, TR 2900 ms; 5 mm slice) demonstrating multiple small periventricular lesions. (Courtesy NMR Research Group, Queen Square.)

evidence for dissemination in space, i.e. evoked responses and MRI; and (3) tests which exclude other conditions.

IgG oligoclonal bands are found in the CSF of over 80% of patients with clinically definite MS. Their presence may be used to 'support' the diagnosis of MS, but it is important to remember that oligoclonal bands may be found in a wide range of neurological disorders many of which produce a similar clinical picture to MS.

Evoked potentials demonstrate a delay in conduction, indicating underlying demyelination. The most useful is the visual evoked potential (VEP), which gives a considerably higher positive yield than either the brain stem auditory evoked potential (BAEP) or the somatosensory evoked potential (SSEP). Results of these tests may be incorporated into the diagnostic criteria.

The development of MRI, allowing for the first time the identification of disease activity as it occurs, has made a major contribution to the diagnosis of MS, both in demonstrating dissemination in space and in the exclusion of conditions mimicking MS, particularly those affecting the posterior fossa, craniocervical function and spinal cord. Abnormalities – areas of high signal – are seen in over 95% of patients with clinically definite MS. The abnormalities are predominantly periventricular but may occur throughout the white matter (Fig. 14.1). They are also seen in a wide range of neurological conditions and in normal controls, particularly over the age of 50 years. Several authors have attempted to identify criteria to improve the specificity of MRI in the diagnosis of MS (Paty *et al.* 1988; Fazekas *et al.* 1988). The Fazekas criteria, which include (1) the presence of lesions adjacent to the ventricles, (2) an infratentorial lesion and (3) lesion size greater than 5 mm, have recently been shown to have a specificity of 96%, though a lower sensitivity of 81% (Offenbacher *et al.* 1993). Use of the contrast agent gadolinium diethylenetripentaacetic acid (Gd-DTPA), which has been shown to indicate blood–brain barrier breakdown in association with inflammation, greatly improves the detection of new disease activity (Miller *et al.* 1993).

Outcome in MS

When it comes to predicting outcome there are two separate questions to be considered: (1) what proportion of patients who present with a clinically isolated syndrome suggestive of MS will subsequently develop the condition and (2) is it possible to predict the rate of development of irreversible disability in patients with clinically definite MS? Until recently predictions for both groups of patients have relied heavily on clinical features with limited input from immunological and neurophysiological findings. Given the knowledge, both pathological and more recently from MRI studies (Thompson *et al.* 1991*b*), that much of the disease activity in MS is clinically silent (in some cases it is only seen post mortem: Gilbert & Sadler 1983; Phadke & Best 1983) it is perhaps not surprising that attempts to predict outcome have not been very successful.

Predicting development of MS

The presentation which has been most extensively studied in terms of progression to MS has been optic neuritis. There has been considerable discrepancy in the results of clinical studies, ranging from a predictive likelihood of developing MS of 8% in Japan (Isayama *et al.* 1982) to 75% in the UK after a 15 year follow-up (Francis *et al.* 1987). A number of factors, including patient selection, racial origin, geographical location and particularly duration of follow-up may contribute to these variations (McDonald & Barnes 1992). The risk of developing MS appears more likely for women (Rizzo & Lessell 1988), for those who present between 21 and 40 years (Hely *et al.* 1986) and for patients with IgG oligoclonal bands in their CSF (Sandberg-Wollheim *et al.* 1990). It is reduced in areas in lower latitudes. The influence of HLA is unclear though it has been suggested that HLADR3 in association with HLADR2 may increase risk (Francis *et al.* 1987). MRI studies have demonstrated that two-thirds of patients with optic neuritis have areas of high signal on cerebral MRI, and that their presence indicates a relative risk of developing MS of 68% within 1 year of follow-up (Miller *et al.* 1988).

There have been few clinical studies looking at brain stem and spinal cord syndromes but, as with optic neuritis, abnormal cerebral MRI findings increase the risk of developing MS by as much as 36-fold in the case of non-compressive cord lesions at follow-up. This risk is further increased by the presence of IgG oligoclonal bands in the CSF (Miller *et al.* 1989). A 5 year follow-up study looking at isolated syndromes (Morrissey *et al.* 1993) has confirmed the power of MRI in predicting the developments of MS. Of the 87 patients studied, 80% of those with abnormal MRI findings developed MS, while only 3% of those with normal scans did so. This finding has been supported by a 10 year follow-up of the same cohort (O'Riordan *et al.* 1996*b*). The presence of oligo-

Table 14.1. *Reported prognostic factors in multiple sclerosis*

Factor	Effects on prognosis
Age of onset	Late onset: poor prognosis (1–4, 12) No effect (5–7)
Sex	Male worse (1,5,6) No effect (2,3)
Symptoms at onset	Good: optic neuritis (5,8,12) sensory (4,9,12) diplopia (9) Poor: limb weakness (3,4,5,9) incoordination (1,3) No effect (2,7,10)
Length of first remission	Long: good prognosis (2,4,5,10,11,12) No effect (6)
Relapse frequency	Increased in benign MS (2,13) Low associated with good prognosis (11) No effect (7)
CSF IgG	No association (2,4) Correlation with disability (14)

From Thompson *et al.* (1986), by kind permission of Oxford University Press.
Figures in brackets indicate references listed below: (1) Leibowitz *et al.* 1969, (2) Confavreux *et al.* 1980, (3) Visscher *et al.* 1984, (4) Thompson *et al.* 1986, (5) McAlpine 1961, (6) Lhermitte *et al.* 1973, (7) Kurtzke *et al.* 1977, (8) Poser *et al.* 1982, (9) Poser *et al.* 1986, (10) Shepperd 1979, (11) Weinshenker *et al.* 1989, (12) Phadke 1990, (13) Bonduelle *et al.* 1979, (14) Stendahl-Brodin & Link 1980.

clonal bands and abnormal evoked potentials indicating subclinical involvement of another area are also of predictive value, but this is less strong than for MRI abnormalities (Kempster *et al.* 1987).

Predicting the course of disease

Once the diagnosis of MS has been firmly established one of the central questions is the rate of development of disability, particularly in relation to becoming wheelchair-bound. Factors including age and mode of onset, duration of first remission and relapse frequency have all been studied. There is a suggestion that early age of onset and presentation with either optic neuritis or pure sensory disturbance may be associated with a better prognosis (Table 14.1). Poor prognosis was associated with paresis, bladder dysfunction or cerebral disturbance at presentation. The evidence that the duration of first remission is a more accurate predictor of outcome is slightly stronger and there is a suggestion that polysymptomatic onset may be associated with a poor prognosis. In one of the most rigorous studies, carried out by Weinshenker *et al.* (1989*b*), increased relapse frequency in the early stages of the condition was found to be associated with increased disability, though this was not found in Runmarker and Andersen's recent study which had the benefit of 35 years of follow-up (Runmarker & Andersen 1993).

Immunological abnormalities including the CSF IgG index and oligoclonal bands do not appear to have any relationship with disease activity in MS and consequently are of no value in predicting outcome (Thompson *et al.* 1986; Zeeman *et al.* 1996). There is a growing consensus that a number of cytokines, notably interleukin-2 (IL2), its soluble receptor (IL2-SR) and tumour necrosis factor (TNFα), may correlate with disease activity, though their role in long-term prognosis is unclear (Sharief & Hentges 1991; Sharief & Thompson 1993). Similarly the relationship of adhesion molecules, such as E-selectin, to clinical activity needs to be evaluated (Giovannoni *et al.* 1996).

In contrast, there is a suggestion that an MRI scan at initial presentation gives an indication of the development of disability (Morrissey *et al.* 1993) in that patients who have many lesions at the clinical onset of the disease are likely to have more disability than those who had only a few lesions after a 5 year follow-up period. The predictive value of the initial MRI scan was even greater when the extent of abnormality was assessed by a semi-automated quantitative method (Filippi *et al.* 1994). The role of MRI in predicting disability in patients with established disease is less clear. There is some evidence to suggest that serial scans over a period of time may allow some useful prediction, but this is not very strong (Paty *et al.* 1992; Losseff *et al.* 1996a).

Progression

It is evident that in the majority of patients the onset of the progressive phase is the main determinant of disability (Confavreux *et al.* 1980; Thompson *et al.* 1986; Phadke 1990; Runmarker & Andersen 1993) and this is supported by the observation that patients whose disease is progressive from onset (primary progressive) have the worst prognosis in terms of developing disability. Recent serial MRI studies have suggested that primary progressive patients develop relatively few new lesions over time, with considerably less associated inflammation (gadolinium enhancement) when compared with the secondary progressive group (Thompson *et al.* 1991). Those findings prompted a pathological study addressing the issue of inflammation in the two forms of progressive MS, which demonstrated less inflammation in the primary group but nonetheless established clearly that inflammation did occur (Kidd *et al.* 1993).

As this has such a crucial bearing on the patient's outcome it is relevant to consider what is known about the nature of progression and the development of irreversible deficit in MS from pathological and, more recently, MRI data. It is well established that acute functional deficit results from demyelination and it has recently been demonstrated that inflammation itself can produce symptoms (Youl *et al.* 1991). In a study of acute optic neuritis the clinical syndrome was associated temporally with enhancement of the optic nerve on MRI, implying blood–brain barrier breakdown in association with inflammation. The acute phase was also associated with an abnormal VEP

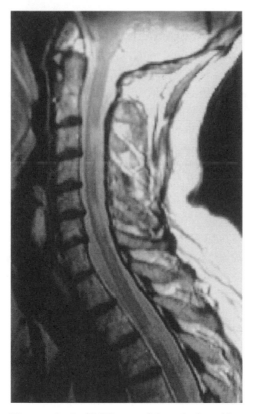

Fig. 14.2. Sagittal MRI scan of the spinal cord in a patient with MS (fast spin echo with TE$_{\text{eff}}$ 102 ms, TR 2500 ms; 3 mm slice thickness) demonstrating lesions at C4 and T1.

which was both delayed and of reduced amplitude, the latter suggesting conduction block. Both the conduction block and clinical symptoms resolved with the resolution of enhancement on MRI.

The cause of irreversible disability remains unclear, as does its relationship to the areas of abnormality seen on MRI. There is a discrepancy between the extent of MRI abnormality and the patient's disability (Thompson *et al.* 1990). Possible explanations for this discrepancy include:

1. the site of the lesion: e.g. involvement of the brain stem is more likely to cause disability than abnormality in the periventricular area.
2. Involvement of the spinal cord – until recently poorly visualized on MRI.
3. The known pathological heterogeneity of lesions.

Recent advances in technology, together with faster methods of imaging, have made it possible to look at the spinal cord (Thorpe *et al.* 1993) (Fig. 14.2). A cross-sectional study of 80 patients with MS has failed to demonstrate any relationship between the number of spinal cord lesions seen on MRI and the patient's disability (Kidd *et al.* 1993). This focuses the explanation onto the pathological heterogeneity of the lesion. In a study of chronic lesions in MS Barnes and colleagues (1991) demonstrated two distinct types of lesions: those with marked gliosis with relative sparing of axons, and those with markedly expanded extracellular space associated with extensive axonal loss. It would be reasonable to assume that the latter lesion would tend to be associated with more severe and irrecoverable disability. In his pathological study Barnes also showed that an MRI technique based on T2 relaxation measurements was able to demonstrate differences between these two lesions as a result of the presence of extracellular water. Lesions with expanded extracellular space showed a bi-exponential curve while in the remainder it was mono-exponential. Further MRI evidence to support the role of axonal loss in the production of irrecoverable disability can be found in the previously mentioned study of the spinal cord (Kidd *et al.* 1993), which showed a clear correlation between atrophy in the cervical cord (presumed to indicate axonal loss) and disability. This has been supported by a serial study which showed a relationship between progressive atrophy and increasing disability (Kidd *et al.* 1996) and a cross-sectional study at the C2 level using a more reproducible methodology (Losseff *et al.* 1996b). A study using T2 relaxation measurements demonstrated that chronic lesions in patients with secondary progressive MS tend to have greater expansion of extracellular space (and therefore by implication axonal loss) than lesions seen in patients with benign MS (Filippi *et al.* 1994). Proton spectroscopy, which looks at the biochemical content of the lesions, has also suggested changes which may indicate axonal loss, i.e. the reduction of the *N*-acetyl aspartate (NAA) peak (Arnold *et al.* 1992). A study by Davie *et al.* (1995) has shown a correlation between levels of NAA in the cerebellum and the degree of ataxia in MS patients. Another new technique, known as magnetization transfer imaging (Dousset *et al.* 1992), which essentially measures the structural integrity of tissue, has shown that the greater the loss of underlying structure the more severe the functional deficit. This has been supported by a clinical study showing a significant correlation between the magnetization transfer ratio and the level of disability in MS (Gass *et al.* 1994).

A related but simpler technique is the measurement of areas of low signal (so-called black holes) on T1-weighted scans. The volume of these abnormalities correlates well with disability (Van Walderveen *et al.* 1995) and they have recently been shown pathologically to represent 'burnt-out' destructive lesions. (Van Waldeween *et al.* 1966).

The second factor in the development of irreversible disability is the capacity for remyelination, which may become severely compromised following prolonged or frequent episodes of demyelination at the same site, or affecting the same tract (Johnson & Ludwin 1981). It is also possible that prolonged/recurrent inflammation at the same site, or at different levels of the same fibres, may predispose towards axonal disruption (Prineas *et al.* 1993).

The effect of environmental factors

A wide range of environmental factors have been implicated either in precipitating relapse or in the progression of disability. These include emotional stress, pregnancy, physical exertion, trauma, immunization and climate and seasonal variation. The only one of these factors which has been shown to influence disease activity has been infection (Sibley *et al.* 1985; Panitch 1994).

A number of studies have failed to demonstrate a relationship between trauma and disease activity (Sibley *et al.* 1991; Siva *et al.* 1993; Sibley 1993). In relation to pregnancy, although an increase in relapse rate has been shown to occur during the puerperium there is reduced relapse rate during the course of pregnancy and when both periods are combined there is no overall increase in relapse rate and no evidence of disease progression (Hutchinson 1993). One report has suggested that pregnancy may be associated with a decreased risk of progression (Runmarker & Andersen 1995).

The relationship between stress and disease activity in MS is difficult to evaluate, but an intriguing variation in beta-adrenergic receptor density on suppressor lymphocytes has been demonstrated (Zoukos *et al.* 1992).

Mortality

There is limited literature on mortality in patients with MS but recent studies suggest at worst a mean survival of 25 years (Phadke 1990) as against 76% surviving 25 years in Rochester Minnesota (Weinshenker 1994). In the largest study of its kind (Poser *et al.* 1986) the best prognosis in terms of death rate was seen in patients who presented with diplopia or sensory disturbance rather than optic neuritis. In an extensive population-based study by Phadke (1990) four adverse factors were found to be associated with increased mortality: age of onset, duration of disease, progressive disease and severe disability. The overwhelming majority of deaths relate to complications secondary to immobility, with few resulting directly from the disease itself. An increase in suicide rate in MS has also been reported (Stenager *et al.* 1992; Sadovnik *et al.* 1991; Sadovnik, 1994).

Outcome of treatments

Treatment in MS may be usefully divided into three separate areas:

1. Treatment which influences the course of the disease.
2. Treatment which influences episodes of disease activity, i.e. relapses.
3. Treatments aimed at symptomatic management and improvement of function (neurorehabilitation).

Treatments which influence the course of the disease

While there are still a number of gaps in our understanding of the disease process in MS a combination of immunological and pathological studies and, more recently, MRI has resulted in an improved understanding of the probable steps involved with consequent

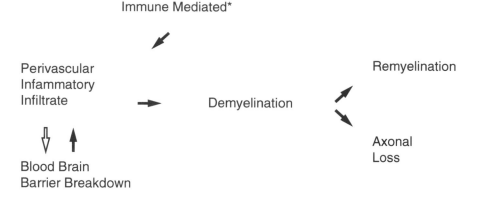

Fig. 14.3. Major steps in the disease process in MS.

identification of sites of possible intervention (Fig. 14.3). These may be broadly divided into: (i) the prevention of demyelination, mainly by interfering with the immunological processes involved, and alternatively (ii) the prevention of axonal loss and/or encouragement of remyelination.

Encouraging remyelination and preventing axonal loss (Compston 1991)
Therapeutic intervention in the area of encouraging remyelination and preventing axonal loss is still very much in the experimental stage, but areas of potential promise include increasing spontaneous remyelination by influencing progenitor cells to become oligodendrocytes rather than the alternative type 2 astrocyte (Raff *et al.* 1983), possibly incorporating the careful use of growth factors (Noble *et al.* 1988). Alternatively, the use of glial repair through transplantation may become a viable therapeutic option (Blakemore *et al.* 1990).

Influencing the immune system
The overwhelming majority of therapeutic approaches over the last 15 years have centred on attempts to influence the immune system. The majority of drugs studied (Table 14.2) have had multiple actions, many of which were poorly understood, and the rational behind their use has rarely been more than to either stimulate or suppress the immune system.

Table 14.2. *Immunotherapy in multiple sclerosis*

Non-specific

Azathioprine: no significant benefit in randomized control trials
Cyclophosphamide: conflicting results but negative randomized control trials
Cyclosporin: side effects outweigh marginal benefit
Deoxyspergualine: no significant benefit
Mitoxantrone: possible benefit but cardiotoxic
Total lymphoid irradiation: no benefit
Alpha interferon: no benefit in trials to date
Interferon beta-1a: reduced relapse rate in relapsing/remitting MS, possible effect on progression
Interferon beta-1b: reduced relapse rate in relapsing/remitting MS
Gamma interferon: increased relapse rate
Copolymer 1: reduced relapse rate in relapsing/remitting MS
IV gamma globulin: possible effect on disability
Linomide: randomized trials abandoned due to cardiotoxicity
Cladribine: randomized trials: no benefit
Oral myelin: randomized control trials under way

Specific

Vaccination: No study to date
CAMPAPTH 1: no clinical data
Anti-CD4 antibody: no benefit in MRI-based phase II trial
Anti-adhesion molecule: pilot study in progress
Anti-cytokines/TNF: studies anticipated

There are a number of factors peculiar to MS which render the interpretation of all but the most carefully designed studies extremely difficult (Noseworthy 1993*a*). These include its unpredictable course, tendency to sudden fluctuations and the level of subclinical activity. A further major difficulty has been the subjective nature of clinical assessment, which has relied heavily on scales devised by Kurtzke – the Kurtzke Scale (Kurtzke 1961) and the Kurtzke Expanded Disability Status Scale (EDSS) which includes eight functional systems (Kurtzke 1983). Both are ordinal, heavily weighted towards mobility, mix impairment and disability, and have considerable interrater and intrarater variability (Noseworthy *et al.* 1990; Francis *et al.* 1991). Apart from some concerns with regard to its reliability this scale is not very responsive to change (Hobart *et al.* 1996), there being a tendency for patients to stay for longer periods at some levels, particularly 6 and 7 (Weinshenker 1994). The difficulties in outcome assessment in MS have been well laid out in a recent paper which summarized the conclusions of a meeting held specifically to address this issue (Whittaker *et al.* 1995) and a Task Force was subsequently constituted to improve clinical outcome measures in MS (Rudick *et al.* 1996).

As discussed earlier, one major advance in this area has been MRI, which allows identification of all new activity while at the same time introducing objectivity in its measurement. The only caveat is that the relationship between MRI activity and clinical activity, particularly in relation to progression, remains unclear. That apart,

MRI must now be seen as an essential component of any further therapeutic trials in MS (Miller *et al.* 1991). Recent work has focused on defining how this might best be done, addressing frequency of scanning, number of patients required, duration of study and data collection and analysis (Barkhof *et al.* 1993; Nauta *et al.* 1994; Miller *et al.* 1996). It is now accepted that MRI is useful in screening new drugs and that using monthly scanning for as short a time as 6 months may detect a significant treatment effect with fewer than 100 patients. However, in any definitive phase III study it is still necessary that a clinical outcome is the primary outcome measure and not the MRI findings.

The MS literature contains data on many drugs that have appeared promising in initial, small open studies but have failed to show benefit when subjected to well-controlled trials involving large numbers of patients. A good example is azathioprine, which despite a number of encouraging pilot studies showed little benefit in a large multicentre trial of 354 MS patients (British & Dutch Azathioprine Trial Group 1988), while a subsequent meta-analysis of all blind randomized trials of azathioprine suggested a slowing in progression: by 0.2 on the EDSS over 3 years (Yudkin *et al.* 1991).

The benefit of the more powerful (and more toxic) immunosuppressant agent cyclophosphamide is less clear. Again, early unblinded studies were promising but no benefit was seen in a large, single-blind Canadian study (Canadian Cooperative Multiple Sclerosis Study Group 1991). A more recent study suggesting that pulse therapy with cyclophosphamide may slow progression has not been corroborated (Weiner *et al.* 1993*a*). Two randomized, blind trials of cyclosporin suggest it may have a therapeutic effect in MS but with unacceptable side effects (Rudge *et al.* 1989; Multiple Sclerosis Study Group 1990). Many studies have used complex regimes, which makes interpretation extremely difficult (Hauser *et al.* 1983). Until recently the only immunomodulating agent which has clearly influenced disease activity in MS was gamma interferon (Panitch *et al.* 1987), which worsened the disease process and increased the relapse rate.

Recently there have been encouraging reports from phase III trials of three compounds: two forms of interferon, beta-1b and -1a, and Copolymer 1 (Thompson & Noseworthy 1996). The first of these, a study of subcutaneous interferon beta-1b, suggested that it reduces both the relapse rate and the frequency of new activity on MRI in patients with early relapsing/remitting MS (IFNB Multiple Sclerosis Study Group 1993; Paty *et al.* 1993). This multicentre study, which was carried out over a 3 year period and involved 372 patients with early relapsing/remitting MS (mean EDSS of 3, mean disease duration < 5 years), was, as far as was possible, placebo-controlled and double-blind. The preparation used had a serine residue at position 17 instead of cysteine to improve stability. Two strengths of interferon beta were given every second day: 1.6 mIU and 8 mIU. The primary end points were the frequency of relapses and the time to the first relapse. One of the secondary end points was change in the EDSS. A small group of 52 patients had MRI scans every 6 weeks for 2 years. The results demonstrated that patients on the higher dose of interferon beta had a 30% reduction in relapse rate over 2 years when compared with controls. In the serial MRI study there was a 70% reduction in the occurrence of new lesions. Furthermore, the accumulation of lesion load differed significantly between the three groups at 1, 2 and 3 year intervals. However, change in disability, as assessed by the EDSS, show no significant difference between any of the three groups. This may be explained by the fact that the early relapsing/remitting patients studied would not be expected to show change over as short a period as 3 years, or that the outcome measure used was not sensitive enough to detect change over this period. It may also suggest that this agent has a more marked effect on the inflammatory stage of the condition rather than processes such as axonal loss which are responsible for progressive disability. The effects on relapse rate and MRI activity were confirmed by an extension study (IFNB Multiple Sclerosis Study Group 1995). Sixty-seven per cent of patients remained in the study for 3 years follow-up and 47% for 4 years. One important and somewhat disconcerting finding reported in this paper was the demonstration of neutralizing antibodies to interferon beta-1b. These were seen in 40% of patients, and those patients who were antibody positive demonstrated a loss of efficacy with relation to relapse frequency. There was some concern raised over the reliability of the viral-based assay which was used, but recently a more robust assay (based on MXA protein) showed similar findings (Sibley *et al.* 1996).

In April 1996 the results of a double-blind, multicentre, placebo-controlled trial of another interferon beta, interferon beta-1a, were published (Jacobs *et al.* 1996). This was a 2 year study of twice-weekly intramuscular interferon beta-1a. The primary end point was time to sustained progression, and using Kaplan–Meier failure time curves the time to sustained progression was greater in the treatment group ($P = 0.02$). This showed a reduction in relapse rate similar to that with interferon beta-1b and also a reduction in new enhancing lesions. Surprisingly, analysis of the MRI data failed to demonstrate a statistically significant reduction in lesion load in those on treatment after 2 years. This study was terminated prematurely when only 57% of patients had completed treatment. This has been the source of some discussion around the interpretation of the effect on progression, casting some concern over the contention that this form of interferon beta may affect disability progression on the EDSS.

It is clear that the interferon betas have some effect on disease activity in MS, possible mechanisms by which they may influence disease including (1) inhibition of gamma interferon production and consequently induction of MHC class II molecules, (2) reduction of cytokine release by macrophages, or (3) increasing suppressor T cell function (Panitch 1992).

Another agent which has been subjected to a phase III study is copolymer 1 (Cop 1) (Johnson *et al.* 1995*a*; Wolinsky 1995). This randomized, double-blind, placebo-controlled trial involved 251 patients in 11 centres. The drug was given by daily subcutaneous injection at a dose of 20 mg over 2 years and the study was restricted to relapsing/remitting MS. The authors reported a significant reduction in mean relapse rate over the 24 months (1.19 in the Cop 1 group versus 1.68 in the placebo group: a 29% reduction). The effects of Cop 1 on the development of disability were less clear cut, and comparing baseline with final EDSS slightly more patients (28.8% in the placebo group) changed by one or more steps on the EDSS than in the Cop 1 group (20.8%). However, when progression to sustained disability was defined as an increase in one or more EDSS steps, maintained for more than 3 months, there was no difference between the two groups. There was only a limited MRI component to this study and this did not show a significant difference between the two groups. A limited extension study was subsequently presented involving 203 patients (Johnson 1995b) which showed a continued effect on relapse rate but no difference on sustained progression in the two groups. An MRI-based study is currently being planned.

Other pivotal trials currently under way include a study of patients with secondary progressive MS with interferon beta-1b (Betaferon) (Polman 1995), a European study of interferon beta-1a (Avonex) in relapsing/remitting and secondary progressive MS and a study of patients presenting with isolated syndromes with interferon beta-1a (Rebif).

Of the other immunomodulating agents under study, results from a multicentre trial of deoxyspergualine have not shown a clinical benefit (Kappos et al. 1995), and the potential role of mitoxantrone is severely limited by its cardiotoxicity (Edan et al. 1995). Initial pilot studies of linomide were encouraging (Andersen et al. 1995), but two phase III trials were discontinued because of previously undetected cardiotoxicity. Although initial studies of Cladribine were encouraging (Sipe et al. 1994) a recent double-blind, placebo-controlled trial was negative. (Rice et al. 1997) A number of studies looking at intravenous immunoglobulin (IVIG) are underway (Noseworthy et al. 1995), and recent results have suggested a beneficial effect as measured by the EDSS (Fazekas et al. 1997).

While the beneficial effect of broad spectrum agents is encouraging, efforts are being made to develop more focused immunomodulating agents. These include antibodies against specific T cell subsets, such as the anti-CD4 antibody which attacks the helper inducer subset (O'Neill et al. 1993). While early uncontrolled studies (Hodgkinson et al. 1992) were encouraging a recent multicentre, double-blind, randomized, placebo-controlled MRI-based study has not shown any benefit with this agent (Van Oosten et al. 1997). Studies of the pan-lymphocyte monoclonal antibody, CAMPATH 1H (Moreau et al. 1994) have shown an effect on MRI activity but clinical data are not yet available. Studies of antibodies against certain cytokines including tumour necrosis factor (TNF) and interleukin-2 (IL2) may also be promising. Other, more radical attempts to influence the immune system include oral tolerance to myelin (Weiner et al. 1993b) and T cell vaccination. Attempts have also been made to block the binding of adhesion molecules and currently a study of monoclonal antibodies to the cell adhesion molecule alpha 4 integran is being undertaken. It is postulated that blocking this adhesion molecule, expressed on T cells and monocytes, from binding with its counter receptor VCAM 1 on brain endothelial cells will prevent transfer of lymphocytes across the blood–brain barrier and the subsequent formation of new lesions. The potential value of tolerization has been stressed by two recent papers which demonstrate the potential effect of intravenous administration of high-dose myelin basic protein (MBP) (Racke et al. 1996) and the beneficial effect of a peptide analogue of MBP in both preventing and reversing the neurological sequelae of experimental allergic encephalitis (Brock *et al.* 1996).

Finally, the potential contribution of diet needs to be mentioned. A number of studies have been carried out assessing the value of a diet low in animal fats and high in polyunsaturates incorporating supplementation with linoleic acid. The results of individual studies have been conflicting, and an attempt to combine all the data in a single meta-analysis has suggested a very slight benefit, though the nature of such an analysis weakens the power considerably (Dworkin *et al.* 1984). Other more stringent diets, including a gluten-free diet, have never been shown to be beneficial. Similarly, therapeutic benefit of high-dose vitamin B_{12}, and a wide range of electrical and physiological measures have never been demonstrated (Sibley 1996*b*). A case in point is the use of hyperbaric oxygen, which it is suggested has been valuable in a number of uncontrolled studies, but this has not been supported in a small placebo-controlled study (Wiles *et al.* 1986). In a recent review of all studies the consensus was that this treatment was not effective in MS (Kleijen & Knipschild 1995).

Treatment of acute relapse

Corticosteroids have an established role in the management of acute relapse in MS though the evidence for their efficacy is far from convincing (Goodin 1991). The initial study (Cooperative Study 1970) looked at the effect of ACTH in a randomized, double-blind, placebo-controlled study involving 197 patients in acute relapse, and reported a significant reduction in relapse duration in the ACTH-treated group, though this only reached a *P* value of < 0.05. In the mid-1980s so-called pulse therapy was introduced which involved high doses of intravenous steroids over 3–5 days. Several small studies suggested a potential benefit (Barnes *et al.* 1985; Durelli *et al.* 1986), which was supported by a larger study carried out in 1987 (Milligan *et al.* 1987) suggesting benefit from 500 mg of methylprednisolone over 5 days ($P < 0.05$). A study comparing 3 days of 1 g of intravenous methylprednisolone against ACTH in 61 patients with relapsing/remitting MS, seen within 4 weeks of onset of symptoms (Thompson *et al.* 1989), showed no difference between the two regimes. A major study on oral steroids, showed equal benefit when compared, double-blind, with I/V methylprednisolone (Barnes *et al.* 1997).

Initial studies looking at the effect of steroids in optic neuritis were no more convincing, with initial conflicting results (Rawson & Liversedge 1979; Bowden *et al.* 1974; Gould *et al.* 1977). In a recent multicentre, placebo-controlled study comparing intravenous steroids followed by oral prednisolone with oral prednisolone alone, the rate of recovery of normal visual fields and colour sensitivity (though not acuity) was significantly faster in the group receiving intravenous steroids at 6 months, though the difference had disappeared by 12 months (Beck *et al.* 1992). A surprising result was that, quite apart from showing no benefit over placebo, patients receiving oral prednisolone alone

Table 14.3. *Symptomatic treatment in multiple sclerosis*

Symptom	Treatment
Spasticity	[a]Baclofen: oral, intrathecal
Therapy input	Dantrolene sodium
	Diazepam
	Vigabatrin
	Local motor nerve blocks with botulinum toxin or phenol
Ataxia	Isoniazid
Therapy input	Carbamazepine
Bladder dysfunction	
Frequency/urgency/hesitancy	[a]Oxybutinin/clean intermittent self-catheterization
Nocturia	[a]Desmopressin
Sexual dysfunction	[a]Papaverine, prostaglandins, yohimbine
Paroxysmal motor and sensory	[a]Carbamazepine
symptoms (including trigeminal neuralgia)	Baclofen
Chronic dysaesthetic pain	Clonazepam
	[a]Tricyclic antidepressants
	Capsaicin analgesic cream
Fatigue	Amantadine
	Pemoline
	Calcium antagonists
Temperature lability	Aminopyridines

[a] Proven clinical value.

appeared to have a greater tendency to further episodes of optic neuritis in the subsequent 2 year follow-up period (Trobe & Arbor 1993).

MRI studies have shown that administration of intravenous methylprednisolone results in a transient cessation of enhancement which returns when steroids are stopped. It is also clear that new lesions occur while patients are on steroids (Miller *et al.* 1992).

Symptomatic management and neurorehabilitation

Symptomatic management (Thompson 1996)

Given the diffuse nature of the disease it is hardly surprising that patients with MS may develop an extensive range of symptoms (Table 14.3). Before discussing these it is important to mention a number of areas which pose major management problems and which tend to be overlooked, notably cognitive impairment, fatigue and thermolability.

Cognitive impairment Recent studies have shown that up to 50% of patients show some impairment of cognitive function, albeit only detectable through comprehensive neuropsychological testing (Rao *et al.* 1991*a*,*b*). While there is great variation in the severity of dysfunction it tends to be more marked in patients with secondary progressive MS compared with those in the early relapsing/remitting stage of the disease. Nonetheless, even in patients with isolated lesions cognitive deficits may be detected (Callanan *et al.* 1989). The most commonly affected areas include memory, sustained concentration, abstract conceptual reasoning and information processing. Studies which seek to clarify the nature of these deficits may result in improvements in cognitive therapy.

Fatigue Fatigue is a common but poorly defined problem in MS (Krupp *et al.* 1988). It is seen in association with acute relapse but may also be of a chronic and severely disabling nature. Definition and quantification are both difficult, though a useful scale has been developed recently. There is a suggestion that two drugs, amantadine and pemoline, may be useful in the management of fatigue (Weinshenker *et al.* 1992), though a recent study comparing these two agents with placebo showed that pemoline was no better than placebo, and the benefit from amantadine was minimal. Not surprisingly there was a large placebo effect (Krupp *et al.* 1995). A practical approach to fatigue management remains an important therapeutic option.

Thermolability The effect of temperature change on MS symptomatology is well documented, particularly deterioration in function with raised temperature (including that which is exercise induced) though also occasionally with cold. This is thought to result from slowing of conduction in partially demyelinated fibres and a number of studies using potassium channel blockers, which enhance conduction, have been undertaken. A recent double-blind, placebo-controlled, crossover study of 4-aminopyridine has shown a beneficial result without the serious side effects, including convulsion, suggested by earlier studies (Vandeman *et al.* 1992) even after prolonged follow-up (Polman *et al.* 1994). A slow-release preparation which may reduce side effects is currently under study (Bever *et al.* 1995).

Spasticity Spasticity is a common problem in patients with MS, particularly in the progressive stage. It tends to be more common in the lower limbs than in the upper, suggesting that it is of spinal origin. In functional terms it interferes with mobility, including transfers in those who are wheelchair-bound, and when severe is associated with spasms which may be flexor, extensor or abductor and which are often painful. The combination of spasticity and spasm may affect sleep pattern and in severely disabled patients interfere with personal hygiene. On occasion spasticity is of functional value, allowing the patient to weight-bear beyond the residual power in the lower limbs. Management involves physiotherapy, medication and, in severe cases, surgical intervention. None of these measures has been subjected to controlled studies.

The mainstay of treatment is the centrally acting GABA agonist baclofen, which should be started at a low level and increased slowly in association with physiotherapy input. Alternative medications include the peripherally acting agent dantrolene sodium, which can occasionally be useful, particularly in conjunction with baclofen, though it is poorly tolerated. Diazepam may have a role but other GABA agonists including vigabatrin have not been found to be of much value. More recently the role of intrathecally administered baclofen has been studied. This has been particularly appropriate for patients with very severe spasticity who show a response to baclofen but are unable to tolerate it in the high doses required; it has been shown to be effective in reducing both spasticity and the frequency of spasms (Penn *et al.* 1989; Ochs *et al.* 1989). Botulinum toxin may also have a limited role in the management of spasticity though its use necessitates large doses given at regular intervals. Intrathecal phenol may still have a role in the treatment of patients who have already lost bladder and bowel function.

Ataxia Ataxia is one of the most frustrating problems in MS, particularly when it becomes a prominent feature in the early stages of the condition and prevents the useful function of reasonably strong limbs. It is an extremely difficult symptom to influence but if any benefit is to be achieved then a combined approach including therapy and medication is best; the former to concentrate on areas such as posture and control of movement and the latter to attempt to dampen the intention tremor. Small studies have been carried out on isoniazid and carbamazepine; the former has been best documented (Sabra *et al.* 1982), though in the author's experience it is only effective in a small proportion of patients. Stereotactic surgery may be useful, particularly when the tremor is unilateral, but electrostimulation of the ventrolateral nucleus of the thalamus may be less invasive (Nguyen 1995). The use of weights is rarely of value.

Bladder dysfunction Bladder symptoms, particularly urgency and frequency of micturition, are extremely common in MS even at an early stage (Betts *et al.* 1993). Of all the areas of symptomatic management this is probably the one in which the greatest achievements have been made in the last decade. A combination of anticholinergic agents, such as oxybutynin, and clean intermittent self-catheterization (CISC) frequently results in excellent bladder control. For patients with nocturia desmopressin (DDAVP) has proved to be effective taken nasally. Finally, for patients in whom bladder control is proving impossible despite these measures, chemical denervation with capsaicin may be useful (Fowler *et al.* 1992).

Sexual dysfunction may also be usefully addressed in the male patient in whom there is failure to have or maintain an erection. This may be managed with intracorporeal papaverine or prostadiol, or, occasionally, oral yohimbine.

Paroxysmal symptoms Paroxysmal symptoms, such as paroxysmal dysarthria, ataxia, dysaesthesia and trigeminal neuralgia, are very effectively managed with carbamazepine.

The long-acting prostoglandin E_1 analogue misoprostol may also be useful in resistant trigeminal neuralgia (Reder & Arnason 1995). Chronic pain is a more difficult symptom. It is frequently related to lower back disturbance as a result of weakness of trunk muscles, spasticity in the lower limbs and poor posture, and is best managed with a combination of analgesia and therapy input. Dysaesthetic pain may respond to clonazepam or tricyclic antidepressants, though is not infrequently resistant to medication.

Dysphagia and respiratory symptoms Difficulty in swallowing as a result of pseudobulbar palsy occurs more frequently than is appreciated in MS. Respiratory involvement, particularly diaphragmatic weakness, although rarely noted is also more frequent than realized and may be life-threatening (Howard *et al.* 1992). It is seen more commonly in advanced stages of MS but may also complicate acute relapses, and although it is associated with poor prognosis a proportion of patients who require ventilation will recover and survive for many years.

Neurorehabilitation

Neurorehabilitation is frequently thought of in terms of the prevention of the secondary complications of neurological impairment, particularly the development of fixed contractures and pressure sores in patients with high tone and immobility. Pressure sores may occur in up to 15% of patients, though with improved management, particularly in relation to pressure relief, reducing spasticity and avoiding incontinence, this may be reduced (Elkin & Scheinberg 1992). While secondary complications are important in MS there are a number of other issues which must be considered in planning long-term management.

First, there is a wide diversity of symptoms in MS and while none of these is unique to the condition their sheer number poses a major management problem, particularly as many of the problems impact on each other. For example, the ability to manage bladder dysfunction with CISC will depend on upper limb coordination, mobility and cognitive state. Neurorehabilitation must be able to embrace all these individual areas but must ensure that this expertise is truly integrated – hence the proposed multidisciplinary team approach which should include a neurologist, nurse specialist/continence advisor, physiotherapist, occupational therapist, speech therapist, neuropsychologist and social worker.

The next issue is how best this multidisciplinary team can be effective in the management of chronic and often progressive disease. This requires clear guidelines as to when intervention is appropriate and crucial to this is assessment which will in turn identify areas of potential functional improvement. Following patient selection the rehabilitation process must be carefully monitored through clinical audit to assess extent and duration of benefit. For this to be done outcome measures addressing disability and handicap must be incorporated into the rehabilitation programme.

The International Federation of MS Societies addressed the issue of measuring impairment, disability and handicap in the early 1980s and agreed on a Minimal Record of Disability (MRD) (Slater & Raun 1984). This consisted of the Kurtzke Scale, the

Incapacity Status Scale and the Environmental Status Scale respectively. There are limitations with all three of these scales and a number of other scales have evolved since that time which may be more appropriate, particularly in the area of disability. These include the Functional Independence Measure (FIM) (Keith *et al.* 1987), derived from the Barthel Index (Mahoney & Barthel 1986), and the Functional Independence Measure/Functional Assessment Measure (FIM + FAM), an expansion of the FIM (Hall *et al.* 1993). Some small studies have suggested that at least in the short term disability and handicap may be improved in the face of stable or even slowly deteriorating impairment following multidisciplinary inpatient input (Bourdette *et al.* 1991; Kidd *et al.* 1995; Freeman *et al.* 1997) and this has been supported by a recent randomized controlled study of rehabilitation in MS (Freeman *et al.* 1996*b*). A preliminary investigation of the factors predicting rehabilitation outcome has suggested that ataxia and severe cognitive impairment have a particularly negative impact (Langdon & Thompson 1995).

It is essential that these outcome measures are incorporated into an overall plan for the patient, and recent work in developing Anticipated Recovery Pathways (ARPs) or Integrated Care Pathways (ICPs) goes some way towards achieving this (Rossiter & Thompson 1995).

The final issue is how this care may best be delivered. The acute hospital setting is usually inappropriate for such management unless investigation is required or the patient is severely ill. The patient may be best managed through a combination of inpatient, outpatient and community rehabilitation (Battaglia 1992). Ideally the last is most appropriate but requires close coordination and well-resourced community support, which is rarely available. Inpatient management has shown good results, at least in the short term, but the issue of carryover and the cost of such Units must be considered. An outpatient service which would offer a bridge between community and inpatient management may be the most appropriate medium, though difficulties with travelling and patient fatigue must also be considered. In summary it may well be that a combination of all three are required, with careful selection of patients according to their needs and disabilities.

References

Allen, I. V. & Kirk, J. (1992). Demyelinating diseases. In *Greenfield's Neuropathology*, 5th edn, ed. J. H. Adams & L. W. Duchen, pp. 447–520. London: Edward Arnold.

Andersen, O. *et al.* (1995). Linomide reduces the rate of active lesions in relapsing–remitting multiple sclerosis. *J. Neuroimmunol.* Suppl. **1**, 26.

Arnold, D. L. *et al.* (1992). Proton magnetic resonance spectroscopic imaging for metabolic characterization of demyelinating plaques. *Ann. Neurol.* **31**, 235–41.

Barkhof, F. *et al.* (1993). Database for serial magnetic resonance imaging in multiple sclerosis. *Neuroradiology* **35**, 362–6.

Barnes, D. *et al.* (1991). The longstanding MS lesion: a quantitative MRI and electron microscopic study. *Brain* **114**, 1271–80.

Barnes, D., Hughes, R. A. C., Morris, R., Wade-Jones, O., Brown, P., Britton, T., Francis, D. A.,

Perkin, D. G., Rudge, P., Swash, M. Katifi, H., Farmer, S. & Frankel, J. (1997). Randomised trial of oral and intravenous steroid in acute relapses of multiple sclerosis. *Lancet* **349**, 902–906.

Barnes, M. P. *et al.* (1995). Intravenous methyl-prednisolone for multiple sclerosis in acute relapse. *J. Neurol. Neurosurg. Psychiatry* **48**, 157–9.

Battaglia, M. A. (1992). Rehabilitation for MS people: the experience of the Italian MS Society. In *Rehabilitation in Multiple Sclerosis (RIMS)*, Proceedings of the First European Workshop, ed. P. Ketelaer & M. A. Battaglia, pp. 80–2. Genoa: AISM Assocazione Italiana Sclerosi Multipla.

Beck, R. W. *et al.* (1992). A randomized, controlled trial of cortico-steroids in the treatment of acute optic neuritis. *N. Engl. J. Med.* **326**, 581–9.

Betts, C. D., D'Mellow, M. T. & Fowler, C. J. (1993). Urinary symptoms and the neurological features of bladder dysfunction in multiple sclerosis. *J. Neurol. Neurosurg. Psychiatry* **56**, 245–50.

Bever, C. T. *et al.* (1995). The pharmacokinetics and tolerability of a slow-release formulation of 4-aminopyridine in multiple sclerosis patients. *Neurology* **45** (Suppl. 4), 684P.

Blakemore, W. F., Crang, A. J. & Franklin, R. J. M. (1990). Transplantation of glial cell cultures into areas of demyelination in the adult CNS. *Prog. Brain Res.* **82**, 225–32.

Bourdette, D. *et al.* (1991). Evidence that a multidisciplinary team care clinic is more effective than standard medical care in treating veterans with multiple sclerosis. *Neurology* **41**, 353.

Bowden, A. N. *et al.* (1974). A trial of corticotrophin gelatin injection in acute optic neuritis. *J. Neurol. Neurosurg. Psychiatry* **37**, 869.

British and Dutch Azathioprine Trial Group (1988). Double-masked trial of azathioprine in multiple sclerosis. *Lancet* **332**, 179–83.

Brock, S. *et al.* (1996). Treatment of experimental encephalomyelitis with a peptide analogue of myelin basic protein. *Nature* **379**, 343–6.

Callanan, M. M. *et al.* (1989). Cognitive impairment in patients with clinically isolated lesions of the type seen in multiple sclerosis. *Brain* **112**, 361–75.

Canadian Cooperative Multiple Sclerosis Study Group (1991). The Canadian cooperative trial of cyclophosphamide and plasma exchange in progressive multiple sclerosis. *Lancet* **337**, 441–6.

Compston, A. (1991). Limiting and repairing the damage in multiple sclerosis. Editorial. *J. Neurol. Neurosurg. Psychiatry* **54**, 945–8.

Confavreux, C., Aimard, G. & Devic, M. (1980). Course and prognosis of multiple sclerosis assessed by the computerised data processing of 349 patients. *Brain* **103**, 281–300.

Cooperative Study (1970). The evaluation of therapy in multiple sclerosis: ACTH versus placebo. Final report. *Neurology* **20**, 1–59.

Davie, C. A. *et al.* (1995). Persistent functional deficit in multiple sclerosis and autosomal dominant cerebellar ataxia is associated with axon loss. *Brain* **118**, 1583–92.

Dousset, V. *et al.* (1992). Experimental allergic encephalomyelitis and multiple sclerosis: lesion characterization with magnetic transfer imaging. *Radiology* **182**, 483–91.

Durelli, L. *et al.* (1986). High dose intravenous methylprednisolone in the treatment of multiple sclerosis: clinico-immunologic correlations. *Neurology* **36**, 238–43.

Dworkin, R. H. *et al.* (1984). Linoleic acid and multiple sclerosis: a reanalysis of three double blind trials. *Neurology* **34**, 1441–5.

Edan, G. *et al.* (1995). Demonstration of the efficacy of Mitoxantrone (MTX) in MS patients with very active disease. *J. Neuroimmunol.* Suppl. **1**, 16.

Elin, R. & Scheinberg, L. C. (1992). Multiple sclerosis: treatment and rehabilitation. In *Principles and Practice of Restorative Neurology*, ed. R. R. Young & P. J. Delwaide, pp. 136–44. Oxford: Butterworth.

Fazekas, F. *et al.* (1988). Criteria for an increased specificity of MRI interpretation in elderly subjects with suspected multiple sclerosis. *Neurology* **38**, 1822–1825.

Fazekas, F., Deisenhammer, F., Strasser-Fuchs, S., Nahler, G. & Mamoli, B. for the Austrian Immunoglobulin in Multiple Sclerosis Study Group (1997). Randomised placebo-controlled trial of monthly intravenous immunoglobulin therapy in relapsing-remitting multiple sclerosis. *Lancet* **349**, 589–93.

Filippi, M. *et al.* (1994). Quantitative brain MRI lesion load predicts the course of clinically isolated syndromes suggestive of multiple sclerosis. *Neurology* **44**, 635–41.

Fowler, C. J. *et al.* (1992). Intravesical capsaicin for neurogenic bladder dysfunction. *Lancet* **339**, 1239.

Francis, D. A. *et al.* (1987). A reassessment of the risk of multiple sclerosis developing in patients with optic neuritis after extended follow-up. *J. Neurol. Neurosurg. Psychiatry* **50**, 758–65.

Francis, D. A. *et al.* (1991). An assessment of disability rating scales used in multiple sclerosis. *Arch. Neurol.* **48**, 299–301.

Freeman, J. A. *et al.* (1996*a*). A neurological rehabilitation unit: audit of activity and outcome. *J. R. Soc. Med.* **30**, 21–6.

Freeman, J. A., Langdon, D. W., Hobart, J. C. & Thompson, A. J. (1997). The impact of inpatient rehabilitation on progressive multiple sclerosis. *Ann. Neurol.* **42**, 236–44.

Gass, A. *et al.* (1994). Correlation of magnetisation transfer ratio with clinical disability in multiple sclerosis. *Ann. Neurol.* **36**, 62–7.

Gilbert, J. J. & Sadler, M. (1983). Unexpected multiple sclerosis. *Arch. Neurol.* **40**, 533–6.

Giovannoni, G. *et al.* (1996). Soluble E-selectin in multiple sclerosis: raised concentrations in patients with primary progressive disease. *J. Neurol. Neurosurg. Psychiatry* **60**, 20–6.

Goodkin, D. S. (1991). The use of immunosuppressive agents in the treatment of multiple sclerosis: a critical review. *Neurology* **41**, 980–5.

Gould, E. S. *et al.* (1977). Treatment of optic neuritis by retrobulbar injection of triamcinolone. *BMJ* I, 1495–7.

Hall, K. M. *et al.* (1993). Characteristics and comparisons of functional assessment indices: Disability Rating Scale, FIM, Functional Assessment Measure. *J. Head Trauma Rehabil.* **8**, 60–74.

Hauser, S. L. *et al.* (1983). Intensive immunosuppression in progressive multiple sclerosis: a randomized, three-arm study of high-dose intravenous cyclophosphamide, plasma exchange, and ACTH. *N. Eng. J. Med.* **308**, 173–80.

Hely, M. A. *et al.* (1986). Acute optic neuritis: a prospective study of risk factors for multiple sclerosis. *J. Neurol. Neurosurg. Psychiatry* **49**, 1125–30.

Hobart, J. C. *et al.* (1996). Evaluating neurological outcome measures: the bare essentials. *J. Neurol. Neurosurg. Psychiatry* **60**, 127–30.

Hodgkinson, S. *et al.* (1992). Phase 1 study of chimeric anti-CD4 monoclonal antibody in multiple sclerosis. *Neurology* **42** (Suppl. 3), 209.

Holmes, J., Madgwick, T. & Bates, D. (1995). The cost of multiple sclerosis. *Br. J. Med. Econ.* **8**, 181–93.

Howard, R. S. *et al.* (1992). Respiratory involvement in multiple sclerosis. *Brain* **115**, 479–94.

Hutchinson, M. (1993). Pregnancy in multiple sclerosis. *J. Neurol. Neurosurg. Psychiatry* **56**, 1043–5.

IFNB Multiple Sclerosis Study Group (1993). Interferon beta-1b is effective in relapsing–remitting multiple sclerosis. I. Clinical results of a multicenter, randomized, double-blind, placebo-controlled trial. *Neurology* **43**, 655–61.

IFNB Multiple Sclerosis Study Group (1995). Interferon beta-1b in the treatment of MS: final outcome of the randomised controlled trial. *Neurology* **45**, 1277–85.

Inman, R. P. (1984) Disability indices, the economic costs of illness, and social insurance: the case of multiple sclerosis. *Acta Neurol. Scand.* **70**, 46–55.

Isayama, Y. *et al.* (1982). Acute optic neuritis and multiple sclerosis. *Neurology* **32**, 73–6.

Jacobs, L. D. *et al.* (1996). Intramuscular interferon beta-1a for disease progression in relapsing multiple sclerosis. *Ann. Neurol.* **39**, 285–94.

Johnson, E. S. & Ludwin, S. K. (1981). The demonstration of recurrent demyelination and remyelination of axons in the central nervous system. *Acta Neuropathol.* **53**, 93–8.

Johnson, K. P. *et al.* (1995*a*). Copolymer 1 reduces relapse rate and improves disability in relapsing–remitting multiple sclerosis: results of a phase III multicentre, double-blind, placebo-controlled trial. *Neurology* **45**, 1268–76.

Johnson, K. P. and the US Phase III Copolymer 1 Study Group (1995*b*). Copolymer 1: multicentre multiple sclerosis trial extension shows improved effects on relapse rate and disability. *Ann. Neurol.* **38**, 973.

Kappos, L. *et al.* (1995). Deoxyspergualine (DSG) in MS: second interim analysis of the European multicentre study. *J. Neurol.* **242**, S23.

Keith, R. A. *et al.* (1987). The Functional Independence Measure: a new tool for rehabilitation. In *Advances in Clinical Rehabilitation*, ed. M. G. Eisenberg & R. C. Grzesiak, Pp. 6–18. New York: Springer-Verlag.

Kempster, P. A. *et al.* (1987). Value of visual evoked response and oligoclonal bands in cerebrospinal fluid in diagnosis of spinal multiple sclerosis. *Lancet* **I**, 769–71.

Kidd, D. *et al.* (1993). Spinal cord MRI using multi-array coils and fast spin echo. II. Findings in multiple sclerosis. *Neurology* **43**, 2632–7.

Kidd, D. *et al.* (1995). The benefit of inpatient neurorehabilitation in multiple sclerosis. *Clin. Rehabil.* **9**, 198–203.

Kidd, D. *et al.* (1996). MRI dynamics of brain and spinal cord in progressive multiple sclerosis. *J. Neurol. Neurosurg. Psychiatry* **60**, 15–19.

Kleijen, J. & Knipschild, P. (1995). Hyperbaric oxygen for multiple sclerosis: review of controlled trials. *Acta Neurol. Scand.* **91**, 330–1.

Krupp, L. B. *et al.* (1988). Fatigue in multiple sclerosis. *Arch. Neurol.* **45**, 435–7.

Krupp, L. B. *et al.* (1995). Fatigue therapy in multiple sclerosis: results of a double-blind, randomised, parallel trial of amantadine, pemoline and placebo. *Neurology* **45**, 1956–61.

Kurtzke, J. F. (1961). Further notes on disability evaluation in multiple sclerosis with scale modifications. *Neurology* **15**, 654–61.

Kurtzke, J. F. (1983). Rating neurologic impairment in multiple sclerosis: an expanded disability status scale (EDSS). *Neurology* **33**, 1444–52.

Kurtzke, J. F. *et al.* (1977). Studies on the natural history of multiple sclerosis. 8. Early prognostic features of the later course of the illness. *J. Chron. Dis.* **30**, 819–30.

Langdon, D. W. & Thompson, A. J. (1995). Variables affecting the outcome of neurorehabilitation of patients with multiple sclerosis. *J. Neurol.* **242**, S38.

Leibowitz, U. *et al.* (1969). Survival and death in multiple sclerosis. *Brain* **92**, 115–30.

Lhermitte, F. *et al.* (1973). The frequency of relapse in multiple sclerosis: a study based on 245 cases. *J. Neurol.* **205**, 47–59.

Losseff, N. A. *et al.* (1996*a*). Clinical and magnetic resonance imaging predictors in primary and secondary progressive MS. *Multiple Sclerosis* **1**, 218–22.

Losseff, N. A. *et al.* (1996*b*). Spinal cord atrophy and disability in multiple sclerosis: a new reproducible and sensitive MRI method with potential to monitor disease progression. *Brain* **119**, 701–8.

Lublin, F. & Reingold, S. (1996). Defining the clinical course of multiple sclerosis: results of an international survey. *Neurology* **46**, 907–10.

McAlpine, D. (1961). The benign form of multiple sclerosis: a study based on 241 cases seen within three years of onset and followed up until the tenth year or more of the disease. *Brain* **84**, 186–203.

McDonald, W. I. & Barnes, D. (1992). Disease of the optic nerve. In *Diseases of the Nervous System: Clinical Neurobiology*, ed. A. K. Asbury, G. M. McKhann & W. I. Mcdonald, pp. 421–33. Philadelphia: W. B. Saunders.

Mahoney, F. I. & Barthel, D. W. (1986). Functional evaluation: the Barthel Index. *Maryland State Med. J.* **14**, 61–5.

Miller, D. H. *et al.* (1988). The early risk of multiple sclerosis after optic neuritis. *J. Neurol. Neurosurg. Psychiatry* **51**, 1569–71.

Miller, D. H. *et al.* (1989). The early risk of multiple sclerosis following isolated acute syndromes of the brainstem and spinal cord. *Ann. Neurol.* **26**, 635–9.

Miller, D. H. *et al.* (1991). Magnetic resonance imaging in monitoring the treatment of multiple sclerosis: CEC guide-lines. *J. Neurol. Neurosurg. Psyiatry* **54**, 683–8.

Miller, D. H. *et al.* (1992). High dose steroids in acute relapses of multiple sclerosis: MRI evidence for a possible mechanism of therapeutic effect. *J. Neurol. Neurosurg. Psychiatry* **55**, 450–3.

Miller, D. H., Barkhof, F. & Nauta, J. J. (1993). Gadolinium enhancement increases the sensitivity of MRI in detecting disease activity in multiple sclerosis. *Brain* **116**, 1077–94.

Miller, D. H. *et al.* (1996). Guidelines for the use of magnetic resonance techniques in monitoring the treatment of multiple sclerosis. *Ann. Neurol.* **39**, 6–16.

Milligan, N. M., Newcombe, R. & Compston, D. A. S. (1987). A double blind controlled trial of high dose methylprednisolone in patients with multiple sclerosis. I. Clinical effects. *J. Neurol. Neurosurg. Psychiatry* **50**, 511–16.

Moreau, T. *et al.* (1994). Preliminary evidence from magnetic resonance imaging for reduction in disease activity after lymphocyte depletion in multiple sclerosis. *Lancet* **344**, 298–301.

Morrissey, S. P. *et al.* (1993). The significance of brain magnetic resonance imaging abnormalities at presentation with clinically isolated syndromes suggestive of multiple sclerosis: a five year follow up study. *Brain* **116**, 135–46.

Multiple Sclerosis Study Group (1990). Efficacy and toxicity of cyclosporine in chronic progressive multiple sclerosis: a randomized, double-blind, placebo-controlled clinical trial. *Ann. Neurol.* **27**, 591–605.

Nauta, J. J. P. (1994). Magnetic resonance imaging in monitoring the treatment of multiple sclerosis patients: statistical power of parallel-groups and crossover designs. *J. Neurol. Sci.* **122**, 6–14.

Nguyen, J. P. *et al.* (1995). Treatment of severe tremor by chronic thalamic stimulation in 25 patients with multiple sclerosis. *J. Neuroimmunol.* Suppl. **1**, 30.

Noble, M. *et al.* (1988). Platelet derived growth factor promotes division and motility and inhibits premature differentiation of the oligodendrocyte/type 2 astrocyte progenitor cell. *Nature* **333**, 560–2.

Noseworthy, J. H. (1993). Clinical trials in multiple sclerosis. *Curr. Opin. Neurol. Neurosurg.* **6**, 209–15.

Noseworthy, J. *et al.* (1983). Multiple sclerosis after age 50. *Neurology* **33**, 1537–44.

Noseworthy, J. H. *et al.* (1990). Interrater variability with the expanded disability status scale

(EDSS) and functional systems (FS) in multiple sclerosis clinical trial. *Neurology* **40**, 971–5.

Noseworthy, J. H. *et al.* (1994). Intravenous immunoglobulin therapy in multiple sclerosis: progress from remyelination in the Theiler's virus model to a randomised, double-blind, placebo-controlled clinical trial. *J. Neurol. Neurosurg. Psychiatry* **57**, S11–17.

Ochs, G. *et al.* (1989). Intrathecal baclofen for long-term treatment of spasticity: a multi-centre study. *J. Neurol. Neurosurg. Psychiatry* **52**, 933–9.

Offenbacher, H. *et al.* (1993). Assessment of MRI criteria for a diagnosis of MS. *Neurology* **43**, 905–9.

O'Neil, J. K. *et al.* (1993). Control of immune-mediated disease of the central nervous system with monoclonal (CD4-specific) antibodies. *J. Neuroimmunol.* **45**, 1–11.

O'Riordan, J. I. *et al.* (1996*a*). Clinical, CSF, and MRI findings in Devic's neuromyelitis optica. *J. Neurol. Neurosurg. Psychiatry* **60**, 382–7.

O'Riordan, J. I. *et al.* (1996*b*). The long term risk of multiple sclerosis following clinically isolated syndromes of the central nervous system. *J. Neurol.* **243**, S33.

Panitch, H. S. *et al.* (1987). Exacerbations of multiple sclerosis in patients treated with gamma interferon. *Lancet* **I**, 893–4.

Panitch, H. S. (1992). Interferons in multiple sclerosis: a review of the evidence. *Drugs* **44**, 946–62.

Panitch, H. S. (1994). Influence of infection on exacerbations of multiple sclerosis. *Ann. Neurol.* **36**, S25–8.

Paty, D. W. *et al.* (1988). MRI in the diagnosis of MS: a prospective study with comparison of clinical evaluation, evoked potentials, oligoclonal banding, and CT. *Neurology* **38**, 180–5.

Paty, D. W. *et al.* (1992). Does the MRI activity rate predict the clinical course of MS? *Neurology* **42** (Suppl. 3), 427.

Paty, D. W. *et al.* (1993). Interferon beta-1b is effective in relapsing–remitting multiple sclerosis. 2. MRI analysis results of a multicenter, randomized, double-blind, placebo-controlled trial. *Neurology* **43**, 662–7.

Penn, R. D. *et al.* (1989). Intrathecal baclofen for severe spinal spasticity. *N. Engl. J. Med.* **320**, 1517–21.

Phadke, J. G. (1990). Clinical aspects of multiple sclerosis in North-East Scotland with particular reference to its course and prognosis. *Brain* **113**, 1597–628.

Phadke, J. G. & Best, P. V. (1983). Atypical and clinically silent multiple sclerosis: a report of 12 cases discovered unexpectedly at necropsy. *J. Neurol. Neurosurg. Psychiatry* **46**, 414–20.

Polman, C. H. *et al.* (1994). 4-Aminopyridine in the treatment of patients with MS: long term efficacy and safety. *Arch. Neurol.* **51**, 292–6.

Polman, C. H. (1995). Interferon beta-1b in secondary progressive multiple sclerosis: outline of the clinical trial. *Multiple Sclerosis* **1**, S51–4.

Poser, S. *et al.* (1982). Age at onset, initial symptomatology, and the course of multiple sclerosis. *Acta Neurol. Scand.* **66**, 355–62.

Poser, C. M. *et al.* (1983). New diagnostic criteria for multiple sclerosis: guidelines for research protocols. *Ann. Neurol.* **13**, 227–31.

Poser, S. *et al.* (1986). Prognostic indicators in multiple sclerosis. *Acta Neurol. Scand.* **74**, 387–92.

Prineas, J. W. *et al.* (1993). Multiple sclerosis: pathology of recurrent lesions. *Brain* **116**, 681–93.

Racke, M. K. *et al.* (1996). Intravenous antigen administration as a therapy for autoimmune demyelinating disease. *Ann. Neurol.* **39**, 46–56.

Raff, M. C., Miller, R. H. & Noble, M. (1983). A glial progenitor that develops *in vitro* into an astrocyte or an oligodendrocyte depending on culture medium. *Nature* **303**, 390–6.

Rao, S. M. *et al.* (1991*a*). Cognitive dysfunction in multiple sclerosis. I. Frequency patterns and prediction. *Neurology* **41**, 685–91.

Rao, S. M. *et al.* (1991*b*). Cognitive dysfunction in multiple sclerosis. II. Impact on employment and social functioning. *Neurology* **41**, 692–6.

Rawson, M. D. & Liversedge, L. A. (1969). Treatment of retrobulbar neuritis with corticotrophin. *Lancet* **II**, 222.

Reder, A. T. & Arnason, B. G. W. (1995). Trigeminal neuralgia in multiple sclerosis relieved by a prostaglandin E analogue. *Neurology* **45**, 1097–100.

Revesz, T. *et al.* (1994). A comparison of the pathology of primary and secondary progressive multiple sclerosis. *Brain* **117**, 756–65.

Rice, G. and the Cladribine Group (1997). Cladribine and chronic progressive multiple sclerosis: the results of a multi-centre trial. Minneapolis, MN: American Academy of Neurology; LBN9.

Rizzo, J. F. & Lessell, S. (1988). Risk of developing multiple sclerosis after uncomplicated optic neuritis: a long term prospective study. *Neurology* **38**, 185–90.

Rossiter, D. & Thompson, A. J. (1995). The introduction of integrated care pathways for patients with multiple sclerosis in an inpatient neurorehabilitation setting. *Disabil. Rehabil.* **17**, 443–8.

Rudge, P. *et al.* (1989). Randomised double-blind controlled trial of cyclosporin in multiple sclerosis. *J. Neurol. Neurosurg. Psychiatry* **52**, 559–65.

Rudick, R. *et al.* (1996). Clinical outcomes assessment in multiple sclerosis. *Ann. Neurol.* **49**, 1237–42.

Runmarker, B. & Andersen, O. (1993). Prognostic factors in a multiple sclerosis incidence cohort with twenty-five years of follow-up. *Brain* **116**, 117–34.

Runmarker, B. & Andersen, O. (1995). Pregnancy is associated with a lower risk of onset and a better prognosis in multiple sclerosis. *Brain* **118**, 253–62.

Sabra, A. F. *et al.* (1982). Treatment of action tremor in multiple sclerosis with isoniazid. *Neurology* **32**, 912–13.

Sadovnik, A. D. *et al.* (1991). Cause of death in patients attending multiple sclerosis clinics. *Neurology* **41**, 1193–6.

Sadovnick, A. D. (1994). Genetic epidemiology of multiple sclerosis: a survey. *Ann. Neurol.* **36**, S194–230.

Sandberg-Wollheim, M. *et al.* (1990). A long term prospective study of optic neuritis: evaluation of risk factors. *Ann. Neurol.* **27**, 386–93.

Sharief, M. K. & Hentges, R. (1991). Association between tumour necrosis factor-alpha and disease progression in patients with multiple sclerosis. *N. Engl. J. Med.* **325**, 467–72.

Sharief, M. K. & Thompson, E. J. (1993). Correlation of interleukin-2 and soluble interleukin-2 receptor with clinical activity of multiple sclerosis. *J. Neurol. Neurosurg. Psychiatry* **56**, 169–74.

Shepperd, D. I. (1979). Clinical features in multiple sclerosis in north east Scotland. *Acta Neurol. Scand.* **60**, 218–30.

Sibley, W. A. (1993). Physical trauma and multiple sclerosis. *Neurology* **43**, 1871–4.

Sibley, W. A. (1996). *Therapeutic Claims in Multiple Sclerosis: A Guide to Treatments*. New York: Demos Vermande.

Sibley, W. A., Bamford, C. R. & Clark, K. (1985). Clinical viral infections and multiple sclerosis. *Lancet* **I**, 1313–15.

Sibley, W. A. *et al.* (1991). A prospective study of physical trauma and multiple sclerosis. *J. Neurol. Neurosurg. Psychiatry* **54**, 584–8.

Sipe, J. C. *et al.* (1994). Cladribine in treatment of chronic progressive multiple sclerosis. *Lancet* **344**, 9–13.

Siva, A. *et al.* (1993). Trauma and multiple sclerosis: a population-based cohort study from Olmsted County, Minnesota. *Neurology* **43**, 1878–82.

Skegg, D. C. G. (1991). Multiple sclerosis: nature or nurture? *BMJ* **302**, 247–8.

Slater, R. J. & Raun, N. E. (eds.) (1984). Symposium on the Minimal Record of Disability for multiple sclerosis. *Acta Neurol. Scand.* **70** (Suppl. 101).

Stenager, E. N. *et al.* (1992). Suicide and multiple sclerosis: an epidemiological investigation. *J. Neurol. Neurosurg. Psychiatry* **55**, 542–5.

Stendahl-Brodin, L. & Link, H. (1980). Relation between benign course of multiple sclerosis and low grade humoral immune response in cerebrospinal fluid. *J. Neurol. Neurosurg. Psychiatry* **43**, 102–5.

The IFNB Multiple Sclerosis Study Group and the University of British Columbia MS MRI Analysis Group (1996). Neutralizing antibodies during treatment of multiple sclerosis with interferon beta-1b. Experience during the first three years. *Neurology* **47**, 889–94.

Thompson, A. J. (1996). Multiple sclerosis: symptomatic treatment. *J. Neurol.* **243**, 559–65.

Thompson, A. J. & Noseworthy, J. H. (1996). New treatments for multiple sclerosis: a clinical perspective. *Curr. Opin. Neurol.* **9**, 187–98.

Thompson, A. J. *et al.* (1986). A clinical and laboratory study of benign multiple sclerosis. *Q. J. Med.* **225**, 69–80.

Thompson, A. J. *et al.* (1989). Relative efficacy of intravenous methylprednisolone and ACTH in the treatment of acute relapse in MS. *Neurology* **39**, 969–71.

Thompson, A. J. *et al.* (1990). Patterns of disease activity in multiple sclerosis: a clinical and magnetic resonance imaging study. *BMJ* **300**, 631–4.

Thompson, A. J. & McDonald, W. I. (1991). The diagnosis of primary progressive multiple sclerosis. In *Current Concepts in Multiple Sclerosis*, Excerpta Medica International Congress Series 960, ed. H. Wiethölter, J. Dichgans & J. Mertin, pp. 43–6. Amsterdam: Elsevier.

Thompson, A. J. *et al.* (1991). Major differences in the dynamics of primary and secondary progressive multiple sclerosis. *Ann. Neurol.* **29**, 53–62.

Thompson, A. J. *et al.* (1993). Brain MRI changes in phenylketonuria: associations with dietary status. *Brain* **116**, 811–21.

Thompson, A. J., Polman, C. H., Miller, D. H., McDonald, W. I., Brochet, B., Filippi, M., Montalban, X. & de Sá, J. (1997). Primary progressive multiple sclerosis (review article). *Brain* **120**, 1085–96.

Thorpe, J. W. *et al.* (1993). Spinal cord MRI using multi-array coils and fast spin echo. I. Technical aspects and findings in healthy adults. *Neurology* **43**, 2625–31.

Trobe, J. D. & Arbor, A. (1993). One-year results in the optic neuritis treatment trial. *Neurology* **43**, A280.

Vandeman, H. A. M. *et al.* (1992). The effect of 4-aminopyridine on the clinical signs in MS: a randomised, placebo controlled, double blind crossover study. *Ann. Neurol.* **32**, 123–30.

Van Oosten, B. W., Lai, M., Hodgkinson, S., Barkhof, F., Miller, D. H., Moseley, I. F. *et al.* (1997). Treatment of multiple sclerosis with the monoclonal anti-CD4 antibody cM-T412: results of a randomized, double-blind, placebo-controlled, MR-monitored phase II trial. *Neurology* **49**, 351–7.

Van Walderveen, M. A. A. *et al.* (1995). Correlating MRI and clinical disease activity in multiple sclerosis: relevance of hypointense lesions on short-TR/short-TE (T_1-weighted) spin-echo images. *Neurology* **45**, 1684–90.

Van Walderveen, M. A. A. *et al.* (1966). Histopathological correlates of hypointense lesions on T_1-weighted SE MR images in multiple sclerosis. *J. Neurol.* **243**, S18.

Visscher, B. R. *et al.* (1984). Onset symptoms as predictors of mortality and disability in multiple sclerosis. *Acta Neurol. Scand.* **70**, 321–8.

Weiner, H. L. *et al.* (1993*a*). Intermittent cyclophosphamide pulse therapy in progressive multiple sclerosis: final report of the Northeast Cooperative Multiple Sclerosis Treatment Group. *Neurology* **43**, 910–18.

Weiner, H. L. *et al.* (1993*b*). Double-blind pilot trial of oral tolerization with myelin antigens in multiple sclerosis. *Science* **259**, 1321–4.

Weinshenker, B. G. (1994). Natural history of multiple sclerosis. *Ann. Neurol.* **36**, S6–11.

Weinshenker, B. G. *et al.* (1989*a*). The natural history of multiple sclerosis: a geographically based study. 1. Clinical course and disability. *Brain* **112**, 133–46.

Weinshenker, B. G., Bass, B. & Rice, G. P. A. (1989*b*). The natural history of multiple sclerosis: a geographically based study. 2. Predictive value of the early clinical course. *Brain* **112**, 1419–28.

Weinshenker, B. G. *et al.* (1992). A double-blind, randomized crossover trial of pemoline in fatigue associated with multiple sclerosis. *Neurology* **42**, 1468–71.

Whitaker, J. N. *et al.* (1995). Outcome assessment in multiple sclerosis clinical trials: a critical analysis. *Multiple Sclerosis* **1**, 37–47.

Wiles, C. M. *et al.* (1986). Hyperbaric oxygen in multiple sclerosis: a double blind trial. *BMJ* **292**, 367–71.

Wolinsky, J. S. (1995). Copolymer 1: a most reasonable alternative therapy for early relapsing–remitting multiple sclerosis with mild disability. Editorial. *Neurology* **45**, 1245–7.

Youl, B. D. *et al.* (1991). The pathophysiology of acute optic neuritis: an association of gadolinium leakage with clinical and electrophysiological deficits. *Brain* **114**, 2437–50.

Yudkin, P. L. *et al.* (1991). An overview of randomised controlled trials of azathioprine in the treatment of multiple sclerosis. *Lancet* **338**, 1051–5.

Zeeman, A. Z. J. *et al.* (1966). A study of oligoclonal band negative multiple sclerosis. *J. Neurol. Neurosurg. Psychiatry* **60**, 27–30.

Zoukos, Y. *et al.* (1992). Lymphocyte β-adrenergic receptor density and function are increased in multiple sclerosis; a regulatory role for cortisol and interleukin-1. *Ann. Neurol.* **31**, 627–32.

15 Mechanical disorders of the spine

HOWARD L. WEINER AND PAUL R. COOPER

Mechanical disorders of the spine are defined as degenerative spinal conditions, such as disc degeneration and spondylosis, which are frequent causes of radiculopathy and myelopathy, and which are not associated with trauma or neoplasm. These conditions are among the most commonly treated diseases in neurosurgical practice. Lumbar discectomy represents the most common neurosurgical procedure performed in the United States. Lumbar stenosis is the most commonly diagnosed condition in adults, older than 65 years, undergoing lumbar spine surgery (Turner *et al.* 1992). Similarly, cervical spondylotic myelopathy is said to be 'the most common spinal cord disorder in persons over 55' (Rengachary & Redford 1991). The operative treatment of mechanical disorders of the spine has undergone unparalleled technical advancement during the past 10 years. However, the reported outcome of surgery for these conditions is highly variable. The majority of outcome studies are retrospective analyses which are methodologically imperfect. A critical review of the literature reveals several consistent flaws in the study design as well as in the analysis and reporting of outcome data (Turner *et al.* 1992).

This chapter is divided into four sections. We have reviewed the outcome of surgical treatment of four common mechanical disorders of the spine: cervical spondylotic myelopathy, herniated lumbar disc, lumbar stenosis and degenerative lumbar instability. A critical analysis of the results reported in the literature is undertaken.

Cervical spondylotic myelopathy

Cervical spondylosis is extremely common in the adult population (Rengachary & Redford 1991). Radiographic spondylosis is present in 25 –50% of the population by age 50 years and increases to 75–85% by age 65 years (Montgomery & Brower 1992). Cervical spondylotic myelopathy (CSM) is the most serious consequence of degenerative disease of the cervical spine and is the most common cause of acquired spastic paraparesis in middle and later life (Rengachary & Redford 1991; Whitecloud 1991; Montgomery & Brower 1992). Surgical management is indicated for those patients with persistent or progressive neurological deficit, intractable pain and, in certain circumstances, neurodiagnostic imaging demonstrating spinal cord compression with the risk of further cord damage (Sypert 1992).

A debate persists in the literature as to the best operative management of CSM. A variety of surgical strategies, in various combinations, have been advocated (Cloward 1958; Epstein *et al.* 1969; Fager 1973; Piepgras 1977; Sypert 1992). Anterior removal of compressive osteophytes and laminectomy are the two commonly utilized techniques (Robinson & Smith 1955, Bailey & Badgley 1960; Bohlman & Emery 1988; Simeone 1989; Klara & Foley 1993). Numerous reports of outcome following various surgical procedures have been published (Yonenobu *et al.* 1985). Although anterior decompression is believed to be superior to laminectomy (Verbiest 1973), the literature offers no general consensus or statistical evidence that any one surgical procedure yields a superior outcome compared with another (Yonenobu *et al.* 1985). Some authors recommend anterior or posterior decompression exclusively, while others individualize their decision based on several criteria, including the number of vertebral levels involved as well as the anteroposterior spinal canal diameter (Epstein *et al.* 1969; Guidetti & Fortuna 1969; Fager 1973; Phillips 1973; Bohlman 1977; Crandall & Gregorius 1977; Yonenobu *et al.* 1985). However, none of these recommendations has been scientifically substantiated.

The results of surgery for CSM reported in the literature are difficult to interpret (Cooper 1992). Although several reports have shown that the outcome is significantly better for patients with radicular symptoms than for those with myelopathy, many studies have failed to distinguish between outcome in patients with radiculopathy and myelopathy and have included patients with both syndromes (Bertalanffy & Eggert, 1988; Cooper 1992). There is frequently failure to distinguish myelopathy caused by soft disc herniation from that caused by bony osteophytes. Often, the outcome measures are not clearly defined. Moreover, the relationship of outcome to factors such as age, duration and severity of preoperative symptoms, levels of involvement and length of follow-up are not clearly defined. A shorter duration of follow-up has clearly been shown to favour a better outcome (Turner *et al.* 1992).

Natural history

There are no studies of the natural history of this disorder in the era of CT and MRI. The results of current treatment modalities, which utilize modern imaging, cannot be compared with outcome reported in the past, prior to CT and MRI (Snow & Weiner 1993). Moreover, older studies, which found no significant difference between operative and non-operative treatment, had compared natural history with posterior surgical decompression, a procedure which, in our opinion, is not the optimal treatment of the disease (Lees & Turner 1963). These studies have shown that the natural course of the disease is one of stepwise deterioration over time (Montgomery & Brower 1992). Episodic worsening is the expected course in untreated individuals, with symptoms remaining generally static between the worsening periods. Complete recovery or improvement in disability status is extremely rare. However, only a small group of patients will ever experience a rapidly deteriorating course (Whitecloud 1991). Unfortunately, natural history studies have been unable to demonstrate factors identifying the rare patients at risk for rapid deterioration (Montgomery & Brower 1992).

Clarke & Robinson (1956) found that no patient ever returned to a normal state. Of the 120 patients they studied, 75% had episodic worsening, 20% showed slow, steady progression, and 5% had a rapid onset followed by a lengthy disability (Montgomery & Brower 1992). Spontaneous regression was highly uncommon (Montgomery & Brower 1992). Lees & Turner (1963) studied 44 patients with myelopathy and cervical spondylosis on myelography for 3–40 years. Of 28 patients treated with a cervical collar, 7 showed no change, 17 improved and 4 were worse at follow-up. Twenty-five of the 44 patients had severe disability at some time, and in most instances the disability remained (Montgomery & Brower 1992). Of those who improved, in many the gains were slight and did not result in an alteration in disability level (Snow & Weiner 1993). Most patients experienced a stepwise deterioration, with repeated episodes of progression, followed by quiescent periods (Montgomery & Brower 1992). Because few of their patients experienced steady, progressive deterioration, they concluded that the disease has a benign course, and recommended conservative management. However, this study is difficult to evaluate because no information is available regarding the number of levels of cord compression present on myelography (Snow & Weiner 1993). Like Lees & Turner, Nurick described a period of worsening followed by static periods, often lasting several years (Nurick 1972; Montgomery & Brower 1992). Disability remained static, except in older patients, in whom it progressed. Bradshaw (1957), in a 2 year follow-up of patients with myelopathy who were treated conservatively, reported that 12 had improved, 6 showed no change and 8 deteriorated. However, all patients who improved had evidence of only single-level spondylosis. Of patients with multilevel spondylosis – the most prevalent pattern of the disease – 7 were substantially worse, 4 unchanged and 1 dead (Snow & Weiner 1993). These data suggest that patients with generalized spondylosis do worse when treated conservatively than when treated surgically. Similarly, Roberts, studying 24 patients with multilevel myelographic defects, found that 29% of patients with motor disability improved when treated with a cervical collar, compared with the 38% whose condition remained unchanged, and the 33% who deteriorated (Roberts 1966; Snow & Weiner 1993). Similarly, Symon & Lavender (1967; Montgomery & Brower 1992) concluded that CSM is unlikely to have a benign course over the life of an individual patient. They found that 67% of patients who were managed non-operatively showed a steady progressive deterioration.

Cervical laminectomy

During the 1960s and 1970s, cervical laminectomy was the preferred method of treating CSM (Scoville 1961; Stoops & King 1965; Epstein *et al.* 1969, 1982; Guidetti & Fortuna 1969; Fager 1973; Casotto & Buoncristiani 1981; Sypert 1992). However, a critical review of the literature reveals that cervical laminectomy, the oldest and previously the most frequently utilized procedure, seems to offer the least favourable outcome of the available operative procedures (Rengachary & Redford 1991). While some enthusiastic reports have claimed that 70–80% of patients improve after laminectomy (Epstein 1988; Snow & Weiner 1993; Zeidman & Ducker 1993), a review of the current literature reveals that good to excellent results are, on average, obtained in only 60% of patients (Schmidek & Smith 1988). Furthermore, a substantial number of patients remain disabled from this disorder postoperatively, and 10–15% of patients become worse immediately after surgery (Schmidek & Smith 1988; Snow & Weiner 1993). Moreover, a group of patients deteriorate following initial improvement, if followed for a long enough period of time (Snow & Weiner 1993; Whitecloud 1991).

Similarly, the results reported in the older literature were generally less than satisfactory (Whitecloud 1991). Improvement was noted in approximately 50% of patients undergoing laminectomy, and progression of myelopathy postoperatively was well documented (Whitecloud 1991). Overall, delayed loss of neurological function, in addition to perioperative neurological deficit, was estimated to occur in 19–53% of cases (Whitecloud 1991). Additional technical manoeuvres intended to enhance the favourable results, such as sectioning of dentate ligaments, durotomy with duroplasty, and foraminotomy have not led to a significantly better outcome (Rengachary & Redford 1991). Recently, Snow & Weiner (1993) found that 77% of patients improved after laminectomy. However, in one-quarter of this group the improvement was minimal, and their study population was heterogeneous and only two-thirds of the patients had true myelopathy.

Several explanations have been given for the limited benefit of cervical laminectomy seen in patients with CSM. In general, the poor outcome can be related to inadequate decompression and late-onset instability. First, anterior compressive osteophytes are not removed by laminectomy, and continue to compress the cord. While the spinal cord may migrate posteriorly, away from the anterior compressive lesions, following laminectomy, this is not always the case (Allen *et al.* 1987; Rengachary & Redford 1991). Second, instability may be increased following extensive decompressive laminectomy, leading to dynamic mechanical compression of the cord, kyphotic deformities and delayed neurological deterioration (Herkowitz 1988; Rengachary & Redford 1991; Sypert 1992). Third, radiculopathy often persists because the nerve roots remain stretched over a ventral mass (Sypert 1992).

Anterior cervical decompression

The relatively poor results from posterior procedures led to the interest in anterior operative intervention in patients with CSM (Guidetti & Fortuna 1969; Phillips 1973; Bohlman 1977; Moussa *et al.* 1983; Yonenobu *et al.* 1985; Hanai *et al.* 1986; Bernard & Whitecloud 1987; Zdeblick & Bohlmann 1989; Whitecloud 1991). The anterior approach for the treatment of cervical spondylosis has become the recognized treatment of choice because it provides a direct approach to the pathological lesion (Eriksen *et al.* 1984) and yields a successful outcome in the majority of patients, provided they are carefully selected for surgery (Moussa *et al.* 1983). Anterior cervical decompression and interbody fusion (ACDF) is probably the most frequently performed surgical procedure for the treatment of this condition (Cooper 1992). For single-level spondylotic myelopathy this procedure has been widely accepted (Yonenobu *et al.* 1985). However, debate continues as to the optimal approach for multisegmental cervical spondylosis, particularly when it is associated with a congenitally narrowed spinal canal. Several authors now recommend multilevel vertebrectomy and fusion in this situation (Rengachar & Redford 1991; Saunders *et al.* 1991; Seifert & Stolke 1991; Whitecloud 1991). In contrast, although there is little scientific data to support its superiority, multilevel decompressive laminectomy remains the favoured operation for this condition by some groups (Zeidman & Ducker 1993).

It is difficult to compare the various studies reporting outcome following anterior surgery for CSM (Whitecloud 1991). Nevertheless, a review of the literature reveals that, on average, anterior decompressive surgery improves patients in approximately 70–95% of cases (Whitecloud 1991; Cooper 1992; Sypert 1992). In the original operation described by Robinson & Smith (1955), neither osteophytes nor the posterior longitudinal ligament were removed (Cooper 1992). Although Bohlman, and subsequently Zhang, reported that discectomy and simple stabilization of the pathological segment, without removal of osteophytes, benefited most patients, the vast majority of authors now advocate both decompression and stabilization (Crandall & Batzdorf 1966; Guidetti & Fortuna 1969; Phillips 1973; Crandall & Gregorius 1977; Moussa *et al.* 1983; Yonenobu *et al.* 1985; Hanai *et al.* 1986; Zdeblick & Bohlmann 1989; Whitecloud 1991; Cooper 1992). Crandall & Batzdorf noted a 71% improvement in 21 patients with CSM treated by the Cloward technique, which calls for the removal of compressive osteophytes (Cloward 1958; Crandall & Batzdorf 1966; Whitecloud 1991). Utilizing the same operative procedure, Guidetti & Fortuna, and Phillips, reported 82% and 74% rates of improvement, respectively, concluding that anterior surgery was markedly superior to laminectomy or conservative treatment (Guidetti & Fortuna 1969; Phillips 1973; Whitecloud 1991). Comparing the results of laminectomy with those of anterior decompression and Cloward fusion, Crandall & Gregorius (1977) found that a significantly greater number of patients deteriorated following laminectomy. Other authors have reported a rate of improvement ranging from 64% to 82% using the Cloward technique (Crandall & Batzdorf 1966; Guidetti & Fortuna 1969; Phillips 1973; Hanal *et al.* 1986; Bertalanffy & Eggert 1988; Cooper 1992). Recent studies have been similarly encouraging. Irvine & Strachan (1987) evaluated 46 patients at a mean of 10 years postoperatively, and found that 78% remained improved. Moussa *et al.* (1983) reported that 70% of 125 patients were improved by surgery after an average follow-up of 2.3 years. Mann *et al.* (1984) treated 50 patients with a variation of Cloward's technique and found that all patients experienced improvement of at least one neurological grade. Emphasizing the importance of adequate spinal cord decompression, several investigators have advocated radical anterior microsurgical osteophytectomy (Kadoya *et al.* 1984; Mann *et al.* 1984; Sypert 1992). In a recent prospective study of 60 patients treated with radical anterior microsurgical decompression and reconstruction, Sypert reported that 95% of patients demonstrated some recovery of spinal cord function (Kadoya *et al.* 1984; Mann *et al.* 1984; Sypert 1992). Nearly two-thirds of his patients improved two to three neurological grades.

Not all reports of anterior decompression have been optimistic (Whitecloud 1991). Lunsford *et al.* (1980) found that half the patients who underwent a variety of anterior decompressive procedures were either unimproved or worse following surgery. They could not identify any predictive indices, nor could they correlate outcome with the severity of myelopathy, the number of levels operated on, or the presence of canal stenosis (Schmidek & Smith 1988). Similarly, Galera & Tovi (1968) found only a 39% improvement rate as well as a significant number of patients who had deteriorated with long-term follow-up. It is possible that the decompression was inadequate in these series of patients, although this was not directly analysed (Cooper 1992).

Some authors have recommended anterior cervical discectomy without fusion for the treatment of cervical spondylosis (Bertalanffy & Eggert 1988). However, the literature contains no data to support the superiority of this technique over anterior decompression with fusion (Martins 1976; Rosenorn *et al.* 1983; Kadoya *et al.* 1984). Although few studies have included patients who were treated both with and without fusion, the available studies suggest that the outcome for these two groups is comparable (Cooper 1992). Decompression without fusion is a reasonable strategy only if minimal bone removal is undertaken. However, fusion is strongly advocated in those cases in which bone removal is extensive, to prevent instability and kyphotic deformity (Cooper 1992).

Corpectomy

The proponents of corpectomy believe that incomplete removal of bony compressive lesions is responsible for the high rate of poor outcome reported in many studies and that multilevel osteophytectomy inadequately decompresses the spinal cord (Cooper 1992). Partial vertebrectomy, followed by stabilization with a variety of graft configurations, has been advocated because it simultaneously provides stabilization and radical decompression of the entire longitudinal extent of the diseased cervical spine (Rengachary & Redford 1991). This procedure has been utilized for patients with either multilevel spondylosis, constitutive spinal stenosis, or anterior compressive lesions located directly posterior to the vertebral body. Saunders (1991) has argued that it is the single surgical procedure which simultaneously addresses the complex pathophysiological features of CSM: compression, instability and cord distortion.

In general, the reported outcome following this procedure is excellent (Kojima *et al.* 1989; Saunders 1991; Seifert & Stolke 1991; Cooper 1992). Several authors have reported improvement in 73–100% of patients (Hanai 1986; Bernard & Whitecloud 1987; Kojima 1989; Saunders 1991; Seifert & Stolke 1991). Saunders *et al.* (1991) found that over 87% of patients with CSM were significantly improved after central corpectomy, while 54% of the entire series were considered completely cured. Similarly, Seifert & Stolke (1991) found that 14 of 19 patients with severe myelopathy were symptom-free or had only minor residual symptoms. In a comparative study, Yonenobu *et al.* (1985) concluded that subtotal vertebrectomy was significantly superior to either the Cloward or Smith–Robinson techniques.

Anterior and posterior approaches compared

In general, the few studies which have directly compared anterior and posterior approaches to the cervical spine, in patients with CSM, are methodologically problematic. In Yonenobu's comparison of laminectomy with anterior decompression, posterior decompression was empirically chosen for all patients with four or more levels of spondylosis, thus rendering direct comparison between surgical groups invalid (Yonenobu *et al.* 1985). Similarly, Hukuda *et al.* (1985), in a retrospective analysis of 269 patients treated with either anterior or posterior procedures, performed a laminectomy only when three or more levels were involved pathologically. Therefore, their finding of no significant difference between the two approaches is confounded by selection bias. Epstein found that 85% of patients improved after laminectomy and removal of osteophytes, compared with the 73% and 68% who improved after anterior surgery and laminectomy, respectively (Epstein 1988; Rowland 1992). However, the methods utilized to assess outcome were not clearly indicated (Rowland 1992).

There are still no clear-cut criteria for determining which patients will predictably experience a successful outcome following surgery for CSM (Whitecloud 1991). Although several factors have been reported to influence outcome, including age at operation, duration of symptoms, pattern of onset of symptoms, severity of myelopathy, number of segmental levels involved, and the anteroposterior spinal canal diameter (Bertalanffy & Eggert 1988; Yonenobu *et al.* 1985), only a shorter duration of symptoms preoperatively has been consistently associated with a more favourable outcome (Bertalanffy & Eggert 1988; Whitecloud 1991; Snow & Weiner 1993). Poor outcome following technically successful decompressive surgery has been attributed to errors in diagnosis (e.g. patients with motor neuron disease), poor patient selection and irreversible intrinsic cord damage (Snow & Weiner 1993). Mehalic *et al.* (1990) found persistent intrinsic cord hyperintensity on T2-weighted MRI images in those patients not improving postoperatively.

Extent of decompression and outcome

Although no study to date has directly related outcome to the adequacy of decompression, a critical review of the literature indicates that the extent of anterior osteophyte decompression clearly correlates with outcome (Seifert & Stolke 1991; Cooper 1992). In fact, the adequacy of spinal cord decompression is probably the most important factor in determining outcome (Cooper 1992). Some earlier investigators had argued against removal of osteophytes, claiming that sufficient bony fusion and immobility of the degenerative cervical segment would result in resorption of posterior osteophytes (Sugar 1981; Gore & Sepic 1984). However, there is no evidence that cervical osteophytes resorb, and incomplete removal of osteophytes has been clearly associated with poor outcome, accounting for progresive myelopathy as well as the necessity for reoperation in several patients (Bertalanffy & Eggert 1988).

Radical anterior cervical decompression and fusion appears to be the most direct and rational approach to CSM (Sypert 1992). Nevertheless, the literature is replete with statistically unfounded arguments as to why one operative approach is superior to another (Klara & Foley 1993). As some have argued (Lunsford *et al.* 1980; Rowland 1992), only a randomized, prospective study comparing the various surgical procedures with one another, as well as with non-operative treatment, with matched patient groups, can scientifically resolve the existing controversy.

Herniated lumbar disc

The outcome following lumbar discectomy has improved as surgical techniques have been refined and patient selection criteria have become more precise (Pappas *et al.* 1992). A recent study reported that the vast majority of patients undergoing surgery for herniated lumbar disc (HLD) have a good-to-excellent outcome (Pappas *et al.* 1992). However, a critical review of the literature reveals that the percentage of 'excellent' outcomes actually reported varies from 46% to 90% (Spengler & Frymoyer 1991). This wide range in reported outcome reflects the variability in patient selection criteria, surgical technique, neuroradiological investigation, outcome rating scales and length of follow-up.

Controversy exists regarding the best method of surgical decompression of the lumbar herniated nucleus pulposas: standard open discectomy, microdiscectomy, chemonucleolysis, or other percutaneous methods. However, most investigators have emphasized that the key element for a successful outcome is appropriate patient selection rather than the actual surgical technique employed (Andersen & Burchiel 1991; McCulloch 1991).

Natural history

No treatment method can be evaluated without knowledge of the natural history of the disease as well as a comparison of surgical intervention with conservative therapy. Of all patients presenting to surgeons for evaluation of sciatica, more than 80% can be managed by non-operative treatment (Spengler & Frymoyer 1991). In fact, over half the patients with classical HLD will recover within 1 month without intervention, and an even larger percentage will be asymptomatic in 3 months (Long 1991).

There have been two prospective studies comparing long-term outcome of standard laminectomy for HLD with non-operative treatment. Weber (1983) followed 280 patients over a 10 year period to determine the short- and long-term outcome in two randomized groups. He found that, although the surgical group had statistically significantly better results at 1 year following surgery, at 4 years the difference in symptom relief between the two groups did not achieve significance, and that at 10 year follow-up, neither subjective nor objective differences existed between the two groups (Andersen & Burchiel 1991). The author suggested that, if the length of follow-up is sufficiently long, surgery had no beneficial effect over conservative therapy in patients with 'doubtful surgical indications' (Weber 1983). However, this study was confounded by the lack of radiographic confirmation of disc herniation in any of its subjects and, therefore, compared treatment in patients with uncertain indications for surgery. In contrast, Lewis *et al.* (1987) compared 10 year follow-up data on two such cohorts, 99% of whom had significant preoperative myelographic defects, and found that 86% of patients reported an improvement in pain following surgery. Taken together, the two studies indicate that lumbar discectomy has the beneficial effect of earlier relief of sciatica and of reducing the initial period of disability in patients with clear radiographic and physical indications for surgery. These reports illustrate that, in order to demonstrate a beneficial effect from surgical intervention, proper patient selection is critical (Andersen & Burchiel 1991; Spengler & Frymoyer 1991).

Patient selection

If patients are carefully selected for operative intervention, the rate of successful outcome following lumbar discectomy should be between 80% and 95% (Wilson & Harbaugh 1981; Lewis *et al.* 1987; Pappas *et al.* 1992; Dvorak *et al.* 1988; Frymoyer 1988; Rogers 1988; Silver 1988; Andrews & Lavyne 1990; Abramovitz & Neff 1991; Spengler & Frymoyer 1991; Delashaw *et al.* 1992). Patients undergoing surgery should have a history and physical examination consistent with HLD, with radiographic confirmation of nerve root compression (Delashaw *et al.* 1992). Factors associated with good outcome include lower extremity radicular pain rather than back pain alone, radicular pain with straight leg raising, decreased reflexes on the affected side, evidence of herniation on imaging studies, absence of worker's compensation, and absence of psychosocial abnormalities (Errico & Lowell 1993). Patients with the predominant complaint of low back pain, as opposed to radiculopathy, as well as those whose imaging studies fail to reveal the corresponding cause of their radicular pain, will not have a satisfactory outcome following lumbar discectomy (Delashaw *et al.* 1992). Furthermore, several investigators have emphasized the importance of carefully evaluating patients preoperatively for existing co-morbidities such as personality dysfunction, drug history, personal injury litigation, or history of a work-related injury (Long 1991). Patients with compensation or ligation cases have clearly been shown to have poorer outcomes from surgery (Delashaw *et al.* 1992; Pappas *et al.* 1992).

Evaluation of outcome

The method utilized to evaluate outcome can have a significant effect on results. It has been shown that patient questionnaire design significantly influences the rate of 'successful' outcomes (Howe & Frymoyer 1984). Howe & Frymoyer compared the use of different questionnaires and were able to alter the apparent 'effectiveness' of treatment by the design of the questionnaire (Dunsker 1987). The lack of a generally accepted, systematic outcome rating scale has precluded the objective comparison of results among disparate groups of patients. Most studies rate outcome in vague terminology such as excellent, good or satisfactory. The results of these operations in different hands are difficult, if not impossible, to compare (Dunsker 1987). Moreover, in most cases, the individual rater who scores patient outcome is frequently a member of the operating team rather than an unbiased third party. A recent study advocated the use of a simple rating scale, the Functional–Economic Outcome Rating Scale or Prolo Scale, to evaluate the outcome of lumbar spine procedures, and to compare the economic and functional status of patients both pre- and postoperatively (Pappas *et al.* 1992). The authors of the study state that future studies should require both patients and physicians to evaluate surgical outcome simultaneously, to determine any differences between the groups of reviewers (Pappas *et al.* 1992).

Conventional laminotomy

Conventional laminotomy and open surgical discectomy allow direct visualization of the pathology as well as decompression of the nerve root and thecal sac. It is the gold standard with which all other treatment modalities are to be compared (Delashaw *et al.* 1992; Errico & Lowell 1993). Standard discectomy has had good or excellent results in nearly 90% of procedures (Errico & Lowell 1993).

Microsurgical discectomy

Microsurgical discectomy was introduced to improve visualization and minimize tissue dissection. Its advocates cite a smaller incision, reduced operative time, decreased time in the hospital and more rapid return to work as benefits of this procedure (Caspar *et al.* 1991; Errico & Lowell 1993). However, the term 'microdiscectomy' carries as many technical definitions as there are surgeons employing it as a technique for disc removal (Wilson & Harbaugh 1981; Rogers 1988; Silver 1988; Andersen & Burchiel 1991; Caspar *et al.* 1991; Delashaw *et al.* 1992). Whereas Caspar has advocated a standard subtotal discectomy performed under the microscope, Williams performs only a conservative discectomy without any bone removal and with preservation of the supposed normal, functioning disc (Williams 1978; Caspar *et al.* 1991; Errico & Lowell 1993). Successful outcome has been reported to occur in 80–95% of patients treated by this method (Williams 1978; Wilson & Harbaugh 1981; Rogers 1988; Silvers 1988; Andrews & Lavyne

1990; Caspar *et al.* 1991; Delashaw *et al.* 1992). However, a review of several studies comparing outcome from standard laminectomy and the discectomy with that of microdiscectomy reveals that the only appreciable difference between the two groups was length of postoperative hospitalization: 4 days for microsurgery versus 7 days for standard discectomy (Williams 1978; Wilson & Harbaugh 1981; Rogers 1988; Silvers 1988; Andrews & Lavyne 1990; Caspar *et al.* 1991; Delashaw *et al.* 1992; Hadley 1992). These studies indicate that the decision facing the surgeon is, therefore, not between types of surgical procedures, but rather whether the microscope is used or not (Long 1991).

Chemonucleolysis

Although popular at one time, the safety and efficacy of chemonucleolysis have recently come to be questioned. Comparative studies have demonstrated open surgical discectomy to be more efficacious (Day *et al.* 1985; Maroon & Abla 1985; van Alphen *et al.* 1989; Delashaw *et al.* 1992). In addition to its ineffectiveness in treating sequestered disc fragments, percutaneous chymopapain injection has been associated with anaphylactic reactions in about 0.5% of patients. Intracerebral haemorrhage, seizures, subarachnoid haemorrhage and transverse myelitis may result if the enzyme is inadvertently introduced into the subarachnoid space (Delashaw *et al.* 1992).

Percutaneous discectomy

Percutaneous discectomy was introduced in the 1960s to alleviate sciatica while sparing the patient a full operative procedure (Errico & Lowell 1993). In general, advocates of this technique accept reduced efficacy in return for diminished invasiveness. Furthermore, because only contained disc fragments are amenable to this technique, it has a very limited range of clinical applications (Errico & Lowell 1993). Although studies have reported a 75% success rate with percutaneous discectomy in carefully selected patients, the role of this procedure currently remains poorly defined (Davis *et al.* 1991; Delashaw *et al.* 1992; Koutrouvelis *et al.* 1993).

Conclusions

The literature on outcome of treatment for HLD reflects the vast array of procedures available to the surgeon. However, it is now well known that successful outcome is dependent on proper patient selection for surgery rather than on the specific operative procedure. Most studies utilize varying criteria for operative intervention as well as different rating systems to score results. Future studies will need to address these shortcomings in order to elucidate the relative efficacy of a specific treatment.

Lumbar stenosis

Degenerative lumbar stenosis is a common condition that may require decompressive surgery when conservative measures fail to relieve pain discomfort and incapacitation (Silvers *et al.* 1993). However, the natural history of lumbar stenosis is largely unknown (Turner *et al.* 1992), and little has been published concerning the response of patients to conservative measures. Moreover, no randomized trial comparing surgery with non-operative treatment has been conducted, and therefore no conclusions can be drawn as to the relative benefits and risks of surgery versus conservative treatment (Turner *et al.* 1992). Wide decompressive laminectomy, usually combined with medial facetectomy and foraminotomy at the symptomatic level, is the recognized standard of surgical treatment for this disease (Aryanpur & Ducker 1990). Despite the widespread use of laminectomy in the treatment of lumbar stenosis, questions remain regarding diagnostic criteria, indications for surgery, optimal surgical procedure and patient characteristics associated with a favourable outcome (Turner *et al.* 1992).

An extensive review of the literature reveals that there is considerable variability in the reported results for treatment of degenerative lumbar stenosis (Getty 1980; Hall *et al.* 1985; Ganz 1990; Spengler 1991; Caputy & Luessenhop 1992; Turner *et al.* 1992). Several large series published in the last decade have reported success rates ranging between 60% and 95% for patients undergoing operative intervention (Getty 1980; Weir & de Leo 1981; Hall *et al.* 1985; Nasca 1987; Andersen & Burchiel 1991; Katz *et al.* 1991). In fact, one recent review found that the range of good-to-excellent outcomes reported by different authors, at long-term follow-up, was 26–100% (Turner *et al.* 1992). Rather than differences in surgical technique, the most likely factors accounting for variable results are patient selection criteria, length of follow-up, patient age and varying methodology in analysing outcome (Caputy & Luessenhop 1992). Moreover, many of these studies lack explicit criteria for 'success', omit important details, such as the number of levels decompressed, fail to incorporate the patients' assessment of outcome, and do not require a minimum duration of follow-up, thereby biasing the results towards short-term successes (Katz *et al.* 1991; Turner *et al.* 1992).

Long-term outcome

Whereas most studies indicate very high short-term success rates, recent reports have shown that the long-term outcome is more variable, with a progressive deterioration in results over time (Hall *et al.* 1985; Nasca 1987; Ganz 1990; Katz *et al.* 1991; Caputy & Luessenhop 1992; Silvers *et al.* 1993). Caputy & Leussenhop (1992) recently reported that approximately 25% of their patients suffered symptomatic recurrences at 5 year follow-up, and they anticipated that 50% or more of patients would be in this category within 10–15 years. They attributed the poor later outcome to the progressive nature of this degenerative condition. Most of the late surgical failures were due to renewed neurological involvement secondary to either restenosis at decompressed levels or progression of stenosis at adjacent levels. They found that reoperation resulted in a high level of surgical success (Caputy & Leussenhop 1992). Similarly, others (Katz *et al.* 1991; Silvers *et al.* 1993) have found that, although the outcome 1 year after surgery was highly successful, the initial therapeutic benefit did not persist through the 5 year follow-up period.

Patient population

Much of the discrepancy in the published results can be attributed to the fact that the definition of lumbar stenosis is broad, and that most studies include a heterogeneous group of patients. Patients with lumbar stenosis can be subdivided into those with a congenital narrowing of the spinal canal and those who have degenerative changes (Hall *et al.* 1985). However, these categories are not mutually exclusive, and underlying congenital stenosis predisposes a patient to symptomatic narrowing of the spinal canal as degenerative changes occur with ageing (Hall *et al.* 1985). In fact, many studies have included patients with lumbar stenosis associated with degenerative spondylolisthesis in their study cohort, despite the fact this is a distinct pathological entity with a different optimal treatment. The inclusion of such patients in studies analysing the outcome of decompressive laminectomy for lumbar stenosis merely confounds the outcome data. Several investigators have reported a less favourable outcome in patients with stenosis associated with spondylolisthesis who undergo decompressive laminectomy alone and have recommended simultaneous decompression and fusion in these patients (Grabias 1980; Hopp & Tsou 1988; Aryanpur & Ducker 1990; Caputy & Luessenhop 1992; Silvers *et al.* 1993). A recent prospective study found a significantly better outcome in patients with spondylolisthetic stenosis who underwent concomitant intertransverse-process arthrodesis and decompression (Herkowitz & Kurz 1991) compared with those undergoing decompression alone. In contrast, although fusion is recommended in those cases in which near-total facet removal is performed for decompression, simple degenerative lumbar stenosis with spondylolisthesis seldom requires a fusion (Grabias 1980).

Extent of decompression

Inadequate decompression at initial surgery has been clearly associated with a poor outcome (Getty 1980; Hall *et al.* 1985; Katz *et al.* 1991). Conversely, a positive correlation has been found between the extent of decompression of the lateral recess and the outcome of surgery (Johnsson *et al.* 1981). However, the actual extent of decompression that yields the best outcome has been debated in the literature (Katz *et al.* 1991). Decompressive lumbar laminectomy is the generally accepted surgical treatment for degenerative lumbar stenosis. However, some have argued that this procedure, with its extensive ligamentous and bony/articular decompression, is associated with a higher risk of failure as a result of instability (Hopp & Tsou 1988; Aryanpur & Ducker 1990; Katz *et al.* 1991). Therefore, several alternative surgical treatments have been proposed (Aryanpur & Ducker 1990). A recent study proposed a more limited decompression, namely, multilevel laminotomies and foraminotomies, as an equal or superior procedure to conventional wide decompressive laminectomy (Aryanpur & Ducker 1990). These authors reported a 90% excellent short-term outcome, claiming that this procedure is less disruptive, and requires less operating time. However, there have been no prospective studies comparing this procedure with standard laminectomy, and the long-term outcome following multilevel laminotomy is unknown. In contrast, others have not found a higher incidence of instability following decompressive laminectomy (Katz *et al.* 1991). Claiming that lumbar stenosis is a progressive disease and that symptomatic recurrence can be expected with time, these authors have advocated the more extensive decompressive laminectomy (Hall *et al.* 1985). In fact, some have even suggested decompressing all levels shown to be radiographically stenotic, rather than only those which are clinically symptomatic, in order to minimize the potential for progressive stenosis at adjacent levels (Katz *et al.* 1991; Caputy & Luessenhop 1992). However, no long-term outcome studies have substantiated this recommendation.

Patient selection for surgery

Several studies have shown that patient selection factors have a significant effect on outcome of surgery for lumbar stenosis (Johnsson *et al.* 1981; Hall *et al.* 1985; Aryanpur & Ducker 1990; Conley *et al.* 1990; Ganz 1990; Herkowitz & Kurz 1991; Katz *et al.* 1991; Caputy & Luessenhop 1992; Silvers *et al.* 1993). The overall experience suggests that patients with segmental compression treated with adequate decompression have a successful outcome, whereas patients with more generalized disease have less predictable results (Grabias 1980). Patients with radiculopathy or neurogenic claudication have a significantly better outcome than those whose predominant symptom is low back pain (Grabias 1980; Hall *et al.* 1985; Ganz 1990; Silvers *et al.* 1993). In one study, all patients whose preoperative myelograms revealed a sagittal spinal canal diameter of less than 11 mm had a good outcome. Others have correlated successful outcome with the presence of posture-related symptoms. They emphasized the importance of functional myelography as well as the significance of changes in the sagittal diameter of the spinal canal between flexion and extension (Ganz 1990). Conversely, several other patient factors have been associated with a poor outcome: a history of multiple operations, involvement of three or more spinal levels, the presence of psychosomatic disorders and insurance or medicolegal issues, and coexisting chronic illness (such as osteoarthritis, cardiac disease, rheumatoid arthritis or chronic pulmonary disease) (Grabias 1980; Katz *et al.* 1991). However, advanced age has not been found to be an independent predictor of poor outcome.

Conclusion

Turner *et al.* (1992), in a critical review of 74 published articles on the outcome of surgery for lumbar stenosis, concluded that the most definitive finding in the literature was its poor scientific quality. Major deficits in study design, analysis and reporting were the rule. Given the wide discrepancy in reported outcome for the surgical treatment of degenerative lumbar stenosis, it is obvious that prospective, multicentre longitudinal studies, comparing decompressive laminectomy with multilevel laminotomies as well as with non operative management, are needed to address the controversies remaining in the literature.

Fusion for degenerative lumbar instability

Degenerative conditions of the lumbar spine which are associated with abnormal spinal movement require operative stabilization. Lumbar spine fusion is indicated in the setting of pathological spine motion, often associated with neural compression, or when the spine is destabilized during neural decompressive procedures (Dickman *et al.* 1992). Fusions can be anterior, posterior, posterolateral, and by posterior interbody techniques (Zindrick 1991). The posterolateral intertransverse-process fusion has previously been the generally accepted primary fusion procedure for lumbosacral spine instability (Hanley *et al.* 1991). It is associated with an acceptable rate of arthrodesis and few complications (Dickman *et al.* 1992).

The use of internal fixation for the lumbosacral spine was initiated to enhance fusion rates in cases of degenerative spondylolisthesis and segmental instability (Lorenz *et al.* 1993). The three goals of spinal fusion, namely deformity correction, arthrodesis and patient mobilization, were felt to be best accomplished with internal fixation (Hanley *et al.* 1991; Dickman *et al.* 1992; Haid & Dickman 1993). The development of instrumentation for internal spinal fixation has evolved rapidly during the last 30 years (Dickman *et al.* 1992). Transpedicular screw fixation has become an important method for internal fixation in a variety of degenerative conditions of the lumbar spine (Dickman *et al.* 1992). Many pedicular fixation systems are currently available. However, no studies have demonstrated a significant advantage of any one system (Lorenz *et al.* 1993).

Intertransverse-process fusion alone

Although few studies have directly compared the outcome of patients who had instrumentation with those who did not, most of the recent data indicate that pedicle screw fixation and intertransverse-process fusion yields a superior outcome when compared with intertransverse-process fusion alone. Studies of non-instrumental fusions in the lumbar spine have reported fusion rates of single levels between 60% and 80% (Zindrick 1991). Attempts to fuse more than one level further reduce the success rate. The incidence of pseudarthrosis following attempted posterolateral fusion ranges from 5%

to 20% for fusions of one or two motion segments (Stillerman & Maiman 1990; Lorenz *et al*. 1993). Posterior fusions have yielded pseudarthrosis rates as high as 55% (Stillerman & Maiman 1990). Herkowitz & Kurz (1991) recently reported a 36% rate of pseudarthrosis in patients undergoing intertransverse-process arthrodesis without instrumentation for degenerative spondylolisthesis. Pseudarthrosis is considered the most common cause of failure in spinal fusion and frequently precludes a successful outcome following subsequent stabilizations (Kostuik & Frymoyer 1991).

Pedicle screw fixation

In contrast, recent clinical and experimental studies have found a significantly improved outcome following transpedicular screw-rod fixation. Dickman *et al*. (1992) recently reported a 96% fusion rate, and an 88% improvement in neurological deficits, in 104 patients treated with this procedure, even in those patients with prior pseudarthrosis. West *et al*. (1991) reported 30 month follow-up results for arthrodesis using pedicle screw implants. Fusion rates for painful degenerative disease, spondylolisthesis and pseudarthrosis were 90%, 93% and 65%, respectively. Most patients experienced a marked decrease in pain, and two-thirds eventually returned to work (Lorenz *et al*. 1993). Similarly, *in vivo* laboratory experiments have demonstrated a significantly enhanced fusion rate following spinal instrumentation when compared with posterolateral bone grafting alone (McAfee *et al*. 1989).

Comparative studies

Several retrospective as well as prospective studies comparing instrumentation using pedicle screws with non-instrumented fusion have supported these findings (Lorenz *et al*. 1991; Zindrick 1991). In general, instrumentation has decreased the pseudarthrosis rate from 20% to 5% (Harrison & Sundaresan 1991). Dean *et al*. reported an 80% symptomatic improvement with VSP instrumentation compared with 63% in patients who were fused without instrumentation (Zindrick 1991). Pseudarthrosis occurred in 31% of the non-instrumented group compared with only 5% of those undergoing one- and two-level fusion with pedicle screws. Grubb and Lipscomb reported a 35% pseudarthrosis rate following standard posterolateral fusion, in contrast to 6% following instrumentation (Zindrick 1991). In a prospective, randomized, comparative study, Lorenz *et al*. (1991) found a significantly better outcome in the group undergoing adjunctive pedicular fixation with regard to pseudarthrosis, symptomatic relief and return to work.

However, not every comparative study has found a significant difference between pedicle screw internal fixation and intertransverse-process bony fusion. For example, Bernhardt *et al*. in a retrospective analysis, found no significant difference in the rate of fusion or pain relief between a group of instrumented and non-instrumented fusion patients (Zindrick 1991). As this technique continues to evolve, it is clear that further well-designed, prospective studies are necessary to establish conclusively the effectiveness, safety and indications of the various transpedicular fixation systems (Zindrick 1991).

Conclusion

The potential for markedly improving patient outcome following surgery for mechanical disorders of the spine has increased dramatically in recent years. The pathophysiology and natural history of these conditions are better understood, and signifi cant recent advances have been made in neuroimaging, surgical technique and spinal instrumentation. It is now time for clinical investigators to adopt more rigorous standards in order to address the existing controversies regarding the relative benefits and risks of various surgical procedures versus conservative treatment, for objectively defined patient groups (Turner *et al.* 1992). A comprehensive review of the literature indicates that there is a critical need to publish uniform, standardized methodological information on patient characteristics, surgical interventions and outcome assessment.

Acknowledgement
The authors would like to thank Drs Thomas J. Errico and Gordon Engler for their assistance in preparing this chapter.

References

Abramovitz, J. & Neff, S. (1991). Lumbar disc surgery: results of the prospective lumbar discectomy study of the joint section on disorders of the spine and peripheral nerves of the American Association of Neurological Surgeons and Congress of Neurological Surgeons. *Neurosurgery* **29**, 301–8.

Allen, B. L., Jr, Tencer, A. F. & Ferguson, R. L. (1987). The biomechanics of decompressive laminectomy. *Spine* **12**, 803–8.

Andersen, B. J. & Burchiel, K. J. (1991). Surgical treatment of low back pain and sciatica. *Neurosurg. Clin. North Am.* **2**, 921–31.

Andrews, D. W. & Lavyne, M. H. (1990). Retrospective analysis of microsurgical and standard lumbar discectomy. *Spine* **15**, 329–55.

Aryanpur, J. & Ducker, T. (1990). Multilevel lumbar laminotomies: an alternative to laminectomy in the treatment of lumbar stenosis. *Neurosurgery* **26**, 429–33.

Bailey, R. W. & Badgley, C. E. (1960). Stabilization of the cervical spine by anterior fusion. *J. Bone Joint Surg. Am.* **42**, 565–94.

Bernard, T. N. J. & Whitecloud, T. S. I. (1987). Cervical spondylotic myelopathy and myeloradiculopathy: anterior decompression and stabilization with autogenous fibula strut graft. *Clin. Orthop.* **221**, 149–60.

Bertalanffy, H. & Eggert, H.-R. (1988). Clinical long-term results of anterior cervical discectomy without fusion for treatment of cervical radiculopathy and myelopathy: a follow-up of 164 cases. *Acta Neurochir. (Wien)* **90**, 127–35.

Bohlman, H. H. (1977). Cervical spondylosis with moderate to severe myelopathy: a report of seventeen cases treated by Robinson anterior cervical discectomy and fusion. *Spine* 2, 151–62.

Bohlman, H. & Emery, S. E. (1988). The pathophysiology of cervical spondylosis and myelopathy. *Spine* 13, 843–6.

Bradshaw, P. (1957). Some aspects of cervical spondylosis. *Q. J. Med.* 26, 177–208.

Caputy, A. J. & Luessenhop, A. J. (1992). Long-term evaluation of decompressive surgery for degenerative lumbar stenosis. *J. Neurosurg.* 77, 669–76.

Casotto, A. & Buoncritiani, P. (1981). Posterior approach in cervical spondylotic myeloradidulopathy. *Acta Neurochir. (Wien)* 57, 275–85.

Caspar, W., Campbell, B., Barbier, D. D. *et al.* (1991). The Caspar microsurgical discectomy and comparison with a conventional standard lumbar disc procedure. *Neurosurgery* 28, 78–87.

Clarke, E. & Robinson, P. K. (1956). Cervical myelopathy: a complication of cervical spondylosis. *Brain* 79, 483–510.

Cloward, R. B. (1958). The anterior approach for removal of ruptured cervical disks. *J. Neurosurg.* 15, 602–17.

Conley, F. K., Cady, C. T. & Lieberson, R. E. (1990). Decompression of lumbar spinal stenosis and stabilization with Knodt rods in the elderly patient. *Neurosurgery* 26, 758–63.

Cooper, P. R. (1992). Cervical spondylotic myelopathy: management with anterior operation. In *Degenerative Disease of the Cervical Spine*. New York: American Association of Neurological Surgeons.

Crandall, P. H. & Batzdorf, U. (1966). Cervical spondylotic myelopathy. *J. Neurosurg.* 25, 57–66.

Crandall, P. H. & Gregorius, F. K. (1977). Long-term follow-up of surgical treatment of cervical spondylotic myelopathy. *Spine* 2, 139–46.

Davis, G. W., Onik, G. & Helms, C. (1991). Automated percutaneous discectomy. *Spine* 16, 359–63.

Day, A. L., Savage, D. F., Friedman, W. A. *et al.* (1985). Chemonucleolysis versus open discectomy: the case against chymopapain. *Clin. Neurosurg.* 33, 385–94.

Delashaw, J. B., Knego, R. S. & Jane, J. A. (1992). Lumbar disc disease. *Perspect. Neurol. Surg.* 3, 1–35.

Dickman, C. A., Fessler, R. G., MacMillan, M. *et al.* (1992). Transpedicular screw-rod fixation of the lumbar spine: operative technique and outcome in 104 cases. *J. Neurosurg.* 77, 860–70.

Dunsker, S. B. (1987). Alternatives in the surgical treatment of herniated lumbar disks. *Clin. Neurosurg.* 35, 459–73.

Dvorak, J., Gauchat, M.-H. & Valach, L. (1988). The outcome of surgery for lumbar disc herniation. 1. A 4–17 years' follow-up with emphasis on somatic aspects. *Spine* 13, 1418–22.

Epstein, J. (1988). The surgical management of cervical spinal stenosis, spondylosis, and myeloradiculopathy by means of the posterior approach. *Spine* 13, 864–9.

Epstein, J. A., Carras, R., Lavine, L. S. *et al.* (1969). The importance of removing osteophytes as part of the surgical treatment of myeloradiculopathy in cervical spondylosis. *J. Neurosurg.* 30, 219–26.

Epstein, J. A., Janin, Y., Carras, R. *et al.* (1982). A comparative study of the treatment of cervical spondylotic myelopathy. *Acta Neurochirur. (Wien)* 61, 89–104.

Eriksen, E. F., Buhl, M., Fode, K. *et al.* (1984). Treatment of cervical disc disease using Cloward's technique: the prognostic value of clinical preoperative data in 1106 patients. *Acta Neurochirur. (Wien)* 70, 181–97.

Errico, T. J. & Lowell, T. D. (1993). The operative treatment of lumbar herniated nucleus pulposus. *Curr. Opin. Orthop.* 4, 115–24.

Fager, C. A. (1973). Results of adequate posterior decompression in the relief of spondylotic cervical myelopathy. *J. Neurosurg.* **38**, 684–92.

Frymoyer, J. W. (1988). Back pain and sciatica. *N. Engl. J. Med.* **318**, 291–300.

Galera, R. & Tovi, D. (1968). Anterior disc excision with interbody fusion in cervical spondylotic myelopathy and rhizopathy. *J. Neurosurg.* **28**, 305–10.

Ganz, J. C. (1990). Lumbar spinal stenosis: postoperative results in terms of preoperative posture-related pain. *J. Neurosurg.* **72**, 71–4.

Getty, C. J. M. (1980). Lumbar spinal stenosis: the clinical spectrum and the results of operation. *J. Bone Joint Surg. Br.* **62**, 481–5.

Goro, D. R. & Sopio, S. B. (1904). Anterior cervical fusion for degenerated or protruded discs. a review of one hundred forty-six patients. *Spine* **9**, 667–71.

Grabias, S. (1980). The treatment of spinal stenosis. *J. Bone Joint Surg. Am.* **62**, 308–13.

Guidetti, B. & Fortuna, A. (1969). Long-term results of surgical treatment of myelopathy due to cervical spondylosis. *J. Neurosurg.* **30**, 714–21.

Hadley, M. N. (1992). Expert commentary on Delashaw, J. B., Knego, R. B. & Jane, J. A.: Lumbar disc disease. *Perspect. Neurol. Surg.* **3**, 36–7.

Haid, R. W., Jr & Dickman, C. A. (1993). Instrumentation and fusion for discogenic disease of the lumbosacral spine. *Neurosurg. Clin. North Am.* **4**, 135–48.

Hall, S., Bartleson, J. D., Onofrio, B. M. *et al.* (1985). Lumbar spinal stenosis: clinical features, diagnostic procedures, and results of surgical treatment in 68 patients. *Ann. Intern. Med.* **103**, 271–5.

Hanai, K., Fujiyoshi, F. & Kamei, K. (1986). Subtotal vertebrectomy and spinal fusion for cervical spondylotic myelopathy. *Spine* **11**, 310–15.

Hanley, E. N., Jr, Phillips, E. D. & Kostuik, J. P. (1991). Who should be fused? In *The Adult Spine: Principles and Practice.* New York: Raven Press.

Harrison, M. J. & Sundaresan, N. (1991). Spinal instrumentation for degenerative disease of the lumbar spine. *Mt. Sinai J. Med.* **58**, 169–76.

Herkowitz, H. N. (1988). A comparison of anterior cervical fusion, cervical laminectomy, and cervical laminoplasty for the surgical management of multiple level spondylotic radiculopathy. *Spine* **13**, 774–80.

Herkowitz, H. N. & Kurz, L. T. (1991). Degenerative lumbar spondylolisthesis with spinal stenosis: a prospective study comparing decompression with decompression and intertransverse process arthrodesis. *J. Bone Joint Surg. Am.* **73**, 802–8.

Hopp, E. & Tsou, P. M. (1988). Postdecompression lumbar instability. *Clin. Orthop.* **227**, 143–50.

Howe, J. & Frymoyer, J. W. (1984). The effects of questionnaire design on the determination of end results in lumbar spinal surgery. *Spine* **10**, 804–5.

Hukuda, S., Mocizuki, T., Ogata, M. *et al.* (1985). Operations for cervical spondylotic myelopathy: a comparison of the results of anterior and posterior procedures. *J. Bone and Joint Surg. Br.* **67**, 609–15.

Irvine, G. B. & Strachan, W. E. (1987). The long-term results of localized anterior cervical decompression and fusion in spondylotic myelopathy. *Paraplegia* **25**, 18–22.

Johnsson, K.-E., Willner, S. & Pettersson, H. (1981). Analysis of operated cases with lumbar spinal stenosis. *Acta Orthop. Scand.* **52**, 427–33.

Kadoya, S., Nakamura, T. & Kwak, R. (1984). A microsurgical anterior osteophytectomy for cervical spondylotic myelopathy. *Spine* **9**, 437–41.

Katz, J. N., Lipson, S. J., Larson, M. G. *et al.* (1991). The outcome of decompressive laminectomy for degenerative lumbar stenosis. *J. Bone Joint Surg. Am.* **73**, 809–16.

Klara, P. M. & Foley, K. (1993). Surgical treatment of osteophytes and calcified discs of the cervical spine. *Neurosurg. Clin. North Am.* **4**, 53–60.

Kojima, T., Waga, S., Kubo, Y. *et al.* (1989). Anterior cervical vertebrectomy and interbody fusion for multi-level spondylosis and ossification of the posterior longitudinal ligament. *Neurosurgery* **24**, 864–72.

Kostuik, J. P. & Frymoyer, J. W. (1991). Failures after spinal fusion: causes and surgical treatment results. In *The Adult Spine: Principles and Practice.* New York: Raven Press.

Koutrouvelis, P. G., Lang, E., Heilen R. *et al.* (1993). Stereotactic percutaneous lumbar discectomy. *Neurosurgery* **32**, 582–6.

Lees, F. & Turner, J. W. A. (1963). Natural history and prognosis of cervical spondylosis. *BMT* **2**, 1607–10.

Lewis, P. J., Weir, B. K. A. & Broad, R. W. (1987). Long-term prospective study of lumbosacral discectomy. *J. Neurosurg.* **67**, 49–53.

Long, D. M. (1991). Decision making in lumbar disc disease. *Clin. Neurosurg.* **39**, 36–51.

Lorenz, M., Zindrick, M., Schwaegler, P. *et al.* (1991). A comparison of single-level fusions with and without hardware. *Spine* **16** (Suppl.), S455–8.

Lorenz, M. A., Hodges, S. & Vrbos, L. (1993). Spinal fixation. *Curr. Opin. Orthop.* **4**, 192–204.

Lunsford, L. D., Bissonette, D. J. & Zorub, D. S. (1980). Anterior surgery for cervical disc disease. II. Treatment of cervical spondylotic myelopathy in 32 cases. *J. Neurosurg.* **53**, 12–19.

Mann, K. S., Khosla, V. K. & Gulati, D. R. (1984). Cervical spondylotic myelopathy by single-stage multilevel anterior decompression. *J. Neurosurg.* **60**, 81–7.

Maroon, J. C. & Abla, A. (1985). Microdiscectomy versus chemonucleolysis. *Neurosurgery* **16**, 644–9.

Martins, A. N. (1976). Anterior cervical discectomy with and without interbody bone graft. *J. Neurosurg.* **44**, 290–5.

McAfee, P. C., Farey, I. D., Sutterlin, C. E. *et al.* (1989). Device-related osteoporosis with spinal instrumentation. *Spine* **14**, 919–26.

McCulloch, J. A. (1991). Microdiscectomy. In *The Adult Spine: Principles and Practice.* New York: Raven Press.

Mehalic, T. F., Pezzuti, R. T. & Applebaum, B. I. (1990). Magnetic resonance imaging and cervical spondylotic myelopathy. *Neurosurgery* **26**, 217–27.

Montgomery, D. M. & Brower, R. S. (1992). Cervical spondylotic myelopathy: clinical syndrome and natural history. *Orthop. Clin. North Am.* **23**, 487–93.

Moussa, A. H., Nitta, M. & Symon, L. (1983). The results of anterior cervical fusion in cervical spondylosis: review of 125 cases. *Acta Neurochir. (Wien)* **68**, 277–88.

Nasca, R. J. (1987). Surgical management of lumbar spinal stenosis. *Spine* **12**, 809–16.

Nurick, S. (1972). The natural history and the results of surgical treatment of the spinal cord disorder associated with cervical spondylosis. *Brain* **95**, 101–8.

Pappas, C. T. E., Harrington, T. & Sonntag, V. K. H. (1992). Outcome analysis in 654 surgically treated lumbar disc herniations. *Neurosurgery* **30**, 862–6.

Phillips, D. G. (1973). Surgical treatment of myelopathy with cervical spondylosis. *J. Neurol. Neurosurg. Psychiatry* **36**, 879–84.

Piepgras, D. G. (1977). Posterior decompression for myelopathy due to cervical spondylosis: laminectomy versus laminectomy with dentate ligament section. *Clin. Neurosurg.* **24**, 508–15.

Rengachary, S. S. & Redford, J. B. (1991). Partial median corpectomy for cervical spondylotic myelopathy. In *Neurosurgery Update II.* New York: McGraw-Hill.

Roberts, A. H. (1966). Myelopathy due to cervical spondylosis treated by collar immobilization. *Neurology* **16**, 951–4.

Robinson, R. A. & Smith, G. W. (1955). Anterolateral cervical disc removal and interbody fusion for cervical disc syndrome. *Bull. Johns Hopkins Hosp.* **96**, 223–4.

Rogers, L. A. (1988). Experience with limited versus extensive disc removal in patients undergoing microsurgical operations for ruptured lumbar discs. *Neurosurgery* **22**, 82–5.

Rosenorn, J., Hansen, E. B. & Rosenorn, M. A. (1983). Anterior cervical discectomy with and without fusion: a prospective study. *J. Neurosurg.* **59**, 252–5.

Rowland, L. P. (1992). Surgical treatment of cervical spondylotic myelopathy: time for a controlled trial. *Neurology* **12**, 5 13.

Saunders, R. L. (1991). Anterior reconstructive procedures in cervical spondylotic myelopathy. *Clin. Neurosurg.* **37**, 682–721.

Saunders, R. L., Bernini, P. M., Shirreffs, T. G. *et al.* (1991). Central corpectomy for cervical spondylotic myelopathy: a consecutive series with long-term follow-up evaluation. *J. Neurosurg.* **74**, 163–70.

Schmidek, H. H. & Smith, D. A. (1988). Anterior cervical disc excision in cervical spondylosis. In *Operative Neurosurgical Techniques,* 2nd edn. Philadelphia: W. B. Saunders.

Scoville, W. B. (1961). Cervical spondylosis treated by bilateral facetectomy and laminectomy. *J. Neurosurg.* **18**, 423–8.

Seifert, V. & Stolke, D. (1991). Multisegmental cervical spondylosis: treatment by spondylectomy, microsurgical decompression, and osteosynthesis. *Neurosurgery* **29**, 498–503.

Silvers, H. R. (1988). Microsurgical versus standard lumbar discectomy. *Neurosurgery* **22**, 837–41.

Silvers, H. R., Lewis, P. J. & Asch, H. L. (1993). Decompressive lumbar laminectomy for lumbar stenosis. *J. Neurosurg.* **78**, 695–701.

Simeone, F. A. (1989). Surgical management of cervical disc disease: posterior approach. *Semin. Spine Surg.* **1**, 239–44.

Snow, R. B. & Weiner, H. (1993). Cervical laminectomy and foraminotomy as surgical treatment of cervical spondylosis: a follow-up study with analysis of failures. *J. Spinal Disord.* **6**, 245–51.

Spengler, D. M. (1991). Lumbar decompression for spinal stenosis: surgical indications and technique. In *The Adult Spine: Principles and Practice.* New York: Raven Press.

Spengler, D. M. & Frymoyer, J. W. (1991). Lumbar discectomy: indications and technique. In *The Adult Spine: Principles and Practice.* New York: Raven Press.

Stillerman, C. B. & Maiman, D. J. (1990). Pedicles screw-plate fixation of the lumbar spine. *Perspect. Neurol. Surg.* **1**, 24–34.

Stoops, W. & King, R. (1965). Chronic myelopathy associated with cervical spondylosis: its response to laminectomy and foraminotomy. *JAMA* **192**, 281–4.

Sugar, O. (1981). Spinal cord malfunction after anterior cervical discectomy. *Surg. Neurol.* **15**, 4–8.

Symon, L. & Lavender, P. (1967). The surgical treatment of cervical spondylotic myelopathy. *Neurology* **17**, 117–26.

Sypert, G. W. (1992). Anterior decompression and fusion for cervical myelopathy. In *Disorders of the Cervical Spine.* Baltimore: Williams and Wilkins.

Turner, J. A., Ersek, M., Herron, L. *et al.* (1992). Surgery for lumbar spinal stenosis: attempted meta-analysis of the literature. *Spine* **17**, 1–8.

van Alphen, H. A. M., Braakman, R., Bezemer, P. D. *et al.* (1989). Chemonucleolysis versus discectomy: a randomized multicenter trial. *J. Neurosurg.* **70**, 869–75.

Verbiest, H. (1973). The management of cervical spondylosis. *Clin. Neurosurg.* **20**, 262–94.

Weber, H. (1983). Lumbar disc herniation: a controlled, prospective study with ten years of observation. *Spine* **8**, 131–40.

Weir, B. & de Leo, R. (1981). Lumbar stenosis: analysis of factors affecting outcome in 81 surgical cases. *Can. J. Neurol. Sci.* **8**, 295–8.

West, J. L. I., Bradford, D. S. & Ogilvie, J. W. (1991). Results of spinal arthrodesis with pedicle screw plate fixation. *J. Bone Joint Surg. Am.* **73**, 1179–84.

Whitecloud, T. S., III (1991). Cervical spondylosis: the anterior approach. In *The Adult Spine: Principles and Practice*. New York: Raven Press.

Williams, R. W. (1978). Microlumbar discectomy: a conservative surgical approach to the virgin herniated disc. *Spine* **3**, 175–82.

Wilson, D. H. & Harbaugh, R. (1981). Microsurgical and standard removal of the protruded lumbar disc: a comparative study. *Neurosurgery* **8**, 422–7.

Yonenobu, K., Fuji, T., Ono, K. *et al.* (1985). Choice of surgical treatment for multisegmental cervical spondylotic myelopathy. *Spine* **10**, 710–16.

Zdeblick, T. A. & Bohlmann, H. H. (1989). Myelopathy, cervical kyphosis, and treatment by anterior corpectomy and strut grafting. *J. Bone Joint Surg. Am.* **71**, 170–82.

Zeidman, S. M. & Ducker, T. B. (1993). Cervical myelopathy due to degenerative changes of disk herniations. *Curr. Opin. Orthop.* **4**, 54–68.

Zindrick, M. R. (1991). The role of transpedicular fixation systems for stabilization of the lumbar spine. *Orthop. Clin. North Am.* **22**, 333–44.

16 Degenerative diseases in the CNS

DONALD B. CALNE AND W. KOLLER

Over the last two decades, increasing interest has been focused upon measuring the progression, impact and outcome of chronic neurological disease. The derivation of quantitative indices is important because such information has a wide range of applications. These include:

1. *Exploration of pathogenesis.* The time course of evolution has been a traditional tool for investigating the nature of the pathological mechanism underlying neurological diseases. The slow but inexorable advance of neurodegenerative processes contrasts substantially with the sudden onset of cerebrovascular disease or the fluctuating natural history of immunologically mediated neuropathology.

2. *Evaluation of therapy.* The need for quantification of symptoms, signs and functional impairment is self-evident in the fields of pharmacotherapy and surgical therapy. A comparison between active treatment and placebo, or between alternative forms of therapy, only becomes possible through the application of measurements of outcome.

3. *Patient care.* Acquisition of measures of disease progression is of value in the education of patients and their caregivers. The correlation of disease duration with disability provides a basis for estimating prognosis. This is of particular significance for planning the future practical needs of the patient.

4. *Planning health care.* Politicians, economists and sociologists must have information upon which to base their decisions when designing and implementing public and private health care systems. Quantitative assessment of outcome is a vital component of the equation that must be used to balance the requirements of society against the resources that are available.

General principles

Crude information on the outcome of disease, such as death, is useful in providing a coarse profile of events. More sensitive indices have been developed to generate a more detailed picture of the evolution of chronic illness. For neurodegenerative disease, measures of change fall into the following categories:

1. An endpoint defined by a major change in (a) lifestyle or (b) medical management.
2. Subjective clinical scoring protocols based upon (a) history and (b) examination.
3. Objective measures of simple tasks taking account of (a) speed and (b) accuracy.
4. Precise physiological testing.
5. Analytic brain imaging.
6. Estimation of the social and economic consequences for the community.

We shall consider each of these in turn.

Major changes in lifestyle or medical management

For patients suffering from neurodegenerative disease, certain changes in lifestyle or medical management have been employed as milestones to record the evolution of disease. Lifestyle examples are loss of employment, the need for a wheelchair, or admission to a facility that provides a sheltered environment.

Important changes in medical treatment have also been considered to represent reference points in the natural history of the disorder. For example, in the case of idiopathic Parkinsonism (IP, Parkinson's disease), the stage of disability that triggers the introduction of levodopa therapy has recently been employed in two large studies on deprenyl. While this endpoint may seem vague and variable, it has proved quite consistent and convenient in the context of large multicentre studies (Parkinson Study Group 1989a). An endpoint of this type allows the application of Kaplan–Meier survival analysis and other classical methods of statistical evaluation, such as the comparison of hazard ratios. It is appropriate to focus attention on how investigators employ a 'soft' endpoint, to obtain a highly consistent result. 'The primary endpoint in the trial occurred when, in the judgement of the enrolling investigator, a subject reached a level of functional disability sufficient to warrant the initiation of levodopa therapy. In arriving at this judgement, the investigator considered several factors: the threat to the subject's employability, the threat to the subject's ability to manage domestic or financial affairs, an appreciable decline in the subject's handling of the activities of daily living, and an appreciable worsening of gait or balance' (Parkinson Study Group 1989).

Subjective clinical scoring protocols

Many clinical scoring protocols have been formulated to generate quantitative measures of the symptoms and signs of neurodegenerative disease. Recently they have received addendums to take account of adverse reactions to medications. Again, IP constitutes a suitable example for analysis. Similar considerations exist for other neurodegenerative disorders, but we shall direct our attention to IP because of the substantial interest and effort focused on this disorder in order to evaluate new approaches to treatment over the last 25 years.

Some of the clinical features of IP, such as tremor, lend themselves so well to recording techniques that semiquantitative assessment can be traced back to the last century. However, strong motivation for the development of quantitative rating scales became evident as stereotactic surgery came into vogue and powerful new forms of pharmacotherapy were introduced after the discovery of dopamine depletion as a key feature of IP.

Two approaches have evolved for clinical scoring: one based upon the history, and the other upon the examination. Both are important, but while there was initially more emphasis placed upon the examination, it has now become apparent that the scores deriving from historical information often give a more meaningful statement because they come from evaluations based upon an averaging process over reasonable periods of time. In contrast, the examination is conducted over a brief period of time, which might be quite unrepresentative because of the increasingly frequent transient, but dramatic changes in mobility that occur in IP (wearing off reactions and on–off phenomena).

Many of the clinical rating scales combine scores obtained from the history with those assigned as a result of examination. Scores determined by the history are often referred to as evaluations of the 'Activities of Daily Living' because they address practical issues such as the patients' ability to feed themselves or dress themselves.

Clinical rating protocols have three major drawbacks:

1. The components do not usually have a direct correlation with any important neurobiological index of the severity of disease. An important exception is bradykinesia, which is linearly related to loss of dopaminergic nigral cells (see below).
2. Numbers assigned have no linear significance: '4' is simply two steps up from '2'; this does not mean that a clinical feature assigned '4' is twice as bad as one assigned '2' in any linear way.
3. Different clinical features are commonly summed to give scores that represent the overall level of disturbed function for the patient. Alternatively, subtotals are often created that supposedly represent different manifestations of the same category of deficit, such as 'bradykinesia'. The addition of inherently disparate quantities gives a somewhat misleading impression of meaningful measurement.

Clinical rating protocols have major advantages over most of the alternative methods for quantifying IP:

1. They are quick.
2. They are cheap.
3. They provide a general summary of the status of the patient, rather than an isolated and circumscribed measure that tends to be obtained from objective quantification.

There are several reviews that give details of the various clinical scoring protocols that have been employed to assess IP (Terravainen & Calne 1980; Lader & Richens 1981;

Ward *et al.* 1983; Kraus *et al.* 1990). The most widely used protocol at the present time is the Unified Parkinson's Disease Rating Scale (UPDRS) (AIMS 1976), which is derived predominantly from the Columbia Rating Scale (Duvoisin 1971) and Schwab's protocol for assessing the Activities of Daily Living (Schwab & England 1969). The main limitation of the UPDRS is the time required to complete it, but it has, nevertheless, gained widespread acceptance, and it is certainly a valuable source for choosing selected portions that are particularly appropriate for a specific study. Because of its importance, this scale is provided in Appendix A.

In addition to the comprehensive clinical rating scales that have been produced, a clinical staging protocol was published at the time when levodopa therapy was being introduced. The severity of disease was broken into five stages by Hoehn & Yahr (1967). This is another widely applied tool, so it is included here as Appendix B. Hoehn and Yahr stages have the advantage of simplicity and brevity.

Studies based upon clinical scoring protocols generally employ an arbitrary endpoint defined as an absolute or relative change in score or stage.

Objective measures of simple tasks

Continuing with the example of IP, some of the earliest approaches to measuring deficits entailed simple motor tasks such as moving a marker between two points and timing the number of hits within a standard period. The velocity and the accuracy of movement can both be measured. A somewhat more sophisticated example of the same type of test is the Purdue Peg Board.

For the lower limbs, walking has been timed over a given distance, including starting, turning around and stopping.

The advantage of these tests is that they provide a compromise in which cost is low and yet the results avoid the inevitable problem of interindividual variation among different observers. Minor changes in the design of tasks allow the difficulty of the test to be adjusted to meet the needs of the particular category of patients under study.

Precise physiological testing

Regarding precise physiological testing, again the example of IP is convenient to pursue. The last two decades have witnessed the creation of a variety of more complex physiological tests designed to measure deficits. These include torque motors to measure rigidity and long-latency reflexes; techniques for recording reaction times that may or may not involve a choice of direction after the 'go' signal; computerized comparisons between movements executed in isolation or in combination with simple or complex movements of the contralateral limb; measures with accelerometers; measures of ocular movement which may or may not be linked to limb movement; measures of visual evoked potentials; and studies of magnetic stimulation of the brain. Many other examples have been undertaken.

Studies that involve precise physiological testing are usually employed to explore the functional disturbances of motor control in IP, but in principle they can also be used to provide rather precise endpoints. For example, some have been included in the battery of screening tests applied to the evaluation of the results of surgical transplant procedures for IP (Widner *et al.* 1992).

Analytic brain imaging

In discussing analytic brain imaging we shall maintain the example of IP. Positron emission tomography (PET) with fluorodopa has been used to assess the outcome of implantation of fetal mesencephalic tissue into the brain of Parkinsonian patients (Sawle *et al.* 1992; Widner *et al.* 1992). PET also has a potential for use in the difficult task of evaluating pharmacotherapy designed to provide neuroprotection.

PET has proved valuable for investigating the normal rate of evolution of the underlying pathology of IP (Bhatt *et al.* 1991), and for demonstrating unexpected progression of nigrostriatal lesions after exposure to the neurotoxin MPTP (Vingerhoets *et al.* 1993).

Recently the fluorodopa uptake constant, derived from PET, has been shown to correlate in a direct and linear fashion with the number of nigral dopaminergic neurons in animals models of Parkinsonism (Pate *et al.* 1993). A similar relationship has been shown to obtain for human subjects with disorders that involve the nigrostriatal pathway. Thus, fluorodopa PET has proved to be an extraordinarily useful tool that allows, in a sense, an *in vivo* biopsy of the substantia nigra to be taken.

Several groups have shown that fluorodopa PET measurements correlate linearly with the UPDRS score for bradykinesia (Eidelberg *et al.* 1990; Snow *et al.* 1991; Vingerhoets *et al.* 1997). This finding allows the inference that the bradykinesia score, in particular, provides an index of the dopaminergic nigral cell count. This finding provides linkage between a clinical rating scale and an important neurobiological variable.

Social and economic consequences

There is no doubt that the chronic degenerative diseases of the nervous system result in major social and economic hardships. Unfortunately, however, there has not been any concerted effort to collect information on this topic. The National Foundation for Brain Research (US) estimates that the annual cost of disorders of the brain and nervous system in the United States is $401.1 billion, of which 103.7 billion is directly due to neurological diseases (National Foundation for Brain Research 1992). The analysis included both what are defined as direct and indirect costs. Direct costs are expenditures on medical and non-medical services, such as physicians, hospital, nursing home, pharmaceuticals, home care, rehabilitation, transportation, medical devices and direct financial assistance. Indirect costs are broadly defined to include lost wages due to illness or disability or death, lost wages of caregivers, and societal expenditures for education and public health. We will use both IP and Alzheimer's disease (AD) as examples.

Idiopathic Parkinsonism

The mean age of onset of IP is approximately 60 years; however, 5–10% of patients will have onset before the age of 40 years (Marttilla 1992). Many individuals receive the diagnosis of IP at the most productive time of their life. They realize that the disease is progressive and that their future is uncertain. The psychological damage can not be estimated in monetary terms. The emotional toll in human suffering and the anguish of family members is certainly immense.

Singer (1973) assessed the social cost of IP in 149 patients who were about to begin levodopa therapy. He concluded that IP was like premature social ageing. IP patients were less likely to work and if working had more absenteeism. Those with IP were less likely to engage in household tasks or to have a close circle of friends. In general, IP patients lived a solitary existence. The social costs were much greater for the younger-onset IP patients. Singer also collected some economic data and found that IP patients received less income from direct earnings and a greater percentage of their income in pension plans and social security than age-matched controls. Kurlan and colleagues (1988) studied the 800 patients who formed the DATATOP cohort (Parkinson Study Group 1989b). They found that 31% of IP patients at Hoehn–Yahr stage I and II who were currently working lost their jobs within a 1-year period. They suggested that a 10% slowing of IP could result in 16–19 additional weeks of employment and postulated that a modestly successful protective therapy for early IP could realize a substantial saving of approximately US $327 million annually.

It is obvious that much more data are needed to document the high economic and social costs of IP with greater precision.

Alzheimer's disease

AD is common. It is estimated that nearly 4 million persons in the United States are afflicted and that by the year 2040 as many as 9 million persons in that country will be affected (Evans 1990). The incidence of AD increases with age. Thus, concomitant with an increase in life span, AD will become more prevalent. AD, which robs individuals of cognition, poses a major economic burden for the patient, their family and society as a whole (May 1993).

The cost of caring for AD patients is clearly substantial. Many patients require constant care whether at home, at adult care centres or in nursing homes. Hu *et al.* (1986) studied 44 patients with dementia who were either in the community or in nursing homes in Pennsylvania or in Washington, DC. They found that the annual costs per person were US $22 248 for a nursing home resident and US $11 735 for an individual cared for at home. Because of inflation these figures would now be much higher. These investigators (Huang *et al.* 1988) also estimated that the national cost of dementia in 1990 is US $20 billion dollars a year for direct medical and social service cost and US $38 billion dollars for informal care costs, making a total of US $58 billion dollars. Hay & Ernst (1987) estimated the societal cost for all persons first diagnosed with AD in 1983 to be between US $27.9 to US $31.2 billion dollars. This study was incidence-based and considered the lifetime cost of those newly diagnosed. Rice *et al.* (1991) developed estimates of the costs of caring for AD patients in northern California by studying 100 nursing home patients and 100 community-based patients. The total societal cost of care per person, whether institutionalized or non-institutionalized, was approximately US $47 000. They also discovered that 60% of the cost of formal care was paid by the family regardless of whether the patients were living in a nursing home. It is evident that AD is a devastating illness that is very costly to society. Unfortunately, this enormous economic burden is likely to increase in the future.

Several measurement instruments have been used to address the issue of quality of life in Parkinson's disease; e.g. the Parkinson's Disease Questionnaire (PDQ-39), the Parkinson's Impact Scale (PIMS), and the Parkinson's Disease Questionnaire and Living scale (PDQL) (Jenkinson *et al.* 1995; Calne *et al.* 1996; de Boer *et al.* 1996). These scales vary in complexity. The PIMS is relatively brief, consisting of questions in 10 areas of a patient's life, that can be completed in 5–10 minutes. It is sensitive to fluctuations in treatment responses, taking into account best and worst scores if appropriate. These Quality of Life measures require assessment of their sensitivity to changes in disease severity over time. They may prove useful in clinical practice as well as in research.

Conclusion

The outcome of neurodegenerative disorders has been studied in terms of the effect of therapy, but not in terms of the effect of the treatment on the patient's sense of well-being. There is not enough information about the consequences for the patient, or for society in terms of disruption of life for caregivers and family, loss of work and the direct and indirect economic burden of these diseases and their treatment.

Appendix A. Unified Parkinson's Disease Rating Scale (UPDRS)

Unified Parkinson's Disease Rating Scale (version 3.0, February 1987): definitions of 0–4 scale.

Subscale I. Mentation, behaviour and mood

1. Intellectual impairment:
   0 = None
   1 = Mild; consistent forgetfulness with partial recollection of events and no other difficulties
   2 = Moderate memory loss, with disorientation and moderate difficulty handling complex problems; mild but definite impairment of function at home, with need of occasional prompting
   3 = Severe memory loss with disorientation for time and often for place, severe impairment in handling problems

4 = Severe memory loss, with orientation preserved to person only; unable to make judgements or solve problems; requires much help with personal care; cannot be left alone at all

2. Thought disorder (due to dementia or drug intoxication):
   0 = None
   1 = Vivid dreaming
   2 = 'Benign' hallucinations with insight retained
   3 = Occasional to frequent hallucinations or delusions without insight; could interfere with daily activities
   4 = Persistent hallucinations, delusions or florid psychosis; not able to care for self

3. Depression:
   0 = Not present
   1 = Periods of sadness or guilt greater than normal but never sustained for days or weeks
   2 = Sustained depression (1 week or more)
   3 = Sustained depression with vegetative symptoms (insomnia, anorexia, weight loss, loss of interest)
   4 = Sustained depression with vegetative symptoms and suicidal thoughts or intent

4. Motivation/initiative:
   0 = Normal
   1 = Less assertive than usual; more passive
   2 = Loss of initiative or interest in elective (non-routine) activities
   3 = Loss of initiative or interest in day-to-day (routine) activities
   4 = Withdrawn; complete loss of motivation

Subscale II. Activities of daily living (determine for 'on'/'off')

5. Speech:
   0 = Normal
   1 = Mildly affected; no difficulty being understood
   2 = Moderately affected; sometimes asked to repeat statements
   3 = Severely affected; frequently asked to repeat statements
   4 = Unintelligible most of the time

6. Salivation:
   0 = Normal
   1 = Slight but definite excess of saliva in mouth; may have night-time drooling
   2 = Moderately excessive saliva; may have minimal drooling
   3 = Marked excess of saliva; some drooling
   4 = Marked drooling; requires constant use of tissue or handkerchief

7. Swallowing:

    0 = Normal

    1 = Rare choking

    2 = Occasional choking

    3 = Requires soft food

    4 = Requires nasogastric tube or gastrostomy feeding

8. Handwriting:

    0 = Normal

    1 = Slightly slow or small

    2 = Moderately slow or small; all words are legible

    3 = Severely affected; not all words are legible

    4 = The majority of words are not legible

9. Cutting food and handling utensils:

    0 = Normal

    1 = Somewhat slow and clumsy, but no help needed

    2 = Can cut most foods, although clumsy and slow; some help needed

    3 = Food must be cut by someone, but can still feed slowly

    4 = Needs to be fed

10. Dressing:

    0 = Normal

    1 = Somewhat slow, but no help needed

    2 = Occasional assistance needed with buttoning, getting arms into sleeves

    3 = Considerable help required, but can do some things alone

    4 = Helpless

11. Hygiene:

    0 = Normal

    1 = Somewhat slow, but no help needed

    2 = Needs help to shower or bathe; very slow in hygienic care

    3 = Requires assistance for washing, brushing teeth, combing hair, going to bathroom

    4 = Needs Foley catheter or other mechanical aids

12. Turning in bed and adjusting bedclothes:

    0 = Normal

    1 = Somewhat slow and clumsy, but no help needed

    2 = Can turn alone or adjust sheets, but with great difficulty

    3 = Can initiate attempt, but cannot turn or adjust sheets alone

    4 = Helpless

13. Falling (unrelated to freezing):

    0 = None

    1 = Rare falling

2 = Occasionally falls, less than once daily

3 = Falls an average of once daily

4 = Falls more than once daily

14. Freezing when walking:

0 = None

1 = Rare freezing when walking; may have start hesitation

2 = Occasional freezing when walking

3 = Frequent freezing; occasionally falls because of freezing

4 = Frequently falls because of freezing

15. Walking:

0 = Normal

1 = Mild difficulty; may not swing arms or may tend to drag leg

2 = Moderate difficulty, but requires little or no assistance

3 = Severe disturbance of walking, requires assistance

4 = Cannot walk at all, even with assistance

16. Tremor:

0 = Absent

1 = Slight and infrequently present, not bothersome to patient

2 = Moderate; bothersome to patient

3 = Severe; interferes with many activities

4 = Marked; interferes with most activities

17. Sensory complaints related to Parkinsonism:

0 = None

1 = Occasionally has numbness, tingling, or mild aching

2 = Frequently has numbness, tingling, or aching; not distressing

3 = Frequent painful sensations

4 = Excruciating pain

Subscale III. Motor examination

18. Speech:

0 = Normal

1 = Slight loss of expression, diction and/or volume

2 = Monotone, slurred but understandable; moderately impaired

3 = Marked impairment, difficult to understand

4 = Unintelligible

19. Facial expression:

0 = Normal

1 = Minimal hypomimia; could be normal 'poker face'

2 = Slight but definitely abnormal diminution of facial expression

3 = Moderate hypomimia; lips parted some of the time

4 = Masked or fixed facies, with severe or complete loss of facial expression; lips parted $\frac{1}{4}$ inch or more

20. Tremor at rest:

0 = Absent

1 = Slight and infrequently present

2 = Mild in amplitude and persistent, or moderate in amplitude but only intermittently present

3 = Moderate in amplitude and present most of the time

4 = Marked in amplitude and present most of the time

21. Action or postural tremor of hands:

0 = Absent

1 = Slight; present with action

2 = Moderate in amplitude; present with action

3 = Moderate in amplitude; present with posture-holding as well as with action

4 = Marked in amplitude; interferes with feeding

22. Rigidity (judged on passive movement of major joints with patient relaxed in sitting position; 'cogwheeling' to be ignored):

0 = Absent

1 = Slight or detectable only when activated by mirror or other movements

2 = Mild to moderate

3 = Marked, but full range of motion easily achieved

4 = Severe; range of motion achieved with difficulty

23. Finger taps (patient taps thumb with index finger in rapid succession with widest amplitude possible, each hand separately):

0 = Normal ($\geq$ 15/5 s)

1 = Mild slowing and/or reduction in amplitude (11–14/5 s)

2 = Moderately impaired; definite and early fatiguing; may have occasional arrests in movement (7–10/5 s)

3 = Severely impaired; frequent hesitation in initiating movements or arrests in ongoing movement (3–6/5 s)

4 = Can barely perform the task (0–2/5 s)

24. Hand movements (patient opens and closes hands in rapid succession with widest amplitude possible, each hand separately):

0 = Normal

1 = Mild slowing and/or reduction in amplitude

2 = Moderately impaired; definite and early fatiguing; may have occasional arrests in movement

3 = Severely impaired; frequent hesitation in initiating movements or arrests in ongoing movement

4 = Can barely perform the task

25. Rapid alternating movements of hand (pronation–supination movements of hands, vertically or horizontally, with as large an amplitude as possible, both hands simultaneously):

    0 = Normal
    1 = Mild slowing and/or reduction in amplitude
    2 = Moderately impaired; definite and early fatiguing; may have occasional arrests in movement
    3 = Severely impaired; frequent hesitation in initiating movements or arrests in ongoing movement
    4 = Can barely perform the task

26. Leg agility (patient taps heel on ground in rapid succession, picking up entire leg; amplitude should be about 3 inches):

    0 = Normal
    1 = Mild slowing and/or reduction in amplitude
    2 = Moderately impaired; definite and early fatiguing; may have occasional arrests in movement
    3 = Severely impaired; frequent hesitation in initiating movements or arrests in ongoing movement
    4 = Can barely perform the task

27. Arising from chair (patient attempts to arise from a straight-backed wood or metal chair, with arms folded across chest):

    0 = Normal
    1 = Slow, or may need more than one attempt
    2 = Pushes self up from arms of seat
    3 = Tends to fall back and may have to try more than one time but can get up without help
    4 = Unable to arise without help

28. Posture:

    0 = Normal erect
    1 = Not quite erect, slightly stooped posture; could be normal for older person
    2 = Moderately stooped posture, definitely abnormal; can be slightly leaning to one side
    3 = Severely stooped posture with kyphosis; can be moderately leaning to one side
    4 = Marked flexion, with extreme abnormality of posture

29. Gait:

    0 = Normal
    1 = Walks slowly; may shuffle with short steps, but no festination or propulsion
    2 = Walks with difficulty but requires little or no assistance; may have some

festination, short steps or propulsion

3 = Severe disturbance of gait; requires assistance

4 = Cannot walk at all, even with assistance

30. Postural stability (response to sudden posterior displacement produced by pull on shoulders while patient is erect, with eyes open and feet slightly apart; patient is prepared):

0 = Normal

1 = Retropulsion, but recovers unaided

2 = Absence of postural response; would fall if not caught by examiner

3 = Very unstable; tends to lose balance spontaneously

4 = Unable to stand without assistance

31. Body bradykinesia and hypokinesia (combining slowness, hesitancy, decreased arm swing, small amplitude, and poverty of movement in general):

0 = None

1 – Minimal slowness, giving movement a deliberate character; could be normal for some persons; possibly reduced amplitude

2 = Mild degree of slowness and poverty of movement that is definitely abnormal; alternatively, some reduced amplitude

3 = Moderate slowness; poverty or small amplitude of movement

4 = Marked slowness; poverty or small amplitude of movement

Subscale IV. Complications of therapy (in the past week)

A. Dyskinesias

32. Duration: What proportion of the waking day are dyskinesias present? (historical information):

0 = None

1 = 1–25% of day

2 = 26–50% of day

3 = 51–75% of day

4 = 76–100% of day

33. Disability: How disabling are the dyskinesias? (historical information; may be modified by office examination):

0 = Not disabling

1 = Mildly disabling

2 = Moderately disabling

3 = Severely disabling

4 = Completely disabling

34. Painful dyskinesias: How painful are the dyskinesias?

0 = No painful dyskinesias

1 = Slightly
2 = Moderately
3 = Severely
4 = Markedly

35. Presence of early morning dystonia (historical information):
    0 = No
    1 = Yes

B. Clinical fluctuations

36. Are any 'off' periods predictable as to timing after a dose of medication?
    0 = No
    1 = Yes

37. Are any 'off' periods unpredictable as to timing after a dose of medication?
    0 = No
    1 = Yes

38. Do any 'off' periods come on suddenly (e.g. within a few seconds)?
    0 = No
    1 = Yes

39. What proportion of the waking day is the patient 'off', on average?
    0 = None
    1 = 1–25% of day
    2 = 26–50% of day
    3 = 51–75% of day
    4 = 76–100% of day

C. Other complications

40. Does the patient have anorexia, nausea or vomiting?
    0 = No
    1 = Yes

41. Does the patient have any sleep disturbances (e.g. insomnia or hypersomnolence)?
    0 = No
    1 = Yes

42. Does the patient have symptomatic orthostatis?
    0 = No
    1 = Yes

Appendix B. Modified Hoehn and Yahr staging

Stage 0.0 = No signs of disease

Stage 1.0 = Unilateral involvement only

Stage 1.5 = Unilateral and axial involvement

Stage 2.0 = Bilateral involvement without impairment of balance

Stage 2.5 = Mild bilateral involvement with recovery on retropulsion (pull) test

Stage 3.0 = Mild to moderate bilateral involvement; some postural instability but
physically independent

Stage 4.0 = Severe disability; still able to walk or stand unassisted

Stage 5.0 = Wheelchair-bound or bedridden unless aided

References

AIMS (1976). *ECDEU Assessment Manual*, pp. 534–7. Rochville: US Department of Health, Education and Welfare.

Bhatt, M. H., Snow, B. J., Martin, W. R. W., Pate, B., Ruth, T. & Calne, D. B. (1991). Positron emission tomography suggests the rate of progression of idiopathic parkinsonism is slow. *Ann. Neurol.* **29**, 673–7.

Calne, S., Schulzer, M., Mak, E. *et al.* (1996). Validating a quality of life rating scale for idiopathic parkinsonism: Parkinson's Impact Scale (PIMS). *Parkinsonism and Related Disorders*, vol. 2, 55–61.

de Boer, A. G., Wijker, W., Speelman, J. D., De Haes, J. C. *et al.* (1996). Quality of life in patients with Parkinson's disease: development of a questionnaire. *J. Neurol. Neurosurg. Psychiatry* **61**, 70–4.

Duvoisin, R. C. (1971). The evaluation of extrapyramidal disease. In *Monoamines noyaux gris centraux et syndrome de Parkinson*, ed. J. de Ajuriaguerra & G. Gauthier, pp. 313–25. Geneva: Georg et Cie.

Eidelberg, D., Moeller, J. R., Dhawan, V. *et al.* (1990). The metabolic anatomy of Parkinson's disease: complementary [^{18}F]fluorodeoxyglucose and [^{18}F]fluorodopa positron emission tomographic studies. *Mov. Disord.* **5**, 203–13.

Evans, D. (1990). Estimated prevalence of Alzheimer's disease in the United States. *Milbank Q* **68**, 267–89.

Hay, J. W. & Ernst, R. L. (1987). The economic costs of Alzheimer's disease. *Am. J. Public Health* **77**, 1169–75.

Hoehn, M. M. & Yahr, M. D. (1967). Parkinsonism: onset, progression and mortality. *Neurology* **17**, 427–42.

Hu, T., Huang, L. & Cartwright, W. (1986). Evaluation of the costs of caring for the senile demented elderly: a pilot study. *Gerontologist* **26**, 158–63.

Huang, L., Cartwright, W. & Hu, T. (1988). The economic cost of senile dementia in the United States, 1985. *Public Health Rep.* **103**, 3–7.

Jenkinson, C., Peto, V., Fitzpatrick, R., Greenhall, R. & Hyman, N. (1995). Self-reported functioning and well-being in patients with Parkinson's disease; comparison of the short-form health survey (SF-36) and the Parkinson's Disease Questionnaire (PDQ-39). *Age Ageing* **24**, 505–9.

Kraus, P. H., Klotz, P., Steinberg, R. & Przuntek, H. (1990). Contribution of motor performance tests to the early diagnosis of Parkinson's disease. In *Early Markers in Parkinson's and Alzheimer's Diseases*. Ed. P. Doskert, P. Reiderer, S. Benedetti, R. Roncucci, pp. 41–49. Vienna: Springer-Verlag.

Kurlan, R., Clark, S., Shoulson, I., Penney, J. B. & the Parkinson Study Group (1988). Economic impact of protective therapy for early Parkinson's disease. *Ann. Neurol.* **24**, 153.

Lader, M. & Richens, A. (eds.) (1981). In *Central Nervous System*, pp. 1–164. London & Basingstoke: Macmillan.

Marttila, R. J. (1992). Epidemiology. In *Handbook of Parkinson's Disease*, ed. W. C. Koller, pp. 35–58. New York: Marcel Dekker.

May, W. (1993). The economic impact of Alzheimer's disease. *Neurology* **43** (Suppl. 4), S6–10.

National Foundation for Brain Research (1992). *The Cost of Disorders of the Brain*, vol. 2. National Foundation for Brain Research.

Parkinson Study Group (1989*a*). Effect of deprenyl on the progression of disability in early Parkinson disease. *N. Engl. J. Med.* **321**, 1364–71.

Parkinson Study Group (1989). DATATOP: a multicenter controlled clinical trial in early Parkinson's disease. *Arch. Neurol.* **46**, 1052–60.

Pate, B. D., Kawamata, T., Yamada, T., McGeer, E. F., Hewitt, K. A., Snow, B. J., Ruth, T. J. & Calne, D. B. (1993). Correlation of striatal fluorodopa uptake in MPTP monkey with dopaminergic indices. *Ann. Neurol.* **34**, 331–8.

Rice, D. P., Fox, P., Hauck, W. *et al.* (1991). The burden of caring for Alzheimer's disease patients. National Center for Health Statistics. Proceedings of the 1991 Public Health Conference on Records and Statistics, pp. 119–24. Washington, DC: US Department of Health and Human Services.

Sawle, G., Bloomfield, P. M., Bjorklund, A., Brooks, D. J., Brundin, P., Leenders, K. L., Lindvall, O., Marsden, C. D., Rehncrona, S., Widner, H. & Frackowiak, S. J. (1992). Transplantation of fetal dopamine neurons in Parkinson's disease: positron emission tomography [^{18}F]-6-fluorodopa studies in two patients with putaminal implants. *Ann. Neurol.* **31**, 166–73.

Schwab, R. S. & England, A. C. Jr (1969). Projection technique for evaluating surgery in Parkinson's disease. In *Third Symposium on Parkinson's Disease*, ed. F. J. Gillingham & I. M. L. Donaldson, pp. 152–5. Edinburgh: E. & S. Livingstone.

Singer, E. (1973). Social costs of Parkinson's disease. *J. Chron. Dis.* **26**, 243–54.

Snow, B. J., Schulzer, M., Martin, W. R. W., Tsui, J. K. & Calne, D. B. (1991). PET studies on the relationship between dopaminergic deficit and motor performance in Parkinson's disease. *Neurology* **41** (Suppl. 1), 359.

Teravainen, H. T. & Calne, D. B. (1980). Quantitative assessment of parkinsonian deficits. In *Parkinson's Disease: Current Progress, Problems and Management*, ed. U. K. Rinne, M. Klinger & G. Stamm, pp. 145–64. Amsterdam: Elsevier/North-Holland.

Vingerhoets, F. J. G., Snow, B. J., Langston, J. W., Tetrud, J. M., Schulzer, M. & Calne, D. B. (1993). Evolution of subclinical dopaminergic lesions in MPTP-exposed humans. *Neurology* **43**, A389.

Vingerhoets, J., Schulzer, M., Calne, D. B. & Snow, B. J. (1997). Which clinical sign of Parkinson's disease best reflects the nigrostriatal lesion? *Neurology* **41**, 58–64.

Ward, C. D., Sanes, J. N., Dambrosia, J. M. & Calne, D. B. (1983). Methods for evaluating treatment in Parkinson disease. *Adv. Neurol.* **37**, 1–7.

Widner, H., Tetrud, J. W., Rehncrona, S., Snow, B. J., Brundin, P., Gustavii, B., Bjorklund, A., Lindvall, O. & Langston, J. W. (1992). Bilateral fetal mesencephalic grafting in two patients with MPTP-induced parkinsonism. *N. Engl. J. Med.* **327**, 1556–63.

17 Neuromuscular disease

W. J. K. CUMMING

The outcome of interventional therapy in the field of neuromuscular disease has to be set against the natural history of the underlying condition.

For many, if not most, of neuromuscular disorders, such information is either scanty or just beginning to emerge. The majority of neuromuscular disorders have in the past been considered untreatable and attention has been paid more to management than to interventional therapy. Such therapies have applied mainly to the areas of inflammatory myopathy and myasthenia gravis. However, in these disorders, where treatment has been available for a very considerable time, there is no consensus as to which treatment modality is most appropriate.

The neuromuscular disorders considered in this chapter are those which are encountered frequently, i.e. anterior horn cell disease, diseases of the myoneural junction, inflammatory myopathy, Xp21 deletional myopathies, myotonic dystrophy, congenital myopathies and the metabolic myopathies (Table 17.1). Within the latter only those in which therapeutic intervention has been shown to be of benefit will be considered since in many of them, particularly the mitochondrial disorders, the natural history is as yet poorly understood.

Motor neurone disease (amyotrophic lateral sclerosis)

The term motor neurone disease (MND) is often used interchangeably with amyotrophic lateral sclerosis (ALS). However, ALS is one subdivision of MND, which also encompasses progressive bulbar palsy (PBP), progressive muscular atrophy (PMA) and primary lateral sclerosis (PLS).

ALS, the combination of upper and lower motor neurone signs and symptoms with the development of bulbar symptomatology, is the most common of these conditions. PBP, with patients presenting initially with difficulty in speech and swallowing and then progressing to generalized involvement, is the next most common. PMA, where the initial signs are in lower motor neurones only, is relatively uncommon, and PLS, the presence of upper motor neurone involvement alone, is rare (80% ALS, 10% PBP, 7% PMA and 2% PLS: Caroscio *et al.* 1987; Norris *et al.* 1993).

Patients with PBP and ALS appear to have a similar prognosis, although the disease is

Table 17.1. *Studies on the natural history and therapy of neuromuscular diseases*

Disorder	Natural history	Therapy
Motor neurone disease	Norris *et al.* (1993), Rinsel *et al.* (1993)	Brooks *et al.* (1991)
Myoneural junction disorders		
Myasthenia gravis	Engel (1992), Grob *et al.* (1981)	Evoli *et al.* (1988, 1992), Fonseca & Havard (1990)
Myasthenic syndrome (LEMS)	O'Neill *et al.* (1988)	Bird (1992)
Inflammatory myopathy Polymyositis/		
dermatomyositis	Banker & Engel (1986)	Cumming (1989), Dalakas (1989)
Inclusion body myositis	Chou (1993)	Mastaglia *et al.* (1993), Leff *et al.* (1993)
Dystrophinopathies		
Duchenne dystrophy	Emery (1993), Gardner-Medwin (1977)	Bach *et al.* (1987)
Becker dystrophy	Emery (1993)	Kakulas (1990)
Myotonic dystrophy	Harper (1989)	Harper (1989)
Metabolic disorders	DiMauro *et al.* (1992)	Slonim & Goans (1985)

somewhat more benign in those who present with PMA and PLS. However, given that the onset of symptoms only occurs when there has been approximately 80% loss of motor neurones (Brookes *et al.* 1991), the disease is always well established by the time of presentation, when the patient will for the first time become aware of functional weakness. Trials of treatment are therefore only addressing the final stages of the disease. Future trials should conform to the criteria recently established (Brooks *et al.* 1991).

The incidence of MND is 1–2 per 100 000, with a prevalence of 5–7 per 100 000 (Annegers *et al.* 1991*a*; Chancellor & Warlow 1992). The disease is twice as common in men as in women and has a mean age of onset in the mid-fifties. In the cohort of patients studied by Appel (Appel *et al.* 1987), speech impairment was the initial manifestation of ALS in 21% of patients and weakness of the extremities in 66%. Of the patients presenting with limb weakness 44% had weakness or fatiguability of the right extremity, 36% of the left extremity and 20% in both extremities at the onset. Some 12% of patients had sensory complaints, of pain or paraesthesiae, at the onset. The subsequent course of this group of patients was characteristically weakness starting in the right lower extremity and then involving the left lower extremity. When the onset was in the upper limb the next area of involvement in most patients was the contralateral upper limb. If the presentation was bulbar, the next area of involvement was the upper limb.

Sequential studies of muscle strength in large groups of patients (Appel *et al.* 1987; Brooks *et al.* 1991; Munsat *et al.* 1991; Ringel *et al.* 1993) have shown that loss of function is linear with time.

There appear to be different rates of progression defined by Appel *et al.* as slow, intermediate and rapid. Some 20% of their patients progressed relatively slowly, 77% at an intermediate rate and 3–4% rapidly. This variation in rate of progression has been confirmed by others (Annegers *et al.* 1991*b*; Chio *et al.* 1993). There is some suggestion that patients who present with PBP progress more quickly than patients presenting initially with limb weakness, leading to death within $1\frac{1}{2}$–2 years in about two-thirds of all patients with this type of presentation.

Some 20–30% of patients presenting with ALS succumb within 2 years of the onset of symptoms and 20% survive for 5–6 years. No form of interventional therapy has changed the course of disease progression in MND (Roufs 1991; Askmark *et al.* 1993; Eisen *et al.* 1993; Smith *et al.* 1993; Westarp *et al.* 1993), until the advent of riluzole (Lacomblez *et al.* 1996).

In patients presenting with PBP the use of enteral feeding techniques has improved the quality of life, but has made no difference to the underlying course of the disorder. Attempts at treatment with thyrotrophin releasing hormone (TRH) have, despite initial enthusiasm, been shown to be of no benefit to patients (Brooke 1989; Eckland *et al.* 1990; Munsat *et al.* 1992). The use of long-term ventilation is a major ethical issue than rather a therapy in this condition (Hayashi & Kato, 1989; Howard *et al.* 1989; Gay *et al.* 1991; Hayashi *et al.* 1991; Silverstein *et al.* 1991).

The recent identification of immune and excitatory amino acid disturbances in MND (Drachman Kuncl 1989; Appel 1993; Appel *et al.* 1993) has provided the basis for more rational therapy. A dose-ranging study of riluzole, an anti-glutamate, anti-excitotoxic medication in 959 patients with El Escorial definite or probable ALS of less than 5 years' duration showed benefit in increasing longevity. At the end of the study, after a median follow-up of 18 months 50% of placebo-treated and 57% of riluzole-treated patients (100 mg ribizole/day) were alive without tracheostomy (the primary end-joint). Functional strength scales, however, showed no difference in the two groups, a result that could be due to poor sensitivity in these secondary outcome and measures. This study (Lacomblez *et al.* 1996) confirmed the result of an earlier, smaller study of riluzole in ALS (Bensimon *et al.* 1994) but failed to confirm relative benefit to those with bulbar-onset ALS suggested in the earlier study.

Other drugs, including gabapentin, ciliary neurotrophic factor (CNTF) and *L*-cysteine have proved ineffective in clinical trials. Other neurotrophic factors, such as BDNF, IgF-1 and GDNF are undergoing evaluation. A trial of intravenous immune globulin showed no benefit in any subgroup of patients (Saad *et al.* 1994).

Myoneural junction disorders

Myasthenia gravis

Myasthenia is a model of an autoimmune disorder in which the target organ, the motor end plate of the skeletal muscle fibres, is rendered abnormal by complement-mediated lysis triggered by specific autoantibodies against the acetylcholine receptor (Engel 1992; Nakano & Engel 1993). The result is fatiguable weakness of muscles characteristically in the younger age group (under 45 years), presenting initially as ocular involvement, then oropharyngeal involvement, then limb involvement and at any stage the supervention of respiratory involvement. In the older age group (45 + years) the clinical presentation is more varied and often limb presentation precedes oropharyngeal or ocular involvement (Grobb 1983).

In the younger age group females are more commonly affected than males, whereas in the older age group males are more commonly affected. Each group showed differences in HLA correlates (Carlsson *et al.* 1990).

The disease may remain confined to the eye muscles (ocular myasthenia gravis). If the disease remains ocular for a period of 2 years, only some 10% of patients will progress to generalized myasthenia (Oosterhuis 1989).

Studies of untreated myasthenia, where the diagnosis was achieved with precision, are relatively few (Rowland *et al.* 1956; Simpson & Thomaides 1987). It would appear that in those patients who are destined to develop generalized myasthenia gravis the disease will reach its maximum severity over a period of 3–5 years. Spontaneous remission rates in early studies remain around 12%. There is, however, a general consensus that intervention in terms of thymectomy (Lanska 1990) and/or immunosuppressive therapy (Fonseca & Havard 1990; Evoli *et al.* 1992; Shah & Lisak 1993) leads to a better outcome of the disease than for those in whom no therapy was ever undertaken (Grob *et al.* 1981, 1987; Valli *et al.* 1987; Beghi *et al.* 1991; Engel 1992). Most studies would suggest that some 65–85% of treated patients will remit or substantially improve (Rowland 1987).

It has been noted that assessing the effects of individual therapies is difficult in myasthenia gravis because of the paucity of prospective controlled trials (Martin & Ringel 1992). Most retrospective studies have suffered from the common limitations of being poorly controlled, with patients receiving multiple therapies. There is little doubt that the improvement in managing patients with respiratory failure, as a consequence of their myasthenia, has had a dramatic impact on outcome.

Anticholinesterase as a medication will improve the symptoms in the majority of patients. However, this is symptomatic therapy only and makes no attempt to control the underlying mechanism of the disease.

Thymectomy has now become standard therapy in most centres, being performed earlier rather than later (Scadding *et al.* 1985; Evoli *et al.* 1988; Durelli *et al.* 1991; Nussbaum *et al.* 1992; Blossom *et al.* 1993). Olanow and colleagues (1982, 1987) demonstrated that early thymectomy, following symptom reduction to Osserman grade 0 or 1 with plasmapheresis, led to 80% of patients having an excellent response at 3 years, with 55% off all medication, and 38% never requiring medical therapy. Long-term follow-up in that group of patients (A. Roses, personal communication 1994) confirms the original figures.

Steroid therapy will also reduce the symptoms or induce remission in some 80% of patients (Johns 1987; Scherpbier & Oosterhuis 1987; Miano *et al.* 1991; Evoli *et al.* 1992). There appears to be no difference in clinical response rate amongst those patients who did or did not have a thymectomy associated with steroid therapy.

Pretreatment with plasmapheresis (Seybold 1987; Cumming & Hudgson 1986; Cumming 1992), which induces short-term improvement lasting some 3–6 weeks in most patients, followed by thymectomy, would seem to produce comparable remission rates to that seen with corticosteroids (Tindall *et al.* 1987, 1993). This approach would appear to have the advantage in therapy in that it is not associated with the long-term side effects of steroid therapy.

Immunoglobulin therapy has been increasingly used in the treatment of myasthenia and appears to have its maximal role in the relief of residual symptoms following thymectomy (Liblau *et al.* 1991; Ferrero *et al.* 1993). Azathioprine has proved of value in the management of ocular disease and in refractory generalized disease (Hohfeld *et al.* 1988; Fonseca & Havard 1990; Kuks *et al.* 1991; Wilensky *et al.* 1993).

Transient neonatal myasthenia occurs in some 10–15% of infants born to mothers who have myasthenia gravis irrespective of the state of activity of the mother's disease (Morel *et al.* 1988). These children present with poor respiratory effort and poor sucking; they respond to short-term treatment with anticholinesterases.

Lambert–Eaton myasthenic syndrome

Patients with Lambert–Eaton myasthenic syndrome (LEMS) characteristically present with fatiguability and/or weakness in the lower limb girdle musculature which appears to improve rather than worsen with persistent activity. Involvement of the ocular and bulbar musculature is infrequent and mild when it does occur. There are also features of autonomic dysfunction including dry mouth, impotence and abnormal sweating. Although initially thought to be uniquely associated with underlying small cell carcinoma of the lung, the incidence of non-small cell carcinoma LEMS is steadily increasing and most studies would now suggest that 50% of patients would have carcinoma-associated disease (O'Neill *et al.* 1988).

If such a carcinoma is present, then treatment is directed to the underlying condition. However, there is evidence that significant improvement may be brought about by using 3,4-diaminopyridine, steroids, plasmapheresis and intravenous immunoglobulin (Bird 1992; Sanders *et al.* 1993).

Inflammatory myopathies

The inflammatory myopathies may be either infective or non-infective in aetiology. The infective myositides constitute a major management problem in Third World countries, particularly where pyrogenic myositis is a frequent complication of pre-existing bowel or parasitic infection of skeletal musculature (Gambhir *et al.* 1992; Fam *et al.* 1993). Similar findings are now occurring increasingly in patients who are immunocompromised, particularly those who are HIV-positive (Nitta & Kuritzkes 1991; Christin & Sarosi 1992).

Viral myositis is the commonest form of inflammatory muscle disease in the developed world but does not contribute a major management problem since the vast majority of cases are self-limiting, complete functional recovery being the rule rather than the exception (Naylor *et al.* 1987).

The non-infective inflammatory myopathies constitute polymyositis (PM), dermatomyositis (DM) and inclusion body myositis (IBM). These are the commonest primary muscle disorders seen in clinical practice in either children or adults. They form a group of disorders that are amenable to therapy and which have a potentially satisfactory outcome (Mader & Keystone 1993).

Patients with PM or DM usually present with a slowly progressive painful limb girdle syndrome with, in the DM type, a heliotrope rash around the eyes, the malar region and extensor aspects of the limbs (Banker & Engel 1986; Bohan 1988; Byrne & Dennett 1993).

In childhood, the commonest condition seen is DM (Banker & Victor 1966). Both PM and DM are seen in association with neoplastic disorders (Callan 1984, 1991; Haftel *et al.* 1992).

In PM, pathologically there are inflammatory infiltrates with predominant endomysial scattered necrosis; immunologically the disease is mediated by T-cells (CD8[+]) and there is expression of MHC class 1 antigens. In DM, the pathological findings are inflammatory infiltrate which is predominantly perifascicular, and necrosis that tends to be grouped, with single necrotic cells scattered throughout the biopsy. There is perfascicular atrophy and microvascular changes are common in the childhood form of the disease. CD4[+] cells are common, CD8[+] cells are rare. B-cells (CD22) are common and MAC antigens are expressed (Targoff & Reichlin 1988; Targoff 1989; Karpati & Carpenter 1993).

The serum creatine kinase level is elevated in the majority of cases and electromyography demonstrates short-duration, small-amplitude polyphasic motor potentials in some 90% of patients, fibrillation potentials and positive sharp waves in about 75% of patients and complex repetitive discharges in about 33% of patients (Bertorini 1988).

About a quarter of all patients seen with PM/DM have an underlying definable connective tissue disorder, usually systemic lupus erythematosus, progressive systemic sclerosis, Sjogren's syndrome, rheumatoid arthritis or mixed connective tissue disease (Rosenberg *et al.* 1988).

Symptomatic cardiac involvement is relatively uncommon (Henderson *et al.* 1981), but cardiac assessment will reveal evidence of subclinical disease in some two-thirds or more of patients. Involvement ranges from cardiac conduction defects to cardiomyopathy (Askari 1984).

Pulmonary function testing will reveal evidence of diaphragmatic and intercostal muscle weakness in about a third of patients (symptomatic in about 10% of patients); presence of anti-Jol antibody is a marker for symptomatic lung involvement.

In childhood DM unique complications occur including subcutaneous calcifications (calcinosis) and gastrointestinal haemorrhage. Calcinosis occurs in between 20% and 50% of children and is refractory to therapy (Ostrov *et al.* 1991).

In untreated DM or PM the clinical course is that of progressive deterioration, with a mortality of up to 50% (Hudgson & Walton 1979).

Although there has never been a controlled trial of immunosuppressive therapy (commonly with prednisolone and azathioprine) in PM/DM, it has been accepted therapy since the concept was first introduced by Walton & Adams (1958). Numerous series have reported varying success rates with such therapy, although it has been accepted that between 10% and 30% of patients will remain refractory to high-dose steroids taken over a long period of time (Bunch *et al.* 1980; Bunch 1981, 1990; Hudgson 1984).

Recent advances in immunopathology suggest that the response to corticosteroids may be influenced by the expression of MHC antigens on the muscle cell membrane (McDouall *et al.* 1989). However, this research is in its infancy and requires large-scale (probably multinational) studies before its validity can be established.

It is currently recommended that prednisolone 1.5 mg/kg body weight is instituted as first line of therapy once the diagnosis has been established (Mastaglia & Ojeda 1985*a, b*; Mastaglia & Walton 1992; Mastaglia *et al.* 1993). Some groups would use azathioprine (2.5–3 mg/kg body weight per day, up to a maximum 150 mg per day) in combination with prednisolone from the introduction of therapy in view of the evidence that it decreases the duration of steroid therapy in the long term (Cumming 1989).

This dose of steroid is maintained for 6–8 weeks until a clinical response (depending on return of muscle strength, not laboratory values) is shown and then the dose is 'tailed', aiming to have the patient on between 5 and 10 mg prednisolone on alternate days at 12 months, the total duration of therapy being up to 3 years (Dalakas 1988, 1989, 1992*a, b*; Cumming 1989; Lane *et al.* 1989; Henriksson & Lindvall 1990; Joffe *et al.* 1993). On such a regime over two-thirds of patients will show a response to the point where they do not require walking aids (Cumming 1989; Koh *et al.* 1993).

In the patient resistant to the regime described above, other treatments may prove effective, including methotrexate (Miller *et al.* 1992*d*), cyclophosphamide (Al-Janadi *et al.* 1989), cyclosporin A (Danko & Szegedi 1991) total-body irradiation (Kelly *et al.* 1988), total lymphoid irradiation, thymectomy, plasma exchange (Dau 1992; Herson *et al.* 1992; Miller *et al.* 1992*a,c*) and, more recently, intravenous immunoglobulin (Bodemer *et al.* 1990; Cherin *et al.* 1990, 1991*a,b*; Lang *et al.* 1991; Barron *et al.* 1992; Jann *et al.* 1992) although there has been only one controlled study (Dalakas *et al.* 1993).

In patients with malignancy-associated PM/DM the prognosis is that of the underlying malignancy irrespective of treatment.

There are some suggestions that an acute fulminant course (Venables *et al.* 1982), dysphagia, symptomatic cardiac involvement (Bahn *et al.* 1990), pulmonary infiltration (Arsura & Greenberg 1988) and black race are all associated with a poor prognosis (Rosenberg & Ringel 1988).

Inclusion body myositis

IBM was first described by Chou in 1967 (Chou 1993), when it was characterized by a slowly progressive inflammatory myopathy, seen much more commonly in the older age group (greater than 55 years) and in males rather than females. The lower limbs tend to be affected more than the upper limbs. Pathologically the condition is characterized by basophilic rimmed vacuoles in muscle fibres, which are seen on electron microscopy to be filamentous, and eosinophilic cytoplasmic areas.

It has become increasingly recognized that patients who 'fail' on treatment for previously presumed idiopathic PM/DM may have, on repeat muscle biopsy, evidence of IBM. The inclusions in this condition contain amyloid (Albrecht & Bilbao 1993; Askanas *et al.* 1993; Leclerc *et al.* 1993) and apolipoprotein (Askanas *et al.* 1994).

It would appear that inclusion body myositis is relatively refractory to therapy (Wortmann 1992; Leff *et al.* 1993). However, it has been suggested that a trial of immunosuppressive therapy with steroids and azathioprine should be embarked upon in all patients (Mastaglia *et al.* 1993). If there is no evidence of improvement at 3 months, then therapy should be abandoned. A controlled trial of intravenous immunoglobulin in IBM suggested possible benefit (Salvarani *et al.* 1993; Soueidan & Dalakas 1993).

Xp21 deletional myopathies (dystrophinopathies)

The Duchenne and Becker muscular dystrophy syndromes were formerly delineated on the rather arbitrary basis that if a boy lost the ability to walk before the age of 15 years he had Duchenne dystrophy and one who was still walking at that age had Becker dystrophy (Emery 1993). The distinction is now much more scientifically based in that it has been shown that in Duchenne dystrophy, dystrophin, the protein product of the Xp21 gene, is absent at the muscle membrane, whereas in Becker dystrophy, dystrophin is reduced or shows patchy distribution and immunoblot analysis reveals dystrophin of abnormal size and/or quantity (Anderson & Kunkel 1992). Dystrophin is a subsarcolemmal protein which, in association with a complex of other sarcolemmal proteins, the dystrophin–glycoprotein complex (DCG), provides a linkage to the extracellular matrix component, laminin. In Duchenne dystrophy the lack of dystrophin is associated with absence of, or marked reduction in, the various components of the glycoprotein complex (Matsumura & Campbell 1994).

This molecular analysis has made little practical difference to patients with Duchenne dystrophy (Dubowitz 1989), the majority of boys having, since the original description of the disease, followed a relatively typical clinical course (Emery 1993). However, the changes in the area of Becker dystrophy are much more striking (see below).

Despite these advances in molecular analysis, as yet no clear genotype/phenotype correlations can be drawn (Comi *et al.* 1994, Ballo *et al.* 1994; Angelini *et al.* 1994; Hoffman 1993; Nicholson *et al.* 1993*a–c*; Cumming 1994).

Duchenne dystrophy

Unless born to a family where the disease has already been manifest, in which case the earliest signs of delay in crawling and walking will be recognized, the usual age of presentation for a boy with Duchenne dystrophy is between the ages of 3 and 5 years. Boys are usually then seen because they fail to keep up with their peer group in physical activities. At that time the family will usually give a history of delay in learning to walk. In 50% of boys this is delayed until 18 months of age and some 25% do not walk until they are beyond their second year (Schmalbruch 1992; Emery 1993)

At that stage muscle weakness is often more pronounced in the lower than the upper limbs and affects the proximal more than the distal muscles. Hypertrophy of calf muscles is an early feature; muscles are often said to feel firm or woody. The gait is abnormal and the boys employ the so-called Gowers' manoeuvre when rising from the floor (Wallace & Newton 1989; Emery 1993).

Although there is a variation in the loss of functional ability (Allsop & Ziter 1981), there is evidence from Brooke et al. (1989) that the individual muscles continue to decline in strength at a fairly uniform rate of 0.4 units/year on a 0–10 scale. Some children will, however, appear to improve their functional ability even when they are clearly shown to be losing muscle strength, and these periods of apparent arrest underline the need to assess the efficacy of any suggested treatment with considerable care.

Eventually all boys will require a wheelchair for mobility and in 95% of cases this will occur by the age of 12 years. Although not significantly correlated with the age of onset of the disease, the age of going into a wheelchair remains correlated with the age of death: the age of death after 15 years increases roughly by 1 year for each year that the boy remained ambulant after the age of 7 years (Emery 1993). In general terms, the earlier a boy becomes wheelchair-confined, the poorer the prognosis.

In the later stages of the disease contractures develop, particularly flexion of elbows, knees and hips and, unless there is intervention, scoliosis.

There is an independent loss of ventilatory function which is compounded by scoliosis, so that ventilatory function progressively declines (Cooper et al. 1988). There is developing cardiac abnormality which is masked by immobility (Nigro et al. 1990). Death usually occurs in the early twenties (Riggs 1990; Patterson et al. 1991).

It is understandable that with such a progressive disease, attempts at therapeutic intervention with a long list of compounds have been attempted (Kakulas 1990), including vitamin E, growth hormone, calcium antagonists (Moxley et al. 1987; Backman et al. 1988; Bertorini et al.1988, 1991; Coakley et al. 1988; Heckmatt et al. 1988; Merlini et al. 1988; Griggs et al. 1990; Scott et al. 1990; Sugita 1991; Zupan 1992) and most recently corticosteroids (DeSilva et al. 1987; Angelini et al. 1991; Dubowitz 1991; Fenichel et al. 1991; Griggs et al. 1991; Mesa et al. 1991).

The American Cooperative Study (Griggs et al. 1993) suggested that prednisolone may delay weakness and it is now suggested that corticosteroids are given to boys with Duchenne dystrophy. It has to be pointed out, however, that the original study of steroids ran for a little over 2 years and the 3 and 4 year figures are just becoming available. It would not be the author's practice to start a 4- or 5-year old boy on prednisolone with the expectation of continuing that therapy until the age of death (around 20 years), and the status of therapy with prednisolone must be further evaluated in the long term (Khan 1993).

The aim of therapy (Gardner-Medwin 1977) is to prolong walking and thence wheelchair life, which it was thought would delay the onset of scoliosis and subsequent ventilatory dysfunction. Recent studies have produced conflicting results in terms of overall benefit to ventilatory function (Colbert & Craig 1987; Miller *et al.* 1992*b*; Shapiro *et al.* 1992). The protagonists of the Luqúe's procedure have not been able to confirm initial high expectations that this procedure delays the onset of respiratory insufficiency (Heckmatt *et al.* 1990; Galasko *et al.* 1992). The use of assisted ventilation, whether started at the first hint of a decrease in vital capacity or delayed until the onset of hypercapnia, raises more ethical problems than it provides answers (Baydur *et al.* 1990; Mohr & Hill 1990; Fukunaga *et al.* 1993), and the management of the terminal respiratory event in all boys with Duchenne dystrophy must be one for discussion between the family and the physician (Curran & Colbert 1989; Gilgoff *et al.* 1989; Miller *et al.* 1990; Hill *et al.* 1992). It is usual practice to treat respiratory infections aggressively provided there is no significant hypercapnia or hypoxaemia between infections (Bach *et al.* 1987; Hilton *et al.* 1993).

The advent of molecular techniques has led to novel therapies for Duchenne dystrophy (Engel 1993), particularly myoblast transfer (Karpati *et al.* 1989; Partridge *et al.* 1989; Morgan *et al.* 1990; Partridge 1991; Houzelstein *et al.* 1992). The concept of this therapy is to introduce sufficient dystrophin molecules into affected muscle by transplanting normal muscle cells from either a related or an unrelated donor. Despite enthusiasm in some quarters (Law *et al.* 1990, 1991), the results of formal trials have revealed that this therapy is not beneficial (Kurland & Molgaard 1982; Dubowitz 1992).

At present the concept of introducing a dystrophin 'mini gene' (Morandi *et al.* 1993) into the muscle fibres by viral methods is feasible in animal models (Dunckley *et al.* 1992), but as yet no clinical trials have been undertaken (Acsadi *et al.* 1991; Lee *et al.* 1991; Wells *et al.* 1992; Dunckley *et al.*1993; Ragot *et al.* 1993; Vincent *et al.* 1993). For these therapies to be effective, not only must dystrophin be reintroduced into the muscle fibre, but also the glycoprotein complex would have to be recreated (absence of one of the glycoprotein components, 50DAG, is associated with severe autosomal recessive muscular dystrophy (Matsumura *et al.* 1992) which clinically mimicks Duchenne dystrophy) and there is as yet no proof that this is possible (Higuchi *et al.* 1993).

Becker muscular dystrophy

The realization that Becker dystrophy presents not only as a limb girdle myopathy but may also manifest only as cardiomyopathy, muscle pain and cramps on exercise (Gospe *et al.* 1989), unilateral muscle hypertrophy without weakness, or hyperckaemia

(Servidei *et al.* 1993) has greatly broadened the spectrum of the clinical phenotype of the genotypic expression of partial dystrophin deletion (Hoffman 1993).

The management for the 'typical' case of Becker dystrophy in which ambulation is prolonged until after the teens and hence there is little or no risk of scoliosis, is somewhat different to that of Duchenne dystrophy in that prolonged survival, albeit in a wheelchair, is well recognized. However, the cardiac effects of dystrophinopathy become of increasing importance in long-term survivors in Becker dystrophy and the need for cardiac transplantation, on the basis of advancing cardiomyopathy, is becoming increasingly recognized (Casazza *et al.* 1988; De *et al.* 1992; Quinlivan & Dubowitz 1992; Steare *et al.* 1992). It has to be stressed that the mode of death in many patients with Becker dystrophy is cardiac and that transplantation is therefore an effective method of prolonging survival.

In the 'atypical' presentations of Becker dystrophy the importance of genetic counselling cannot be over-stressed (Laing 1993).

Myotonic dystrophy

Myotonic dystrophy is the commonest dystrophy in the general population, with a prevalence of 5 in 100 000 (Harper 1989).

It is now recognized that myotonic dystrophy is a multi-system disorder, with marked clinical variability (Bouchard 1989), the neuromuscular manifestations of which (distal muscle weakness and myotonia; facial, temporalis and sternomastoid wasting) are only one of the important features of the disease. Anticipation, in which symptom severity increases and age of onset decreases in each generation, is not uncommon in myotonic dystrophy. The mutation underlying myotonic dystrophy is an expansion of a CTG repeat in the 3' untranslated region of a predicted cAMP-dependent protein kinase gene on chrosome 19q13.3 (Carey *et al.* 1994).

Involvement of the heart is seen in well over 90% of patients at some stage of the illness. Progressive conduction defects and cardiac arrhythmias are seen in some 50% of patients, and form one of the commonest causes of sudden death in the condition (Fragola *et al.* 1991; Graf & Podczeck 1992; Badano *et al.* 1993). Involvement of the oropharyngeal musculature leads to progressive dysphagia with subsequent 'overflow' into the respiratory tract, with attendant complications (Bhutani 1993).

Pulmonary hypoventilation from respiratory muscle weakness and an impaired central ventilatory response leads to sleep disturbance, particularly sleep apnoea (Cirignotta *et al.* 1987). Disturbance of gut motility leads to gastric dilatation and particularly to the development of gall stones. Cataracts are common (Reardon *et al.* 1993). Gonadal involvement in the female leads to subfertility and frequent spontaneous abortions (Marinkovic *et al.* 1990). In those females affected by the disorder who do carry to term, polyhydramnios is common.

There is no evidence that any form of drug therapy will improve the long-term outlook in myotonic dystrophy. Some drugs, such as phenytoin, clomipramine and nifedipine (Grant *et al.* 1987; Antonini *et al.* 1990), may reduce myotonia; however, many patients are so accustomed to their myotonia that any attempt to relieve it is resented. Attention to detail with respect to cardiac arrhythmias will improve the quality of life. Similarly, attention to cataracts (with early lens implantation), cholelithiasis and swallowing difficulties markedly improves the quality of life.

Metabolic myopathies

Disorders of glycogen, lipid and mitochondrial function all lead to disorder of neuromuscular function which presents either as a progressive proximal myopathy or as attacks of muscle pain on exercise, with or without the subsequent development of muscle weakness.

From the disorders of metabolism thus far identified, only in two – that is lipid myopathy due to carnitine deficiency and McArdle's disease – have rational forms of therapy been identified. In McArdle's disease, Slonim (Slonim & Goans 1985) introduced the concept of modifying the diet to present energy in a form which the muscle cell could metabolize rather than being dependent on glycogen. The so-called Slonim diet has produced considerable relief for patients with McArdle's disease in many instances, and to a lesser extent for patients with other forms of glycogen storage disease.

In children, and to a lesser extent adults, who have evidence of lipid myopathy due to carnitine deficiency, supplemental carnitine leads to improvement in the underlying myopathy in childhood and, in the adult, at least appears to arrest progression of the myopathy (DiMauro *et al.* 1992; Shapiro *et al.* 1993).

References

Acsadi, G. *et al.* (1991). Human dystrophin expression in *mdx* mice after intramuscular injection of DNA constructs. *Nature* **352**, 815 –18.

Albrecht, S. & Bilbao, J. M. (1993). Ubiquitin expression in inclusion body myositis: an immunohistochemical study. *Arch. Pathol. Lab. Med.* **117**, 789–93.

Al-Janadi, M., Smith, C. D. & Karsh, J. (1989). Cyclophosphamide treatment of interstitial pulmonary fibrosis in polymyositis/dermatomyositis. *J. Rheumatol.* **16**, 1592–6.

Allsop, K. G. & Ziter, F. A. (1981). Loss of strength and functional decline in Duchenne's dystrophy. *Arch. Neurol.* **38**, 406–11.

Anderson, M. S. & Kunkel, L. M. (1992). The molecular and biochemical basis of Duchenne muscular dystrophy. *Trends Biochem. Sci.* **17**, 289–92.

Angelini C. *et al.* (1991). A trial with a new steroid in Duchenne muscular dystrophy. In *Muscular Dystrophy Research: From Molecular Diagnosis Toward Therapy*, ed. C. Angelini, G. A. Danieli & D. Fontanari, pp. 173–9. Amsterdam: Elsevier.

Angelini, C. *et al.* (1994). Clinical–molecular correlation in 104 mild X-linked muscular dystrophy patients: characterization of sub-clinical phenotypes. *Neuromusc. Discord.* **4**, 349–58.

Annegers, J. F., Appel, S., Lee, J. R.-J. & Perkins, P. (1991*a*). Incidence and prevalence of amyotrophic lateral sclerosis in Harris County, Texas, 1985–1988. *Arch. Neurol.* **48**, 589–93.

Annegers, J. F., Appel, S. H., Perkins, P. & Lee, J. (1991b). Amyotrophic lateral sclerosis mortality rates in Harris County, Texas. *Adv. Neurol.* **56**, 239–43.

Antonini, G. *et al.* (1990). Effect of clomipramine on myotonia: a placebo-controlled, double-blind, crossover trial. *Neurology* **40**, 1473–4.

Appel, S. H. (1993). Excitotoxic neuronal cell death in amyotrophic lateral sclerosis. *Trends Neurosci* **16**, 3–5.

Appel, S. H., Smith, R. G., Engelhardt, J. I. & Stefani, E. (1993). Evidence for autoimmunity in amyotrophic lateral sclerosis. *J. Neurol. Sci.* **118**, 169–74.

Appel, V., Stewart, S. S., Smith, G. & Appel, S. H. (1987). A rating scale for amyotrophic lateral sclerosis: description and preliminary experience. *Ann. Neurol.* **22**, 320–33.

Arsura, E. L. & Greenberg, A. S. (1988). Adverse impact of interstitial pulmonary fibrosis on prognosis in polymyositis and dermatomyositis. *Semin. Arthritis Rheum.* **18**, 29–37.

Askanas, V., Alvarez, R. B. & Engel, W. K. (1993). Beta-amyloid precursor epitopes in muscle fibers of inclusion body myositis. *Ann. Neurol.* **34**, 551–60.

Askanas, V. *et al.* (1994). Apolipoprotein E immunoreactive deposits in inclusion-body muscle diseases. *Lancet* **343**, 364–5.

Askari, A. D. (1984). Cardiac abnormalities. In *Inflammatory Disorders of Muscle* **10**, ed. B. M. Ansell, pp. 131–49. Philadelphia: W. B. Saunders.

Askmark, H. *et al.* (1993). A pilot trial of dextromethorphan in amyotrophic lateral sclerosis. *J. Neurol. Neurosurg. Psychiatry* **56**, 197–200.

Bach, J. R., O'Brien, J., Krotenberg, R. & Alba, A. S. (1987). Management of end stage respiratory failure in Duchenne muscular dystrophy. *Muscle Nerve* **10**, 177–82.

Backman, E. *et al.* (1988). Selenium and vitamin E treatment of Duchenne muscular dystrophy: no effect on muscle function. *Acta Neurol. Scand.* **78**, 429–35.

Badano, L. *et al.* (1993). Left ventricular myocardial function in myotonic dystrophy. *Am. J. Cardiol.* **71**, 987–91.

Ballo, R., Viljoen, D. & Beighton, P. (1994). Duchenne and Becker muscular dystrophy prevalence in South Africa and molecular findings in 128 persons affected. *S. Afr. Med. J.* **84**, 494–7.

Banker, B. Q. & Engel, A. G. (1986). The polymyositis and dermatomyositis syndromes. In *Myology*, vol. 2, ed. A. G. Engel & B. Q. Banker, pp. 1385–422. New York: McGraw-Hill.

Banker, B. Q. & Victor, M. (1966). Dermatomyositis (systemic angiopathy), of childhood. *Medicine* **45**, 261–89.

Barron, K. S., Sher, M. R. & Silverman, E. D. (1992). Intravenous immunoglobulin therapy: magic or black magic? *J. Rheumatol.* **19**, 94–7.

Baydur, A. *et al.* (1990). Decline in respiratory function and experience with long-term assisted ventilation in advanced Duchenne's muscular dystrophy. *Chest* **97**, 884–9.

Beghi, E. *et al.* (1991). Prognosis of myasthenia gravis: a multicenter follow-up study of 844 patients. *J. Neurol. Sci.* **106**, 213–20.

Bensimon, G., Lacomblez, L., Meininger, V., ALS/Ribizole study group (1994). A controlled trial of ribizole in angiopathic lateral sclerosis. *N. Engl. J. Med.* **330**, 585–91.

Bertorini, T. E. (1988). Electromyography in polymyositis and dermatomyositis (PM/DM). In *Polymyositis and Dermatomyositis*, ed. M. C. Dalakas, pp. 217–34. Boston: Butterworth.

Bertorini, T. E. *et al.* (1988). Effect of chronic treatment with the calcium antagonist diltiazem in Duchenne muscular dystrophy. *Neurology* **38**, 609–13.

Bertorini, T. E. *et al.* (1991). Effect of dantrolene in Duchenne muscular dystrophy. *Muscle Nerve* **14**, 503–7.

Bhan, A., Baithun, S. I., Kopelman, P. & Swash, M. (1990). Fatal myocarditis with acute polymyositis in a young adult. *Postgrad. Med. J.* **66**, 229–31.

Bhutani, M. S. (1993). Dysphagia in myotonic dystrophy. *Am. J. Gastroenterol.* **88**, 974–5.

Bird, S. J. (1992). Clinical and electrophysiologic improvement in Lambert–Eaton syndrome with intravenous immunoglobulin therapy. *Neurology* **42**, 1422–3.

Blossom, G. B. *et al.* (1993). Thymectomy for myasthenia gravis. *Arch. Surg.* **128**, 855–62.

Bodemer, C. *et al.* (1990). Efficacy of intravenous immunoglobulins in sclerodermatomyositis. *Br. J. Dermatol.* **123**, 545–6.

Bohan, A. (1988). Clinical presentation and diagnosis of polymyositis and dermatomyositis. In *Polymyositis and Dermatomyositis*, ed. M. C. Dalakas, pp. 19–36. Boston: Butterworth.

Bouchard, J. P. (1989). Phenotype variability in myotonic dystrophy. *Can. J. Neurol. Sci.* **16**, 93–8.

Brooke, M. H. (1989). A summary of the current position of TRH in ALS therapy. *Ann. N.Y. Acad. Sci.* **553**, 431–61.

Brooke, M. H. *et al.* (1989). Duchenne muscular dystrophy: patterns of clinical progression and effects of supportive therapy. *Neurology* **39**, 475–80.

Brooks, B. R. (1989). Thyrotropin-releasing hormone in ALS. *Ann. N.Y. Acad. Sci.* **553**, 422–30.

Brooks, B. R. *et al.* (1991). Design of clinical therapeutic trials in amyotrophic lateral sclerosis. *Adv. Neurol.* **56**, 521–46.

Bunch, T. W. (1981). Prednisone and azathioprine for polymyositis: long term follow up. *Arthritis Rheum.* **24**, 45–8.

Bunch, T. W. (1990). Polymyositis: a case history approach to the differential diagnosis and treatment. *Mayo Clin. Proc.* **65**, 1480–97.

Bunch, T. W., Worthington, J. W., Combs, J. J., Ilstrup, D. M. & Engel, A. G. (1980). Azathioprine with prednisone for polymyositis: a controlled clinical trial. *Ann. Intern. Med.* **92**, 365–9.

Byrne, E. & Dennett, X. (1993). Idiopathic inflammatory myopathies: clinical aspects. In *Baillière's Clinical Neurology*, vol. 2.3, ed. F. L. Mastaglia, pp. 499–526. London: Baillière Tindall.

Callan, J. P. (1984). Myositis and malignancy. In *Inflammatory Disorders of Muscle*, vol. 10, ed. B. M. Ansell, pp. 117–30. London: W. B. Saunders.

Callen, J. P. (1991). The relationship of dermatomyositis/polymyositis to malignancy. *J. Rheumatol.* **18**, 1645–6.

Carey, N. *et al.* (1994). Meiotic drive at the myotonic dystrophy locus? *Nature Genet.* **6**, 117–18.

Carlsson, B. *et al.* (1990). Different HLA DR-DQ associations in subgroups of idiopathic myasthenia gravis. *Immunogenetics* **31**, 285–90.

Caroscio, J. T., Mulvihill, M. N., Sterling, R. & Abrams, B. (1987). Amyotrophic lateral sclerosis: its natural history. *Neurol. Clin.* **5**, 1–8.

Casazza, F. *et al.* (1988). Cardiac transplantation in Becker muscular dystrophy. *J. Neurol.* **235**, 496–8.

Chancellor, A. M. & Warlow, C. P. (1992). Adult onset motor neuron disease: worldwide mortality, incidence and distribution since 1950. *J. Neurol. Neurosurg. Psychiatry* **55**, 1106–15.

Cherin, P. *et al.* (1990). Intravenous immunoglobulin for polymyositis and dermatomyositis. *Lancet* **336**, 116.

Cherin, P. *et al.* (1991a). Effectiveness of intravenous immunoglobulins in polymyositis and dermatomyositis: an open trial in 15 patients. *Presse Med.* **20**, 244–9.

Cherin, P. *et al.* (1991b). Efficacy of intravenous gammaglobulin therapy in chronic refractory polymyositis and dermatomyositis: an open study with 20 adult patients. *Am. J. Med.* **91**, 162–8.

Chio, A., Magnani, C. & Schiffer, D. (1993). Amyotrophic lateral sclerosis mortality in Italy, 1958 to 1987: a cross-sectional and cohort study. *Neurology* **43**, 927–30.

Chou, S. M. (1993). Inclusion body myositis. In *Baillière's Clinical Neurology*, vol. 2.3, ed. F. L. Mastaglia, pp. 557–77. London: Baillière Tindall.

Christin, L. & Sarosi, G. A. (1992). Pyomyositis in North America: case reports and review. *Clin. Infect. Dis.* **15**, 668–77.

Cirignotta, F. *et al.* (1987). Sleep-related breathing impairment in myotonic dystrophy. *J. Neurol.* **235**, 80–5.

Coakley, J. H. *et al.* (1988). The effect of mazindol on growth hormone secretion in boys with Duchenne muscular dystrophy. *J. Neurol. Neurosurg. Psychiatry* **512**, 1551–7.

Colbert, A. P. & Craig, C. (1987). Scoliosis management in Duchenne muscular dystrophy: prospective study of modified Jewett hyperextension brace. *Arch. Phys. Med. Rehabil.* **68**, 302–4.

Comi, G. P. *et al.* (1994). Clinical variability in Becker muscular dystrophy: genetic, biochemical and immunohistochemical correlates. *Brain* **117**, 1–14.

Cooper, R. G., Stokes, M. J. & Edwards, R. H. T. (1988). Physiological characterisation of the warm up effect of activity in patients with myotonic dystrophy. *J. Neurol. Neurosurg. Psychiatry* **51**, 1134–41.

Cumming, W. J. K. (1989). Steroids in polymyositis. In Steroids in Diseases of the Central Nervous System, ed. R. Capildeo, pp. 247–57. London: Wiley.

Cumming, W. J. K. (1992). Disorders of neuromuscular transmission. In *Textbook of Geriatric Medicine and Gerontology*, 4th edn, ed. J. C. Brocklehurst, R. C. Tallis & H. M. Fillit, pp. 430–2. Edinburgh: Churchill Livingstone.

Cumming, W. J. K. (1994). Clinical diagnosis of the dystrophinopathies. *Muscle Nerve* **17**, S36.

Cumming, W. J. K. & Hudgson, P. (1986). The role of plasmaphoresis in preparing patients with myasthenia for thymectomy. *Muscle Nerve* **9** (Suppl.), 155.

Curran, F. J. & Colbert, A. P. (1989). Ventilation management in Duchenne muscular dystrophy and postpoliomyelitis syndrome: twelve years' experience. *Arch. Phys. Med. Rehabil.* **70**, 180–5.

Dalakas, M. C. (1988). Treatment of polymyositis and dermatomyositis with corticosteroids: a first therapeutic approach. In *Polymyositis and Dermatomyositis*, ed. M. C. Dalakas, pp. 235–53. Boston: Butterworth.

Dalakas, M. (1989). Treatment of polymyositis and dermatomyositis. *Curr. Opin. Rheumatol.* **1**, 443–9.

Dalakas, M. C. (1992*a*). Clinical, immunopathologic, and therapeutic considerations of inflammatory myopathies. *Clin. Neuropharmacol.* **15**, 327–51.

Dalakas, M. C. (1992*b*). Inflammatory myopathies. In *Handbook of Clinical Neurology*, vol. 62, ed. P. J. Vinken, G. W. Bruyn & H. L. Klawans, pp. 369–90. Amsterdam: Elsevier.

Dalakas, M. C. *et al.* (1993). A controlled trial of high-dose intravenous immune globulin infusions as treatment for dermatomyositis. *N. Engl. J. Med.* **329**, 1993–2000.

Danko, K. & Szegedi, G. (1991). Cyclosporin A treatment of dermatomyositis. *Arthritis Rheum.* **34**, 933–4.

Dau, P. C. (1992). Plasma exchange in polymyositis and dermatomyositis. *N. Engl. J. Med.* **327**, 1030.

De, V. M., De, V. W. G. & La, R. G. V. (1992). The heart in Becker muscular dystrophy, facioscapulohumeral dystrophy, and Bethlem myopathy. *Muscle Nerve* **15**, 591–6.

DeSilva, S., Drachman, D. B., Mellits, D. & Kuncl, R. W. (1987). Prednisone treatment in Duchenne muscular dystrophy: long-term benefit. *Arch. Neurol.* **44**, 818–22.

DiMauro, S., Tonin, P. & Servidei, S. (1992). Metabolic myopathies. In *Handbook of Clinical Neurology*, vol. 62, ed. P. J. Vinken, G. W. Bruyn & H. L. Klawans, pp. 479–526. Amsterdam: Elsevier.

Drachman, D. B. & Kuncl, R. W. (1989). Amyotrophic lateral sclerosis: an unconventional autoimmune disease? *Ann. Neurol.* **26**, 269–74.

Dubowitz, V. (1989). The Duchenne dystrophy story: from phenotype to gene and potential treatment. *J. Child Neurol.* **4**, 240–50.

Dubowitz, V. (1991). Prednisone in Duchenne dystrophy. *Neuromuscul. Disord.* **1**, 161–3.

Dubowitz, V. (1992). Transferring myoblasts in Duchenne dystrophy. *BMJ* **305**, 844–5.

Dunckley, M. G. *et al.* (1992). Retroviral-mediated transfer of a dystrophin minigene into *mdx* mouse myoblasts *in vitro*. *FEBS Lett.* **296**, 128–34.

Dunckley, M. G., Wells, D. J., Walsh, F. S. & Dickson, G. (1993). Direct retroviral-mediated transfer of a dystrophin minigene into *mdx* mouse muscle *in vivo*. *Hum. Mol. Genet.* **2**, 717–23.

Durelli, L. *et al.* (1991). Actuarial analysis of the occurrence of remissions following thymectomy for myasthenia gravis in 400 patients. *J. Neurol. Neurosurg. Psychiatry* **54**, 406–11.

Eckland, D. J. A., Modarres-Sadeghi, H., Lightman, S. L. & Guiloff, R. J. (1990). The effects of repeated administration of a long acting TRH analogue (RX77368), on TSH, T4, T3 and prolactin in patients with motor neuron disease. *J. Neurol. Neurosurg. Psychiatry* **53**, 803–4.

Eisen, A., Stewart, H., Schulzer, M. & Cameron, D. (1993). Anti-glutamate therapy in amyotrophic lateral sclerosis: A trial using lamotrigine. *Can. J. Neurol. Sci.* **20**, 297–301.

Emery, A. E. H. (1993). *Duchenne Muscular Dystrophy*. Oxford: Oxford Medical Publications.

Engel, A. G. (1992). Myasthenia gravis and myasthenic syndromes. In *Handbook of Clinical Neurology*, vol. 62, eds. P. J. Vinken, G. W. Bruyn & H. L. Klawans, pp. 391–455. Amsterdam: Elsevier.

Engel, A. G. (1993). Gene therapy for Duchenne dystrophy. *Ann. Neurol.* **34**, 3–4.

Evoli, A. *et al.* (1988). Thymectomy in the treatment of myasthenia gravis: report of 247 patients. *J. Neurol.* **235**, 272–6.

Evoli, A. *et al.* (1992). Long-term results of corticosteroid therapy in patients with myasthenia gravis. *Eur. Neurol.* **32**, 37–43.

Fam, A. G., Rubenstein, J. & Saibil, F. (1993). Pyomyositis: early detection and treatment. *J. Rheumatol.* **20**, 521–4.

Fenichel, G. M. *et al.* (1991). A comparison of daily and alternate-day prednisone therapy in the treatment of Duchenne muscular dystrophy. *Arch. Neurol.* **48**, 575–9.

Ferrero, B. *et al.* (1993). Therapies for exacerbation of myasthenia gravis. The mechanism of action of intravenous high-dose immunoglobulin G. *Ann. N.Y. Acad. Sci.* **681**, 563–6.

Fonseca, V. & Havard, C. W. H. (1990). Long-term treatment of myasthenia gravis with azathioprine. *Postgrad. Med. J.* **66**, 102–5.

Fragola, P. V. *et al.* (1991). The natural course of cardiac conduction disturbances in myotonic dystrophy. *Cardiology* **79**, 93–8.

Fukunaga, H. *et al.* (1993). Long-term follow-up of patients with Duchenne muscular dystrophy receiving ventilatory support. *Muscle Nerve* **16**, 554–8.

Galasko, C. S. B., Delaney, C. & Morris, P. (1992). Spinal stabilisation in Duchenne muscular dystrophy. *J. Bone. Joint. Surg. [Br.].* **74B**, 210–14.

Gambhir, I. S. *et al.* (1992). Tropical pyomyositis in India: A clinico-histopathological study. *J. Trop. Med. Hygiene* **95**, 42–6.

Gardner-Medwin, D. (1977). Objectives in the management of Duchenne muscular dystrophy . *Isr. J. Med. Sci.* **13**, 229–34.

Gay, P. C. *et al.* (1991). Effects of alterations in pulmonary function and sleep variables on survival in patients with amyotrophic lateral sclerosis. *Mayo Clin. Proc.* **66**, 686–94.

Gilgoff, I., Prentice, W. & Baydur, A. (1989). Patient and family participation in the management of respiratory failure in Duchenne's muscular dystrophy. *Chest*, **95**, 519–24.

Gospe, S. M. *et al.* (1989). Familial X-linked myalgia and cramps: a non-progressive myopathy associated with a deletion in the dystrophin gene. *Neurology.* **39**, 1277–80.

Graf, M. & Podczeck, A. (1992). Myotonic heart disease. *Neurology.* **42**, 700.

Grant, R., Sutton, D. L., Behan, P. O. & Ballantyne, J. P. (1987). Nifedipine in the treatment of myotonia in myotonic dystrophy. *JNNP*, **50**, 199–206.

Griggs, R. C. *et al.* (1990). Randomized double blind trial of mazindol in Duchenne dystrophy. *Muscle Nerve* **13**, 1169–73.

Griggs, R. C. *et al.* (1991). Prednisone in Duchenne dystrophy: a randomized, controlled trial defining the time course and dose response. *Arch. Neurol.* **48**, 383–8.

Griggs, R. C. *et al.* (1993). Duchenne dystrophy: Randomized, controlled trial of prednisone (18 months) and azathioprine (12 months). *Neurology.* **43**, 520–7.

Grob, D., Brunner, N. G. & Namba, T. (1981). The natural course of myasthenia gravis and effect of therapeutic measures. *Ann. N.Y. Acad. Sci.* **377**, 652–69.

Grob, D., Arsura, E. L., Brunner, N. G. & Namba, T. (1987). The course of myasthenia gravis and therapies affecting outcome. *Ann. N.Y. Acad. Sci.* **505**, 472–99.

Grob, D. (1983). Clinical manifestations of myasthenia gravis. In *Myasthenia Gravis*, eds. E. X. Albuquerque & A. T. Eldefrawi, pp. 319–45. London: Chapman & Hall.

Haftel, H. M., McCune, W. J. & Sullivan, D. B. (1992). Risk of cancer in dermatomyositis or polymyositis. *N. Engl. J. Med.* **327**, 207–8.

Harper, P. S. (1989). Myotonic dystrophy: the clinical picture. In *Myotonic Dystrophy*, 2nd edn, ed. P. S. Harper, pp. 13–36. London: Saunders.

Hayashi, H. & Kato, S. (1989). Total manifestations of amyotrophic lateral sclerosis (ALS) in the totally locked-in state. *JNS* **93**, 19–35.

Hayashi, H., Kato, S. & Kawada, A. (1991). Amyotrophic lateral sclerosis patients living beyond respiratory failure. *JNS* **105**, 73–8.

Heckmatt, J. Z., Loh, L. & Dubowitz, V. (1990). Nighttime nasal ventilation in neuromuscular disease. *Lancet* **i**, 579–81.

Heckmatt, J. Z., Hyde, S. A., Gabain, A. & Dubowitz, V. (1988). Therapeutic trial of isazonine in Duchenne muscular dystrophy. *Muscle Nerve* **11**, 836–47.

Henderson, A., Cumming, W. J. K., Williams, D. O. & Hodgson, P. (1981). Cardiac complications of polymyositis. *JNS* **47**, 425–8.

Henriksson, K. G. & Lindvall, B. (1990). Polymyositis and dermatomyositis 1990: Diagnosis, treatment and prognosis. *Prog. Neurobiol.* **35**, 181–93.

Herson, S., Cherin, P. & Coutellier, A. (1992). The association of plasma exchange synchronized with intravenous gamma globulin therapy in severe intractable polymyositis. *J. Rheumatol.* **19**, 828–9.

Higuchi, I. *et al.* (1993). Histochemical and ultrastructural pathology of skeletal muscle in a patient with abetalipoproteinemia. *Acta. Neuropathology (Berl.)* **86**, 529–31.

Hill, N. S. *et al.* (1992). Sleep-disordered breathing in patients with Duchenne muscular dystrophy using negative pressure ventilators. *Chest* **102**, 1656–62.

Hilton, T., Orr, R. D., Perkin, R. M. & Ashwal, S. (1993). End of life care in Duchenne muscular dystrophy. *Pediatr. Neurol.* **9**, 165–77.

Hoffman, E. P. (1993). Genotype/phenotype correlations in Duchenne/Becker dystrophy. In

Molecular and Cell Biology of Muscular Dystrophy, ed. T. Partridge, pp. 12 –36. London: Chapman & Hall.

Hohlfeld, R. *et al.* (1988). Azathioprine toxicity during long-term immunosuppression of generalized Myasthenia gravis. *Neurology* **38**, 258–61.

Houzelstein, D., Lyons, G. E., Chamberlain, J. & Buckingham, M. E. (1992). Localization of dystrophin gene transcripts during mouse embryogenesis. *J. Cell. Biol.* **119**, 811–21.

Howard, R. S., Wiles, C. M. & Loh, L. (1989). Respiratory complications and their management in motor neuron disease. *Brain* **112**, 1155–70.

Hudgson, P. (1984). Polymyositis and Dermatomyositis in adults. In *Inflammatory Disorders of Muscle*, 10th edn, ed. B. M. Ansell, pp. 85–93. London: Saunders.

Hudgson, P. & Walton, J. N. (1979). Polymyositis and other inflammatory myopathies. In *Handbook of Clinical Neurology*, eds. P. J. Vinken & G. W. Bruyn, pp. 51–93. Amsterdam: North-Holland.

Jann, S. *et al.* (1992). High-dose intravenous human immunoglobulin in polymyositis resistant to treatment. *JNNP* **55**, 60–2.

Joffe, M. M. *et al.* (1993). Drug therapy of the idiopathic inflammatory myopathies: Predictors of response to prednisone, azathioprine, and methotrexate and a comparison of their efficacy. *Am. J. Med.* **94**, 379–87.

Johns T. R. (1987). Long-term corticosteroid treatment of myasthenia gravis. *Ann. N.Y. Acad. Sci.* **505**, 568–83.

Kakulas, B. A. (1990). A consideration of therapeutic interventions in the light of the muscle pathology and likely pathogenesis of the XP21.2 muscular dystrophies. In *Pathogenesis and Therapy of Duchenne and Becker Muscular Dystrophy*, eds. B. A. Kakulas & F. L. Mastaglia, pp. 47–58. New York: Raven Press.

Karpati, G. & Carpenter, S. (1993). Pathology of the inflammatory myopathies. In *Baillière's Clinical Neurology*, 2, ed. F. L. Mastaglia, pp. 527–56. London: Baillière Tindall.

Karpati, G. *et al.* (1989). Dystrophin is expressed in mdx skeletal muscle fibers after normal myoblast implantation. *Am. J. Pathol.* **135**, 27–32.

Kelly, J. J. *et al.* (1988). Response to total body irradiation in dermatomyositis. *Muscle Nerve*, **11**, 120–3.

Khan, M. A. (1993). Corticosteroid therapy in Duchenne muscular dystrophy. *JNS* **120**, 8–14.

Koh, E. T. *et al.* (1993). Adult onset polymyositis/dermatomyositis: clinical and laboratory features and treatment response in 75 patients. *Ann. Rheum. Dis.* **52**, 857–61.

Kuks, J. B. M., Djojoatmodjo, S. & Oosterhuis, H. J. H. G. (1991). Azathioprine in myasthenia gravis: observations in 41 patients and a review of literature. *Neuromusc. Disord.* **1**, 423–32.

Kurland, L. T. & Molgaard, C. A. (1982). Guammanian ALS: hereditary or acquired? In *Human Motor Neurone Diseases*, Advances in Neurology 36, ed. L. P. Rowland, pp. 165–72. New York: Raven Press.

Lacomblez, L., Bensimon, G., Leigh, P. N., Guillet, P., Meininger, V. For the Amyotrophic Lateral Sclerosis/Ribizole Study Group II. (1996). *Lancet* **347**, 1425–31.

Laing, N. G. (1993). Molecular genetics and genetic counselling for Duchenne/Becker muscular dystrophy. In *Molecular and cell biology of muscular dystrophy*, ed. T. Partridge, pp. 37–84. London: Chapman Hall.

Lane, R. J. M., Emslie-Smith, A., Mosquera, I. E. & Hudgson, P. (1989). Clinical, biochemical and histological responses to treatment in polymyositis: a prospective study. *J. R. Soc. Med.* **82**, 333–8.

Lang, B. A. *et al.* (1991). Treatment of dermatomyositis with intravenous gammaglobulin. *Am. J. Med.* **91**, 169–72.

Lanska, D. J. (1990). Indications for thymectomy in myasthenia gravis. *Neurology* **40**, 1828–9.

Law, P. K. *et al.* (1990). Dystrophin production induced by myoblast transfer therapy in Duchenne muscular dystrophy. *Lancet* **336**, 114–15.

Law, P. *et al.* (1991). Pioneering development of myoblast transfer therapy. In *Muscular dystrophy research: from molecular diagnosis toward therapy*, eds. C. Angelini, G. A. Danieli & D. Fontanari, pp. 109–16. Amsterdam: Elsevier.

Leclerc, A., Tome, F. M. S. & Fardeau, M. (1993). Ubiquitin and Beta-amyloid-protein in Inclusion body myositis (IBM), familial IBM-like disorder and oculopharyngeal muscular dystrophy: an immunocytochemical study. *Neuromusc. Disord.* **3**, 283–91.

Lee, C. C., Pearlman, J. A., Chamberlain, J. S. & Caskey, C. T. (1991). Expression of recombinant dystrophin and its localization to the cell membrane. *Nature* **349**, 334–6.

Leff, R. L. *et al.* (1993). The treatment of inclusion body myositis: a retrospective review and a randomized, prospective trial of immunosuppressive therapy. *Medicine. (Baltimore)* **72**, 225–35.

Liblau, R. *et al.* (1991). Intravenous gamma-globulin in myasthenia gravis: interaction with anti-acetylcholine receptor autoantibodies. *J. Clin. Immunol.* **11**, 128–31.

Mader, R. & Keystone, E. C. (1993). Inflammatory myopathy: do we have adequate measures of the treatment response? *J. Rheumatol.* **20**, 1105–7.

Marinkovic, Z., Prelevic, G., Wuerzburger, M. & Nogic, S. (1990). Gonadal dysfunction in patients with myotonic dystrophy. *Exp. Clin. Endocrinol.* **96**, 37–44.

Martin, A. W. & Ringel, S. P. (1992). Neuromuscular junction and muscle disease. In *Prognosis of neurological disorders*, eds. R. W. Evans, D. S. Baskin & F. M. Yatsu, pp. 359–74. Oxford: Oxford University Press.

Mastaglia, F. L., Laing, B. A. & Zilko, P. (1993). Treatment of inflammatory myopathies. In *Baillière's Clinical Neurology*, 2, ed. F. L. Mastaglia, pp. 717–40. London: Baillière Tindall.

Mastaglia, F. L. & Ojeda, V. J. (1985*a*). Inflammatory myopathies, part 1. *Ann. Neurol.* **17**, 215–27.

Mastaglia, F. L. & Ojeda, V. J. (1985*b*). Inflammatory myopathies, part 2. *Ann. Neurol.* **17**, 317–23.

Mastaglia, F. L. & Walton, J. N. (1992). Inflammatory myopathies. In *Skeletal Muscle Pathology*, 2nd edn, eds. F. L. Mastaglia & Lord Walton of Detchant, pp. 453–92. Edinburgh: Churchill Livingstone.

Matsumura, K. & Campbell, K. P. (1994). Dystrophin-glycogen complex: its role in the molecular pathogenesis of muscular dystrophies. *Muscle Nerve* **17**, 2–15.

Matsumura, K. *et al.* (1992). Deficiency of the 50K dystrophin-associated glycoprotein in severe childhood autosomal recessive muscular dystrophy. *Nature* **359**, 320–2.

McDouall, R. M., Dunn, M. J. & Dubowitz, V. (1989). Expression of class I and class II MHC antigens in neuromuscular diseases. *JNS* **89**, 213–26.

Merlini, L. *et al.* (1988). Growth hormone evaluation in Duchenne muscular dystrophy. *Ital. J. Neurol. Sci.* **9**, 471–6.

Mesa, L. E. *et al.* (1991). Steroids in Duchenne muscular dystrophy: Deflazacort trial. *Neuromusc. Disord.* **1**, 261–6.

Miano, M. A. *et al.* (1991). Factors influencing outcome of prednisone dose reduction in myasthenia gravis. *Neurology* **41**, 919–21.

Miller, J. R., Colbert, A. P. & Osberg, J. S. (1990). Ventilator dependency: decision making; daily functioning and quality of life for patients with Duchenne muscular dystrophy. *Dev. Med. Child Neurol.* **32**, 1079–86.

Miller, F. W., Leitman, S. F. & Plotz, P. H. (1992*a*). Plasma exchange in polymyositis and dermatomyositis. Reply. *N. Engl. J. Med.* **327**, 1030–1.

Miller, F., Moseley, C. F. & Koreska, J. (1992*b*). Spinal fusion in Duchenne muscular dystrophy. *Dev. Med. Child Neurol.* **34**, 775–86.

Miller, F. W. *et al.* (1992*c*). Controlled trial of plasma exchange and leukapheresis in polymyositis and dermatomyositis. *N. Engl. J. Med.* **326**, 1380–84.

Miller, L. C. *et al.* (1992*d*). Methotrexate treatment of recalcitrant childhood dermatomyositis. *Arthritis Rheum.* **35**, 1143–9.

Mohr, C. H. & Hill, N. S. (1990). Long-term follow-up of nocturnal ventilatory assistance in patients with respiratory failure due to Duchenne-type muscular dystrophy. *Chest* **97**, 91–6.

Morandi, L. *et al.* (1993). Very small dystrophin molecule in a family with a mild form of Becker muscular dystrophy. *Neuromusc. Disord.* **3**, 65–70.

Morel, E. *et al.* (1988). Neonatal myasthenia gravis: a new clinical and immunologic appraisal on 30 cases. *Neurology* **38**, 138–42.

Morgan, J. E., Hoffman, E. P. & Partridge, T. A. (1990). Normal myogenic cells from newborn mice restore normal histology to degenerating muscles of the mdx mouse. *J. Cell. Biol.* **111**, 2437–49.

Moxley, R. T. III, Brooke, M. H., Fenichel, G. M., Mendell, J. R., Griggs, R. C., Miller, J. P., Province, M. A., Patterson, V., CIDD Group (1987). Clinical investigation in Duchenne dystrophy. VI. Double-blind controlled trial of nifedipine. *Muscle Nerve* **10**, 22–33.

Munsat, T. L., Hollander, D., Andres, P. & Finison, L. (1991). Clinical trials in ALS: measurement and natural history. *Adv. Neurol.* **56**, 515–19.

Munsat, T. L. *et al.* (1992). Intrathecal thyrotropin-releasing hormone does not alter the progressive course of ALS: experience with an intrathecal drug delivery system. *Neurology* **42**, 1049–53.

Nakano, S. & Engel, A. G. (1993). Myasthenia gravis: quantitative immunocytochemical analysis of inflammatory cells and detection of complement membrane attack complex at the end-plate in 30 patients. *Neurology* **43**, 1167–72.

Naylor, C. D., Jevnikar, A. M. & Witt, N. L. (1987). Sporadic viral myositis in two adults. *Can. Med. Assoc. J.* **137**, 819–22.

Nicholson, L. V. B. *et al.* (1993*a*). Integrated study of 100 patients with Xp21 linked muscular dystrophy using clinical, genetic, immunochemical, and histopathological data, part 1, trends across the clinical groups. *J. Med. Genet.* **30**, 728–36.

Nicholson, L. V. B. *et al.* (1993*b*). Integrated study of 100 patients with Xp21 linked muscular dystrophy using clinical, genetic, immunochemical, and histopathological data, part 2, correlations within individual patients. *J. Med. Genet.* **30**, 737–44.

Nicholson, L. V. B. *et al.* (1993*c*). Integrated study of 100 patients with Xp21 linked muscular dystrophy using clinical, genetic, immunochemical, and histopathological data, part 3, differential diagnosis and prognosis. *J. Med. Genet.* **30**, 745–51.

Nigro, G., Comi, L. I., Politano, L. & Bain, R. J. I. (1990). The incidence and evolution of cardiomyopathy in Duchenne muscular dystrophy. *Int. J. Cardiol.* **26**, 271–7.

Nitta, A. T. & Kuritzkes, D. R. (1991). Pyomyositis due to group C streptococci in a patient with AIDS. *Rev. Infect. Dis.* **13**, 1254–5.

Norris, F. *et al.* (1993). Onset, natural history and outcome in idiopathic adult motor neuron disease. *JNS* **118**, 48–55.

Nussbaum, M. S. *et al.* (1992). Management of myasthenia gravis by extended thymectomy with anterior mediastinal dissection. *Surgery* 112, 681–8.

Olanow, C. W., Lane, R. J. M. & Roses, A. D. (1982). Thymectomy in late onset myasthenia gravis. *Arch. Neurol.* 39, 82–3.

Olanow, C. W. *et al.* (1987). Thymectomy as primary therapy in myasthenia gravis. *Ann. N.Y. Acad. Sci.* 505, 595–606.

O'Neill, J. H., Murray, N. M. F. & Newsom-Davis, J. (1988). The Lambert-Eaton myasthenic syndrome. A review of 50 cases. *Brain* 111, 577–96.

Oosterhuis, H. J. G. H. (1989). The natural course of myasthenia gravis; a long-term follow-up study. *JNNP* 52, 1121–7

Ostrov, B. E., Goldsmith, D. P., Eichenfield, A. H. & Athreya, B. H. (1991). Hypercalcemia during the resolution of calcinosis universalis in juvenile dermatomyositis. *J. Rheumatol.* 18, 1730–4.

Partridge, T. A. (1991). Myoblast transfer: a possible therapy for inherited myopathies? *Muscle Nerve* 14, 197–212.

Partridge, T. A. *et al.* (1989). Conversion of mdx myofibres from dystrophin-negative to -positive by injection of normal myoblasts. *Nature* 337, 176–8.

Patterson, V., Morrison, O. & Hicks, E. (1991). Mode of death in Duchenne muscular dystrophy. *Lancet* 337, 801–2.

Quinlivan, R. M. & Dubowitz, V. (1992). Cardiac transplantation in Becker muscular dystrophy. *Neuromusc. Disord.* 2, 165–7.

Ragot, T. *et al.* (1993). Efficient adenovirus-mediated transfer of a human minidystrophin gene to skeletal muscle of mdx mice. *Nature* 361, 647–50.

Reardon, W. *et al.* (1993). Cataract and myotonic dystrophy: the role of molecular diagnosis. *Br. J. Ophthalmol.* 77, 579–83.

Riggs, T. (1990). Cardiomyopathy and pulmonary emboli in terminal Duchenne's muscular dystrophy. *Am. Heart. J.* 119, 690–3.

Ringel, S. P. *et al.* (1993). The natural history of amyotrophic lateral sclerosis. *Neurology* 43, 1316–22.

Rosenberg, N. L., Carry, M. R. & Ringel, S. P. (1988). Association of inflammatory myopathies with other connective tissue disorders and malignancies. In *Polymyositis and Dermatomyositis*, ed. M. C. Dalakas, pp. 37–69. Boston: Butterworth.

Rosenberg, N. L. & Ringel, S. P. (1988). Adult polymyositis and dermatomyositis. In *Inflammatory Diseases of Muscle*, ed. F. L. Mastaglia, pp. 87–106. Oxford: Blackwell Scientific Publications.

Roufs, J. B. (1991). L-threonine as a symptomatic treatment for amytrophic lateral sclerosis (ALS). *Med. Hypotheses* 34, 20–3.

Rowland, L. P. (1987). Therapy in myasthenia gravis: introduction. *Ann. N.Y. Acad. Sci.* 505, 566–7.

Rowland, L. P., Hoefer, P. F. A., Aranow, H. & Merritt, H. H. (1956). Fatalities in myasthenia gravis. A review of 39 cases with 29 autopsies. *Neurology* 6, 307–26.

Saad, F. A., Vita, G., Toffolatti, L. & Danieli, G. A. (1994). A possible missense mutation detected in the dystrophin gene by double strand conformation analysis (DSCA). *Neuromusc. Disord.* 4, 335–41.

Salvarani, C. *et al.* (1993). High-dose immunoglobulin therapy in a case of inclusion body myositis: clinical and immunologic aspects. *J. Rheumatol.* 20, 1455–6.

Sanders, D. B., Howard, J. F. Jr. & Massey, J. M. (1993). 3,4-Diaminopyridine in Lambert-Eaton myasthenic syndrome and myasthenia gravis. *Ann. N.Y. Acad. Sci.* 681, 588–90.

Scadding, G. K., Havard, C. W. H., Lange, M. J. & Domb, I. (1985). The long term experience of thymectomy for myasthenia gravis. *JNNP* **48**, 401–6.

Scherpbier, H. J. & Oosterhuis, H. J. G. H. (1987). Factors influencing the relapse risk of steroid dose reduction in myasthenia gravis. *Clin. Neurol. Neurosurg.* **89**, 145–50.

Schmalbruch, H. (1992). The muscular dystrophies. In *Skeletal Muscle Pathology*, 2nd edn, eds. F. L. Mastaglia & Lord Walton of Detchant, pp. 283–318. Edinburgh: Churchill Livingstone.

Scott, O. M., Hyde, S. A., Vrbova, G. & Dubowitz, V. (1990). Therapeutic possibilities of chronic low frequency electrical stimulation in children with Duchenne muscular dystrophy. *JNS*, **95**, 171–82.

Servidei, S. *et al.* (1993). Familial hyperCKaemia can be a varient of Becker muscular dystrophy. *Neurology* **43**, A293.

Seybold, M. E. (1987). Plasmapheresis in myasthenia gravis. *Ann. N.Y. Acad. Sci.* **505**, 584–7.

Shah, A. & Lisak, R. P. (1993). Immunopharmacologic therapy in myasthenia gravis. *Clin. Neuropharmacol.* **16**, 97–103.

Shapira, Y. *et al.* (1993). Infantile idiopathic myopathic carnitine deficiency: Treatment with L-carnitine. *Pediatrics* **9**, 35–8.

Shapiro, F. *et al.* (1992). Spinal fusion in Duchenne muscular dystrophy: a multidisciplinary approach. *Muscle Nerve* **15**, 604–14.

Silverstein, M. D. *et al.* (1991). Amyotrophic lateral sclerosis and life-sustaining therapy: patients' desires for information, participation in decision making, and life-sustaining therapy. *Mayo Clin. Proc.* **66**, 906–13.

Simpson, J. A. & Thomaides, T. (1987). Treatment of myasthenia gravis: an adult. *Q. J. Med.* **64**, 693.

Slonim, A. E. & Goans, P. J. (1985). Myopathy in McArdle's syndrome. Improvement with a high-protein diet. *N. Engl. J. Med.* **312**, 355–9.

Smith, R. A. *et al.* (1993). Recombinant growth hormone treatment of amyotrophic lateral sclerosis. *Muscle Nerve* **16**, 624–33.

Soueidan, S. A. & Dalakas, M. C. (1993). Treatment of inclusion-body myositis with high-dose intravenous immunoglobulin. *Neurology* **43**, 876–9.

Steare, S. E., Dubowitz, V. & Benatar, A. (1992). Subclinical cardiomyopathy in Becker muscular dystrophy. *Br. Heart. J.* **68**, 304–8.

Sugita, H. (1991). Advances in drug therapy, with special emphasis on protease inhibitors. In *Muscular dystrophy research: from molecular diagnosis toward therapy*, eds. C. Angelini, G. A. Danieli & D. Fontanari, pp. 181–90. Amsterdam: Elsevier.

Targoff, I. N. (1989). Immunologic aspects of myositis. *Curr. Opin. Rheumatol.* **1**, 432–42.

Targoff, I. N. & Reichlin, M. (1988). Immunological aspects. In *Inflammatory Diseases of Muscle*, ed. F. L. Mastaglia, pp. 37–70. Oxford: Blackwell Scientific Publications.

Tindall, R. S. A. *et al.* (1987). Preliminary results of a double-blind; randomized; placebo-controlled trial of cyclosporine in myasthenia gravis. *N. Engl. J. Med.* **316**, 719–24.

Tindall, R. S. A. *et al.* (1993). A clinical therapeutic trial of cyclosporine in myasthenia gravis. *Ann. N.Y. Acad. Sci.* **681**, 539–51.

Valli, G., Jann, S., Premoselli, S. & Scarlato, G. (1987). Myasthenia gravis treatment: twelve years experience in 110 patients. *Ital. J. Neurol. Sci.* **8**, 593–604.

Venables, G. S., Bates, D., Cartlidge, N. E. F. & Hudgson, P. (1982). Acute polymyositis with subcutaneous oedema. *JNS* **55**, 161–4.

Vincent, N. *et al.* (1993). Long-term correction of mouse dystrophic degeneration by adenovirus-mediated transfer of a minidystrophin gene. *Nature (Genet.)* **5**, 130–4.

Wallace, G. B. & Newton, R. W. (1989). Gowers' sign revisited. *Arch. Dis. Child.* **64**, 1317–19.

Walton, J. N. & Adams, R. D. (1958). *Polymyositis.* Edinburgh: Livingstone.

Wells, D. J. *et al.* (1992). Human dystrophin expression corrects the myopathic phenotype in transgenic *mdx* mice. *Hum. Molec. Genet.* **1**, 35–40.

Westarp, M. E. *et al.* (1993). Antiretroviral therapy in sporadic adult amyotrophic lateral sclerosis. *Neuroreport* **4**, 819–22.

Wilensky, R., Dwyer, B. & Mayer, R. F. (1993). Relapses in patients with myasthenia gravis treated with azathioprine. *Ann. N.Y. Acad. Sci.* **681**, 591–3.

Wortmann, R. L. (1992). The dilemma of treating patients with inclusion body myositis. *J. Rheumatol* **19**, 1327–9

Zupan, A. (1992). Long-term electrical stimulation of muscles in children with Duchenne and Becker muscular dystrophy. *Muscle Nerve* **15**, 362–7.

18 Outcome of polyneuropathies and mononeuropathies

L. H. VAN DEN BERG, J. H. J. WOKKE AND
F. G. I. JENNEKENS

Introduction

Peripheral neuropathies are a heterogeneous group of diseases of the peripheral nervous system. It is useful to distinguish three categories based upon the pattern of involvement: polyneuropathy, mononeuropathy and plexopathy. The typical polyneuropathy is a symmetrical disorder, resulting in distal weakness of limb muscles and sensory loss. Mononeuropathies are isolated lesions of peripheral nerves, which may be multifocal (multiple mononeuropathies or mononeuritis multiplex). Plexopathies are lesions affecting the brachial or lumbar plexus, and the presenting symptoms involve one limb or part of a limb.

Diagnosing a neuropathy is relatively simple, but establishing its aetiology can often be cumbersome (Dyck *et al.* 1981; Notermans *et al.* 1991; Schaumberg *et al.* 1991*a*). Many acquired, and a few hereditary neuropathies can be treated. Most neuropathies have a good prognosis for life expectancy; some may eventually prove to be incapacitating.

First we shall present a brief discussion of some factors which play a role in the outcome of a neuropathy. This will be followed by a review of current knowledge on the outcome of different neuropathies or groups of neuropathies.

Factors which play a role in the outcome

Gene defects

Neuropathies of a similar phenotype can be caused by defects in different genes. This may explain some of the variation in time of onset and course of the neuropathies. The nature of a gene defect may have consequences for the phenotype, the severity and the course of a neuropathy. This is exemplified by recent discoveries concerning the genetic basis of hereditary motor and sensory neuropathy (HMSN) type I and hereditary neuropathy with liability to pressure palsies (HNPP); these will be discussed in more detail below. It follows that at least in the case of HMSN type I, certain predictions about the onset and course can be reached on the basis of findings obtained during DNA investigation. A similar development may be expected for other hereditary neuropathies.

Underlying pathology

In broad terms, two types of nerve degeneration should be distinguished: demyelination and axonal degeneration. Recovery from a demyelinating disorder is possible if ongoing demyelination can be halted and the cause eliminated. Demyelination acts as a stimulus for the proliferation of Schwann cells. These new Schwann cells tend to remyelinate the demyelinated axons, thus allowing the return of conduction. Remyelination is basically a rapid process and so recovery from an extensive demyelinating neuropathy is feasible within a matter of weeks.

Recovery from axonal neuropathy generally takes much more time. Axonal degeneration is often of the dying back type: dying back implies that distal parts of axons disappear whilst the proximal parts and cell bodies are preserved. Recovery under these circumstances first requires the elimination of the cause of the neuropathy and then the growth of damaged axons to their targets. Under optimal experimental conditions a lesioned axon will elongate by 1 or 2 mm per day, but conditions in humans are often far from optimal. The rate of growth depends on the presence in the distal parts of the peripheral nerves of Schwann cells and basal lamina tubes: these stimulate growth and assist in pathfinding. The longer the period before the onset of regeneration, the greater the number of Schwann cells and basal lamina tubes which will have disappeared (Vuorinen *et al.* 1995) and the poorer the prognosis. Furthermore the greater the distance grown by the regenerating axons, the greater the decrease in rate of growth (Sunderland 1978). Growth of neurites is an age-related process: it is fast in young individuals and decreases with age. For these and other reasons, recovery from axonal neuropathies often remains incomplete.

Recovery from partial nerve lesions (loss of some nerve fibres whilst others are preserved without damage) occurs at least in part by collateral sprouting and reinnervation. In such cases there is collateral branching of intact nerve fibres in the target organ of the lesioned nerve and these branches grow towards the denervated muscle fibres or parts of the skin, and reinnervate the denervated cells. Collateral reinnervation often occurs much sooner than regrowth of lesioned nerve fibres because the distance that has to be bridged by the collateral branches is short. Another factor may be that collateral branches originate from healthy nerve fibres.

In practice, recovery often depends not on one of the three aforementioned processes but on a combination of two or even all three of them. Demyelinating neuropathies, for example the inflammatory disorders, usually include some degree of axonal degeneration. Recovery depends in part on remyelination and in part on regeneration of damaged axons. If the latter is only partially successful, reinnervation may also be accomplished by collateral branching of healthy remyelinated nerve fibres in the target organs.

Experimental investigations of recombinant human neurotrophic factors that influence growth of axons and collateral branching and reinnervation are in progress; some of these are the subject of clinical trials. There is a fair chance that one or several of these compounds will become available in the not too distant future for therapeutic purposes (Kerkhoff & Jennekens 1993).

The nature of the clinical symptoms and the course of a peripheral neuropathy

Some peripheral neuropathies are predominantly motor or sensory and rarely autonomic; others are mixed. A progressive motor neuropathy leads to paralysis and a progressive sensory neuropathy to analgesia or an incapacitating form of sensory ataxia (Dalakas 1986). Autonomic neuropathies cause hypo- or hyperhidrosis, orthostatic hypotension and dysfunction of internal organs, the last including impotence, gastrointestinal motility disorders, urine retention, sinus tachycardia, bradycardia and sinus arrest or asystole (Appenzeller & Kornfeld 1973; Feldman & Schiller 1983; McLeod et al. 1987a,b; Mulligan & Katz 1989; Ingall et al. 1990).

The clinical course of a neuropathy may be acute or subacute (evolving over weeks or a few months), slowly progressive (evolving over years) or relapsing. Spontaneous recovery is a feature of some of the acute neuropathies.

Prevention and treatment

Genetic counselling may help to prevent hereditary neuropathies, while measures concerning food intake or medication may prevent some of the acquired neuropathies. Early recognition of a treatable neuropathy will in some cases allow for onset of treatment before severe damage to the peripheral nervous system has developed. Adequate treatment is available for some severe or chronic neuropathies. Surgical intervention may facilitate nerve regeneration in certain mononeuropathies.

Rehabilitation and treatment of complications

The major goals for rehabilitation are to maximize residual function, to adjust the home or working environment, to maintain adequate joint mobility, to treat the consequences of autonomic dysfunction, and to relieve pain (Berger & Schaumburg 1988). Splinting may be required to prevent contractures and muscle overstretch or to support a limb in a position of maximum function. Lower-extremity orthoses may be required to prevent foot drop. Patients with acute neuropathies are usually bedridden, leading to complications caused by immobilization; they may require treatment for ventilatory and autonomic failure.

Hereditary neuropathies

The hereditary neuropathies are a complex and heterogeneous group of disorders. In some syndromes the neuropathy is one manifestation of a multisystem disease; in others, it is the only expression of a gene mutation. The metabolic basis of several of these neuropathies is known; for some others elucidation of the pathophysiological mechanism can be expected in the near future on the basis of recent genetic findings.

A series of discoveries has provided new insights into the genetic mutations for several types of hereditary neuropathy. These developments entail great consequences for early diagnosis and prevention but not (yet) for therapy.

The hereditary motor and sensory neuropathies (HMSNs)

A classification of the most common hereditary neuropathies was proposed by Dyck and Lambert in 1968. Major changes in this classification system are now necessary due to the identification of underlying gene mutations encoding myelin and other proteins (Harding 1995). Some authors prefer, therefore, the acronyms CMT (Charcot–Marie–Tooth) and DS (Dejerine–Sottas) instead of HMSN types I and II and HMSN type III respectively. The natural history of these 'HMSNs' is usually one of slowly progressive distal limb weakness and atrophy, and distal sensory loss. Foot deformities (pes cavus and hammer toes) are frequent (Harding & Thomas 1980; Dyck *et al.* 1993*a*). The variation in clinical presentation is wide, ranging from pes cavus as the only clinical abnormality to wheelchair dependency. Onset may occur in early infancy but is more usual in the second half of the first decade or in the second decade, or even later (Bird & Kraft 1978). Early onset of the neuropathy is generally associated with a more severe phenotype.

The HMSNs can be classified on the basis of clinical, genetic, neurophysiological and pathological features. Types I and III are demyelinating, hypertrophic neuropathies with marked slowing of nerve conduction; type II is an axonal neuropathy. Type III differs from type I in being more severe. Types I and II can be subdivided into autosomal dominant and recessive varieties (Gabreëls-Festen *et al.* 1991, 1992*a*). There is also an X-linked form (Fryns & Van den Berghe 1980). Type III was previously thought to be autosomal recessive but appears now to be genetically heterogeneous and in at least some cases autosomal dominant.

HMSN type I

Dominant HMSN type I is genetically heterogeneous. Type IA is linked to chromosome 17 and is either due to a duplication of 1.5 megabase in 17p11.2–p12, which includes the gene for peripheral myelin protein 22 (*pmp* 22), or rarely to a point mutation in the *pmp* 22 gene. Gene duplication seems to cause a less severe phenotype than point mutation (Raymakers *et al.* 1991; Lupski *et al.* 1991; Valentijn *et al.* 1992; Hoogendijk *et al.* 1993; Roa *et al.* 1993). Type IA occurs much more frequently than IB. IB is linked to chromosome 1 and has now been related convincingly to the gene for peripheral myelin protein *Po* (Kulkens *et al.* 1993). Clinical, neurophysiological and morphological studies indicate that HMSN type IB is more severe than the form of HMSN type IA due to duplication in 17p11.2–p12 (Dyck *et al.* 1989). Some families have been described in which no evidence has been found for linkage to either chromosome 1 or chromosome 17, indicating that dominantly inherited HMSN type I consists of at least three genetically distinct diseases (Chance *et al.* 1990). A somewhat milder phenotype of dominant HMSN type I would seem most often to be related to a duplication of the *pmp* 22 gene and the more severe forms to point mutations in the *pmp* 22 gene or to a defect in the *Po* gene.

Longitudinal, clinical and electrophysiological studies of HMSN type IA have revealed that slowing of motor nerve conduction scarcely increases after the first decade. Secondary axonal damage is therefore considered the most likely cause for the variable, most often slight, progress in muscle weakness after the first decade (Killian *et al.* 1996). Data on life expectancy are not available but it is expected to be normal in the large majority of patients.

An autosomal recessive form of HMSN type I was mapped to chromosome 8q in Tunisian families. The phenotype was an early-onset severe neuropathy, and nerve biopsies showed loss of myelinated fibres and hypomyelination (Ben Othmane *et al.* 1993). However, in other (Tunisian) families this syndrome did not map to this locus, suggesting genetic heterogeneity.

HMSN type II

Dominant HMSN type II is also genetically heterogeneous. Two loci have been reported: one on chromosome 1 and one on chromosome 3 (Hentati *et al.* 1992; Kwon *et al.* 1995). Age at onset varies and may even be during middle age (Harding & Thomas 1980). The course of the disease is often mild and, although actual data are not available, life expectancy may be presumed to be in the normal range in most patients.

There are several reports on an autosomal recessive form of HMSN type II (Ouvrier *et al.* 1981; Gabreëls-Festen *et al.* 1991). Onset of muscle weakness is at the distal parts of the lower and upper limbs. Many of these patients become wheelchair-dependent in their teens and experience major loss of hand function.

HMSN type III

The entity of HMSN type III, or Dejerine–Sottas (DS) disease, is disputed. It is defined as a severe demyelinating/hypomyelinating neuropathy with very slow motor nerve conduction velocities (< 10 m/s), presenting in infancy with delayed motor development. Inheritance has been suggested (but not proven) to be autosomal recessive (Gabreëls-Festen *et al.* 1993). Patients are often short in stature, kyphoscoliotic, and have severe deformities of the hands and feet. Many of these patients do not learn to walk independently or become wheelchair-dependent in the course of the first or second decade. We have observed several patients who developed respiratory insufficiency due to muscle weakness and kyphoscoliosis in their third or fourth decade. There is now evidence for substantial pathological and genetic heterogeneity in this syndrome (Gabreëls-Festen *et al.* 1993). Fresh heterozygous (dominant) mutations of the *pmp*-22 and *Po* genes have been detected in patients with the clinical picture of HMSN type III (Harding 1995; Ionasescu *et al.* 1995; Roa *et al.* 1993).

X-linked HMSN (HMSN X)

In X-linked HMSN male patients tend to be more severely affected than female patients, who have a mild neuropathy or are asymptomatic (Harding 1995). The neurophysiological features in males may resemble those of HMSN type I, whereas in females they are more axonal in type. The locus for X-linked HMSN maps to Xq13.1. Several families with X-linked HMSN have been described with point mutations in the gene coding for the protein connexin 32, which is localized in the Xq13.1 region.

Hereditary neuropathy with liability to pressure palsies (HNPP)

In the currently used classification of 'hereditary motor and sensory neuropathies', HNPP does not qualify as a type of HMSN. It does, however, appear to be associated with a deletion of the 1.5 megabase region on chromosome 17 p11.2–p12, the region that is duplicated in most HMSN type IA patients (Chance *et al.* 1993; Gouider *et al.* 1995). HNPP is an autosomal dominant disorder usually presenting as recurrent, transient, pressure-induced mononeuropathies (Staal *et al.* 1965; Debruyne *et al.* 1980). Laboratory examination of affected individuals reveals a subclinical generalized neuropathy. The first mononeuropathy usually presents in the second decade. Palsies may follow relatively minor trauma to the peripheral nerves. In older age groups the mononeuropathies are often no longer fully transient and clinical signs of an asymmetric polyneuropathy may develop. Exceptionally, some members of affected families present the phenotype of a polyneuropathy from the onset (Gabreëls-Fasten *et al.* 1992*b*).

Hereditary sensory and autonomic neuropathies (HSANs)

The hereditary sensory and autonomic neuropathies (HSAN type I–V according to Dyck's classification) are a heterogeneous group of disorders which have in common predominant involvement of thin sensory and equally thin autonomic nerve fibres (Swanson 1963; Pearson 1979; Dyck 1993). A progressive autosomal dominant disorder with clinical manifestations in the second decade or thereafter should be distinguished from autosomal recessive disorders with congenital onset and no obvious progression. HSAN type III is related to a gene localized on chromosome 9 (Blumenfeld *et al.* 1993); the genetic basis of the other types has not been elucidated. HSAN may be associated with sensorineural deafness and early-onset dementia (Wright & Dyck 1995) or with cataracts, mental retardation and skin lesions (Heckmann *et al.* 1995). Characteristic features of many of these neuropathies are acral mutilation, painless arthropathy and unrecognized fractures of the hand, foot or distal parts of the limbs. Acral mutilation starts with plantar ulceration or whitlow and may progress to osteomyelitis and osteolysis and finally amputation. Adequate daily care of the distal parts of the limbs, in most patients especially the feet, can completely prevent ulceration and its consequences. The soles of the feet and the interior of the shoes should be inspected daily and creases in the socks prevented. The feet should be hydrated daily in case of anhidrosis.

Table 18.1. *Drugs and chemicals in acute hepatic prophyrias*[a]

Reported to exacerbate disease	Theoretically risky	Believed to be safe
Barbiturates	Alcuronium	Aspirin
Bemegride	Alkyl-containing compounds	Atropine
Chloramphenicol	Bupivacaine	Bromides
Chlordiazepoxide	Clonazepam (large doses)	Calcium salts
Chloroquine	Clonidine	Chlorpromazine
Chloropropamide	Etidocaine	Chloral hydrate
Danazol	Hydralazine	Corticosteroids
Diazepam	Lidocaine	Cyclopropane
Ergot preparations	Mepivacaine	Dicumarol
Estrogens	Methychlothiazide	Droperidol
Ethanol excess	Pargyline	Ether
Eucalyptol (in mouthwash)	Phenoxybenzamine	Fentanyl
Glutethimide	Prilocaine	Gallamine
Griseofulvin	Pyrocaine	Guanethidine
Halothane	Spironolactone	Mefenamic acid
Hydantoins		Meperidine
Imipramine	All agents known to induce	Methadone
Ketamine	cytochrome P450 or to increase	Morphine
Meprobamate	hepatic haem turnover	Neostigmine
Methsuximide		Nitrous oxide
Methyldopa		Oxylate/sodium
Methyprylone		Pancuronium
Nikethamide		Paraldehyde
Oral contraceptives		Penicillin
Pentazocine		Pentamethonium
Phensuximide		Procaine
Phenylbutazone		Promazine
Progestogens		Promethazine
Pyrazinamide		Propoxyphene
Pyrazolone derivatives		Propranolol
Sulphonamides		Reserpine
Theophylline derivatives		Succinylcholine
Tolbutamide		Tetracycline
Troxidone		*d*-Tubocurarine
Valproate		Vitamins A, B, C, D and E

[a] Among agents reported to exacerbate disease, those underlined are incriminated most often. Those listed as theoretically risky have not been incriminated clearly in humans, but experimental studies indicate a potential for damage. Those believed to be safe have been used in humans without ill effects, are not theoretically risky, and have not been reported to exacerbate porphyria (Windebank & Bonkovky, 1993).

The porphyrias

The porphyrias are a group of rare autosomal dominant disorders (acute intermittent porphyria, variegate porphyria and coproporphyria) characterized by disturbances in haem biosynthesis and associated with an axonal type of peripheral neuropathy and mental disturbance. Porphyric neuropathy occurs in acute episodes and should be distinguished from Guillain–Barré syndrome. Attacks usually start with abdominal pain. Weakness is acute and localized at proximal or distal portions of any extremity, both symmetric and asymmetric. The clinical picture is often complicated by signs of autonomic neuropathy. Attacks are induced by the use of drugs which activate the cytochrome P450 system in the liver (Table 18.1) and by starvation (Windebank & Bonkovski 1993). Prevention of acute attacks can usually be achieved by ensuring adequate food intake and by not taking porphyrogenic drugs. Intravenous administration of haem (haematin) is an effective treatment for acute attacks and results in a rapid and reproducible remission of symptoms (Windebank & Bonkovski 1993; Pierach 1982). Mortality from acute attacks of porphyria was once approximately 30% but is now low. Most patients with porphyric neuropathy recover and gradually regain strength and sensation. Autonomic features recover rapidly. Since the neuropathic porphyrias are dominantly inherited, all at-risk relatives should be screened for latent disease.

Peripheral neuropathy in some rare hereditary metabolic disorders

Peripheral nerves are involved in a number of rare lysosomal, peroxisomal and lipid disorders; neuropathy is not usually the predominant feature of these diseases (Jennekens 1987). Some disorders which are exceptional in this respect are listed in Table 18.2, which also gives details on characteristic features, treatment and prognosis (Zlotogora *et al.* 1981; Jennekens 1987; Skjeldal *et al.* 1987; Filling-Katz *et al.* 1989; Donaghy *et al.* 1990; Kolodney *et al.* 1991; Yao & Herbert 1993).

Familial amyloid polyneuropathy (FAP)

FAP in its most frequent form is a very characteristic polyneuropathy which presents in the third or fourth decade or at older ages with autonomic dysfunction and small sensory nerve fibre changes (Andrade 1952; Kyle & Dyck 1993). Loss of temperature and pain sensation first becomes apparent in the feet and is followed at later stages by thick sensory nerve fibre changes and muscle weakness. Amyloid is deposited in nerves, and also in cardiac and skeletal muscle, carpal ligament, ocular vitreous and other tissues. Among the autonomic changes, impotence, diarrhoea and orthostatic hypotension are prominent. In this disease, a mutated form of the plasma protein transthyretin is deposited in the tissue as amyloid. The clinical picture varies dependent on the type of mutation in transthyretin (Mascarenhas Saraiva 1991). This neuropathy is disabling and relentlessly progressive. Survival time after onset is 10–15 years.

Recently an entirely new development created some hope for FAP patients. More than 90% of transthyretin is produced in the liver. Liver transplantation was suggested to normalize transthyretin production and this was attempted in patients with the Portuguese form of FAP (FAP met 30). The effect on neuropathy was favourable. Progression was halted and some improvement was observed (Skinner *et al.* 1994). Liver

Table 18.2. *Peripheral neuropathy in some rare hereditary metabolic disorders*

Type	Inheritance	Clinical features	Outcome
Metachromatic leukodystrophy	AR	Hypotonia, weakness. Infantile, juvenile and adult forms	CNS involvement leads to mental deterioration and vegetative state until death 5–10 years later
Krabbe's disease	AR	Motor and mental deterioration. Hypertonicity. Blindness, deafness. Infantile (3–6 months or 2–8 years) and adult forms.	Death within 2 years of onset. Later onset cases have a more protracted course
Fabry's disease	X-linked	Attacks of painful hands or feet. Autonomic dysfunction. Renal (and other organs) dysfunction. Onset in childhood or adolescence	Phenytoin or carbamazepine relieves pain. Renal transplantation helps renal failure and neuralgia. Attacks may be induced by fatigue, temperature change or exercise. Course is slowly progressive
Refsum's disease	AR	Symmetric distal weakness and sensory loss. Ataxia. Night blindness, retinitis pigmentosa. Onset early childhood to third or fourth decade	Initially gradual progression, sometimes fluctuating course. A phytanic-acid-free diet (and plasmapheresis) stops progression of the disease. Untreated patients have a poor prognosis (half die before age 30 years)
A-beta-lipoproteinaemia	AR	Growth retardation, ataxia, tremor, dysarthria, distal weakness and sensory loss. Proprioceptive dysfunction. Onset from birth	Patients may live until middle age. Effect of vitamin E supplementation: neurological symptoms are prevented, but neurological changes that are already present do not disappear
Tangier disease	AR	Variable. Multiple mononeuropathy (relapsing). Distal weakness and sensory loss. Autonomic dysfunction	Variable. Slowly progressive disability. Neurological defects have no consequences for life expectancy
Cerebrotendinous xanthomatosis	AR	Ataxia, dementia, spasticity, palatal myoclonus, pseudo-bulbar palsy. Onset usually late childhood or adolescence	Slowly progressive. Death occurs in fourth decade. Successful treatment with chenodeoxycholic acid has been reported

AR, autosomal recessive.

transplantation is, however, a major intervention and not without risks, particular in patients with autonomic neuropathy (Harding & Reilly 1995).

Neuropathy associated with systemic diseases

Diabetic neuropathy

Many different neuropathies may occur in diabetes mellitus (Dyck *et al.* 1985, 1993*b*). These can be subdivided into symmetrical polyneuropathies and mononeuropathies, but mixed syndromes are common. The type of neuropathy bears little correlation to the type of diabetes. Most patients with long-standing diabetes, either insulin-dependent or non-insulin-dependent, will develop some degree of polyneuropathy. Strict control of blood sugar concentration is important and may prevent neuropathy (Dyck *et al.* 1986*a*). In several patients with diabetic neuropathy, inflammatory infiltration and vasculitis was found in nerve biopsies. In these patients a good response to anti-inflammatory and/or anti-immune therapy was observed; a recent study showed a good response in patients with (1) multifocal axonal neuropathy caused by inflammatory vasculopathy, predominantly in patients with non-insulin-dependent diabetes mellitus, indistinguishable from diabetic proximal neuropathy or mononeuropathy multiplex, and (2) demyelinating neuropathy indistinguishable from chronic inflammatory demyelinating polyradiculoneuropathy (CIDP), predominantly in patients with insulin-dependent diabetes mellitus (Said *et al.* 1994; Krendel *et al.* 1995).

Symmetrical polyneuropathy
Distal sensory/autonomic neuropathy A distal, predominantly sensory polyneuropathy is the commonest type of diabetic peripheral nerve disorder. It remains mild in most patients though some of them may experience numbness and tingling or aching and lancinating pain, particularly at night. Occasionally the neuropathy follows a progressive course and in these patients symptoms and signs may extend from the feet upwards, to the legs, the hands and even the trunk. Sensory neuropathy occasionally presents as burning sensations in the soles of the feet and impairment of function predominantly in thin sensory nerve fibres.

Autonomic neuropathy is usually associated with symmetrical sensory neuropathy. The most frequent manifestation is probably distal hypohidrosis or anhidrosis. The risk of foot ulceration is present in all patients with hypalgesia and hypohidrosis (Archer *et al.* 1983; Parkhouse & LeQuesne 1988). Impotence is another frequent sign of diabetes in males and is characterized initially by loss of erections with preserved ejaculation and orgasm (McCulloch & Wu 1982). Diabetic impotence may also be caused by sensory and vascular dysfunction; this requires urological evaluation, since therapy may be available in some of these cases (Melman 1988). Postural hypotension is much less frequent and is sometimes aggravated by medication (Sheps 1976). A high resting heart rate and sinus arrythmia may occur. Genitourinary dysfunction may result – eventually

– in bladder atonia, overflow incontinence and urinary tract infections. The most common gastrointestinal symptom of autonomic diabetic neuropathy is constipation. It usually responds to symptomatic therapy. Nocturnal diarrhoea is infrequent and usually episodic and severe. Autonomic neuropathy has great potential consequences for the well-being of patients and is associated with an increased mortality rate (Ewing *et al.* 1980; Sampson *et al.* 1990).

Treatment has little influence on symmetrical distal sensory and autonomic neuropathy. Rigid control of glycaemia with an insulin pump has been shown to retard deterioration in comparison with conventional insulin treatment but does not improve neuropathy (Dyck *et al.* 1986*a*; DCCT Research Trial 1995). Pancreatic transplantation may slow the progression of diabetic neuropathy (Kennedy *et al.* 1990). Symptomatic treatment is required for pain and signs of autonomic neuropathy.

Symmetrical proximal lower extremity motor neuropathy (diabetic amyotrophy) Initial symptoms are low back or thigh pain, followed by weakness of hip and thigh muscles (Casey & Harrison 1972; Subramony & Wilburn 1982). Progression of weakness often continues over a period of weeks or months. This neuropathy usually develops in individuals over 50 years of age with poorly controlled or undetected diabetes. In cases of insidious onset, recovery is often disappointing. When the course is more rapid, satisfactory recovery may occur following good diabetic control.

Focal and multifocal neuropathy

Mononeuropathies The mononeuropathies are less common than the polyneuropathies and occur mostly in elderly patients. They may appear earlier in the course of the disease than the symmetric polyneuropathies. Cranial nerves (the occulomotor nerve in particular), practically all limb nerves and truncal nerves may become involved (Zorilla & Kozak 1967; Thomas & Tomlinson 1993). The cranial and truncal neuropathies present with loss of sensory or motor function and are often associated with pain. These neuropathies have an acute onset and a relatively good prognosis. The mononeuropathies in the limbs are most often due to pressure or entrapment. Diabetic nerves respond less favourably to decompression than is customary for normal nerves.

Asymmetric proximal lower limb motor neuropathy (diabetic amyotrophy) This neuropathy usually occurs in individuals over the age of 50 years. Typical clinical features are pain (most prominent at night) and asymmetric proximal weakness. Most patients improve slowly and recover partially or wholly (Casey & Harrison 1972; Thomas & Tomlinson 1993). It is doubtful whether this syndrome really has to be distinguished from symmetric proximal motor neuropathy.

Uraemic neuropathy

In the 1960s and early 1970s, polyneuropathy proved to be a frequent and sometimes severe complication of endstage renal failure and an important problem in the management of patients treated with intermittent haemodialysis (Jennekens & Jennekens-Schinkel 1989; Asbury 1993). Nowadays, dialysis treatment of patients with chronic renal failure is initiated before clinical signs of neuropathy have developed. If dialysis treatment is adequate, be it long-term intermittent haemodialysis or continuous ambulatory peritoneal dialysis, neuropathy is only a problem in exceptional cases (Dazzi *et al.* 1991; Ropper 1993). Successful transplantation restores renal function and in most patients leads to full clinical recovery from neuropathy, at least if clinical manifestations of neuropathy are present. Nerve conduction also improves (Bolton & Young 1990).

Polyneuropathy due to nutritional deficiency and alcoholism

Alcoholic polyneuropathy

Neuropathy in alcoholism is always associated with inadequate nutrition leading to vitamin deficiency. It is not known whether the neuropathy is due to a toxic effect of alcohol, to malnutrition, or to both. The neuropathy is a distal, symmetrical syndrome of the lower limbs which is initially mainly sensory. At later stages, this is complicated by sensory (and cerebellar) ataxia, distal weakness and autonomic symptoms (Behse & Buchthal 1977). Treatment includes abstinence from alcohol, a high-calorie, protein-rich diet, multiple vitamin supplements and intramuscular injections of thiamine. The prognosis is good when the neuropathy is moderate or mild, but recovery takes a few months. Treatment initiated in the later stages of neuropathy may rapidly alleviate paraesthesiae, but improvement in strength may not appear until much later. The prognosis of untreated alcohol-nutritional deficiency neuropathy is poor (Hawley *et al.* 1982; Hillbom & Wennberg 1984).

Vitamin B and E deficiency

In the Western world thiamine deficiency is generally associated with alcoholism, but can also occur when a thiamine-poor diet is used for other reasons. The symptoms, signs, course and prognosis are closely similar to those described in alcohol-nutritional deficiency polyneuropathy. Treatment consists of intramuscular injection of 50 mg thiamine daily for 2 weeks, followed by 5 mg per day orally. Pyridoxine deficiency may cause a mild sensory polyneuropathy. Deficiency may be induced by treatment with the antituberculous drug isonicotinic acid hydrazide and the antihypertensive drug hydralazine. Oral pyridoxine supplementation at 100 mg/day prevents neuropathy. Vitamin B_{12} (cobalamin) deficiency may develop in patients with a malabsorption syndrome due to pernicious anaemia. It causes a peripheral sensory neuropathy with decreased tendon reflexes and abnormal conduction of sensory nerves and a more severe disorder of long tracts in the spinal cord. Prevention is possible by monthly intramuscular injections of approximately 300 μg. Vitamin E deficiency is a feature of lipid malabsorption syndromes, i.e. abetalipoproteinaemia, cystic fibrosis and congenital biliary atresia. It results in a mixed sensory and spinocerebellar syndrome. It can be prevented by administering high oral doses of vitamin E, while checking serum levels.

Inflammatory, infective and immune neuropathies

Guillain–Barré syndrome

Guillain–Barré syndrome (GBS) is a predominantly motor neuropathy with a subacute onset, but several variants of the syndrome have been described. The degree of paralysis is variable, ranging from a mild footdrop to paralysis of the limbs with facial and even oculomotor weakness. Respiratory insufficiency often occurs and patients may require artificial ventilation. Sensory symptoms, usually paraesthesiae in the hands and feet, are mild in most cases, but more severe sensory loss or ataxia may be present. Autonomic dysfunction occurs in many cases and may lead to life-threatening complications.

The course of the disease is usually subdivided into a progressive, a plateau and a recovery phase. Symptom progression is complete after 2 weeks in over 50% of cases, after 3 weeks in over 80%, and after 4 weeks in over 90% (Loffel et al. 1977; Mascucci & Kurzke 1971; Ropper et al. 1991). The plateau phase is of variable but usually short duration. Recovery over a period of weeks or months is typical of GBS, but most patients have some residual deficit. Three to 8 per cent die due to complications such as sepsis, adult respiratory distress syndrome, pulmonary emboli or cardiac arrest (Pleasure et al. 1968; Winer et al. 1985; Ropper 1986, 1992). Many survivors continue to have minor problems, such as footdrop or distal numbness, that do not impair the conduct of everyday life. Permanent disabling weakness, ataxia, paraesthesiae or sensory loss occurs in 5–10%, occasionally leading to wheelchair dependency (Sobue et al. 1983; Winer et al. 1985; Ropper 1986, 1992). Muscle strength may take up to 2 years to reach its optimum (Pleasure et al. 1968). GBS itself does not result in chronic fatigue, but mild depression, indicated by persistent mental fatigue, is common. A few men have suffered residual impotence (Ropper 1992).

Some features of the initial clinical illness are of help in predicting the eventual outcome (Loffel et al. 1977; McKann et al. 1988). In general, individuals who experience only mild distal extremity weakness and begin to improve within weeks of the onset enjoy excellent recovery. Poor outcome is associated with old age, rapid onset of neurological deficit, need for ventilatory support, and mean amplitude of compound muscle action potentials following distal nerve stimulation < 20% of normal. Recent studies suggest a poor outcome in patients with high antibody titres to the GM1 ganglioside, sometimes preceded by a *Campylobacter jejuni* infection (Yuki *et al.* 1990; Van den Berg *et al.* 1992). Children have a better prognosis and the electrodiagnostic prognostic factors may not apply in children (Bradshaw & Jones 1992).

When started within 2 weeks of the disease, plasma exchange has proved to be beneficial to the outcome of GBS (Guillain–Barré Study Group 1984; Osterman *et al.* 1984; French Cooperative Group 1987). The time before patients were able to walk unassisted and the duration of mechanical ventilation were halved by plasma exchange, and the outcome at 6 months was improved. In a randomized trial, intravenous infusion of immunoglobulin (IVIg) was found to be at least as effective as plasma exchange (Van der Meché & Schmitz 1992). In patients with GBS without sensory loss it was shown that treatment with IVIg was significantly better than plasma exchange (Visser *et al.* 1995). Good respiratory and medical care in the intensive care unit has also proved to be important in the treatment of GBS. The prevention of infection and other complications is a central feature of treatment, since 25% of patients acquire pneumonia and 30% develop urinary tract infections (Pleasure *et al.* 1968; Hughes 1990; Ropper 1992).

Chronic inflammatory demyelinating polyradiculoneuropathy (CIDP)

CIDP is a demyelinating polyneuropathy whose course differs from GBS in that its progression is measured in months or years. Generally it is not a self-limiting disease. CIDP is a sensorimotor neuropathy with a variable motor predominance. There are two major types of the disease – a chronic progressive and a relapsing–remitting type – with considerable overlap (Thomas *et al.* 1969; Dyck *et al.* 1975; McCombe *et al.* 1987c; Barohn *et al.* 1989a). The duration of progression, number of relapses and severity are unpredictable at onset. The course of the relapsing type displays a considerable range in the interval between relapses, the severity of an episode, and the rate and degree of recovery. When adequately treated, improvement between episodes is generally satisfactory. Many relapsing cases resolve after a few years (Prineas & McLeod 1976). Patients with a relapsing course are considered to have a more favourable prognosis than those with the progressive form, but one study found the differences in disability were not significant in prolonged follow-up (McCombe *et al.* 1987c).

The course of the non-relapsing form is either stepwise or gradual. If untreated this condition may become disabling or fatal. With treatment the prognosis significantly improves (Dyck *et al.* 1982, 1986b). In two large series, up to 30% of patients eventually made a complete recovery with steroid treatment, plasma exchange, or both. IVIg has proved beneficial in some cases (Vermeulen *et al.* 1993). One series of 92 cases with a mean follow up of 6.5 years disclosed that 34% had minimal or no disability, 31% had mild motor and sensory signs, 24% were moderately disabled, 3% required assistance in daily activities, and 7% died (McCombe *et al.* 1987c). Several authors have suggested that pregnancy initiates relapses (McCombe *et al.* 1987b). In some patients CIDP is associated with HIV infections (see below), systemic lupus erythematosus, lymphoma or Castleman's disease (Brunet *et al.* 1981; Rechthand *et al.* 1984; McCombe *et al.* 1987*a*; Donaghy *et al.* 1989).

Multifocal motor neuropathy

Multifocal motor neuropathy (MMN) is a recently recognized neuropathy with the clinical presentation of asymmetrical progressive muscular atrophy: progressive asymmetrical weakness and muscle wasting without sensory loss (Krarup *et al.* 1990; Lange *et al.* 1992). The diagnosis is made by the presence of conduction block on electrophysiological examination. MMN may be associated with raised IgM anti-GM1 antibodies. The identification of MMN in patients presenting with a lower motor neuron disease is important, as MMN is a potentially treatable disease. Treatment with cyclophosphamide or high-dose intravenous immunoglobulins may lead to improvement in muscle strength (Pestronk *et al.* 1988; Chaudry *et al.* 1993; Nobile-Orazio *et al.* 1993; Azulay *et al.* 1994; Van den Berg *et al.* 1995*a,b*). Little is known of the prognosis and long-term effect of treatment of MMN (Van den Berg *et al.* 1994; Elliott *et al.* 1994).

Inflammatory sensory neuronopathy (ganglionitis)

Pathological examination has shown that *inflammatory sensory neuronopathy* is an inflammatory disorder, predominantly of the dorsal root ganglia. Small inflammatory cell infiltrates have, however, also been seen in sural nerve biopsies. The onset of this syndrome is often acute or subacute, but it may be chronic (Griffin *et al.* 1990; Windebank *et al.* 1990). Presenting symptoms are numbness, pain and insufficient coordination, mainly in the lower limbs, or in upper and lower limbs. Examination reveals a symmetric or occasionally asymmetric syndrome with loss of all sensory modalities and often a severe form of sensory ataxia. Symptoms of autonomic neuropathy have been reported. There is no muscle weakness. The syndrome may be associated with other diseases: carcinoma of the lung and other malignancies (Horwich *et al.* 1977; McLeod 1993), Sjögren syndrome (Hull *et al.* 1984; Smith *et al.* 1993), paraproteinaemia, coeliac disease. Treatment with immunosuppressive agents is not clearly effective, either when onset is acute or subacute or in the more chronic varieties. The course is usually chronic. Some degree of spontaneous improvement has been observed. In one of our patients sensory ataxia largely disappeared and weakness with marked slowing of nerve conduction, compatible with CIDP, developed gradually.

Trigeminal neuropathy is another pure sensory syndrome, numbness and pain being the main complaints, with loss of pain and touch sensation at examination. The syndrome is mostly bilateral and often asymmetric. It is probably a special form of ganglionitis. It may occur in Sjögren syndrome, systemic sclerosis, mixed connective tissue disease or undifferentiated connective tissue disease (Hagen *et al.* 1990). A few patients experience some improvement over a period of years.

Vasculitic neuropathy

Vasculitic neuropathy is a disease usually occurring in adults. Patients typically present with the clinical syndrome of multiple mononeuropathies, in which many single peripheral or cranial nerves are affected. Onset is often sudden, with local prickling paraesthesiae and pain, and weakness and sensory loss. The course may, however, be more chronic and in these cases the patient may present with a symmetric or asymmetric sensorimotor polyneuropathy (Chang *et al.* 1984; Bouche *et al.* 1986; Kisell *et al.* 1985; Chalk *et al.* 1993). Vasculitis may preferentially affect small vessels (hypersensitivity angiitis; usually without neuropathy), medium-sized vessels (polyarteritis nodosa or PAN, Churg–Strauss syndrome, Wegener granulomatosis; often without peripheral neuropathy) or large vessels (temporal arteritis and Takayasu arteritis; occasionally with neuropathy). Vasculitic neuropathy may complicate the connective tissue diseases, in particular rheumatoid arthritis and Sjögren syndrome, but is very unusual in systemic sclerosis. Vasculitic neuropathy may also occur on its own, without involvement of any other organ (non-systemic vasculitic neuropathy) (Dyck *et al.* 1987).

Acute vasculitic neuropathy can result in a dramatic loss of all myelinated nerve fibres and many Schwann cells from a peripheral nerve within a matter of days or weeks; it is difficult to recover from such a condition. Early diagnosis and treatment with high doses of corticosteroids is required in these cases and the outcome is often good. Controlled trials, however, have never been performed. When corticosteroids are not effective, cyclophosphamide should be considered (Fauci *et al.* 1979; Enevoldson & Wiles 1991). The prognosis for life is less favourable in systemic than in non-systemic vasculitic neuropathy (Dyck *et al.* 1987).

HIV-related peripheral neuropathy

HIV-related neuropathies include acute and chronic inflammatory demyelinating neuropathies, cranial neuropathies, mononeuropathy multiplex, progressive radiculopathy, dorsal root ganglioneuritis, distal symmetric sensorimotor neuropathy (DSPN) and an autonomic neuropathy (De la Monte *et al.* 1988; So *et al.* 1988; Vishnubhakat & Beresford 1988; Barohn *et al.* 1989*b*). With time, the majority of AIDS patients develop some degree of symptomatic neuropathy (Winer *et al.* 1992; Husstedt *et al.* 1993). In contrast, AIDS in childhood is usually not complicated by peripheral neuropathy (Koch *et al.* 1989). All types of neuropathy can occur at any stage of infection, but the inflammatory demyelinating neuropathies are associated with relative immunocompetence in the early stages of HIV infection and the later-onset DSPN with AIDS. The course and prognosis of the inflammatory demyelinating neuropathies with or without HIV infection is similar. The neuropathy responds well to treatment with plasma exchange or immunoglobulin (Miller *et al.* 1986; Cornblath 1988). The most common form of neuropathy in HIV-infected patients is a distal symmetric sensory or sensorimotor neuropathy. Sensory impairment such as numbness and painful dysaesthesiae is usually much more prominent than weakness. The hands are rarely involved. The course of the neuropathy is slowly progressive or occasionally non-progressive. Spontaneous remissions are rare; in one case, treatment with AZT resulted in mild improvement (Dalakas *et al.* 1988). The pathogenesis of DSPN is unknown. Treatment is symptomatic.

Lyme disease

Within weeks of inoculation the spirochaete causing the infection of Lyme disease spreads from the skin to other parts of the body and from that time on patients may present with various types of peripheral neuropathy, including cranial neuropathy (most often facial nerve weakness mimicking Bell's palsy), radiculoneuropathy, plexopathy, meningoradiculopathy, symmetric or asymmetric polyneuropathy and a syndrome resembling GBS (Clark *et al.* 1985; Steere 1989). Antibiotics improve symptoms, prevent progression to later stages, and can eradicate the infection in nearly all patients (Garcia-Monco & Benach 1995; Steere 1989; Luft *et al.* 1989; Halperin *et al.* 1990). The role of corticosteroids has not been clearly established. A randomized study showed steroids as efficacious as penicillin in relieving pain in lymphocytic meningoradiculitis/polyneuritis. In a long-term follow-up, patients treated with steroids and antibiotics tended to recover faster than did those treated with antibiotics alone (Garcia-Monco & Benach 1995).

Leprosy

Leprosy is predominantly, though not exclusively, a disease of nerves. *Mycobacterium leprae* invades the peripheral nerves and shows a preference for cutaneous nerves in cool parts of the body (earlobes, nose, scrotum, distal parts of the limbs). Currently, the number of patients registered with leprosy is approximately 1.7 million (Noordeen, 1995). Worldwide, the disease is on the retreat and optimists foresee the possibility of its total eradication. This prospect is based on the favourable effects obtained with the drug regimens recommended by the World Health Organization in 1982 (Sabin *et al.* 1993; Jamil *et al.* 1993). Until that time monotherapy with dapsone was customary for all forms of leprosy. Dapsone is bacteriostatic and weakly bactericidal. For patients with paucibacillary forms of leprosy (indeterminate, tuberculoid leprosy and borderline tuberculoid leprosy), monotherapy was probably sufficient to eliminate all viable bacilli, but this aim was not achieved in the multibacillary forms (borderline-borderline, borderline lepromatous and lepromatous leprosy). In addition, monotherapy appeared to result in drug resistance to dapsone. Combination therapy with two or three drugs, each with a different mechanism of action and including at least one bactericidal drug, seemed an attractive alternative, as it would allow for shorter treatment periods and would reduce the chance of drug resistance. Multi-drug therapy is now widely applied, using dapsone, rifampicin, clofazimin and other compounds.

Patients are non-infectious from a few days after initiation of therapy and can no longer spread the infection. Therapy is continued for at least 2 years, and until no viable bacilli can be demonstrated in skin smears. The infection has then been conquered and relapses are rare. As far as the individual patient is concerned, however, deformities, mutilations and insensitive skin areas with the risk of ulcers remain. The patient needs advice with a view to rehabilitation, but this is often not available in less developed countries where the disease is endemic.

Neuropathy associated with monoclonal gammopathy

Peripheral neuropathy may be associated with monoclonal gammopathy, which can be benign or result from a haematological malignancy (Kelly *et al.* 1987). A better term for a benign monoclonal gammopathy is monoclonal gammopathy of undetermined significance (MGUS), as a malignancy may subsequently develop (Kyle 1978). Practically all types of neuropathy have been described in association with monoclonal gammopathy. MGUS, however, occurs in about 1% of the healthy population over the age of 50 years and in 3% of those over the age of 70 years. Therefore it is not always clear whether the monoclonal gammopathy is coincidental or the cause of neuropathy. It is has been shown that half the patients with neuropathy associated with IgM monoclonal gammopathies have antibodies to the myelin associated glycoprotein (MAG). The course of the neuropathy associated with anti-MAG antibodies is slowly progressive, but may be static for years. Immunosuppressive treatment and/or plasmapheresis may lead to clinical improvement in patients with neuropathy associated with monoclonal gammopathy (Pestronk 1995). Neuropathy associated with IgG or IgA monoclonal gammopathy generally responds better to treatment than IgM monoclonal gammopathy (Kyle & Dyck 1993). A prospective study of polyneuropathy associated with MGUS showed that polyneuropathy in IgM-MGUS is more progressive with significantly more weakness and sensory signs (Notermans *et al.* 1994*b*). These studies indicate that the neuropathies associated with IgM-MGUS and IgG/A-MGUS may be two different entities. However, more studies are necessary on the long-term outcome, treatment and predictive features in neuropathy associated with monoclonal gammopathy.

Critical illness polyneuropathy

Patients suffering from sepsis and multi-organ failure or polytrauma may react by developing a 'systemic inflammatory response syndrome' (SIRS). Among the complications of this syndrome are different types of myopathy and a so-called critical illness polyneuropathy. Once the underlying condition that has caused SIRS is under control, it may appear that there are difficulties in weaning the patient from the ventilator. This is most often due to cardiac and pulmonary causes, but when these are excluded a neuromuscular origin should be considered. Diagnosis of the neuropathy is usually not possible on clinical examination alone. The limbs are weak and atrophic, due either to the myopathy or neuropathy, and the tendon reflexes may be reduced. A reliable investigation of sensibility is often impossible. Neurophysiological tests of motor nerves and of muscle may not be helpful. The best method of establishing that weakness is at least in part due to neuropathy is to examine the sensory nerve conduction and to demonstrate depression of sensory nerve action potentials (SNAPs) or, even better, progressive decrease of SNAPs by serial examinations. The neuropathy is primarily axonal and predominantly distal. Dependent on its severity, recovery follows in weeks or months but may remain partial in the most serious cases (Bolton 1995; Leijten *et al.* 1995).

Toxic neuropathies

A number of pharmaceutical compounds and some occupational, biological and environmental agents may produce a mostly distal axonopathy (Schaumberg *et al.* 1991*b*). Complete or partial recovery often occurs if therapy or exposure is stopped, but there are striking differences between agents. This can be illustrated by two examples. Thalidomide was initially used as a hypnotic, in relatively high doses, and produced a predominantly sensory axonal neuropathy in some patients. Recovery was poor and patients complained for years of painful paraesthesiae (Fullerton & O'Sullivan 1968). However, a patient with vincristine neuropathy following, the use of this drug in cancer, which is also axonal though probably not neuronal, can recover rapidly (Casey *et al.* 1973). Other agents each have their own characteristic pattern of recovery.

Idiopathic polyneuropathy

The percentage of patients with idiopathic neuropathies has decreased markedly (from 50–70% in the 1950s to 10–15% in more recent studies) following the recognition of new entities such as CIDP and neuropathy associated with monoclonal gammopathy, and from improved classification systems as in hereditary neuropathies (Notermans *et al.* 1993). Nevertheless, a group of patients remains in whom a diagnosis cannot be made. A recent study has identified most of these patients as suffering from chronic idiopathic axonal polyneuropathy (CIAP) (Notermans *et al.* 1993). The neuropathy was pure sensory or sensorimotor and a 5 year follow-up study of 75 patients showed that the overall clinical course was slowly progressive and handicap, if present, not severe (Notermans *et al.* 1994*a*).

Mononeuropathies

Idiopathic facial paralysis (Bell's palsy)

Idiopathic facial paralysis appears in all age groups (Katusic *et al.* 1986; Hauser *et al.* 1971). Rarely the disorder is recurrent, bilateral or familial (Yanagihara *et al.* 1984; Pitts *et al.* 1988). Facial weakness usually develops within a few hours or evolves over 1 or 2 days. Recovery can be rapid and complete, or it can be delayed and partial. About half the patients recover completely. Ten to fifteen per cent of the patients are dissatisfied with their recovery (Hauser *et al.* 1971). Incomplete paralysis predicts a favourable outcome. Patients who start to show improvement in an average of 10 days, recover completely in approximately 2 months. When recovery has not yet started 2 months after onset, there is likely to be some residual abnormality. Treatment with cortico-steroids is advocated by some authors, but its effectiveness in shortening the period of recovery or the percentage of patients with incomplete recovery has not been convinc-ingly demonstrated.

Entrapment neuropathies: carpal tunnel syndrome

The most common entrapment neuropathy is compression of the median nerve at the wrist, carpal tunnel syndrome (CTS). It usually presents with numbness, tingling and burning sensations in the first three digits (Steward 1987; Dawson *et al.* 1990). The majority of patients are healthy middle-aged women or people who use their hands in repetitive stereotypical fashion. In some patients, however, carpal tunnel syndrome is related to pregnancy, diabetes mellitus, hypothyroidism, acromegaly, or amyloid in the carpal tunnel (in amyloid neuropathy and in patients treated by long-term intermittent haemodialysis). Corticosteroid injections into the carpal tunnel may alleviate mild symptoms. Surgery is indicated when entrapment is permanent, the cause of entrap-ment cannot be eliminated, conservative therapy fails to alleviate abnormal sensations or when thenar weakness or atrophy (evidence of axonal injury) develops. Surgery is effective in relieving pain and stopping the progression of weakness in almost all cases. Mild weakness disappears, but more severe loss of muscle power and bulk recovers incompletely or not at all.

Traumatic injury of peripheral nerves

The outcome of peripheral nerve injury can vary greatly, depending on factors such as the level of injury (distal or proximal), the type of nerve lesion (lesions in continuity or lesions disrupting continuity), the type of wound (laceration of nerve with associated soft tissue trauma or sharp clean-cut nerve lesions), the age of the patient, associated injuries and medical or surgical management (Sunderland, 1978; Lundborg, 1988). Some nerves recover better than others. For example, in the upper extremity the radial and median nerve have a better prognosis than the ulnar nerve and in the lower extremity injury of the tibial nerve has a good prognosis but recovery of the peroneal nerve is reputed to be poor. Children have a better prognosis than adults. For theoreti-cal reasons, primary suturing of lesioned nerves is to be preferred, but when there is considerable soft tissue trauma, nerve repair should be postponed until adequate excision of scar tissue can be performed. Whatever type of nerve suture is chosen – epineurial or fascicular – a considerable misdirection of axons at the site of the suture is unavoidable and a number of axons will reinnervate incorrect target cells. The brain has to adapt to an altered pattern of innervation.

Brachial plexus injuries

Brachial plexus injuries may be acute or develop slowly, and may affect the plexus diffusely or in a restricted manner. Severe traction injuries commonly result in combined plexus and root damage (avulsions) and offer little hope of recovery (Leffert, 1985; Thomeer & Marani, 1993). Multiple distal peripheral nerve injuries may coexist, confusing the initial assessment and complicating recovery. Avulsions involve ventral roots more than dorsal roots, resulting in greater motor than sensory impairment. Implantation of the ventral roots into the ventral horns of the spinal cord allows for entry of regenerating axons into the roots; this technique may prove to be of interest from the therapeutic viewpoint (Carlstedt, 1993). Brachial plexus lesions, secondary to fractures and dislocations around the shoulder, generally recover well.

References

Andrade, C. (1952). A peculiar form of peripheral neuropathy: familial atypical generalized amyloidosis with special involvement of the peripheral nerves. *Brain* **75**, 408–27.

Appenzeller, O. & Kornfeld, M. (1973). Acute pandysautonomia. Clinical and morphological study. *Arch. Neurol.* **29**, 334–49.

Archer, A. G., Watkins, P. J., Thomas, P. K. *et al.* (1983). The natural history of acute painful neuropathy in diabetes mellitus. *J. Neurol. Neurosurg. Psychiatry* **46**, 491–7.

Asbury, A. K. (1993). Neuropathies with renal failure, hepatic disorders, chronic respiratory insufficiency and critical illness. In: *Peripheral Neuropathy*, 3rd edn, vol. 2, eds. P. C. Dyck, P. K. Thomas, pp. 1251–65. Philadelphia: Saunders.

Azulay, J. P., Blin, O., Pouget, J. *et al.* (1994). Intravenous immunoglobulin treatment in patients with motor neuron syndromes associated with anti-GM1 antibodies: a double-blind, placebo-controlled study. *Neurology* **44**, 429–32.

Barohn, R., Kissel, J. T., Warmolts, J. R. & Mendell, J. R. (1989*a*). Chronic inflammatory polyradiculoneuropathy. Clinical characteristics, course, and recommendations for diagnositic criteria. *Arch. Neurol.* **46**, 878–84.

Barohn, R. J., LeForce, B. R., McVey, A. L. *et al.* (1989*b*). Peripheral nervous system involvement in human immunodeficiency virus (HIV) infection: a prospective study of a large cohort of HIV-seropositive individuals. *Muscle Nerve* **12**, 762–9.

Barohn, R. J., Gronseth, E., LeForce, B. R. *et al.* (1993). Peripheral nervous system involvement in a large cohort of HIV-infected individuals. *Arch. Neurol.* **50**, 167–71.

Bazzi, C., Pagani, C., Sorgato, G. *et al.* (1991). Uremic polyneuropathy: a clinical and electrophysiological study in 135 short- and long-term hemodialyzed patients. *Clin. Nephrol.* **35**, 176–81.

Behse, F. & Buchthal, F. (1977). Alcoholic neuropathy: clinical, electrophysiological and biopsy findings. *Ann. Neurol.* **2**, 95–101.

Ben Othmane, K. B., Hentati, F., Lennon, F. *et al.* (1993). Linkage of a locus (CMT4A) for autosomal recessive Charcot-Marie-Tooth disease to chromosome 8q. *Hum. Molec. Genet.* **2**, 1625–8.

Berger, A. R. & Schaumburg, H. H. (1988). Rehabilitation of peripheral neuropathies. *J. Neurol. Rehabil.* **2**, 25–6.

Bird, T. D. & Kraft, G. K. (1978). Charcot-Marie-Tooth disease: data for genetic counselling. *Clin. Genet.* **14**, 43–9.

Blume, G., Pestronk, A. & Goodnough, L. T. (1995). Anti-MAG antibody associated polyneuropathy: improvement following immunotherapy with monthly plasma exchange and i.v. cyclophosphamide. *Neurology* **45**, 1577–80.

Blumenfeld, A., Slaugenhaupt, S. A., Axelrod, F. B. *et al.* (1993). Localization of the gene for familial dysautonomia on chromosome 9 and definition of DNA markers for genetic diagnosis. *Nature (Genet)* **4**, 160–4.

Bolton, C. F. (1995). Critical illness polyneuropathy. In *Peripheral Nerve Disorders* 2, eds. A. K. Asbury, P. K. Thomas, pp. 262–80. Oxford: Butterworth Heinemann.

Bolton, C. F. & Young, G. B. (1990). *Neurological Complications of Renal Disease*, pp. 1–250. Stoneham: Butterworth.

Bouche, P., Leger, J. M., Travers, M. A. *et al.* (1986). Peripheral neuropathy in systemic vasculitis: clinical and electrophysiological study of 22 patients. *Neurology* **36**, 1598–602.

Bradshaw, D. Y. & Jones, H. R. (1992). Guillain-Barré syndrome in children: clinical course, electrodiagnosis, and prognosis. *Muscle Nerve* **15**, 500–6.

Brunet, P., Binet, J. L., Saxce, H. *et al.* (1981). Neuropathies au cours de lay lymphadenopathie angio-immunoblastique. *Rev. Neurol.* **137**, 503–15.

Carlstedt, T. (1993). Functional recovery after ventral root avulsion. *Clin. Neurol. Neurosurg.* **95** (Suppl.), S109–S111.

Casey, E. B. & Harrison, M. J. G. (1972). Diabetic amyotrophy: a follow-up study. *BMJ* I, 656–61.

Casey, E. B., Jeliffe, A. M., Le Quesne, P. M. *et al.* (1973). Vincristine neuropathy: clinical and electrophysiological observations. *Brain* **96**, 69–75.

Chalk, C. H., Dyck, P. J. & Conn, D. L. (1993). Vasculitic neuropathy. In: *Peripheral Neuropathy*, 3rd edn, vol. 2, eds. P. C. Dyck & P. K. Thomas, pp. 1424–36, Philadelphia: Saunders.

Chance, P. F., Bird, T. D., O'Connell, P. *et al.* (1990). Genetic linkage and heterogeneity in type I Charcot-Marie-Tooth disease (hereditary motor and sensory neuropathy type I). *Am. J. Hum. Genet.* **47**, 915–25.

Chance, P. F., Alderson, M. K., Leppig, K. A. *et al.* (1993). DNA deletion associated with hereditary neuropathy with liability to pressure palsies. *Cell* **72**, 143–51.

Chang, R. W., Bell, C. L. & Hallett, M. (1984). Clinical characteristics and prognosis of vasculitic mononeuropathy multiplex. *Arch. Neurol.* **41**, 618–24.

Chaudhry, V., Corse, A. M., Cornblath, D. R. *et al.* (1993). Multifocal motor neuropathy: response to human immune globulin. *Ann. Neurol.* **33**, 237–42.

Clark, J. R., Carlson, R. D., Sasaki, C. T. *et al.* (1985). Facial paralysis in Lyme disease. *Laryngoscope* **95**, 1341–7.

Cornblath, D. R. (1988). The treatment of the neuromuscular complications of human immunodeficiency virus infection. *Ann. Neurol.* **23**, S88–S91.

Dalakas, M. C. (1986). Chronic idiopathic ataxic neuropathy. *Ann. Neurol.* **19**, 545–54.

Dalakas, M. C., Yarchoan, R., Spitzer, R. *et al.* (1988). Treatment of human immunodeficiency virus-related polyneuropathy with 3'-azido-2',3'-dideoxythymidine. *Ann. Neurol.* **23**, S92–7.

Dawson, D., Hallett, M., Millender, L. (1990). *Entrapment Neuropathies*, 2nd edn. Boston: Little, Brown.

DCCT Research Trial (1995). Effect of intensive diabetes treatment on nerve conduction in the diabetes control and complications trial. *Ann. Neurol.* **38**, 869–80.

Debruyne, J., Dehaene, I. & Martin, J. J. (1980). Hereditary pressure-sensitive neuropathy. *J. Neurol. Sci.* **47**, 385–94.

De la Monte, S. M., Gabuzda, D. H., Ho, D. D. *et al.* (1988). Peripheral neuropathy in the acquired immunodeficiency syndrome. *Ann. Neurol.* **23**, 485–92.

Donaghy, M., Hall, P., Gawler, J. *et al.* (1989). Peripheral neuropathy associated with Castleman's disease. *Journal of Neurological Sciences* **89**, 253–67.

Donaghy, M., King, R. H., McKeran, R. O. *et al.* (1990). Cerebrotendinous xanthomatosis: clinical, electrophysiological and nerve biopsy findings, and response to treatment with chenodeoxylcholic acid. *J. Neurol.* **237**, 216–19.

Dyck, P. J. (1993). Neuronal atrophy and degeneration predominantly affecting peripheral sensory and autonomic neurons. In: *Peripheral Neuropathy*, 3rd edn, vol. 2, eds. P. C. Dyck & P. K. Thomas, pp. 1065–93. Philadelphia: Saunders.

Dyck, P. J., Benstead, T. J., Conn, D. L. *et al.* (1987). Nonsystemic vasculitic neuropathy. *Brain* **110**, 843–53.

Dyck, P. J., Brown, M., Greene, D. *et al.* (1986*a*). Does improved control of glycemia prevent or ameliorate diabetic polyneuropathy? *Ann. Neurol.* **19**, 288–93.

Dyck, P. J., Chance, P., Lebo, R. & Carney, J. A. (1993*a*). Hereditary motor and sensory neuropathies. In: *Peripheral Neuropathy*, 3rd edn, vol. 2, eds. P. C. Dyck & P. K. Thomas, pp. 1094–136. Philadelphia: Saunders.

Dyck, P. J., Daube, J. R., O'Brien, P. C. *et al.* (1986*b*). Plasma exchange in chronic inflammatory demyelinating polyradiculoneuropathy. *N. Engl. J. Med.* **314**, 416–25.

Dyck, P. J., Karnes, J. L., Daube, J. *et al.* (1985). Clinical and neuropathological criteria for the diagnosis and staging of diabetic polyneuropathy. *Brain* **108**, 861–9.

Dyck, P. J., Karnes, J. L. & Lambert, E. H. (1989). Longitudinal study of neuropathic deficits and nerve conduction abnormalities in hereditary motor and sensory neuropathy type 1. *Neurology* **39**, 1302–8.

Dyck, P. J., Kratz, K. M., Karnes, J. L. *et al.* (1993*b*). The prevalence by staged severity of various types of diabetic neuropathy, retinopathy, and nephropathy in a population-based cohort: The Rochester Diabetic Neuropathy Study. *Neurology* **43**, 817–24.

Dyck, P. J., Lais, A. C., Ohta, M. *et al.* (1975). Chronic inflammatory polyradiculoneuropathy. *Mayo Clin. Proc.* **50**, 621–8.

Dyck, P. J., O'Brien, P. C., Oviatt, K. F. *et al.* (1982). Prednisone improves chronic inflammatory demyelinating polyradiculoneuropathy more than no treatment. *Ann. Neurol.* **11**, 136–41.

Dyck, P. J., Oviatt, K. F. & Lambert, E. H. (1981). Intensive evaluation of unclassified neuropathies yields improved diagnosis. *Ann. Neurol.* **10**, 222–9.

Elliott, J. L. & Pestronk, A. (1994). Progression of multifocal motor neuropathy during apparently successful treatment with human immunoglobulin. *Neurology* **44**, 967–8.

Enevoldson, T. P. & Wiles, C. M. (1991). Severe vasculitic neuropathy in systemic lupus erythematosus and response to cyclophosphamide. *J. Neurol. Neurosurg. Psychiatry* **54**, 468–9.

Ewing, D. J., Campbell, I. W. & Clarke, B. F. (1980). The natural history of diabetic autonomic neuropathy. *Q. J. Med.* **193**, 95–100.

Fauci, A. S., Katz, P., Haynes, B. F. & Wolff, S. M. (1979). Cyclophosphamide therapy of severe systemic necrotizing vasculitis. *N. Engl. J. Med.* **301**, 235–41.

Feldman, M. & Schiller, L. R. (1983). Disorders of gastrointestinal motility associated with diabetes mellitus. *Am. J. Intern. Med.* **98**, 378–84.

Filling-Katz, M. R., Merrick, H. F., Fink, J. K. *et al.* (1989). Carbamazepine in Fabry's disease: effective analgesia with dose-dependent exacerbation of autonomic dysfunction. *Neurology* **39**, 598–603.

French Cooperative Group on Plasma Exchange in Guillain-Barre Syndrome (1987). Efficiency of plasma-exchange in Guillain-Barre syndrome: role of replacement fluids. *Ann. Neurol.* **22**, 753–61.

Fryns, J. P. & Van den Berghe, H. (1980). Sex-linked recessive inheritance in Charcot-Marie-Tooth disease with partial manifestations in female carriers. *Hum. Genet.* **55**, 413–15.

Fullerton, P. M., O'Sullivan, D. J. (1968). Thalidomide neuropathy: a clinical, electrophysiological and histological follow-up. *J. Neurol. Neurosurg. Psychiatry* **31**, 543–8.

Gabreëls-Festen, A. A. W. M., Gabreëls, F. J. M., Jennekens, F. G. I. *et al.* (1991). Hereditary motor and sensory neuropathy of neuronal type with onset in early childhood. *Brain* **114**, 855–70.

Gabreëls, F. J. M., Jennekens, F. G. I. *et al.* (1992*a*). Autosomal recessive form of motor and sensory neuropathy type I. *Neurology* **42**, 1755–61.

Gabreëls-Festen, A. A. W. M., Gabreëls, F. J. M., Joosten, E. M. G. *et al.* (1992). Hereditary neuropathy with liability to pressure palsies in childhood. *Neuropaediatrics* **23**, 138–43.

Gabreëls-Festen, A. A. W. M., Gabreëls, F. J. M., Jennekens, F. G. I. & Jansen-van Kempen, T. W. (1993). The status of HMSN TYPE III. *Neuromusc. Disord.* **4**, 63–9.

Garcia-Monco, J. C. & Benach, J. L. (1995). Lyme borreliosis. *Ann. Neurol.* **37**, 691–702.

Goulder, R., LeGuern, E., Gugenheim, M. *et al.* (1995). Clinical, electrophysiologic, and molecular correlations in 13 families with hereditary neuropathy with liability to pressure palsies and a chromosome 17p11.2 deletion. *Neurology* **45**, 2018–23.

Griffin, J. W., Cornblath, D. R., Alexander, E. *et al.* (1990). Ataxic sensory neuropathy and dorsal root ganglionitis associated with Sjogren's syndrome. *Ann. Neurol.* **27**, 304–10.

Guillian-Barre Syndrome Study Group (1984). Plasmapheresis and acute Guillian-Barre syndrome. *Neurology* **35**, 1096–104.

Hagen, N. A., Stevens, J. C. & Michet, C. J. (1990). Trigeminal sensory neuropathy associated with connective tissue disease. *Neurology* **40**, 891–6.

Halperin, J. J., Luft, B. J., Volman, J. J. *et al.* (1990). Lyme borreliosis: peripheral nervous system and manifestations. *Brain* **113**, 1207–21.

Harding, A. E. (1995). From the syndrome of Charcot-Marie and Tooth to disorders of peripheral myelin proteins. *Brain* **118**, 809–18.

Harding, A. E. & Reilly, M. M. (1995). Molecular genetics of inherited neuropathies. In: *Peripheral Nerve Disorders 2*, eds. A. K. Asbury & P. K. Thomas, pp. 118–39. Oxford: Butterworth Heinemann.

Harding, A. E. & Thomas, P. K. (1980). The clinical features of hereditary motor and sensory neuropathy types I and II. *Brain* **103**, 259–80.

Hauser, W. A., Karnes, W. E., Annis, J. & Kurland, L. T. (1971). Incidence and prognosis of Bell's palsy in the population of Rochester, Minnesota. *Mayo Clin. Proc.* **46**, 258–66.

Hawley, R., Kurtze, J. F., Armbrustmacher, V. W. *et al.* (1982). The course of alcoholic-nutritional peripheral neuropathy. *Acta Neurol. Scand.* **66**, 582–7.

Heckmann, J. M., Carr, J. A. & Bell, N. (1995). Hereditary sensory and autonomic neuropathy with cataract, mental retardation and skin lesions: five cases. *Neurology* **45**, 1405–8.

Hentati, A., Lamy, C., Melki, J. *et al.* (1992). Clinical and genetic heterogeneity of Charcot-Marie-tooth disease. *Genomics* **12**, 155–7.

Hillbom, M. & Wenneberg, A. (1984). Prognosis of alcoholic peripheral neuropathy. *J. Neurol. Neurosurg. Psychiatry* **47**, 699–706.

Hoogendijk, J. E., Jansen, E. A. M., Gabreëls-Festen, A. A. W. M. *et al.* (1993). Allelic heterogeneity in hereditary motor and sensory neuropathy type Ia (Charcot-Marie-Tooth type 1a). *Neurology* **43**, 1010–15.

Horwich, M. S., Cho, L., Posner, R. S. *et al.* (1977). Subacute sensory neuropathy: a remote effect of carcinoma. *Ann. Neurol.* **2**, 7–13.

Hughes, R. A. C. (1990). Guillain-Barré syndrome. London: Springer-Verlag.

Hull, R. G., Morgan, S. H., Harding, A. E. & Hughes, G. R. V. (1984). Sjögren's syndrome presenting as a severe sensory neuropathy including involvement of the trigeminal nerve. *Br. J. Rheumatol.* **23**, 301–9.

Husstedt, I. W., Grotemeyer, K. H., Busch, H. & Zidek, W. (1993). Progression of distal-symmetric polyneuropathy in HIV infection: a prospective study. *AIDS* **7**, 1069–73.

Ingall, T. J., McLeod, J. G. & Tamura, N. (1990). Autonomic function and unmyelinated fibres in chronic inflammatory demyelinating polyradiculoneuropathy. *Muscle Nerve* **13**, 70–6.

Ionasescu, V. V., Ionasesce, R., Searby, Ch. & Neahring, R. (1995). Dejerine-Sottas disease with de novo dominant point mutation of PMP22 gene. *Neurology* **46**, 1766–7.

Jamil, S., Keer, J. T., Lucas, B. *et al.* (1993). Use of polymerase chain reaction to assess efficacy of leprosy. *Lancet* **342**, 264–8.

Jennekens, F. G. I. (1987). Peripheral neuropathy in enzyme deficiencies and some other metabolic disorders. In: *Handbook of Clinical Neurology*, vol. 7, ed. W. B. Matthews, pp. 367–411. Amsterdam: Elsevier.

Jennekens, F. G. I. & Jennekens-Schinkel, A. (1989). Neurological aspects of dialysis patients. In: *Replacement of Renal Function by Dialysis*, 3rd edn, ed. J. F. Maher, pp. 978–86. Dordrecht: Kluwer.

Katusic, S. K., Beard, M., Widerholt, W. C. *et al.* (1986). Incidence, clinical features, and prognosis in Bell's palsy, Rochester, Minnesota, 1968–82. *Ann. Neurol.* **20**, 622–7.

Kelly, J. J., Kyle, R. A. & Latov, N. (1987). Polyneuropathies associated with plasma cell dyscrasias. Boston: Martinus Hijhoff.

Kennedy, W. R., Navarro, X., Goetz, F. C. *et al.* (1990). Effect of pancreatic transplantation on diabetic neuropathy. *N. Engl. J. Med.* **322**, 1031–7.

Kerkhoff, H. & Jennekens, F. G. I. (1993). Peripheral nerve lesions: the neuropharmacological outlook. *Clin. Neurol. Neurosurg.* **95** (Suppl.), S103–8.

Killian, J. M., Tiwari, P. S., Jacobson, S. *et al.* (1996). Longitudinal studies of the duplication of C.M.T. polyneuropathy. *Muscle Nerve* **19**, 74–8.

Kissel, J. T., Slivka, A. P., Warmolz, J. R. *et al.* (1985). The clinical spectrum of necrotizing angiopathy of the peripheral nervous system. *Ann. Neurol.* **18**, 251–7.

Kolodney, E. H., Raghavan, S. & Krivit, W. (1991). Late-onset Krabbe disease (globoid cell leukodystrophy): clinical and biochemical features of 15 cases. *Dev. Neurosci.* **13**, 232–9.

Krarup, C., Steward, J. B., Sumner, A. J. *et al.* (1990). A syndrome of asymmetric limb weakness with motor conduction block. *Neurology* **40**, 118–27.

Krendel, D. A., Costigan, D. A. & Hopkins, L. C. (1995). Successful treatment of neuropathies in patients with diabetes mellitus. *Arch. Neurol.* **52**, 1053–61.

Kulkens, T., Bolhuis, P. A., Wolterman, R. A. *et al.* (1993). Deletion of the codon for serine 34 from the major peripheral myelin protein P0 gene in Charcot-Marie-Tooth disease IB. *Nature Genet.* **5**, 35–9.

Kwon, J. M., Elliot, J. L., Yee, W. C. *et al.* (1995). Assignment of a second Charcot-Marie-Tooth type II locus to chromosome 3q. *Am. J. Hum. Genet.* **57**, 853–8.

Kyle, R. H. (1978). Monoclonal gammopathy of undetermined significance: natural history of 241 cases. *Am. J. Med.* **64**, 814–21.

Kyle, R. H. & Dyck, P. J. (1993). Neuropathy associated with the monoclonal gammopathies. In: *Peripheral Neuropathy*, 3rd edn, vol. 2, eds. P. C. Dyck & P. K. Thomas, pp. 1275–1287. Philadelphia: Saunders.

Lange, D. J., Trojaborg, W., Latov, N. *et al.* (1992). Multifocal motor neuropathy with conduction block: is it a distinct clinical entity? *Neurology* **42**, 497–505.

Leijten, F. S. S., Harinck, J. E., Poortvliet, D. C. J. & de Weerd, A. W. (1995). The role of polyneuropathy in motor convalescence after prolonged mechanical ventilation. *JAMA* **274**, 1221–5.

Leffert, R. D. (1985). *Brachial Plexus Injuries*. New York: Churchill-Livingstone.

Loffel, N., Roooi, L. N., Mumenthaler, M. *et al.* (1977). The Laundry-Guillain-Barre syndrome. complications, prognosis, and natural history in 123 cases. *J. Neurol. Sci.* **33**, 71–81.

Luft, B. J., Gorevic, P. C. & Halperin, J. J. (1989). A perspective on the treatment of Lyme borreliosis. *Rev. Infect. Dis.* **11**, 1518–25.

Lundborg, G. (1988). *Nerve Injury and Repair*. Edinburgh: Churchill Livingstone.

Lupski, J. R., Montes de Oca-Luna, R., Slangenhaupt, S. *et al.* (1991). DNA duplication associated with Charcot-Marie-Tooth disease 1a. *Cell* **66**, 219–32.

Mascarenhas Saraiva, M. J. (1991). Recent advances in the molecular pathology of familial amyloid polyneuropathy. *Neuromusc. Disord.* **1**, 3–6.

Masucci, E. F. & Kurzke, J. G. (1971). Diagnostic criteria for the Guillain-Barre syndrome. An analysis of 50 cases. *J. Neurol. Sci.* **13**, 483–90.

McCombe, P. A., McLeod, J. G., Pollard, J. D. *et al.* (1987*a*). Peripheral sensorimotor and autonomous neuropathy associated with systemic lupus erythematosus. *Brain* **110**, 533–49.

McCombe, P. A., McManis, P. G., Frith, J. A. *et al.* (1987*b*). Chronic inflammatory demyelinating polyradiculoneuropathy associated with pregnancy. *Ann. Neurol.* **21**, 102–4.

McCombe, P. A., Pollard, J. D., McLeod, J. G. (1987*c*). Chronic inflammatory demyelinating polyradiculoneuropathy. A clinical and electrophysiological study of 92 cases. *Brain* **110**, 1617–30.

McKann, G. M., Griffin, J. W., Cornblath, D. R. *et al.* (1988). Plasmapheresis and Guillain-Barre syndrome: analysis of prognostic factors and the effect of plasmapheresis. *Ann. Neurol.* **23**, 347–53.

McLeod, J. G. (1993). Paraneoplastic neuropathies. In *Peripheral Neuropathy*, 3rd edn, vol. 2, ed. P. C. Dyck & P. K. Thomas, pp. 1583–1590. Philadelphia: Saunders.

McLeod, J. G., Phil, D. & Tuck, R. R. (1987*a*). Disorders of the autonomic nervous system, part I, pathophysiology and clinical features. *Ann. Neurol.* **21**, 419–30.

McLeod, J. G., Phil, D. & Tuck, R. R. (1987*b*). Disorders of the autonomic nervous system, part II, investigation and treatment. *Ann. Neurol.* **21**, 519–29.

Melman, A. (1988). The evaluation of erectile dysfunction. *Urol. Radiol.* **10**, 119–26.

Miller, R. G., Parry, G., Larry, W. *et al.* (1986). AIDS-related inflammatory polyradiculopathy: successful treatment with plasma exchange. *Neurology* **36**, S206–11.

Mulligan, T. & Katz, P. G. (1989). Why aged men become impotent. *Arch. Inter. Med.* **149**, 1365–6.

Nobile-Orazio, E., Meucci, N., Barbieri, S., Carpo, M. & Scarlato, G. (1993). High-dose intravenous immunoglobulin therapy in multifocal motor neuropathy. *Neurology* **43**, 537–44.

Noordeen, S. K. (1995). Elimination of leprosy as a public health problem: progress and prospects. *Bull. WHO* **73**, 1–6.

Notermans, N. C., Wokke, J. H. J., Jennekens, F. G. I. (1991). Clinical work-up of the patient with a polyneuropathy. In: *Handbook of Clinical Neurology*, vol. 16, *Hereditary Neuropathies and Spinocerebellar Atrophies*, ed. J. M. B. V. De Long, pp. 253–270. Amsterdam: Elsevier.

Notermans, N. C., Wokke, J. H. J., Franssen, H. *et al.* (1993). Chronic idiopathic polyneuropathy presenting in middle or old age. A clinical and electrophysiological study of 75 patients. *J. Neurol. Neurosurg. Psychiatry* **56**, 1066–71.

Notermans, N. C., Wokke, J. H. J., van der Graaf, Y. *et al.* (1994*a*). A 5-year follow-up of patients with chronic idiopathic axonal polyneuropathy. *J. Neurol. Neurosurg. Psychiatry* **57**, 1525–7.

Notermans, N. C., Wokke, J. H. J., Lokhorst, H. *et al.* (1994*b*). A prospective study of polyneuropathy associated with benign gammopathy. Clinical features, laboratory parameters and their prognostic value. *Brain* **117**, 1385–93.

Osterman, P. O., Fagius, J., Lundemo, F. *et al.* (1984). Beneficial effect of plasma exchange in acute inflammatory polyradiculopathy. *Lancet* **II**, 1296–9.

Ouvrier, R. A., McLeod, J. G., Morgan, G. J. *et al.* (1981). Hereditary motor and sensory neuropathy of neuronal type with onset in early childhood. *Brain* **114**, 1855–70.

Parkhouse, N., LeQuesne, P. M. (1988). Impaired vasogenic vascular response in patients with diabetes and neuropathic foot lesions. *N. Engl. J. Med.* **318**, 1306–9.

Pearson, J. (1979). Familial dysautonomia (a review). *J. Autonom. Nerv. Syst.* **39**, 123–30.

Pestronk, A., Cornblath, D. R., Ilyas, A. A. *et al.* (1988). A treatable multifocal motor neuropathy with antibodies to GM1 ganglioside. *Ann. Neurol.* **24**, 73–8.

Pierach, C. A. (1982). Hematin therapy for the acute porphyric attack. *Semin. Liver Dis.* **2**, 125–32.

Pitts, D. B., Adour, K. K. & Hilsinger, R. L. (1988). Recurrent Bell's palsy: analysis of 140 patients. *Laryngoscope* **98**, 535–41.

Pleasure, D. E., Lovelace, R. E. & Duvoisin, R. C. (1968). The prognosis of acute polyradiculoneuritis. *Neurology*, **18**, 1143–8.

Prineas, J. W. & McLeod, J. G. (1976). Chronic relapsing polyneuritis. *J. Neurol. Sci.* **27**, 427–58.

Raymakers, P., Timmerman, V., Nelis, E. *et al.* (1991). Charcot-Marie-Tooth disease is most likely caused by a duplication on chromosome 17p11.2. *Neuromusc. Disord.* **1**, 93–7.

Rechthand, E., Cornblath, D. R., Stern, B. J. *et al.* (1984). Chronic demyelinating polyneuropathy in systemic lupus erythematosus. *Neurology* **34**, 1375–80.

Roa, B. B., Garcia, C. A., Suter, U. *et al.* (1993). Charcot-Marie-Tooth disease type 1A. Assocation with a spontaneous point mutation in the PMP-22 gene. *N. Engl. J. Med.* **329**, 96–101.

Ropper, A. H. (1986). Severe acute Guillain-Barré syndrome. *Neurology* **36**, 543–9.

Ropper, A. H. (1992). The Guillain-Barré syndrome. *N. Engl. J. Med.* **326**, 1130–6.

Ropper, A. H., Wijdicks, E. F. M. & Truax, B. T. (1991). *Guillain-Barré Syndrome*. Philadelphia: Davis.

Sabin, T. D., Swift, T. R., Jacobson, R. R. *et al.* (1993). Leprosy. In *Peripheral Neuropathy*, 3rd edn, vol. 2, eds. P. C. Dyck & P. K. Thomas, pp. 1354–1379. Philadelphia: Saunders.

Said, G., Goulon, C., Lacroix, C. & Moulonguet, A. (1994). Nerve biopsy findings in different patterns of proximal diabetic neuropathy. *Ann. Neurol.* **35**, 559–69.

Sampson, M. J., Wilson, S., Karagianis, P. *et al.* (1990). Progression of diabetic autonomic neuropathy over a decade in insulin-dependent diabetics. *Q. J. Med.* **75**, 635–46.

Schaumburg, H. H., Berger, A. R. & Thomas, P. K. (1991*a*). *Disorders of Peripheral Nerves*, 2nd edn. Contemporary Neurology Series 36. Philadelphia: Davis.

Schaumburg, H. H., Berger, A. R., Thomas, P. K. (1991*b*). Toxic neuropathy. In: *Disorders of Peripheral Nerves*, 2nd edn, pp. 257–302, Contemporary Neurology Series 36. Philadelphia: Davis.

Sheps, S. G. (1976). Use of an elastic garmet in the treatment of orthostatic hypotension. *Cardiology* **61**, 271–7.

Skinner, M., Lewis, W. D., Jones, L. A. *et al.* (1994). Liver transplantation as a treatment for familial amyloidotic polyneuropathy. *Ann. Int. Med.* **120**, 133–4.

Skjeldal, O. H., Stokke, O., Refsum, S. (1987). Clinical and biochemical heterogeneity in conditions with phytanic acid accumulation. *J. Neurol. Sci.* **87**, 77–81.

Smith, B. E., Windebank, A. J. & Dyck, P. J. (1993). Nonmalignant inflammatory sensory polyganglionopathy. In: *Peripheral Neuropathy*, 3rd edn, vol. 2, eds. P. C. Dyck & P. K. Thomas, pp. 1525–1531. Philadelphia: Saunders.

So, Y. T., Holzman, D. M., Abrams, D. I. *et al.* (1988). Peripheral neuropathy associated with acquired immunodeficiency syndrome: prevalence and clinical features from a population-based survey. *Arch. Neurol.* **45**, 945–8.

Sobue, G., Senda, Y., Matsuoka, Y. & Sobue, I. (1983). Sensory ataxia: a residual disability of Guillain-Barré syndrome. *Arch. Neurol.* **40**, 86–0.

Staal, A., de Weerdt, C. J., Went, L. N. (1965). Hereditary compression syndrome of peripheral nerves. *Neurology* **15**, 1008–17.

Steere, A. C. (1989). Lyme disease. *N. Engl. J. Med.* **321**, 586–96.

Steward, J. (1987). *Focal Peripheral Neuropathies.* New York: Elsevier.

Subramony, S. H. & Wilbourn, A. J. (1982). Diabetic proximal neuropathy. Clinical and electromyographic studies. *J. Neurol. Sci.* **53**, 293–9.

Sunderland, S. (1978). *Nerves and Nerve Injuries*, 3rd edn., Baltimore: Williams and Wilkins.

Swanson, A. G. (1963). Congenital insensitivity to pain with anhidrosis. *Arch. Neurol.* **8**, 299–305.

Thomas, P. K. & Tomlinson, D. R. (1993). Diabetic and hypoglycaemic neuropathy. In: *Peripheral Neuropathy*, 3rd edn, vol. 2, eds. P. C. Dyck & P. K. Thomas, pp. 1219–1250. Philadelphia: Saunders.

Thomas, P. K., Lascelles, R. G., Hallpike, J. F. *et al.* (1969). Recurrent and chronic relapsing Guillain-Barré polyneuritis. *Brain* **92**, 589–99.

Thomeer, R. T. W. M. & Marani, E. (1993). Brachial plexus injury. *Clin. Neurol. Neurosurg.* **95**(Suppl.), S1–118.

Valentijn, L. J., Baas, F., Wolterman, R. A. *et al.* (1992). Identical point mutations of PMP-22 in Trembler-J mouse and Charcot-Marie-Tooth disease IA. *Nature Genet.* **2**, 288–91.

Van den Berg, L. H., Marrink, J., De Jager, A. E. J. *et al.* (1992). Anti-GM1 antibodies in patients with Guillain-Barré syndrome. *J. Neurol. Neurosurg. Psychiatry* **55**, 8–11.

Van den Berg, L. H., Lankamp, C. L. A. M., de Jager, A. E. J. *et al.* (1993). Anti-sulphatide antibodies in peripheral neuropathy. *J. Neurol. Neurosurg. Psychiatry* **56**, 1164–8.

Van den Berg, L. H., Franssen, H. & Wokke, J. H. J. (1995a). Improvement of multifocal motor neuropathy during long-term weekly treatment with human immunoglobulin. *Neurology* **45**, 987–8.

Van den Berg, L. H., Kerkhof, H., Oey, P. L. *et al.* (1995). Treatment of multifocal motor neuropathy with high-dose intravenous immunoglobulins: a double-blind, placebo-controlled study. *J. Neurol. Neurosurg. Psychiatry* **59**, 248–52.

Van der Meché, F. G. A., Schmitz, P. I. M. & Dutch Guillain-Barré Study Group (1992). A randomized trial comparing intravenous immune globulin and plasma exchange in Guillain-Barré syndrome. *N. Engl. J. Med.* **326**, 1123–9.

Vermeulen,. M., van Doorn, P. A., Brand, A. *et al.* (1993). Intravenous immunoglobulin treatment in patients with chronic demyelinating polyneuropathy; a double blind, placebo controlled study. *J. Neurol. Neurosurg. Psychiatry* **56**, 36–9.

Vishnubhakat, S. M. & Beresford, R. (1988). Prevalence of peripheral neuropathy in HIV disease: prospective study of 40 patients. *Neurology* **38**, 350–6.

Visser, L. H., van der Meche, A., van Doorn, P. A. *et al.* (1995). Guillain-Barré syndrome without sensory loss (acute motor neuropathy). *Brain* **118**, 841–7.

Vuorinen, V., Siiromen, J. & Roytta, M. (1995). Axonal regeneration into chronically denervated distal stumps. 1. Electron microscope studies. *Acta Neuropathol.* **89**, 209–18.

Windebank, A. J., Blexrud, M. D., Dyck, P. J. *et al.* (1990). The syndrome of acute sensory neuropathy: clinical features and electrophysiologic and pathologic changes. *Neurology* **40**, 584–91.

Windenbank, J. A. & Bonkovski, H. L. (1993). Porphyric neuropathy. In: *Peripheral Neuropathy*, 3rd edn, vol. 2, eds. P. D. Dyck & P. K. Thomas, pp. 1161–1168. Philadelphia: Saunders.

Winer, J. B., Hughes, R. A. C., Greenwood, R. J., Perkin, G. D. & Healy, M. J. R. (1985). Prognosis in Guillian-Barré syndrome. *Lancet* **1**, 1202–3.

Winer, J. B., Bang, B., Clarke, J. R. *et al.* (1992). A study of neuropathy in HIV infection. *Q. J. Med.* **302**, 473–88.

Wright, A. & Dyck, P. J. (1995). Hereditary sensory neuropathy with sensorineural deafness and early onset dementia. *Neurology* **45**, 560–2.

Yanagihara, N., Mori, H., Kozawa, T. *et al.* (1984). Bell's palsy. Nonrecurrent v. recurrent and unilateral v. bilateral. *Arch. Otolaryngol.* **110**, 374–81.

Yao, J. K. & Herbert, P. N. (1993). Lipoprotein deficiency and neuromuscular manifestations. In: *Peripheral Neuropathy*, 3rd edn, vol. 2, eds. P. C. Dyck & P. K. Thomas, pp. 1179–93. Philadelphia: Saunders.

Yuki, N., Yoshimo, H., Sato, S. & Miytake, T. (1990). Acute axonal polyneuropathy associated with anti-GM1 antibodies following *Campylobacter* enteritis. *Neurology* **40**, 1900–2.

Zlotogora, J., Costeff, H. & Elian, E. (1981). Early motor development in metachromatic leukodystrophy. *Arch. Dis. Child.* **51**, 309–10.

Zorilla, E. & Kozak, G. P. (1967). Ophthalmoplegia in diabetes mellitus. *Ann. Intern. Med.* **67**, 968–74.

19 Bacterial meningitis

G. URWIN AND R. A. FELDMAN

Introduction

Bacterial meningitis is associated with substantial morbidity and mortality. The outcome is influenced by host factors including age at the onset of disease, integrity of the dura and underlying immunodeficiencies in particular those of the complement system. In addition, the pathogen causing the disease will have a bearing on the outcome.

Measurement of complication rates of bacterial meningitis is influenced by the follow-up period, as there is a tendency for improvement in complications detected acutely. In a prospective study of children with bacterial meningitis, 37% of cases had an abnormality after 1 month, while only 14% of children had persistent deficits (Pomeroy *et al.* 1990).

The major sequelae of meningitis consist of hearing loss, motor lesions (including seizures, spasticity and paresis) and intellectual deficit. In spite of the advent of potent antimicrobials to treat bacterial meningitis, the incidence of sequelae has not changed greatly over the past 40 years, until recent studies have shown improvement with the use of steroids. Odio *et al.* (1991) demonstrated that early dexamethasone given to children with bacterial meningitis (most of whom had disease due to *H. influenzae*) reduced the rate of sequelae.

The three major pathogens: *Neisseria meningitidis, Haemophilus influenzae* and *Streptococcus pneumoniae*

Epidemiology

Ninety per cent of bacterial meningitis in the post-neonatal period is caused by three pathogens: *Neisseria meningitidis, Haemophilus influenzae* and *Streptococcus pneumoniae*. The remaining 10% of cases are caused by a wide variety of organisms (Table 19.1).

Although the three major causes of bacterial meningitis are all more common in children under the age of 5 years than in adults, the frequency of the pathogens causing disease at different ages will vary (Fig. 19.1). *H. influenzae* type b (Hib) caused 43% of cases in children under the age of 5 years (prior to the introduction of Hib vaccine) and

Table 19.1. *Cases of meningitis collected in the North East Thames Region, UK, during November 1990 to December 1992*

Diagnosis	Per cent
N. meningitidis	38.2
H. influenzae[a]	31.0
S. pneumoniae	20.3
E. coli	1.0
Group B streptococcus	3.2
Streptococcus spp.[b]	1.5
L. monocytogenes	1.6
M. tuberculosis	0.5
S. aureus	0.5
Enterobacteriaceae	1.6
Pseudomonas spp.	0.5
Total	100

Urwin *et al.* (1994).
[a] 95% type b.
[b] Group A streptococci and *S. milleri.*

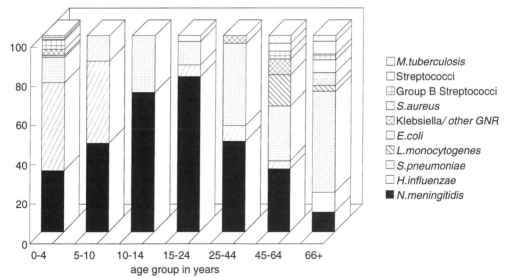

Fig. 19.1. Causes of bacterial meningitis in different age groups in the North East Thames Region UK, 1991–1992 inclusive. (G. Urwin and R. Feldman, unpublished data.)

S. pneumoniae causes 40% of all cases of meningitis in patients over the age of 65 years (Urwin & Feldman 1993, unpublished data).

The incidence of *N. meningitidis* is 2.2/100 000 in the overall population (Table 19.2). In the under-fives, the incidence is 15/100 000. There is a second peak of disease in

Table 19.2. *Incidence of bacterial meningitis in North East Thames Region, UK, 1991*

Pathogen	Cases/100 000 population (number)		
	Overall	Age < 1 year	Age < 5 years
N. meningitidis	2.2 (81)	39 (23)	15 (41)
H. influenzae	1.6 (59)	51 (28)	19 (52)
S. pneumoniae	1.0 (37)	17 (9)	6.7 (18)
Denominator^a	3 756 700	56 800	267 700

(Urwin *et al.* 1994).
^a Denominators from 1991 census results from Office of Population, Census and Statistics.

young teenages and adults of 15–20 years. In the United Kingdom, group B meningococci account for 66% of disease, with group C accounting for 31% of cases. The other groups of meningococci account for a very small proportion of the total disease (Jones & Kaczmarski 1991). More than 90% of *H. influenzae* meningitis is seen in children under the age of 5 years and 95% of invasive *H. influenzae* disease is due to capsular type b. In countries that have introduced Hib vaccine, Hib disease in both children and adults has become substantially less common. In those over the age of 15 years there is an underlying predisposing condition in 74% of cases of *H. influenzae* meningitis (Bol *et al.* 1987). *S. pneumoniae* meningitis is more often seen in children than adults. However, it is the most common cause of meningitis in patients over the age of 65 years.

Mortality

The mortality rate for bacterial meningitis is 10% overall. The age of the patient and the infecting organism have a significant bearing on mortality (Table 19.3). The highest mortality rates are seen in disease due to *S. pneumoniae*, where deaths occur in approximately 30% of cases (Burman *et al.* 1985; Wenger *et al.* 1990). Adults have a substantially higher mortality rate than children with pneumococcal meningitis (Burman *et al.* 1985).

Meningococcal meningitis mortality varies between 3% and 10% (Goldacre 1976; Cartwright *et al.* 1986), but death rates are higher where there is septicaemia. Case fatality ratios vary with the age of the patient; in children under 1 year of age case fatalities were 21.8%, in the 5- to 9-year age group 5.6%, and in those over the age of 25 years 33.8% (Abbott *et al.* 1985). Several studies have reported overall mortality rates of 2–5% in *H. influenzae* type b meningitis (Tudor-Williams *et al.* 1989; Howard *et al.* 1991).

Hearing loss

Bacterial meningitis can cause a range of hearing deficit, both conductive and sensorineural (Kaplan *et al.* 1981). Bacterial meningitis causes 10% of sensorineural deaf-

Table 19.3. *Rates of sequelae by pathogen causing meningitis*

	Per cent		
	N. meningitidis	*S. pneumoniae*	*H. influenza*
Mortality	7.5	30	2–5
Permanent sensorineural hearing loss	7.5	31.8	11.7
Seizures[a]	9	30	47

[a] Seizures during the acute illness.

ness in children (Editorial 1986). Of children with profound hearing loss, meningitis accounts for 27% of cases (Davis & Wood 1992).

A number of mechanisms are thought to result in sensorineural hearing loss. The inner ear may be infected during the haematogenous dissemination of the organism causing meningitis. Direct spread of the organism from the subarachnoid space through the cochlear aqueduct can occur, resulting in the destruction of sensory structures. Toxins produced by the infecting organism may mediate damage to the hair cells and could cause partial hearing loss. Direct nerve damage or secondary ischaemic damage are also possible mechanisms of deafness.

Deafness occurs early in the course of disease. Abnormalities in brainstem auditory evoked responses (BAER) are detectable in the first 48 hours of disease. In a prospective study of 51 children with bacterial meningitis using BAER, Vienny *et al.* (1984) reported 21.6% of children with transient abnormalities in the first 2 weeks of illness. Nearly 10% of children with persistently abnormal BAER during their admission developed persistent deafness. Kaplan *et al.* (1984) reported 37 children with meningitis of whom four had sensorineural hearing loss within 48 hours of admission. Two of these went on to develop permanent bilateral deafness. The other two had complete or nearly complete recovery of their hearing. Partial recovery is more common with initial hearing losses of 2000–3000 Hz; permanent loss is seen with higher frequency loss.

Overall rates of permanent sensorineural hearing loss have been computed from several studies by Fortnum (1992). Hearing losses are most profound in *S. pneumoniae* meningitis, in which 31.8% of children are affected. The rates of hearing loss in disease due to *N. meningitidis* were estimated as 7.5%, and for *H. influenzae* 11.7% (Table 19.3).

Middle ear dysfunction has an over-riding influence on the progress and auditory status of children with hearing impairment following bacterial meningitis. The presence of otitis media is not always associated with conductive deafness. Sensorineural hearing loss was found in six cases with otitis media, but there was no conductive hearing loss (Dodge *et al.* 1984). However, conductive pathology may add to the sensorineural deficit. Conductive deafness persisted in 26% of patients at 6 month follow-up (Smyth *et al.* 1988).

Seizures

Infections of the CNS are an important cause of epilepsy. Prior infection of the CNS is associated with 1–5% of cases of epilepsy (Annegers *et al.* 1988).

Seizures can occur during the acute stages of meningitis, or can continue after the acute illness has resolved. In a prospective study of the neurological sequelae of meningitis, seizures occurred in the acute disease in 31% of cases (Pomeroy *et al.* 1990). Most seizures develop within the first week of illness and resolve within a few days, probably related to the patient's elevated temperature. Late seizures occur in 7% of cases (Pomeroy *et al.* 1990). The pattern of late seizures varies; generalized seizures are more common than focal seizures, although both have been observed. The majority of patients develop seizures within 2 years of the acute illness. Of those who acquire late seizures, a small proportion will have only one seizure. Those who have recurrent seizures are often difficult to control medically, requiring multiple therapy. Annegers *et al.* (1988) identified the 20 year risk of developing seizures following bacterial meningitis as 13% if associated with early seizures. Patients who do not develop early seizures have a lower 20 year risk of developing seizures of 2.4%. Seizures are more commonly associated with meningitis at the extremes of life, i.e. in patients younger than 1 year of age or older than 60 years (Rosman *et al.* 1985).

Seizures during bacterial meningitis are associated with an adverse outcome. The mortality rate is higher in patients who have seizures during their illness. In addition, seizures are often associated with permanent neurological sequelae including deafness and intellectual impairment.

Ataxia

Ataxia may be a presenting sign of bacterial meningitis. In addition it may complicate the illness in approximately 3% of cases. Post-meningitis ataxia is frequently associated with profound deafness, as Schwartz (1972) reported in seven of eight cases. The association of ataxia with deafness suggests that the pathology is labyrinthine rather than cerebellar or brainstem in nature.

Psychological and intellectual sequelae of meningitis

Although bacterial meningitis affects multiple aspects of a child's development, the majority of patients are able to lead normal lives after the disease. Psychological tests performed to measure the degree of disability in cases of meningitis will be influenced by the age at the onset of illness, the age at psychological testing and the socio-economic status of the family. Sibling controls are frequently used to try to eliminate genetic and environmental differences.

In a sibling-matched study of children who had had *H. influenzae* meningitis, index cases had small but significant differences in reading skills. They were more likely than

Table 19.4. *Risk factors for the acquisition of neonatal meningitis*

Prematurity
Low birth weight, especially under 2000 g
Prolonged rupture of membranes
Long and difficult labour
Maternal bacteraemia or septicaemia

controls to receive educational support, particularly the older children and boys, but this may reflect the different demands on these individuals (Feldman & Michaels 1988). In a study of a cohort of 24 children with *H. influenzae* meningitis, Taylor *et al.* (1984) found subjects performed at levels similar to siblings. However, they received more academic support from parents and used more remedial services at school. More frequent educational difficulties were identified by Sell *et al.* (1972); 29% of patients had an IQ 15 points lower than their siblings. Tests on apparently normal survivors indicated that children who have survived bacterial meningitis function less well intellectually than their unaffected peers.

Neonatal meningitis

The predominant organisms that cause neonatal meningitis differ from those which cause disease at other ages.

Epidemiology

Children in the first month of life are particularly susceptible to infection. The incidence of bacterial meningitis is 1.6 per 1000 births (de Louvois *et al.* 1991). Group B streptococcus is the most common bacterial pathogen in this age group, responsible for 28% of cases of neonatal meningitis. *E. coli*, especially capsular antigen type K1, is the second most prominent pathogen. A wide variety of other organisms can cause meningitis at this age, most notably *Listeria monocytogenes*. The three major pathogens, which account for 71% of meningitis in the post-neonatal infant, account for only 10% of disease during the first month of life (Fitzhardinge *et al.* 1974).

Babies are at increased risk of developing bacterial meningitis if they are premature and of low birth weight; when there has been a long and difficult labour; when the membranes have been ruptured for a long time; or if there is evidence of maternal septicaemia or bacteraemia (Table 19.4).

The organisms responsible for meningitis in the first 10 days of life are normally acquired from the mother's genital tract. The route of infection in older neonates is unknown but may be either nosocomial or community acquired. The mother may be the source of the infection, possibly via breast milk (Bingen *et al.* 1992).

Mortality and sequelae

Bacterial meningitis is not only more common in the neonate, but neonates are more likely to develop sequelae and mortality rates are high. In the first 10 days of life the mortality rates from meningitis overall are as high as 56%. In the subsequent days, the mortality is lower, but approaches 25% (Bortolussi *et al.* 1978). Both group B streptococcal and *E. coli* neonatal meningitis have mortality rates of 24–25% (Fitzhardinge *et al.* 1974).

A common acute complication is ventriculitis, generally associated with infection due to enteric Gram-negative bacilli, although it can occur in group B streptococcal infection, and may explain the occasional baby with group B streptococcal disease who has a poor response to therapy. Convulsions or hydrocephalus may occurr in 20–30% of patients (Fitzhardinge *et al.* 1974).

In a prospective study of bacterial meningitis in a birth cohort in Finland, meningitis was responsible for 1.8% of cases of mental retardation, cerebral palsy and/or epilepsy. Long-term sequelae occurred in 30.9% of cases of bacterial meningitis, hearing loss being the most common (Rantakallio *et al.* 1986).

Listeria monocytogenes

Epidemiology

Approximately 40% of patients with *Listeria monocytogenes* infection have involvement of the CNS. It accounts for approximately 2% of bacterial meningitis in adults (Table 19.1) and is the third major cause of neonatal meningitis (Wenger *et al.* 1990). Disease occurs at any age but is most common in the immunocompromised, in the very young and in the elderly.

Mortality and sequelae

The mortality rate for *Listeria* meningitis is high in patients who have underlying immunosuppression or malignancy, and lower in healthy individuals. In a review of 54 cases, Pollock *et al.* (1984) reported a mortality rate of 61% in the susceptible group and 39% in the healthy group (although this is not stratified by age).

In a study of *Listeria* infection in infants and children, two of 21 survivors of neonatal *Listeria* meningitis had neurological sequelae including convulsions, hemiparesis and hydrocephalus. Visintine *et al.* (1977) reported that five of 26 surviving patients had residual defects at discharge including sensorineural deafness (1), recovering monoplegia, unilateral brisk reflexes and cranial nerve palsies (3).

Table 19.5. *MRC staging for tuberculous meningitis*

Stage I	(early) consciousness undisturbed and no focal neurological signs
Stage II	(medium) may have focal neurological signs and/or disturbed consciousness
Stage III	(advanced) patient extremely ill, stuporous or comatose; neurological signs may be present

Medical Research Council (1948).

Tuberculous meningitis

Epidemiology

The CNS can be involved by *Mycobacterium tuberculosis* in a number of different ways. Meningitis is the most common, but encephalopathy without meningitis and cerebral abscesses can also occur. The incidence of tuberculous meningitis (TBM) reflects the incidence of pulmonary tuberculosis in the community. In India (Tripathy 1987) there are 418 cases per 100 000 population, in England 12/100 000 (Medical Research Council 1985). In the UK the majority of cases of TBM occur in children from the Indian subcontinent. In the developed world the recent decline in the incidence of *M. tuberculosis* has slowed and in some parts of the USA reversed. This is related to a number of factors including the AIDS epidemic, immigration from developing countries and homelessness (Snider & Roper 1993).

In a study of infection by the Medical Research Council (1985) pulmonary tuberculosis (TB) accounted for 70% of cases: non-respiratory disease in 24% and both respiratory and non-respiratory in 26% (Medical Research Council 1985). TBM comprises 15% of extrapulmonary TB. Patients with TBM often have evidence of miliary or active pulmonary TB.

Mortality and sequelae

If TBM is left untreated, it is virtually always fatal. However, the advent of chemotherapy has markedly improved this situation. The prognosis depends on the stage of disease at presentation and commencing treatment, and the age of the patient (children under the age of 3 years have a poor prognosis independent of the stage of disease at which they present). The diagnosis may be difficult: patients may not show an initial pleocytosis in the CSF, or may show a marked polymorph response. Occasionally patients with miliary tuberculosis or tuberculomas of the CNS may have a normal CSF on admission and subsequently develop meningitis. Such diagnostic difficulties may delay the starting of therapy (Kocen & Parsons 1970).

The Medical Research Council staging is the most commonly used (Table 19.5) (Medical Research Council 1948): stage I (early), consciousness undisturbed and no focal neurological signs; stage II (medium), may have focal neurological signs and/or disturbed consciousness; stage III (advanced), patients are extremely ill, stuporous or comatose, and focal neurological signs may be present. The mortality rate for Indian children at each stage is: I, 9%; II, 25%, III, 73% (Ramachandran *et al.* 1986). The age of the patient will also have a significant bearing on the mortality rate, with higher mortality rates in young children under 5 years (20%) and in adults over 50 years (60%) (Kennedy & Fallon 1979).

Acute complications are common, such as hydrocephalus, cranial nerve palsies and cerebral infarction. Obstructive hydrocephalus can develop days to months after the commencement of therapy and requires prompt neurosurgical intervention. Seizures can develop at any stage of the illness and may be generalized or focal.

As the disease progresses cerebral vasculitis can cause focal neurological signs: paralysis, of which hemiplegia is the most common; quadriplegia is usually a sign of advanced disease and is associated with a poor prognosis. Cranial nerve palsies occur after the disease is well established and motor nerves are more commonly involved than the optic nerve (Udani *et al.* 1971).

In a study of TBM in New York City, neurological sequelae were present at follow up in 22 of 31 patients. Paraplegia, hemiplegia, gait disorder and cranial nerve palsies were all present. Twenty-three per cent of patients presenting with stage III disease develop severe functional disability, compared with none of the patients presenting with stage I disease (Ogawa *et al.* 1987).

Spirochaetal diseases

Syphilis

Syphilis is a sexually transmitted disease caused by the spirochaete *Treponema pallidum*. Active lesions are found on the mucous membranes and contact with the active lesion will spread the infection. The incidence of syphilis in the USA was falling until 1985 when it started to rise, which may be related to the HIV epidemic.

The CNS can be involved in syphilis at any stage of the disease. In the early stages at least 40% of cases show invasions of the CNS, which may be asymptomatic or manifest as meningitis (Lukehart *et al.* 1988), In the later stages of disease neurosyphilis may be (a) asymptomatic; (b) meningovascular, involving either cerebrum or spine; (c) parenchymal, and manifest as general paresis, tabes dorsalis, optic atrophy and otitis. Gumma may occur within the CNS, usually proximal to the meninges. Before the advent of penicillin, neurosyphilis was found in 6.5% of patients who developed secondary and tertiary disease, of which tabes dorsalis and dementia were the most common manifestations (Clark & Danbolt 1964).

Patients with HIV infection are more at risk of acquiring syphilis than the general population; prevalence was found to be 3% in one cohort. In this group of patients neurosyphilis occurs earlier and syphilitic meningitis is more common. Asymptomatic neurosyphilis is present in a higher proportion of patients co-infected with HIV (Brandon *et al.* 1993).

Lyme disease

Lyme disease is caused by the spirochaete *Borrelia burgdorferi*. The organism is transmitted by tick bite, principally the *Ixodes* species. The disease was first described in Lyme, Connecticut, but is found in many parts of the USA and Europe. It has many features in common with syphilis, including multi-organ involvement. Arthritis is a common manifestation, and both the peripheral and central nervous systems, either alone or together, are frequently involved in the disease from an early stage.

The disease is considered to occur in stages: (a) Primary, with its characteristic skin lesion erythema chronicum migrans at the site of the tick bite. Although there are not usually manifestations of nervous system involvement at this stage, the organisms are thought to disseminate rapidly to the CNS. (b) Secondary, with meningitis, cranial neuropathy and polyneuritis. (c) Tertiary, when the parenchyma of the brain is involved (Pachner 1989).

Early neurological abnormalities include facial palsy, meningitis or radiculoneuritis. Meningitis can occur in 30% of cases (Logigian *et al.* 1990). The meningitis is usually lymphocytic and mild. Aching radicular pain (Bannwarth's syndrome) is a more common manifestation of Lyme disease in Europe than the USA. There is not always a history of a rash. These abnormalities usually resolve within 1–2 months in the majority, although a few patients may be left with residual facial weakness or hearing loss (Logigian *et al.* 1990).

In late-onset Lyme disease the symptoms begin a median of 2 years after the infection, although symptoms can begin earlier or later, after as long as 10 years. A mild encephalopathy is the most common finding, which usually involves memory, sleep and cognition (Halperin *et al.* 1989; Logigian *et al.* 1990). Assessment of the neurological abnormalities is difficult as the manifestations are subtle. The classical skin lesion of erythema migrans is present in 85% of cases with chronic neurological abnormalities.

Treatment does not always result in cure, particularly in late disease. Treatment with ceftriaxone for 14 days improved the CNS involvement of 63% of cases (Logigian *et al.* 1990). The improvement may take several months after therapy has been completed. Up to half the cases may relapse or not improve, and the disease may progress in spite of adequate therapy. Treatment is least successful in patients in whom the illness has been present for a long time.

References

Abbott, J. D., Jones, D. M., Painter, M. J. & Young, S. E. J. (1985). The epidemiology of meningococcal infections in England and Wales 1912–1983. *J. Infect.* **11**, 241–57.

Annegers, J. F., Hauser, W. A., Beghi, E., Nicolosi, A. & Kurland, L. T. (1988). The risk of unprovoked seizures after encephalitis and meningitis. *Neurology* **38**, 1407–9.

Bingen, E., Denamur, E., Lambert-Zechovsky, N. *et al.* (1992). Analysis of DNA restriction fragment length polymorphism extends the evidence for breast milk transmission in *Streptococcus agalactiae* late onset neonatal infection. *J. Infect. Dis.* **165**, 569–73.

Bol, P., Spanjaard, L., van Alpen, L. & Zanen, H. C. (1987). Epidemiology of *Haemophilus influenzae* in patients more than six years of age. *J. Infect.* 15, 81–94.

Bortolussi, R., Krishnan, C., Armstrong, D. & Tovichayathamrong, P. (1978). Prognosis for survival in neonatal meningitis: clinical and pathological review of 52 cases. *Can. Med. Assoc. J.* 118, 165–8.

Brandon, W. R., Boulos, L. M. & Morse, A. (1993). Determining the prevalence of neurosyphilis in a cohort co-infected with HIV. *Int. J. Std Aids* 4, 99–101.

Burman, L. A., Norrby, R. & Trollfers, B. (1985). Invasive pneumococcal infections: Incidence, predisposing factors and prognosis. *Rev. Infect. Dis.* 7, 133–42.

Cartwright, K. A. V., Stuart, J. M. & Noah, N. D. (1986). An outbreak of meningococcal disease in Gloucestershire. *Lancet* II, 558–61

Clark, E. G. & Danbolt, N. (1964). The Oslo Study of the natural course of untreated syphilis. *Med. Clin. North Am.* 48, 613–23.

Davis, A. & Wood, S. (1992). The epidemiology of childhood hearing impairment: factors relevant to planning of services. *Br. J. Audiol.* 26, 77–90.

de Louvois, J., Blackbourn, J., Hurley, R. & Harvey, D. (1991). Infantile meningitis in England and Wales: a two-year study. *Arch. Dis. Child.* 66, 603–7.

Dodge, P. R., Davis, H., Feigin, R. *et al.* (1984). Prospective evaluation of hearing impairment as a sequelae of acute bacterial meningitis. *N. Engl. J. Med.* 311, 869–74.

Editorial (1986). Deafness after meningitis. *Lancet* II, 134–5.

Feldman, H. M. & Michaels, R. H. (1988). Academic achievement in children ten to 12 years after *Haemophilus influenzae* meningitis 81, 339–41.

Fitzhardinge, P. M., Kasemi, M., Ramsey, M. & Stern, M. (1974). Long-term sequelae of neonatal meningitis. *Dev. Med. Child Neurol.* 16, 3–10.

Fortnun, H. M. (1992). Hearing impairment after bacterial meningitis: a review. *Arch. Dis. Child.* 67, 1128–33.

Goldacre, M. J. (1976). Acute bacterial meningitis in childhood. *Lancet* I, 28–31.

Gortvai, P., Delouvois, J. & Hurley, R. (1987). The bacteriology and chemotherapy of acute pyogenic brain abscess. *Br. J. Neurosurg.* 1(2), 189–203.

Halperin, J. J., Luft, B. J. & Anand, A. K. *et al.* (1989). Lyme neuroborreliosis: central nervous system manifestations. *Neurology* 39, 753–9.

Howard, A. J., Dunkin, K. T., Musser, J. M. & Palmer, S. R. (1991). Epidemiology of *Haemophilus influenzae* type b invasive disease in Wales. *BMJ* 303, 441–5.

Jones, D. M. & Kaczmarski, E. B. (1991). Meningococcal infections in England and Wales: report of the Meningococcal Reference Labortory for 1990. *Commun. Dis. Rev.* 1, R76–8.

Kaplan, S. L., Catlin, F. I., Weaver, T. & Feign, R. (1984). Onset of hearing loss in children with bacterial meningitis. *Pediatrics* 74, 575–8.

Kaplan, S. L., Goddard, J., Van Kleeck, M., Catlin, F. I. & Feigin, R. D. (1981). Ataxia and deafness in children due to bacterial meningitis. *Pediatrics* 68, 8–13.

Kennedy, D. H. & Fallon, R. J. (1979). Tuberculous meningitis. *JAMA* 241, 264–8.

Kocen, R. S. & Parsons, M. (1970). Neurologic complications of tuberculosis: some unusual manifestations. *Q. J. Med.* 30, 17–30.

Logigian, E. L., Kaplan, R. F. & Steere, A. (1990). Chronic neurological manifestations of Lyme disease. *N. Engl. J. Med.* 323, 1438–44.

Lukehart, S., Hook, E. W., Baker-Zander, S. H. *et al.* (1988). Invasion of the central nervous system by *Treponema pallidum*. Implications for diagnosis and therapy. *Ann. Intern. Med.* 109, 855–62.

Medical Research Council (1948). Streptomycin treatment of tuberculous meningitis. *Lancet* 1, 582–97.

Medical Research Council (1985). National survey of tuberculosis notifications in England and Wales in 1983. *BMJ* **291**, 658–61.

Odio, C. M., Faingezicht, I., Paris, M. *et al.* (1991). The beneficial effects of early dexamethasone administration in infants and children with bacterial meningitis. *N. Engl. J. Med.* **324**, 1525–31.

Ogawa, S. K., Smith, M. A., Brennessel, D. J. & Lowy, F. D. (1987). Tuberculous meningitis in an urban medical centre. *Medicine* **66**, 317–26.

Pachner, A. R. (1989). Neurologic manifestations of Lyme disease, the new "Great Imitator". *Rev. Infect. Dis.* **11**, S1482–5.

Plotkin, S. A., Daum, R. S. & Giebink, G. S. *et al.* (1988). Treatment of bacterial meningitis. *Pediatrics* **81**, 904–7.

Pollock, S. S., Pollock, T. M. & Harrison, M. J. G. (1984). Infection of the central nervous system by *Listeria monocytogenes*: a review of 54 adult and juvenile cases. *Q. J. Med.* **211**, 331–40.

Pomeroy, S. L., Holmes, S. J., Dodge, P. R. & Feigin, R. D. (1990). Seizures and other neurologic sequelae of bacterial meningitis in children. *N. Eng. J. Med.* **234**, 1651–7.

Ramachandran, P., Duraipandian, M., Nagarajan, M. *et al.* (1986). Three chemotherapy studies of tuberculous meningitis in children. *Tubercle* **67**, 17–29.

Rantakallio, P., Leskinen, M. & Von Wendt, L. (1986). Incidence and prognosis of central nervous system infections in a birth cohort of 12 000 children. *Scand. J. Infect. Dis.* **18**, 287–94.

Rosman, N. P., Peterson, D. B., Kaye, E. M. & Colton, T. (1985). Seizures in bacterial meningitis: prevalence, patterns, pathogenesis and prognosis. *Pediatr. Neurol.* **1**, 278–85.

Schwartz, J. F. (1972). Ataxia in bacterial meningitis. *Neurology* **22**, 1071–4.

Sell, S. H. W., Webb, W. W., Pate, J. E. & Doyne, E. O. (1972). Psychological sequelae to bacterial meningitis: two controlled studies. *Pediatrics* **49**, 212–17.

Smyth, V., O'Connell, B., Pitt, R., O'Callaghan, M. & Scott, J. (1988). Audiological management in the recovery phase of bacterial meningitis. *Int. J. Pediat. Otorhinolaryngol.* **15**, 79–86.

Snider, D. E. Jr. & Roper, W. L. (1993). The new tuberculosis. *N. Engl. J. Med.* **326**, 703–5.

Taylor, H. G., Michaels, R. H., Mazur, P. M., Bauer, R. E. & Liden, C. B. (1984). Intellectual, neuropsychological and achievement outcomes in children six to eight years after recovery from *Haemophilus influenza* meningitis. *Pediatrics* **74**, 198–205.

Tripathy, S. P. (1987). Fifteen-year follow up of the Indian BCG trial. *Proceedings of the XXVI Conference of the International Union Again Tuberculosis and Lung Disease*. Professional Postgraduate Series, Tokyo, pp. 69–72.

Tudor-Williams, G., Frankland, J. & Isaacs, D. *et al.* (1989). *Haemophilus influenzae* type b disease in the Oxford Region. *Arch. Dis. Child.* **64**, 517–19.

Udani, P. M., Parekh, U. C. & Dastur, D. K. (1971). Neurological and related syndromes in CNS tuberculosis, clinical features and pathogenesis. *J. Neurosci.* **14**, 341–57.

Urwin, G., Yuan, M. F. & Feldman, R. A. (1994). Prospective study of bacterial meningitis in North East Thames Region 1991–3, during introduction of *H. influenzae* vaccine. *Br. Med. J.* **309**, 1412–14.

Vienny, H., Despland, P. A., Lutschg, J., Deonna, T., Dutoit-Marco, M. L. & Gander, C. (1984). Early diagnosis and evolution of deafness in childhood bacterial meningitis: a study using brainstem auditory evoked potentials. *Pediatrics* **73**, 579–86.

Visintine, M., Oleske, J. M. & Nahmias, A. J. (1977). *Listeria monocytogenes* infection in infants and children. *Am. J. Dis. Child.* **131**, 393–7.

Wenger, J. D., Hightower, A. W., Facklam, R. R., Gaventa, S. & Broome, C. V. (1990). Bacterial meningitis in the United States 1986: report of a multistate surveillance study. *J. Infect. Dis.* **162**, 1316–23.

20 Brain abscess

R. A. FELDMAN AND G. URWIN

Introduction

Since bacterial brain abscess occurs at rates of 1.2–18 cases per million per year (Table 20.1), large neurological centres may see between 40 and 100 cases in a decade – hardly enough to evaluate interrelations of agent, neurological condition at diagnosis, treatment modality, underlying pathology, and other factors that relate to outcome. Up to the present, outcome has been measured predominantly in terms of mortality rates, expressed as case fatality ratios (CFR).

Outcomes

Between the 1960s and 1980s, CFRs for brain abscesses fell significantly from a range around 40% to 5–10%, a fall associated with the use of computed tomography, magnetic resonance imaging and other methods of visualizing the presence, number and location of intracerebral lesions, the use of more effective culture techniques and treatment for anaerobic organisms, earlier diagnosis, changes in surgical treatment methods and use, and changes in the frequency of underlying pathology (Karandanis & Shulman 1975; Chun *et al.* 1986; Wispelway & Scheld 1987; Arsenia & Ciurea 1988; Harle *et al.* 1988; Schliamser *et al.* 1988; Aebi *et al.* 1991; Sparrow 1991).

A major variable associated with CFR is the neurological status at diagnosis. Using reports from the 1960s through the 1980s, from all age groups and methods of treatment, the CFR for patients comatose at diagnosis was 79/100 compared with a risk of

Table 20.1. *Rates of bacterial brain abscesses*

Author	Country	Cases/million per year	Year
Duel *et al.* 1991	Denmark	1.2–3.6	1963–89
Gortvai *et al.* 1989	England and Wales	3.5–4.3	1978
McClelland *et al.* 1978	Northern Ireland	3–5	1947–76
Nicolosi *et al.* 1991	Olmsted Co., Minnesota	6–18[a]	1935–81
Small & Dale 1984	Scotland	1.6	1968–82
Svanteson *et al.* 1988	Sweden	2.5–3.8	1947–82

[a] Removing epidural and subdural infections.

Table 20.2. *Case fatality ratios and neurological status at diagnosis using Garfield's grading*

Authors	Alert (A)	Drowsy (B)	Pain (C)	None (D)	Year	Comments
Alderson et al. 1981	1/17	7/46	8/19	6/8	1964–78	
Aydin et al. 1988	2/32	3/6	3/4		1979–87	Grade 3 + 4
Basit et al. 1989	1/11	3/9	1/1		1976–84	Multiple abscess
Bradley & Shaw (1983)	19/94	63/143	46/63		1950–79	Grade 3 + 4
Garfield 1969	10/57	23/72	15/23	35/48	1951–67	
Kratimenos & Crockard 1991	0/4	0/7	2/3	0	1975–89	
Miller et al. 1988	6/44	8/40	2/10	4/6	1974–84	
Nielsen et al. 1982	0/33	2/55	36/61	42/51	1935–76	
Richards et al. 1990	0/32	2/30	3/7	2/2	1979–88	
Rosenblum et al. 1978	0/16	4/16	0/2	1/1	1970–77	
Seydoux & Francioli 1992	0/18	3/16	2/3		1977–87	
Shaw & Russell 1975	4/14	7/24	7/8		1950–73	Grade 3 + 4, cerebellar only
Svanteson et al. 1988	1/32	8/35	1/15	5/5	1947–82	Excluding trauma
van Dellen et al. 1987	4/18	1/8	4/7	1/1	1981–85	Cerebellar only
Total (%)	48/422 (**11**)	134/507 (**26**)	130/226 (**58**)	96/122 (**79**)		

Table 20.3. *Case fatality ratios and Glasgow Coma Scores (GCS) at diagnosis of brain abscess*

Authors	GCS 13–15	GCS 8–12	GCS 3–7	Year
Bidzinski & Koszewski 1990	5/51	4/11	3/3	1978–88
Gupta *et al.* 1990	2/50	10/30	0	1980–89
Yildizhan *et al.* 1991	0/5	5/23	10/13	1977–86
Total (%)	7/100 (**7**)	19/64 (**30**)	13/16 (**81**)	

mortality of 11/100 in those alert at diagnosis – an eightfold difference (Table 20.2). Similar difference were seen with Glasgow Coma Scores (GCS) on diagnosis (Table 20.3), where patients with a GCS of 3–7 had a CFR of 81/100 compared with a CFR of 7/100 for those with a GCS of 13–15.

There are several variables associated with improved outcome, including early diagnosis, more accurate localization and adequate microbiological therapy (Rubin & Hooper 1985; Rosenblum *et al.* 1986; Stroobandt *et al.* 1987; Szuwart & Bennefeld 1990). There remains much discussion of the relative values of use of medical or surgical therapy. The results of therapy from many centres (Table 20.4) show a lower CFR for excision (15/100) than aspiration (27/100) or medical therapy (22/100), but these tabulations do not take into account other variables, such as neurological status at diagnosis, or the basis of the choice of therapy, so that the differences cannot be evaluated or compared meaningfully. Post-treatment epilepsy is common (Table 20.5).

The pathology underlying a brain abscess often has a significant effect on the location, to the agent, and relates to an age group (Garfield 1978; Habib *et al.* 1988; Momma *et al.* 1990). As a result, it is difficult to know which of the related factors has the major effect on a CFR. The highest CFR was seen for abscess related to pulmonary pathology (56/100) and the lowest for those following trauma and complicating surgery (19/100) (Table 20.6).

Location of the brain abscess has a relation to underlying pathology, but a higher CFR was only observed for multilobar disease (41/100) (Table 20.7).

Post-treatment epilepsy has been described in relation to location of the brain abscess, but the numbers were too small for meaningful comparisons (Table 20.8).

There has been significant improvement in the microbiological study of brain abscesses since the 1960s (de Louvois 1978; de Louvois 1980; Tabaqchali 1988; Puthucheary & Parasakthi 1990; Brook 1992), with greater awareness of anaerobes, and the associated use of more effective antimicrobial treatment. However, CFRs in relation to infecting agent (Table 20.9) are not often reported in relation to the specific agent identified. The recent decade has witnessed a continuing rise in the number of patients who are immunocompromised, either as a result of immunotherapy for transplantation (Britt *et al.* 1981), depressed immunity following therapy for malignancy, or, increasingly, due to HIV infection. Brain abscesses due to *Listeria* occur in immunosuppressed individuals, especially those receiving organ transplants. In such patients, high CFRs may be common.

Table 20.4. *Case fatality ratios and type of therapy for brain abscess*

Authors	Aspiration	Drainage	Aspiration and excision	Excision	Medical therapy	Year
Bidzinski & Koszewski 1990	3/6	1/14		7/36	1/9	1978–88
Donald et al. 1990	0/11	0/5		0/3	0/4	1985–87
Ferriero et al. 1987	0/2			1/7	0/8	1975–84 children
Gupta et al. 1990	8/25		1/28	0/21	3/6	1980–89
Hirsch et al. 1983	3/27		1/3	0/4		1966–80 children
Jooma et al. 1951	58/95	45/89	15/111	Some		1925–50
Kagawa et al. 1983	6/22		0/17	5/7	12/16	1969–81 CHD only
Kawamoto et al. 1987	3/22	1/1		1/14		1959–83
Leys et al. 1990	2/21			0/15	0/20	1984–87
Mampalam & Rosenblum 1988	2/33			4/46	2/17	1970–86
Miller et al. 1988	10/55	0	0/8	4/22		1974–84
Nielsen 1983	4/11	6/16	0/3	2/11	0/2	1935–76 children
Richards et al. 1990	4/48		0/6	1/13	2/4	1979–88
Rousseaux et al. 1985	0/4			2/12	1/15	1979–82
Saez Llorens et al. 1989	4/18	7/25		7/45		1965–88
Shaw & Russell 1975	5/16		2/4	5/19		1950–73 cerebellar
van Alphen & Dreissen 1976	0/2	9/34	2/10	5/18		1956–73
Westcome et al. 1988	3/19			0/10	3/6	1978–86
Wong et al. (1989)	4/32		2/6	4/26		1978–87 children
Yildizhan et al. 1991	10/17			5/24		1977–86
Total (%)	129/486 (**27**)	69/184 (**38**)	23/196 (**12**)	53/353 (**15**)	24/107 (**22**)	

CHD, congenital heart disease.

Table 20.5. *Mode of therapy for brain abscess and post-treatment epilepsy*

Authors	Aspiration	Drainage	Aspiration and excision	Excision	Medical therapy	Year
Ferreiro et al. 1987	1/2		3/7		0/8	1975–84 children
Hirsch et al. 1983	3/27					1966–80 children
Jooma et al. 1951	15/31	21/38	26/65	10/18		1925–50
Kagawa et al. 1983	0/16		1/17	0/2		1969–81
Leys et al. 1990	8/14			3/14	1/18	1984–87 single
Rousseaux et al. 1985	0/4			2/10	0/12	1979–82
Total (%)	27/94 (29)	21/38 (55)	30/89 (33)	15/46 (33)	1/38 (3)	

Table 20.6. *Case fatality ratios in relation to pathology underlying brain abscess*

Authors	Otogenic	Paranasal	Trauma	CCHD	Post-surgery	Pulmonary	Miscellany	Unknown	Year
Alderson *et al.* 1981	10/45	1/4	2/10					3/14	1964–78
Bradley & Shaw 1983	63/128	14/54	2/17	4/12		37/52	2/12	16/45	1950–79
Chakraborty *et al.* 1989				12/28					1975–88
Chalstrey *et al.* 1991	3/13	2/17	0/11				4/18	1/14	1965–87
Jadavji *et al.* 1985			0/7	6/18	2/6				1960–84
Kagawa *et al.* 1983				23/62					1969–81
Keet 1990	86/233	20/66		6/15		22/60	6/36	21/89	1952–86
McGreal 1962	2/7			3/8			3/8	1/7	1951–60
Miller *et al.* 1988		5/29	1/6	4/18				5/17	1974–84
Nielsen *et al.* 1982	13/42	4/18	8/19	5/13	2/15	24/36	7/14	12/31	1935–76
Wong *et al.* (1989)				9/42					1978–87
Total (%)	177/468 (**38**)	46/188 (**24**)	13/70 (**19**)	72/216 (**33**)	4/21 (**19**)	83/148 (**56**)	22/88 (**55**)	59/217 (**27**)	

CCHD, Cyanotic congenital heart disease.

Table 20.7. Case fatality ratios in relation to location of brain abscess

Authors	Frontal	Parietal	Temporal	Occipital	Cerebellar	Multilobar	Year
Aydin et al. 1988	1/8	0/8	2/10	0		5/6	1979–87
Garfield 1969	18/53	14/38	18/61			10/10	1951–67
Ibrahim et al. 1990	0/5		1/8	0/2	1/3	2/4	1982–88
Kratimenos & Crockard 1991						2/4	1975–89
Miller et al. 1988	4/27	1/6	4/19	0/7		5/7	1974–84
Shaw & Russell 1975					13/41		1950–73
Unnikrishnan et al. 1989					1/29		1968–87
van Alphen & Dreissen 1976	5/22	4/10	13/29	5/10	3/9	2/3	1956–73
Total (%)	28/115 (**24**)	19/62 (**31**)	38/127 (**30**)	5/19 (**26**)	18/82 (**22**)	26/64 (**41**)	

Table 20.8. *Post-treatment epilepsy in relation to location of brain abscess*

Authors	Frontal	Parietal	Temporal	Occipital	Cerebellar	Multilobar	Year
Buonaguro et al. 1989	2/8	1/5	3/10	1/3		0/4	1975–85
Jooma et al. 1951	27/50	8/16	19/56	5/10		13/20	1925–50
Nielsen et al. 1983	17/23	7/11	13/24	0/2	0/7		1935–76
Total (%)	46/81 (**57**)	16/32 (**50**)	35/90 (**39**)	6/15 (**40**)	0/7	13/24 (**54**)	

Table 20.9. *Case fatality ratios in relation to the agent identified in the brain abscess*

Agent	Duel et al. 1991	Jadavji et al. 1985	Dee & Lorber 1986	van Alphen & Dreissen 1976	Iplikcioglu et al. 1991	Nielsen 1983
Actinomyces				1/1		
Bacteroides	1/5	2/7				
Citrobacter koseri		0/1				
E. coli	0/2	0/1				
Fusobacterium	1/1					
H. paraaphrophilus		1/3				
H. aphrophilus	0/5					
H. influenzae	1/2	0/1				
H. parainfluenzae		1/1				
Haemophilus spp.	0/2			1/1		
Klebsiella				1/1		
Lactobacillus	1/2					
Listeria			8/14			
Micrococcus	1/1					
Nocardia	0/1	0/3				
Peptococcus	0/3					
Peptostreptococci	0/6	0/3				
Proteus mirabilis	0/1	1/4		2/5		
Proteus vulgaris	0/2					
Pseudomonas		0/1				
Salmonella typhi					2/6	
Salmonella typhimurium					2/3	
Salmonella enteritidis					1/2	
Staphylococcus aureus	1/7	1/14		2/9		4/6
Anaerobic Streptoccus	0/1	2/11				3/8
α-Haemolytic Streptococcus	1/6	3/17				0/3
Steptococcus dysgalactiae	0/1					
Streptococcus milleri	0/3					
Streptococcus pneumoniae	0/3	1/6		1/5		2/6
Streptococcus pyogenes	0/1			10/30		
Streptococcus sanguis	0/1					

Age relates to several factors concerning CFR, since children have more frequent meningitis, otitis and cyanotic congenital heart disease (Idriss *et al.* 1978; Fischer *et al.* 1981; Nielsen; 1983; Spires *et al.* 1985; Hegde *et al.* 1986; Yang 1989; Ghosh *et al.* 1990; Nunez 1992). For those reports which describe outcome in relation to age (Tables 20.10, 20.11), age does not appear to be a major factor, either for case fatality or for post-treatment epilepsy.

Table 20.10. *Case fatality ratios in relation to age group for brain abscess*

Authors	Age group									Year
	< 1 month	< 1 year	0–4 years	5–14 years	15–19 years	1–19 years	0–19 years	20–59 years	60 + years	
Aydin et al. 1988							0/17	8/23	0/2	1979–87
Garcia-Abeja et al. 1988			0/4	2/8	1/3					1977–85
Jadavji et al. 1985		1/10					11/63			1960–84
Johnson et al. 1988				0/7	0/6					1978–85
McGreal 1962			4/7	6/23						1951–60
Moss et al. 1988			3/23	3/27	1/4		7/54			1958–87
Renier et al. 1988	4/30									1973–85
Saez-Llorens et al. 1989		19/37				11/64				1965–88
Seydoux & Francioli 1992							0/7	3/19	2/13	1977–87
Shaw & Russell 1975							4/15	12/28	3/4	1950–73
Wong et al. (1989)		3/10				13/73				1978–87
Total (%)	4/30 (**13**)	23/57 (**40**)	7/34 (**21**)	11/65 (**17**)	2/13 (**15**)	24/137 (**18**)	22/156 (**14**)	23/70 (**33**)	5/19 (**26**)	

Table 20.11. *Frequency of post-treatment epilepsy following brain abscess in relation to age group*

Authors	Age group (years)							Year
	<1	1–19	1–9	10–19	20–29	30–39	40 +	
Jooma *et al.* 1951			12/28	15/34	25/46	8/15	12/29	1925–50
Nielsen *et al.* 1983[a]					13/21	7/15	5/9	1935–76
Renier *et al.* 1988	12/26	3/33						1973–85
Total (%)	15/26 (58)	3/33 (33)	12/28 (43)	15/34 (44)	38/67 (57)	15/30 (50)	17/38 (45)	

[a] The data from Nielsen *et al.* (1983) are in different age groups from those from Jooma *et al.* (1951) but for purposes of analysis have been placed in the same age categories.

Table 20.12. *Case fatality ratios in relation to number of brain abscesses*

Authors	Single lesion	Multiple lesions	Year
Basit *et al.* 1989		5/21	1976–84
Dyste *et al.* 1988		1/8	1983–85
Kratimenos & Crockard 1991		2/14	1975–89
Kulali *et al.* 1990	2/10	1/4	1988–89
Saez-Llorens *et al.* 1989	9/68	21/33	1965–88
Witzmann *et al.*	5/32	2/6	1975–88
Total (%)	16/110 (15)	32/86 (37)	

The frequency of multiple brain abscesses has ranged widely, averaging 1–15%, and with improved diagnostic procedures the frequency has increased (Uttley 1991). The CFR for multiple brain abscesses (37/100) is higher than for single abscesses (15/100) (Table 20.12), with the outcome also relating to abscess size and location.

Future comparisons of the various individual factors involved in CFRs and in post-treatment, long-term sequelae will be more meaningful if they deal specifically with the major individual factors. This means reporting outcomes in groups relating to neuro-logical status at diagnosis – a major factor – and dealing with the combination of agent, location and underlying pathology, which together may be a significant secondary factor, and separately with age groups. To achieve significance within these groupings, it is probable that only multicentre studies will have sufficient numbers. Within the next decade this should be possible, using computer-held data following carefully defined protocols.

References

Aebi, C., Kaufmann, F. & Schaad, U. B. (1991). Brain abscess in childhood: long-term experiences. *Eur. J. Pediatr.* **150**, 282–6.

Alderson, D., Strong, A. J., Ingham, H. R. & Selkon, T. D. (1981). Fifteen-year review of the mortality of brain abscess. *Neurosurgery* **8**, 1–6.

Arseni, C. & Ciurea, A. V. (1988). Cerebral abscesses secondary to otorhinolaryngological infections. A study of 386 cases. *Zentralbl. Neurochir.* **49**, 22–36.

Aydin, I. H., Aladag, M. A., Kadioglu, H. H. & Onder, A. (1988). Clinical analysis of cerebral abscesses. *Zentralbl. Neurochir.* **49**, 210–19.

Basit, A. S., Ravi, B., Banerji, A. K. & Tandon, P. N. (1989). Multiple pyogenic brain abscesses: an analysis of 21 patients. *J. Neurol. Neurosurg. Psychiatry* **52**, 591–4.

Bidzinski, J. & Koszewski, W. (1990). The value of different methods of treatment of brain abscess in the CT era. *Acta Neurochirurg. Wien* **105**, 117–20.

Bradley, P. J. & Shaw, M. D. M. (1983). Three decades of brain abscess in Merseyside. *J. R. Coll. Surg. Edinb.* **28**, 223–8.

Britt, R. H., Enzmann, D. R. & Remington, J. S. (1981). Intracranial infection in cardiac transplant recipients. *Ann. Neurol.* **9**, 107–19.

Brook, I. (1992). Aerobic and anaerobic bacteriology of intracranial abscesses. *Pediatr. Neurol.* **8**, 210–14.

Buonaguro, A., Colangelo, M., Daniele, B., Cantone, G. & Ambrosio, A. (1989). Neurological and behavioral sequelae in children operated on for brain abscess. *Childs Nerv. Syst.* **5**, 153–5.

Chakraborty, R. N., Bidwai, P. S., Kak, V. K., Banarjee, A. K., Khattri, H. N., Sapru, R. P., Walia, B. N., Kumar, L., Suri, S. & Wahi, P. L. (1989). Brain abscess in cyanotic congenital heart disease. *Ind. Heart J.* **41**, 190–3.

Chalstrey, S., Pfleiderer, A. G. & Moffat, D. A. (1991). Persisting incidence and mortality of sinogenic cerebral abscess: a continuing reflection of late clinical diagnosis. *J. R. S. Med.* **84**, 193–5.

Chun, C. H., Johnson, J. D., Hofstetter, M. & Raff, M. J. (1986). Brain abscess. A study of 45 consecutive cases. *Medicine* **65**, 415–31.

Dee, R. R. & Lorber, B. (1986). Brain abscess due to *Listeria monocytogenes*: case report and literature review. *Rev. Infect. Dis.* **8**, 968–77.

Donald, F. E., Firth, J. L., Holland, I. M., Hope, D. T., Ispahani, P. & Punt, J. A. (1990). Brain abscess in the 1980s. *Br. J. Neurosurg.* **4**, 265–71.

Duel, P., Siboni, K. & Jensen, T. G. (1991). Intracranial abscesses in Odense Hospital. Survey of bacteriology, epidemiology, and treatment with antibiotics, 1963–1989. *Danish Med. Bull.* **38**, 407–10.

Dyste, G. N., Hitchon, P. W., Menezes, A. H., Van Gilder, J. C. & Greene, G. M. (1988). Stereoataxic surgery in the treatment of multiple brain abscesses. *J. Neurosurg.* **69**, 188–94.

Ferriero, D. M., Derechin, M., Edwards, M. S. & Berg, B. O. (1987). Outcome of brain abscess treatment in children: reduced morbidity with neuroimaging. *Pediatr. Neurol.* **3**, 148–52.

Fischer, E. G., McLennan, J. E. & Suzuki, Y. (1981). Cerebral abscess in children. *Am. J. Dis. Child.* **135**, 746–9.

Garcia-Abeja, J. C., Capon Echevarria, I., Rubio Quinones, F., Rodenas Luque, G., Barrionuevo Gallo, B. & Nieto Barrera, M. (1988). [Cerebral abscess in childhood]. *An. Esp. Pediatr.* **29**, 369–73.

Garfield, J. (1969). Management of supratentorial intracranial abscess: a review of 200 cases. *BMJ* **22**, 7–11.

Garfield, J. (1978). Brain abscesses and focal suppurative infections. In: *Infections of the Nervous System*, part I, *Handbook of Clinical Neurology*, vol. 33, eds. G. W. Bruyn & P. J. Vinken, pp. 107–47.

Ghosh, S., Chandy, M. J. & Abraham, J. (1990). Brain abscess and congenital heart disease. *J. Ind. Med. Assoc.* **88**, 312–14.

Gortvai, P., De Louvois, J. & Hurley, R. (1987). Incidence and mortality of abscess of the CNS in England and Wales: results of a survey. *J. Neurol. Neurosurg. Psychiatry* **41**, 1053.

Gupta, S. K., Mohanty, S., Tandon, S. C. & Asthana, S. (1990). Brain abscess: with special reference to infection by *Pseudomonas*. *Br. J. Neurosurg.* **4**, 279–85.

Habib, R. G., Girgis, N. I., Abu el Ella, A. H., Farid, Z. & Woody, J. (1988). The treatment and outcome of intracranial infections of otogenic origin. *J. Trop. Med. Hygiene* **91**, 83–6.

Harle, J. R., Vincentelli, F., Peragut, J. C., Weiller, P. J. & Grisoli, F. (1988). [Cerebral abscess. Analysis of 41 cases over a 10-year period]. *Rev. Med. Interne* **9**, 369–76.

Hegde, A. S., Venkataramana, N. K. & Das, B. S. (1986). Brain abscess in children. *Childs Nerv. System.* **2**, 90–2.

Hirsch, J. F., Roux, F. X., Sainte-Rose, C., Renier, D. & Pierre-Lahn, A. (1983). Brain abscess in child. A study of 34 cases treated by puncture and antibiotics. *Child's Brain* **10**, 251–65.

Ibrahim, A. W., al Rajeh, S. M., Chowdhary, U. M. & Ammar, A. (1990). Brain abscess in Saudi Arabia. *Neurosurg. Rev.* **13**, 103–7.

Idriss, Z. H., Gutman, L. T. & Kronfol, N. M. (1978). Brain abscesses in infants and children. *Clin. Pediatr.* **17**, 738–46.

Iplikcioglu, A. C., Kokes, F., Bayar, M. A., Edebali, N., Gokcek, C. & Buharali, Z. (1991). Brain abscess caused by *Salmonella typhimurium*. Case report and review of the literature. *J. Neurosurg. Sci.* **35**, 165–8.

Jadavji, T. A. J., Humphreys, R. P. & Prober, C. G. (1985). Brain abscesses in infants and children. *Pediatr. Infect. Dis. J.* **4**, 394–8.

Jahn, A. J. & Douglas Snell, G. E. (1980). Otogenic intracranial complications. *J. Otolaryngol.* **9**, 184–93.

Jennett, B. & Bond, M. (1975). Assessment of outcome after severe brain damage. *Lancet* **1**, 480–4.

Johnson, D. L., Markle, B. M., Widermann, B. L. & Hanahan, L. (1988). Treatment of intracranial abscesses associated with sinusitis in children and adolescents. *J. Pediatr.* **113**, 15–23.

Jooma, O. V., Pennybacker, J. B. & Tutton, G. K. (1951). Brain abscess: aspiration drainage, or excision? *J. Neurol. Neurosurg. Psychiatry* **14**, 308–13.

Kagawa, M., Takeshita, M., Yato, S. & Kitamura, K. (1983). Brain abscess in congenital cyanotic heart disease. *J. Neurosurg.* **58**, 913–17.

Karandanis, D. & Shulman, J. A. (1975). Factors associated with mortality in brain abscess. *Arch. Intern. Med.* **135**, 1145–50.

Kawamoto, T., Abe, H., Saito, H. & Kitaoka, K. (1987). [Treatment of brain abscess. Comparison between aspiration and extra-capsular total excision]. *Neurol. Med. Chirurig.* **27**, 429–35.

Keet, P. C. (1990). Cranial intradural abscess management of 641 patients during the 35 years from 1952 to 1986. *Br. J. Neurosurg.* **4**, 273–8.

Koszewski, W. (1991). Epilepsy following brain abscess. The evaluation of possible risk factors with emphasis on new concept of epileptic focus formation. *Acta Neurochirurg. (Wien)* **113**, 110–17.

Kourtopoulus, H., Holme, S. E. & West, K. A. (1981). The management of intracranial abscesses: comparative study between two materials with significantly different rates of mortality. *Acta Neurochirurg. (Wien)* **56**, 127–8.

Kratimenos, G. & Crockard, H. A. (1991). Multiple brain abscess: a review of fourteen cases. *Br. J. Neurosurg.* **5**, 153–61.

Kulali, A., Ozatik, N. & Topcu, I. (1990). Otogenic intracranial abscesses. *Acta Neurochirurg. (Wien)* **107**, 140–6.

Leys, D., Christiaens, J. L., Derambure, P., Hladky, J. P., Lesoin, Rousseaux, M., Jomin, M. & Petit, H. (1990). Management of focal intracranial infections: is medical treatment better than surgery? *J. Neurol. Neurosurg. Psychiatry* **53**, 472–5.

Louvois de, J. (1978). The bacteriology and chemotherapy of brain abscess. *J. Antimicrob. Chemother.* **4**, 395–413.

Louvois de, J. (1980). Bacteriological examination of pus from abscesses of the central nervous system. *J. Clin. Pathol.* **33**, 66–71.

McClelland, C. J., Craig, B. F. & Crockard, H. A. (1978). Brain abscesses in Northern Ireland: a 30-year community review. *J. Neurol. Neurosurg. Psychiatry* **41**, 1043–7.

McGreal, D. A. (1962). Brain abscess in children. *Can. Med. Assoc. J.* **86**, 261–8.

Mampalam, T. J. & Rosenblum, M. L. (1988). Trends in the management of bacterial brain abscesses: a review of 102 cases over 17 years. *Neurosurgery* **23**, 451–8.

Miller, E. S., Dias, P. S. & Uttley, D. (1988). CT scanning in the management of intracranial abscess: a review of 100 cases. *Br. J. Neurosurg.* **2**, 439–46.

Momma, F., Ohara, S., Ohyama, T., Moto, A., Okada, H. & Harada, H. (1990). Brain abscess associated with congenital pulmonary arteriovenous fistula. *Surg. Neurol.* **34**, 439–41.

Moss, S. D., McLone, D. G., Arditi, M. & Yogev, R. (1988). Pediatric cerebral abscess. *Pediatr. Neurosci.* **14**, 291–6.

Nalbone, V. P., Kuruvilla, A. & Gacek, R. R. (1992). Otogenic brain abscess: the Syracuse experience. *Ear Nose Throat J.* **71**, 238–42.

Nicolosi, A., Hauser, W. A., Musicco, M. & Kurland, L. T. (1991). Incidence and prognosis of brain abscess in a defined population: Olmsted County, Minnesota, 1935–1981. *Neuroepidemiology* **10**, 122–31.

Nielsen, H. (1983). Cerebral abscess in children. *Neuropediatrics* **14**, 76–80.

Nielsen, H., Gyldensted, C. & Harmsen, A. (1982). Cerebral abscess. Aetiology and pathogenesis, symptoms, diagnosis and treatment. A review of 200 cases from 1935–1976. *Acta Neurol. Scand.* **65**, 609–22.

Nielsen, H., Harmsen, A. & Gyldensted, C. (1983). Cerebral abscess. A long-term follow-up. *Acta Neurol. Scand.* **67**, 330–7.

Nunez, D. A. (1992). Aetiological role of otolaryngological disease in paediatric intracranial abscess. *J. R. Col. Surg. Edinb.* **37**, 80–2.

Puthucheary, S. D. & Parasakthi, N. (1990). The bacteriology of brain abscess: a local experience in Malaysia. *Trans. R. Soc. Trop. Med. Hygiene* **84**, 589–92.

Rantakallio, P., Leskinen, M. & von Wendt, L. (1986). Incidence and prognosis of central nervous system infections in a birth cohort of 12 000 children. *Scand. J. Infect. Dis.* **18**, 287–94.

Renier, D., Flandin, C., Hirsch, E. & Hirsch, J. F. (1988). Brain abscesses in neonates. A study of 30 cases. *J. Neurosurg.* **69**, 877–82.

Richards, J., Sisson, P. R., Hickman, J. E., Ingham, H. R. & Selkon, J. B. (1990). Microbiology, chemotherapy and mortality of brain abscess in Newcastle-upon-Tyne between 1979 and 1988. *Scand. J. Infect. Dis.* **22**, 511–18.

Rosenblum, M. L., Hoff, J. T., Norman, D., Weinstein, P. R. & Pitts, L. (1978). Decreased mortality from brain abscesses since advent of computerised tomography. *J. Neurosurg.* **49**, 658–68.

Rosenblum, M. L., Mampalam, T. J. & Pons, V. G. (1986). Controversies in the management of brain abscesses. *Clin. Neurosurg.* **33**, 603–32.

Rousseaux, F., Lesoin, F., Destee, A., Jomin, M. & Petit, H. (1985). Long-term sequelae of hemispheric abscesses as a function of the treatment. *Acta Neurochirurg. (Wien)* **740**, 61–7.

Rubin, R. H. & Hooper, D. C. (1985). Central nervous system infection in the compromised host. *Med. Clin. North Am.* **69**, 281–96.

Saez Llorens, X. J., Umana, M. A., Odio, C. M., McCracken, G. H. Jr. & Nelson, J. D. (1989). Brain abscess in infants and children. *Pediatr. Infect. Dis. J.* **8**, 449–58.

Schliamser, S. E., Backman, K. & Norrby, S. R. (1988). Intracranial abscesses in adults: an analysis of 54 consecutive cases. *Scand. J. Infect. Dis.* **20**, 1–9.

Seydoux, C. & Francioli, P. (1992). Bacterial brain abscesses: factors influencing mortality and sequelae. *Clin. Infect. Dis.* **15**, 394–401.

Shaw, M. D. M. & Russell, J. A. (1975). Cerebellar abscess. *J. Neurol. Neurosurg. Psychiatry* **38**, 429–35.

Small, M. & Dale, A. B. (1984). Intracranial suppuration 1968–1982: 1 15-year review. *Clin. Otolaryngol.* **9**, 315–21.

Sparrow, O. C. (1991). The importance of early detection of intracranial suppuration [editorial]. *J. R. Soc. Med.* **84**, 187–9.

Spires, J. R., Smith, R. J. H. & Catlin, F. I. (1985). Brain abscesses in the young. *Otolaryngol. Head Neck Surg.* **93**, 468–74.

Stroobandt, G., Zech, F., Thauvoy, C., Mathurin, P., de Nijs, C. & Gilliard, C. (1987). Treatment by aspiration of brain abscesses. *Acta Neurochirurg. (Wien)* **85**, 138–47.

Svanteson, B., Nordstrom, C. H. & Rausing, A. (1988). Non-traumatic brain abscess. Epidemiology, clinical symptoms and therapeutic results. *Acta Neurochirurg. (Wien)* **94**, 57–65.

Szuwart, U. & Bennefeld, H. (1990). Bacteriological analysis of pyogenic infections of the brain. *Neurosurg. Rev.* **13**, 113–18.

Tabaqchali, S. (1988). Anaerobic infections in the head and neck region. *Scand. J. Infect. Dis.* **57**, (Suppl.), 24–34.

Unnikrishnan, M., Chandy, M. J. & Abraham, J. (1989). Posterior fossa abscesses. A review of 33 cases. *J. Assoc. Phys. India* **37**, 376–8.

Uttley, D. (1991). Multiple cerebral abscesses [editorial]. *Br. J. Neurosurg.* **5**, 119–21.

van Alphen, H. A. M. & Dreissen, J. J. R. (1976). Brain abscess and subdural empyema. *J. Neurol. Neurosurg. Psychiatry* **39**, 481–90.

van Dellen, J. R., Bullock, R. & Postma, M. H. (1987). Cerebellar abscess: the impact of computed tomographic scanning. *Neurosurgery* **21**, 547–50.

Westcombe, D. S., Dorsch, N. W. & Teo, C. (1988). Management of cerebral abscess in adolescents and adults. Experience in the CT-scan era. *Acta Neurochirurg. (Wien)* **95**, 85–9.

Wispelwey, B. & Scheld, W. M. (1987). Brain abscess. *Clin. Neuropharmacol.* **10**, 483–510.

Witzmann, A., Beran, H., Bohm Jurkovic, H., Reisecker, F. & Leblhuber, F. (1989) Brain abscess. Prognostic factors. *Dtsch Med. Wochenschr.* **114**, 85–90.

Wong, T. T., Lee, L. S., Wang, H. S., Shen, E. Y., Jaw, W. C., Chiang, C. H., Chi, C. S., Hung, K. L., Liou, W. Y. & Shen, Y. Z. (1989). Brain abscesses in children – a cooperative study of 83 cases. *Childs Nerv. Syst.* **5**, 19–24.

Yang, S. Y. (1989). Brain abscess associated with congenital heart disease. *Surg. Neurol.* **31**, 129–32.

Yildizhan, A., Pasaoglu, A., Ozkul, M. H., Aral, O. & Ozkul, N. (1991). Clinical analysis and results of operative treatment of 41 brain abscesses. *Neurosurg. Rev.* **14**, 279–82.

21 Viral infections of the nervous system

MOHAMMAD K. SHARIEF AND MICHAEL SWASH

Viral meningitis

Viral meningitis is a common illness, particularly amongst children, and is most often caused by enteroviruses. There is a tendency to equate the syndrome of aseptic meningitis with that of viral meningitis. A distinction should be made, however, since a large number of disorders with varying and sometimes serious outcomes can mimic viral meningitis. On the other hand, the prognosis of viral meningitis is very good, and the disease is rarely fatal, though death due to concurrent myocarditis has been reported in patients with coxsackievirus meningitis. Almost all patients with viral meningitis recover spontaneously; in those who develop serious neurological sequelae, care should be taken to exclude other aetiologies, such as partially treated bacterial meningitis.

The acute illness may be complicated by either complex partial seizures, physical evidence of increased intracranial pressure, or coma in approximately 9.0% of cases. The risk of acute neurological complications is slightly higher in neonates than in older children or adults, but appears to be similar among patients infected with group B coxsackie viruses and echoviruses, the two major enteroviruses causing viral meningitis. Follow-up studies have shown that 5–20% of patients with viral meningitis develop transient post-meningitic disorders, especially prolonged episodes of stress-induced headache. The risk of long-term neurological sequelae, however, is very small indeed (Table 21.1). Long-term prognosis in patients who develop acute complications appears to be as favourable as that for patients who do not experience acute complications.

Although the neurological outcome of viral meningitis is generally good, infection with certain viruses carries a less favourable outcome. For instance, meningitis caused by Epstein–Barr viral infection can result in long-term neurological complications, particularly when a concomitant encephalitic illness is present (Connelly & Dewitt 1994). Meningitis caused by the human immunodeficiency virus (HIV) carries a poor prognosis (see below).

Herpes simplex encephalitis

Herpes simplex virus infection of the central nervous system is a significant cause of mortality and morbidity. The mortality rate from biopsy-proven disease, with either no

Table 21.1. *Acute and long-term neurological complications of viral meningitis*

Authors	No. of patients followed-up	Acute neurological complications	Long-term morbidity	Nature of morbidity
Etter *et al.* 1991	259	26 (10%)	1 (0.4%)	Hydrocephalus
Dufour & Waldvogel 1991	124	8 (6%)	Nil	—
Rorabaugh *et al.* 1993	277	25 (9%)	Nil	—

Table 21.2. *Mortality rates in untreated patients with herpes simplex encephalitis*

Authors	Total no. of patients	No. of deaths	Mortality rate
Whitley *et al.* 1977	10	7	70%
Longstone *et al.* 1980	11	8	73%
Whitley *et al.* 1980	19[a]	14	74%
Kennard & Swash 1981	6	4[b]	67%
Kennedy 1988	19	16	84%
Buttner & Dorndorf 1988	9	8	89%
Ginsberg & Compston 1994	8	6	75%
All patients	82	63	77%

[a] Including infants with disseminated herpes simplex virus disease.
[b] Including one patient treated with vidarabine.

Table 21.3. *Morbidity rates in patients with herpes simplex encephalitis who did not receive vidarabine or acyclovir*

Authors	Total no. of survivors	Patients with residual signs	Morbidity rate
Whitley *et al.* 1977	3	2	
Longson *et al.* 1980	3	3	
Longson *et al.* 1980	4[a]	4	
Kennard & Swash 1981	2	0	
All patients	12	9	75%

[a] Treated with cytarabine.

or ineffective therapy, is at least 70%, with less than 30% of survivors returning to normal function. The introduction of antiviral therapy has improved the outcome, resulting in significantly improved morbidity and mortality rates. The overall mortality rate following antiviral treatment has been reduced to nearly 20%, and almost half the survivors return to normal function.

Mortality following herpes simplex encephalitis

Herpes simplex encephalitis is the most common cause of sporadic acute focal encephalitis. The risk of death (Table 21.2) or severe damage in patients with herpes simplex encephalitis is more than 12-fold that from acute encephalitis of other causes (Rautonen *et al.* 1991). The disease is also associated with high morbidity rate if not treated properly (Table 21.3). A distinction must be made between neonatal infections of the central nervous system, which can be caused by either herpes simplex virus type 1 or type 2, and infection in older children and adults, which is the consequence of herpes simplex virus type 1 in the overwhelming majority of cases. Therefore, the outcome of herpes simplex encephalitis in the newborn will be discussed separately (see below).

Mortality varies according to the level of consciousness at the time of presentation. For instance, the mortality rate amongst comatose patients is much higher than that in semicomatose or lethargic patients. Disoriented patients who flex and respond by eye to pain generally have a low mortality risk, and about half of them will recover completely. Death commonly occurs within a few weeks in patients with prolonged coma, and is usually due to respiratory complications. Prompt treatment of herpes simplex encephalitis with acyclovir, which is highly effective and safe, is essential to avoid a poor outcome.

Herpes simplex encephalitis in fetus and newborn

Although infrequent, untreated neonatal herpes infection results in death in 50–80% of cases and neurological sequelae in about 70% of the survivors (Overall 1994). Neonatal infection is usually acquired from maternal genital herpes, which is asymptomatic or unrecognized in 60–80% of affected women. The greatest risk of neonatal infection occurs when the mother has primary genital herpes involving the cervix at delivery, and the infant is premature and delivered with instrumentation. More than 80% of neonates with herpes will have typical herpetic lesions of the skin, eye or mouth, and most of the remainder will have either encephalitis or a sepsis syndrome with pneumonitis and hepatitis and negative bacterial cultures. Treatment with intravenous acyclovir does reduce mortality and neurological sequelae, but the outcome is still guarded in babies with disseminated disease or encephalitis.

The infecting virus also determines neurological outcome in neonatal herpes simplex encephalitis. The neurological morbidity of patients with herpes simplex virus type 2 encephalitis is much higher than in those with herpes simplex virus type 1 encephalitis. Twenty-four infants treated with acyclovir or vidarabine for neonatal herpes simplex encephalitis were followed for up to 3 years (Corey et al. 1988) to assess neurological and developmental outcome; 15 patients had herpes simplex virus type 2 and 9 had type 1 encephalitis. One patient (7%) with herpes simplex virus type 2 infection died. All 9 herpes simplex virus type 1 patients were normal at follow-up compared with only 4 (23%) of the 14 surviving infants infected with herpes simplex virus type 2.

Effect of treatment on outcome

The influence of treatment on the outcome of herpes simplex encephalitis has evolved over the past three decades. In 1966 iodo-2'-deoxyuridine (IDU) was reported to improve survival, though the natural history and prognosis of the untreated disease was unclear at that time. Subsequently, other drugs were evaluated, and in the early 1970s a controlled trial of IDU, cytosine arabinoside and vidarabine (adenine arabinoside) was undertaken in comparison with placebo. IDU was withdrawn early in the course of that study because of clear-cut toxicity without efficacy. The mortality rate

Table 21.4. *Mortality rates in adults with herpes simplex encephalitis treated with vidarabine or acyclovir*

Authors	Total no. of patients	No. of deaths	Mortality rate
Sköldenberg *et al.* 1984	27[a]	5	19%[c]
Sköldenberg *et al.* 1984	24[b]	12	50%
Whitley *et al.* 1986	32[a]	9	28%[c]
Whitley *et al.* 1986	37[b]	20	54%
Kennedy 1988	12	4	33%
Besser *et al.* 1990	19	5	26%
Rao & Costa 1991	3	1	—

[a] Treated with acyclovir.
[b] Treated with vidarabine.
[c] Statistically significant compared with vidarabine-treated group.

Table 21.5. *Mortality rate following treatment of herpes simplex encephalitis with acyclovir compared with outcome following treatment with vidarabine*

Time after therapy (months)	Mortality rate		
	Acyclovir therapy	Vidarabine therapy	Placebo
1	13–19%	28–45%	≥ 70%
6	18–20%	38–54%	≥ 70%
18	19–28%	50–54%	≥ 70%

Adapted from Whitley (1988).

following treatment with cytosine arabinoside was similar to that in the non-treatment group. In contrast, vidarabine showed a significant improvement in outcome compared with placebo, and by the mid-1970s it became clear that mortality due to herpes simplex encephalitis was significantly reduced by treatment with vidarabine (Table 21.4). Patients who were treated and survived had less severe neurological sequelae, and almost one-third returned to normal function. The results of two further studies, one performed in Sweden and one performed in the United States, showed that recipients of the newer anti-herpes drug, acyclovir, had a lower mortality than those who received vidarabine (Table 21.5).

Neonatal herpes simplex encephalitis also responds to antiherpetic medications (Table 21.6). The mortality and morbidity rates were evaluated in more than 290 babies with neonatal herpes simplex virus infection over a period of 14 years. For patients with biopsy-proven encephalitis, acyclovir therapy was found to be superior to vidarabine therapy. When the outcome in vidarabine-treated patients was compared with that in patients treated with acyclovir, mortality rates were decreased to 20% with acyclovir, and approximately 40% of survivors were evaluated as normal at 1 year after therapy (Whitley 1988). Another study, however, reported no differences in outcome between vidarabine and acyclovir in the treatment of neonatal herpes simplex virus infection (Whitley *et al.* 1991a), but the second study lacked statistical power to determine

Table 21.6. *Mortality rates in infants and children with herpes simplex encephalitis treated with acyclovir or vidarabine*

Authors	Total no. of patients	No. of deaths	Mortality rate
Whitley *et al.* 1986	32[a]	9	28%
Whitley *et al.* 1986	37[b]	20	54%[c]
Whitley *et al.* 1991a	35[a]	5	14%
Whitley *et al.* 1991a	36[a]	5	14%
Mancini *et al.* 1991	10	2	20%
Bigotte *et al.* 1993	10	5	50%

[a] Treated with acyclovir.
[b] Treated with vidarabine.
[c] Statistically significant compared with vidarabine-treated group.

whether there were sizeable differences within the subgroups of those with localized herpes simplex virus infection, encephalitis or disseminated disease.

Nonetheless, the effectiveness of acyclovir has been confirmed by several later studies, and current data indicate that acyclovir is the treatment of choice for neonatal herpes simplex encephalitis, resulting in significantly improved mortality and morbidity rates. Overall, the mortality rate at 1 year is reduced to less than 25%. Despite better outcome with antiviral therapy, improvement does not seem to be dose-related. Bigotte and others (1993) studied the clinical notes of 12 neonates treated for herpes simplex virus infection over a period of 6 years. Acyclovir was given intravenously at doses of 30 mg/kg per 24 hours (5 patients) or 60 mg/kg per 24 hours (7 patients) at an average of 8 days after the first clinical manifestation. The initial dose of 30 mg/kg per 24 hours was increased to 50 or 60 mg/kg per 24 hours in 3 patients, but there was no correlation between outcome and the dose of acyclovir, which was well tolerated in all patients. Five patients died during treatment, and 5 had severe sequelae; follow-up for the 2 remaining patients was not possible.

Predictors of outcome of herpes simplex encephalitis

Previous studies have consistently defined age, level of consciousness on admission or, more objectively, the score on the Glasgow Coma Scale (GCS), and whether or not antiviral agents were administered as being the most important predictors of eventual outcome in herpes simplex encephalitis. Young age at presentation, low score on the GCS, and disruption of oculocephalic responses are significantly associated with poor outcome. When GCS score and age are assessed simultaneously, a GCS score less than or equal to 6 indicates a poor therapeutic outcome. Conversely, with a GCS score in excess of 6, the best outcome is achieved in patients less than 30 years of age. When age is evaluated separately, there appears to be a bimodal curve regarding mortality and morbidity. Older adults do not fare as well as those under 30 years of age, and very young children and neonates, possibly owing to delay in diagnosis, have mortality and morbidity rates higher than expected.

Disease duration also influences outcome. A duration less than 4 days (considering time of onset of fever, disorientation, or any abnormal neurological features as the onset of disease) is associated with the best outcome – a mortality rate of around 7%. If disease duration is greater than 4 days, the mortality rate increases from 7% to 25% despite treatment with acyclovir.

Laboratory parameters predicting outcome

The background EEG activity can be of prognostic value in herpes simplex encephalitis, particularly in neonates (Holmes & Lombroso 1993). Certain abnormalities, such as cerebral electrical inactivity, burst suppression, or prolonged periodic discharges, are highly predictive of poor outcome, whereas other abnormalities of background rhythm, including amplitude, asymmetry and maturation, are associated with more variable outcomes. Outcome, however, cannot be predicted from a single EEG feature, and the prognostic value of the EEG is increased by performing serial studies.

Intracranial pressure (ICP) monitoring in severe encephalitis may also be a useful indicator of prognosis (Barnett et al. 1988). An initial ICP of less than 12 mmHg or a mean daily ICP of less than 20 mmHg usually indicate good prognosis, whereas higher ICP is associated with increased mortality rate. On the other hand, other laboratory investigations, such as concentrations of creatine phosphokinase and procoagulant activity in cerebrospinal fluid, are not predictive of outcome. Similarly, early findings on cranial imaging do not predict outcome, but later serial imaging data showing progression of early findings, such as very extensive low attenuation of cerebral white matter or cortical atrophy, are more accurate in predicting poor prognosis.

Grimm et al. (1991) suggested that the somatosensory evoked potential's short-latency cortical (N20) component may be predictive of outcome in herpes simplex encephalitis. The current role of somatosensory evoked potentials lies in the value of the long-latency (N70) component in detecting focal neurological damage in comatose patients, where clinical evaluation of brain function is difficult, and in monitoring their deterioration.

Neurological sequelae following herpes simplex encephalitis

Of the patients who have survived encephalitis, more than half develop severe debilitating sequelae (Table 21.7), including major motor and sensory deficits, aphasia, seizures, and cognitive and behavioural impairment. The functional outcome of herpes simplex encephalitis has improved following advances in intensive care and, more importantly, the advent of antiviral treatments, notably acyclovir (Table 21.8). In view of its low toxicity, acyclovir should be tried when the disease is clinically suspected, without waiting for the diagnosis to be confirmed by serological tests; treatment can thus be instituted before the patient becomes comatose. If patients survive the acute

Table 21.7. *Rate of neurological complications following herpes simplex encephalitis*

Authors	Range of follow-up (years)	Total no. of patients	No. of patients with neurological deficit	Morbidity rate
Sköldenberg *et al.* 1981	2–4	6	5	83%
Vandvik *et al.* 1982	1–2	5	4	80%
Whitley *et al.* 1986	≤ 1	30	17	57%
Bos *et al.* 1987	≤ 1	11	6	55%
Buge *et al.* 1988	4–8	14	9	64%
Kennedy 1988	9–23	19	14	74%
Whitley 1988	≤ 1	69	52	75%
Mancini *et al.* 1991	2–10	7	6	86%
Whitley *et al.* 1991b	1	58	37	64%
Raroque *et al.* 1993	4–7	13	8	62%

Table 21.8. *Morbidity rates following treatment of herpes simplex encephalitis with acyclovir or vidarabine*

	Morbidity rate	
	Acyclovir therapy	Vidarabine therapy
Severe sequelae or death	33–35%	65–79%
Moderate sequalae	9–11%	8–22%
Normal or minor sequelae	38–56%	13%

Adapted from Whitley (1988).

illness, the factors predicting morbidity include development of seizures at presentation, level of consciousness, duration of disease before the start of therapy, virus type and, in neonates, the presence of a disseminated disease (Table 21.9). Long-term neurological morbidity following herpes simplex encephalitis can be broadly divided into cognitive and focal neurological sequelae.

Cognitive sequelae

Despite antiviral treatment, some patients develop severe neurological and behavioural sequelae, predominantly Korsakoff's psychosis and Kluver–Bucy syndrome. The pattern of cognitive and memory impairment is primarily due to involvement of medial temporal lobe structures. Documentation of the long-term cognitive impairment following herpes simplex encephalitis was presented by Kapur *et al.* (1994). With a dedicated magnetic resonance imaging (MRI) protocol, the major pathological features of post-encephalitic amnesia were: (1) unilateral or bilateral hippocampal damage, accompanied by damage to the parahippocampus, the amygdala and insula; (2) unilateral or asymmetric neocortical temporal lobe damage; (3) predominant damage of anterior and inferior temporal lobe gyri; (4) pronounced abnormality in the substantia innominata, fornix and mammillary bodies; (5) unilateral damage of thalamic nuclei in

Table 21.9. *Prognostic factors influencing morbidity following herpes simplex encephalitis identified by multivariate analysis*

Prognostic factor	Relative risk
Level of consciousness	4.0
Seizures at presentation	3.0
Extent of disease	2.1
Age of onset > 30 years	1.8
Herpes simplex virus type 2[a]	4.9
Recurrent cutaneous lesions[a]	1

Modified from Whitley *et al.* (1991b).
[a] Mainly in neonates.

around 50% of cases; and (6) limited involvement of the cingulate gyrus, parietal and occipital lobes.

The role of MRI of the brain in predicting the severity of memory dysfunction is not clear, but MRI-based volumetry of the hippocampal formation and parahippocampal gyrus may predict cognitive outcome following herpes simplex encephalitis (Yoneda *et al.* 1994). These studies suggest that anterograde and retrograde memory functions involve different neural structures; the former is related to the hippocampal formation and the latter to the parahippocampal gyrus. For lasting amnesia, either severe hippocampal damage or combined damage to the hippocampus and parahippocampal gyrus might be necessary.

Clinically, the long-term neuropsychological impairments following herpes simplex encephalitis are characterized by a dense amnesia in 30–40% of cases, and a less severe but noticeable anterograde memory impairment in about 20%. Naming and problem-solving deficits are found in a small number of cases. The severity of amnesia correlates with severity of damage to medial limbic system structures such as the hippocampus, with bilateral damage being particularly important. By contrast, there is a minimal relation between memory loss and severity of damage to thalamus, to lateral temporal lobe, or to frontal lobes.

Although cognitive disturbances are often severe, improvement can occur over a prolonged interval, and chronic residual sequelae may be relatively mild. For example, extended follow-up of patients with post-encephalitic Kluver–Bucy syndrome suggests that memory disturbances eventually improve, with little residual deficit (Hart *et al.* 1986). Formal neuropsychological assessment is needed in the final determination of the level of disability after herpes simplex encephalitis.

Focal neurological deficits

One-third of patients present with focal neurological deficits. Approximately 80% of patients show a focal EEG abnormality in the acute stage, and 60% a localized abnormality on CT brain scan. Focal neurological signs may persist despite adequate antiviral therapy, due to residual scarring. Herpes simplex virus has the ability to invade, replicate, and induce site-specific damage in the central nervous system. Moreover, viral-induced astrocytic hypertrophy in the central nervous system has been demonstrated by glial fibrillary acidic protein immunoreactivity. Such pathological processes are thought to be responsible for the neurological morbidity of herpes simplex encephalitis.

Chronic partial seizures, sometimes associated with neurological deficits such as hemiparesis and mental retardation, may also follow herpes simplex encephalitis. Post-encephalitic epilepsy occurs in about 15–40% of survivors, and is characteristically associated with olfactory or gustatory aura. High rates of epileptic seizures (70%) and neuro-developmental impairment (80%) have been reported in children, especially when antiviral therapy was given late in the acute phase of the illness. Hemiplegia and aphasia occur in more than 20% of cases, but these abnormalities usually regress within a few months with only mild residual disability.

Morbidity rates are generally high following herpes simplex virus type 2 encephalitis. In a follow-up study of infants infected with this virus, 50% became microcephalic, 57% had seizure disorders, 64% had ophthalmological defects, 64% had cerebral palsy and 57% had mental retardation (Corey *et al.* 1988).

Relapse of herpes simplex encephalitis

Relapse of herpes simplex virus infection of the brain after acyclovir or vidarabine therapy has been documented. The exact incidence of relapse in adults with biopsy-proved herpes simplex encephalitis is unknown, but may be as high as 5%. In studies of neonatal herpes simplex encephalitis, approximately 8% who received acyclovir for 10 days had a documented virological relapse. In addition to early relapse, there may be a syndrome of smouldering central nervous system damage manifested by persistently abnormal CSF and progressive neurological deterioration in children (Gutman *et al.* 1986). Reinstitution of treatment with a higher dose of acyclovir (15 mg/kg every 8 hours) and for a longer course (21 days) or in combination with vidarabine has been attempted in a few patients with early relapse, but the results were inconclusive. Isolates of herpes simplex virus were obtained from some patients who relapsed, and were tested for resistance to acyclovir; they remained sensitive. However, resistant viral mutant strains deficient in thymidine kinase have been identified recently in immunocompromised patients, such as those with AIDS. In these cases, vidarabine can be used instead.

Other viral encephalitides

Mumps, measles and rubella

Encephalitides caused by mumps, measles and rubella have been almost eradicated since the introduction of comprehensive vaccination programmes in 1983. Before the vaccination era, *mumps virus* accounted for approximately 15% of all cases of viral meningitis, and was the commonest cause of mild encephalitis, accounting for about 20% of cases. Death following mumps encephalitis is uncommon: 44 deaths in 10 years were reported by the Centers for Disease Control in the United States. Long-term morbidity is also uncommon following mumps encephalitis, though permanent unilateral hearing loss, optic atrophy, facial paresis, and a sub-acute demyelinating illness have been reported in nearly 2% of cases. Rarely, children can develop hydrocephalus as a result of aqueductal stenosis. Mumps may also cause lower motor neuron features simulating mild paralytic poliomyelitis; sequelae occur in 40% of such cases (Lonnoto *et al.* 1960).

The mortality rate during *measles encephalitis* ranges from 10% to 15%. Death can occur during the acute stage or can be delayed by several weeks. The incidence of neurological sequelae in severe encephalitis averages 20%, but has been as high as 65% in some studies. These sequelae include ataxia, mental retardation, seizures and personality changes. *Subacute sclerosing panencephalitis (SSPE)* is a rare progressive neurological disease caused by the measles virus. In most cases, the disease follows a relentless course leading to death within 1–3 years. A small percentage of patients can survive for up to 10 years with transient remissions.

Central nervous system infection with *rubella virus* is rare. It can be associated with spinal cord, brainstem or peripheral nerve involvement, causing paraplegia, bladder dysfunction and various nerve palsies. Progressive rubella panencephalitis, which in many respects resembles SSPE, occurs following congenital rubella virus infection, but may also complicate postnatal rubella infection. Gradual intellectual deterioration, seizures and corticospinal tract signs develop over a period of several years.

Adenoviruses

The mortality rate following adenovirus encephalitis ranges from 15% to 25% of cases, particularly in those caused by serotype 7 adenovirus. Neurological sequelae are uncommon, but some patients may show necrotic changes on brain CT scans resembling those of herpes encephalitis. The long-term outcome in such patients is poor, with the development of mental retardation and seizures (Riikonen 1993).

Arthropod-borne encephalitis

Exposure to arthropod-borne viruses (arboviruses) is relatively common in some geographical areas, such as Papua New Guinea, Central America and the Amazon region. Arboviruses are also a common cause of sporadic and epidemic encephalitis in the United States, China, Southeast Asia and India. Four major clinical syndromes have been associated with human arbovirus infections: encephalitis, yellow fever, haemorrhagic fevers and undifferentiated tropical fevers. Morbidity and mortality rates of encephalitis caused by these viruses vary, and those related to the common seven viruses are summarized in Table 21.10.

Table 21.10. *Mortality and morbidity rates following arthropod-borne encephalitides*

Type	Mortality rate	Morbidity rate in survivors
Eastern equine encephalitis	50–75%	70–80%
Western equine encephalitis	5–15%	20–50%
St Louis encephalitis	5–20%	15–20%
Japanese B encephalitis	25–40%	60–80%
La Crosse encephalitis	< 1%	< 5%
Venezuelan encephalitis	< 2%	< 2%
California encephalitis	< 1%	5–10%

Enteroviruses

Enteroviruses cause 30–50% of all cases of viral meningitis, most cases of paralytic poliomyelitis and a small number of cases of encephalitis. The outcome of enterovirus meningitis has been presented above. Deaths have been recorded in a small number of patients with acute enterovirus encephalitis, where echoviruses 9, 17 and 21 have been isolated from the brain at necropsy. Fatal myocarditis and encephalitis have been reported after neonatal infection with coxsackievirus group B.

Permanent neurological sequelae following enterovirus encephalitis are rare; however, acute hemiplegia, focal encephalitis with hemichorea, acute cerebellar ataxia and polyradiculitis have been described. An isolated report of a possible cause-and-effect relationship between coxsackievirus B2 and Parkinsonism (Walters 1960) has not been corroborated.

The reported cases of paralytic poliomyelitis have declined steadily following the introduction of live attenuated vaccine, and the disease has been virtually eliminated in Western countries. Long-term morbidity of patients with antecedent poliomyelitis includes respiratory (15–20%), orthopaedic (10–30%) and neurological (5–15%) sequelae. Late neurological complications mainly consist of cervical myelopathies or entrapment neuropathies due to spinal deformity. A recrudescence of paralysis and muscle wasting, the post-polio syndrome, has been repeatedly observed in a small number of patients decades after partial recovery from paralytic poliomyelitis. The current theory that the syndrome is due to physiological and ageing changes in spinal motor neurons has been challenged by a recent report suggesting that the new weakness is associated with persistent or recurrent infection of motor neural cells with polioviruses (Sharief *et al.* 1991). A recurrent or persistent infection might cause a progressive cytopathic effect which would eventually lead to either neuronal cell lysis or alteration of specialized cellular functions which potentially impairs physiological activities. However, further work is needed to support the *persistent virus* theory.

Human T-cell lymphotropic viruses

Human T-cell lymphotropic viruses (HTLV) type I and II, human oncoretroviruses, were first described more than a decade ago. HTLV-I epidemiology and aetiopathology are more defined than those of HTLV-II, but there are some difficulties in discrimination between the two infections. The introduction of advanced serological and molecular assays has recently provided sensitive and specific tools for diagnosis, and the epidemiological and aetiopathological patterns linked to these retroviruses are being more precisely defined.

HTLV-I is the aetiological agent of adult T-cell leukaemia and of a neuromyelopathy that seems to be peculiar to the tropics, known as tropical spastic paraparesis or HTLV-I-associated myelopathy (TSP/HAM). TSP/HAM is a chronic neuromyelopathy characterized by a spastic paraplegia or paraparesis with sphincter disturbances, minimal sensory loss and a chronic progressive evolution without remission. HTLV-I infects 15–25 million individuals in the world in the endemic areas (Japan, intertropical Africa, Caribbean area and south America). In these regions the virus is transmitted by breast feeding, sexual contact and blood transfusion.

The course of TSP/HAM is slowly progressive. The most frequent pattern is a gradual deterioration of gait over 2–10 years to a plateau of moderate or severe disability. Occasionally progression of the gait ceases for a few years before further deterioration occurs. Bladder disturbance is also progressive, with incontinence and impotence occurring relatively late in the course of the disease, and myositis may also occur. Less is known about the pathogenic effects of HTLV-II.

Herpes zoster virus infection

Herpes zoster infection can occur over any sensory dermatome, but thoracic dermatomes are involved in two-thirds of patients; cranial nerve involvement is next in frequency. The development of painful post-herpetic neuralgia is a common complication. The neuralgia is very refractory to usual analgesics, though it often abates over a period of months to years. Acyclovir has been shown to attenuate the course of disseminated cutaneous herpes zoster infections. A meta-analysis of trials with acyclovir, however, failed to detect a significant reduction of pain in the treatment group at 1 or 6 months, although there was a 35% reduction at 3 months (Lancaster *et al.* 1995). Confidence limits were wide, however, and a modest benefit of treatment cannot be ruled out at 1 and 6 months.

Cranial nerve infections with herpes zoster may be followed by otological or ophthalmic sequelae. Otological complications of varicella-zoster virus (Ramsay Hunt syndrome) include facial paralysis, tinnitus, hearing loss, hyperacusis, vertigo, dysgeusia and decreased tear secretion. Cranial nerves, V, IX and X are often affected. Gadolinium-enhanced MRI may demonstrate enhancement of the geniculate ganglion and facial nerve. These manifestations are identical to Bell's palsy but are more severe and carry a graver prognosis. About 8% of Bell's palsy patients eventually are diagnosed as *zoster sine herpete*. Infections of the retina with the varicella-zoster virus can lead to severe visual impairment. Patients with immunodeficiency are particularly predisposed to retinal infection, and the alterations of the immune system may lead to a modified clinical picture.

Herpes zoster is relatively common in advanced HIV infection; the probability of development of infection is about 6% at 1 year and 10% at 2 years. Infection late in the course of illness in patients with advanced HIV disease, but without prior herpes zoster, may indicate improved prognosis. Glesby and colleagues (1993) reported that a first infection with herpes zoster is associated with prolonged survival independent of baseline CD4 cell count and disease stage; however, recurrence tends to be associated with increased mortality.

Herpes zoster infections occur at increased frequency, and cause significant morbidity, in other immunosuppressed patients, particularly those with systemic lupus erythematosus, compared with the general population. Patients who have had severe manifestations of lupus are at greatest risk, though not necessarily at the time of disease flare-up or immunosuppressive therapy. If disease activity allows, a reduction in prednisone dosage may reduce the risk of bacterial superinfection during zoster episodes.

Human immunodeficiency virus infections

Neurological manifestations of HIV infection occur in most adults and children with AIDS. These manifestations may involve any level of the central or peripheral nervous system. Acute encephalitis, aseptic meningitis and acute demyelinating polyneuropathy may occur early in the course of HIV infection, while dementia, central nervous system-related cancer, opportunistic infections and autonomic neuropathy typically present later. Headache and mental status changes are common early manifestations of central nervous system involvement. Most severe headaches are related to an identifiable cause, including a mass lesion, opportunistic cerebral infection and medication side effect. Memory deficits, concentration difficulties and abnormalities on mental status testing may represent early HIV encephalopathy (formerly AIDS–dementia complex), the most common neurological complication. Peripheral neuromuscular disease, including distal symmetric polyneuropathy, autonomic neuropathy, and HIV and chronic zidovudine myopathy, affects 15–40% of all persons with HIV infection or AIDS.

There are several factors that predict mortality in HIV-infected patients, and identify those patients with a particularly bad prognosis. Some predictive factors require complicated laboratory facilities, whereas others are relatively simple and involve easily diagnosed signs and symptoms and inexpensive laboratory tests (Table 21.11).

Progress of HIV encephalopathy

HIV encephalopathy, which is probably caused by direct HIV infection of neuronal cells and was formerly known as AIDS–dementia complex, is the one of the most common neurological disorders in HIV-infected patients. It is more frequent than opportunistic diseases of the central nervous system. It is a common cause of demen-

Table 21.11. *Independent predictors of mortality among HIV-infected women*

Predictive parameter	Relative hazard	95% confidence intervals (%)
Body mass index $\leq 21\,kg/m^2$	2.3	1.1 to 4.8
Low income	2.3	1.1 to 4.5
Erythrocyte sedimentation rate $> 60\,mm/h$	4.9	2.2 to 10.9
Chronic diarrhoea	2.6	1.1 to 5.7
History of herpes zoster	5.3	2.5 to 11.4
Oral candidiasis	7.3	1.6 to 33.3

tia, and is characterized by slowly progressing cognitive impairment, psychomotor slowing and increasing apathy. In demented patients a rapid deterioration is observed, leading to death within about 12 months on average – a markedly shorter survival time than for non-demented HIV-positive individuals. Antiretroviral treatment may improve symptoms and prolong survival in some patients.

In patients with HIV encephalopathy, median time of progression to full-blown AIDS ranges from 800 days in patients with a CD4+ lymphocyte count $\geq 150 \times 10^6/l$ to 300 days in patients with a CD4+ lymphocyte count $< 50 \times 10^6/l$. Other factors associated with poorer survival include the presence of opportunistic central nervous system infections, baseline age ≥ 40 years, haematocrit $< 35\%$ and diminished functional status.

In addition to HIV encephalopathy, there are other primary HIV infections of the central nervous system, including HIV-related meningitis and myelopathy. HIV-related meningitis appears to represent an initial response of the central nervous system to viral invasion. Acute symptoms, such as headache, meningism and cranial neuropathies, are generally self-limiting; however, it is uncertain at present whether the development of symptomatic meningitis is predictive of subsequent progressive neurological involvement. During the final stages of HIV infection some patients develop AIDS-myelopathy, which is characterized by vacuolation and infiltration of the long tracts of the spinal cord by macrophages.

Outcome of opportunistic infections

The prevalence of neurological complications associated with HIV disease has progressively increased as more effective therapies allow persons with AIDS to live longer. Table 21.12 shows average mortality rates in HIV-positive patients who were treated for common central nervous system infections. In addition, a growing number of previously fatal infections related to AIDS are now preventable with relatively specific agents. For instance, pentamidine, dapsone and dapsone–pyrimethamine are used for prophylaxis against *Pneumocystis carinii* pneumonia; rifabutin has been approved to prevent disseminated infection with *Mycobacterium avium* complex; chemoprophylaxis with isoniazid is indicated in patients who are at high risk for *M. tuberculosis* infection; and acyclovir is effective in decreasing recurrences of herpes simplex virus

Table 21.12. *Mortality rate in HIV-positive patients with adequately treated central nervous system infections after a follow-up interval of 4–15 months*

Nature of infection	Administered treatment	Mortality rate	Author
Listeria monocytogenes meningitis	Penicillin, amoxicillin or aminoglycosides	28–33%	Berenguer *et al.* 1991
Coccidioidal meningitis	Fluconazole	25–30%	Galciani *et al.* 1993
Cryptococcal meningitis	Fluconazole	18–25%	Laroche *et al.* 1992
Tuberculous meningitis	Anti-tuberculous therapy	16–24%	Berenguer *et al.* 1992
Toxoplasma encephalitis	Trimethoprim, pyrimethamine or dapsone	42–70%	Oksenhendler *et al.* 1994
Neurosyphilis	Ceftriaxone or benzathine penicillin	23–30%	Dowell *et al.* 1992

infection. Therefore, issues of drug interactions and toxicity have become increasingly important in determining the long-term morbidity and mortality in patients with advanced HIV disease.

Similarly, there have been considerable changes in survival, causes of death, and organ system distribution of major opportunistic infections and neoplasms in patients with AIDS following the widespread use of antiretroviral therapy and prophylaxis for opportunistic infections since 1988. A retrospective review of pathological findings, laboratory data and clinical histories in 565 cases of AIDS (Klatt *et al.* 1994) compared findings from 1982 to 1988 with those from 1989 to 1993. *Pneumocystis carinii* pneumonia remained the most common cause of death, but both the frequency and number of deaths from this disease declined over time. Deaths from cytomegalovirus infection, *Mycobacterium avium* complex infection and toxoplasmosis also declined during this period, but mortality from fungal infections, tuberculosis and HIV-encephalopathy increased. The death rate from malignant lymphoma remained high. Overall, survival of HIV-positive patients increased over time, particularly in those treated with antiretroviral therapy. The lung was the most frequent organ involved by AIDS-associated diseases leading to death, followed by the gastrointestinal tract and the central nervous system.

New goals for treatment of fungal infections

With the rapid increase in cases of AIDS over the past 10 years, certain mycoses have become much more common, particularly those modified by T-cell-mediated mechanisms of host defence. In this clinical setting systemic cryptococcosis, histoplasmosis and coccidioidomycosis pose special therapeutic and prognostic challenges. Compared with fungal infections in general, treatments are seldom curative in AIDS-associated mycoses. These problems have necessitated a redefinition of goals: the aim is now to suppress rather than cure infection in most cases. This change has stimulated trials of new antifungal agents and regimens particularly designed to facilitate long-term outpatient management of mycoses without interfering with treatment of either the HIV infection itself or other concomitant complications.

Opportunistic viral infections

Opportunistic viral infections are detected in more than 70% of HIV-infected patients, comprising cytomegalovirus (60%), herpes simplex virus (15%), JC virus (5%) and adenovirus (5%). The most commonly infected tissues outside the central nervous system are the lungs, adrenals and gastrointestinal tract. Attempts to influence the natural history of these infections by antiviral drugs are not always successful and, at present, most cases are detected post-mortem by histology and cell culture (Pillay *et al.* 1993).

Progress of cerebral lymphomas

Primary lymphomas appear later in the course of AIDS. They are often associated with severe T-cell immunosuppression and with more frequent opportunistic disorders than disseminated lymphomas. Associated Kaposi's sarcomas are surprisingly frequent. There is commonly a time lapse of 1–7 months between the presentation of a cerebral lymphoma and death, and of less than a month between the diagnosis and death. Post-mortem studies frequently show a multicentric involvement, marked gliosis and significant necrosis. Lesions associated with HIV infection, such as toxoplasmosis, cytomegalovirus and HIV encephalitis are also seen in the majority of cases with primary lymphomas.

Neurological outcome of paediatric infection

In infants born to HIV-infected mothers definite diagnosis of perinatal HIV infection by detection of specific antibodies to the virus is not possible during the first 15 months of life since there is transplacental passage of maternal antibodies. Early diagnosis and medical care of paediatric HIV disease often has to rely on recognition of clinical symptoms, particularly those of central nervous system involvement.

Approximately 20–30% of infants born to HIV-infected mothers are infected. From 6 months of age the infected infants show lower mean developmental scores than uninfected infants. Almost two-thirds of the infected infants develop neurological symptoms such as hypo- or hypertonia, corticospinal tract signs and apathy. However, uninfected infants may also exhibit central nervous system dysfunction but, unlike the infected infants, they are usually hypertonic and hyperexcitable. These symptoms are most pronounced in the first weeks of life but completely disappear during the first year. Uninfected infants with neurological abnormalities within the first months commonly suffer from withdrawal symptoms as neonates, due to the narcotic drug abuse of their mothers during pregnancy. Neurological abnormalities and slow achievement of developmental milestones after 6 months are highly suggestive of HIV infection and predate evidence of full-blown encephalopathy.

Among infected infants, there are two patterns of disease progression; in about a fifth of these infants there is a rapid progression to profound immunodeficiency, whereas in the majority the disease progresses much more slowly. The rate of disease progression varies directly with the severity of the disease in the mother at the time of delivery (Blanche *et al.* 1994). The risk of opportunistic infections or encephalopathy in the first 18 months is 50% in the infants of mothers with class IV disease, according to the Centers for Disease Control and Prevention classification, and 15% in the infants of mothers with class II or III disease. Approximately 45% of the former infants and only 10% of the latter die before the age of 18 months. The risk of death correlates inversely with the mother's $CD4^+$ cell count and directly with her HIV p24 antigen level at delivery. There is also a direct correlation between the mother's CD4$^+$ cell count and that of the infant.

Spongiform encephalopathies

Transmissible subacute spongiform encephalopathies are fatal diseases which comprise in humans Creutzfeldt–Jakob disease, Kuru, Gerstmann–Straussler–Scheinker disease, and Fatal Familial Insomnia. Their aetiological agents, prions or transmissible spongiform encephalopathy agents (TSA) are still poorly characterized. TSA/prions resist all the physicochemical procedures that are effective against classical microorganisms. The biochemical hallmark is the post-translational accumulation of a host-encoded protein, the prion protein (PrP). In infected individuals, PrP accumulates under a proteinase K resistant isoform (PrP-res), the amino acid sequence of which does not differ from that of the normal isoform (PrP-c). PrP gene is located on chromosome 20 in humans, and is the major determinant of the susceptibility to TSA/prions. Several hypotheses have been raised to explain the uncommon biological properties of these agents. The prion hypothesis postulates that the agent is only composed of proteins, mainly the PrP-res. Others support the presence of host-independent genetic information of which PrP could be the virulent factor.

Spongiform encephalopathies belong to the group of *slow virus infections* of the nervous system, and are characterized by an incubation period which may be as long as 40 years. Clinically, symptoms are entirely neurological, without signs of immune response in either blood or cerebrospinal fluid. Neuropathologically there is neuronal vacuolization, neuronal death, spongiosis, and gliosis with hyperastrocytosis. These diseases run a protracted course with a universally lethal outcome. No remissions or recoveries have been reported, and the mean duration of illness varies from 2 months to 5 years.

References

Barnett, G. H., Ropper, A. H. & Romeo, J. (1988). Intracranial pressure and outcome in adult encephalitis. *J. Neurosurg.* **68**, 585–8.

Berenguer, J., Solera, J., Diaz, M. D., Moreno, S., Lopezherce, J. A. & Bouza, E. (1991). Listeriosis in patients infected with human immunodeficiency virus. *Rev. Infect. Dis.* **13**, 115–19.

Berenguer, J., Moreno, S. & Laguna, F. (1992). Tuberculous meningitis in patients infected with the human immunodeficiency virus. *N. Eng. J. Med.* **326**, 668–72.

Besser, R., Kramer, G. & Hopf, H. C. (1990). The temporal profile of EEG discharges during the early stage of herpes simplex encephalitis. *EEG EMG* **21**, 243–6.

Bigotte, J., Mselati, J. C., Routon, M. C., Noui Mehidi, F., Lebon, P. & Ponsot, G. (1993). Herpes encephalitis in newborn infants. Retrospective study of 12 cases. *Arch. Fr. Pediatr.* **50**, 209–14.

Blanche, S., Mayaux, M. J., Rouzioux, C. *et al.* (1994). Relation of the course of HIV-infection in children to the severity of the disease in their mothers at delivery. *N. Engl. J. Med.* **330**, 308–12.

Bos, C. A., Olding-Stenkvist, E., Wilterdink, J. B. & Scheffer, A. J. (1987). Detection of viral antigens in cerebrospinal fluid of patients with herpes simplex virus encephalitis. *J. Med. Virol.* **21**, 169–78.

Buge, A., Chamouard, J. M. & Rancurel, G. (1988). Prognosis of herpes simplex encephalitis. Retrospective study of 19 cases. *Prese Med.* **17**, 13–16.

Buttner, T. & Dorndorf, W. (1988). Viral encephalitis. Experiences with 53 patients in Middle Hessia. *Forstchr. Neurol. Psychiatr.* **56**, 315–25.

Connelly, K. P. & Dewitt, L. D. (1994). Neurologic complications of infectious mononucleosis. *Pediatr. Neurol.* **10**, 181–4.

Corey, L., Whitley, R. J., Stone, E. F. & Mohan, K. (1988). Difference between herpes simplex virus type 1 and type 2 neonatal encephalitis in neurological outcome. *Lancet* 1–4.

Dowell, M. E., Ross, P. G., Musher, D. M., Cate, T. R. & Baughn, R. E. (1992). Response of latent syphilis or neurosyphilis to ceftriaxone therapy in persons infected with human immunodeficiency virus. *Am. J. Med.* **93**, 481–8.

Dufour, J. F. & Waldvogel, F. (1991). Meningitis in adults: review of 257 cases. *Schweiz. Med. Wochenschr.* **S35**, 1–37.

Etter, C. G., Wedgwood, J. & Schaad, U. B. (1991). Aseptic meningitis in pediatrics. *Schweiz. Med. Wochenschr.* **121**, 1120–6.

Galgiani, J. N., Catanzaro, A., Cloud, G. A., Higgs, J., Friedman, B. A., Larsen, R. A. & Graybill, J. R. (1993). Fluconazole therapy for coccidioidal meningitis. *Ann. Intern. Med.* **119**, 28–35.

Glesby, M. J., Moore, R. D. & Chaisson, R. E. (1993). Herpes zoster in patients with advanced human immunodeficiency virus infection treated with zidovudine. *J. Infect. Dis.* **168**, 1264–8.

Grimm, G., Madl, C., Oder, W. *et al.* (1991). Evoked potentials in severe herpes simplex encephalitis. *Intensive Care Med.* **17**, 94–7.

Hart, R. P., Kwentus, J. A., Frazier, R. B. & Hormel, T. L. (1986). Natural history of Kluver-Bucy syndrome after treated herpes encephalitis. *South Med. J.* **79**, 1376–8.

Holmes, G. L. & Lombroso, C. T. (1993). Prognostic value of background patterns in the neonatal EEG. *J. Clin. Neurophysiol.* **10**, 323–52.

Kapur, N., Barker, S., Burrows, E. H. *et al.* (1994). Herpes simplex encephalitis: long-term magnetic resonance imaging and neuropsychological profile. *J. Neurol. Neurosurg. Psychiatry* **57**, 1334–42.

Kennard, C. & Swash, M. (1981). Acute viral encephalitis: its diagnosis and outcome. *Brain* **104**, 129–48.

Kennedy, C. R., Duffy, S. W., Smith, R. & Robinson, R. O. (1987). Clinical predictors of outcome in encephalitis. *Arch. Dis. Child* **62**, 1156–62.

Kennedy, P. G. (1988). A retrospective analysis of forty-six cases of herpes simplex encephalitis seen in Glasgow between 1962 and 1985. *Q. J. Med.* **68**, 533–40.

Klatt, E. C., Nichols, L. & Noguch, T. T. (1994). Evolving trends revealed by autopsies of patients with the acquired-immunodeficiency-syndrome: 565 autopsies in adults with the acquired-immunodeficiency-syndrome, Los Angeles, Calif, 1992–1993. *Arch. Pathol. Lab. Med.* **118**, 884–90.

Lancaster, T., Silagy, C. & Gray, S. (1995). Primary care management of acute herpes zoster: systematic review of evidence from randomized controlled trials. *Br. J. Gen. Pract.* **45**, 39–45.

Laroche, R., Dupont, B., Touze, J. E. *et al.* (1992). Cryptococcal meningitis associated with AIDS in African patients: treatment with fluconazole. *J. Med. Vet. Mycol.* **30**, 71–8.

Lennette, E. H., Magoffin, R. L. & Knouf, E. G. (1960). Mumps virus infection simulating paralytic poliomyelitis: a report of 11 cases. *Pediatrics* **25**, 788–97.

Lindan, C. P., Allen, S., Serufilira, A. *et al.* (1992). Predictors of mortality among HIV-infected women in Kigali, Rwanda. *Ann. Intern. Med.* **116**, 320–8.

Longson, M. M., Baily, A. S. & Klapper, P. (1980). Herpes encephalitis. In *Recent Advances in Clinical Virology*, ed. A. Waterson, vol. 2, pp. 147–57. Edinburgh: Churchill Livingstone.

Mancini, J., Chabrol, B., Livet, M. O. & Pinsard, N. (1991). Outcome of herpetic encephalitis. Apropos of 10 cases. *Ann. Pediatr.* **38**, 143–9.

Oksenhendler, E., Charreau, I., Tournerie, C., Azihary, M., Carbon, C. & Aboulker, J. P. (1994). *Toxoplasma gondii* infection in advanced HIV infection. *AIDS* **8**, 483–7.

Overall, J. C. (1994). Herpes simplex virus infection of the fetus and newborn. *Pediatr. Ann.* **23**, 131–6.

Pillay, D., Lipman, M. C. I., Lee, C. A., Johnson, M. A., Griffiths, P. D. & McLaughlin, J. E. A. (1993). A clinicopathological audit of opportunistic viral infections in HIV-infected patients. *AIDS* **7**, 969–74.

Rao, N. & Costa, J. (1991). Rehabilitation of three patients after treatment for herpes encephalitis. *Am. J. Phys. Med. Rehabil.* **70**, 73–5.

Raroque, H. G., Wagner, W., Gonzales, P. C., Leroy, R. F., Karnaze, D., Riela, A. R. & Roach, E. S. (1993). Reassessment of the clinical significance of periodic lateralized epileptiform discharges in pediatric patients. *Epilepsia* **34**, 275–8.

Rautonen, J., Koskiniemi, M. & Vaheri, A. (1991). Prognostic factors in childhood acute encephalitis. *Pediatr. Infect. Dis. J.* **10**, 441–6.

Riikonen, R. (1993). Infantile spasms: infectious disorders. *Neuropediatrics* **24**, 274–80.

Rorabaugh, M. L., Berlin, L. E., Heldrich, F., Roberts, K., Rosenberg, L. A., Doran, T. & Modlin, J. F. (1993). Aseptic meningitis in infants younger than 2 years of age: acute illness and neurologic complications. *Pediatrics* **92**, 206–11.

Sharief, M. K., Hentges, R. & Ciardi, M. (1991). Intrathecal immune response in patients with the post-polio syndrome. *N. Engl. J. Med.* **325**, 729–55.

Sköldenberg, B., Kalimo, K., Carlström, A., Forsgren, M. & Halonen, P. (1981). Herpes simplex encephalitis: a serological follow-up study. *Acta Neurol. Scand.* **63**, 273–85.

Vandvik, B., Vartdal, F. & Norrby, E. (1982). Herpes simplex virus encephalitis: intrathecal synthesis of oligoclonal virus-specific IgG, IgA amd IgM antibodies. *J. Neurol.* **228**, 25–38.

Walters, J. H. (1960). Postencephalitic Parkinson syndrome after meningoencephalitis due to Coxsackie virus group B type 2. *N. Engl. J. Med.* **263**, 744–6.

Whitley, R. J. (1988). Herpes simplex virus infections of the central nervous system: a review. *Am. J. Med.* **85**, 61–7.

Whitley, R. J., Soong, S. J., Dolin, R. *et al.* (1977). Adenine arabinoside therapy of biopsy-proved herpes simplex encephalitis. National Institute of Allergy and Infectious Diseases Collaborative Antiviral Study. *N. Engl. J. Med.* **297**, 289–94.

Whitley, R. J., Alford, C. A., Hirsch, M. S. *et al.* (1986). Vidarabine versus acyclovir therapy in herpes simplex encephalitis. *N. Engl. J. Med.* **314**, 144–9.

Whitley, R., Arvin, A., Prober, C. *et al.* (1991*a*). A controlled trial comparing vidarabine with acyclovir in neonatal herpes simplex virus infection. Infectious Diseases Collaborative Antiviral Study Group. *N. Engl. J. Med.* **324**, 444–9.

Whitley, R., Arvin, A., Prober, C. *et al.* (1991*b*). Predictors of morbidity and mortality in neonates with herpes simplex virus infections. The National Institute of Allergy and Infectious Diseases Collaborative Antiviral Study Group. *N. Engl. J. Med.* **324**, 450–4.

Yoneda, Y., Etsuro, M., Yamashita, H. & Yamadori, A. T. (1994). MRI volumetry of medial temporal lobe structures in amnesia following herpes simplex encephalitis. *Eur. Neurol.* **34**, 243–52.

22 Epilepsy: medical and surgical outcome

TERESA A. TRAN, SUSAN S. SPENCER AND
DENNIS D. SPENCER

Introduction

Epilepsy was first described as a clinical entity by Hippocrates (462–357 B.C.). In his monograph, 'On the Sacred Disease', he considered epilepsy a disease of the brain due to natural, rather than supernatural causes. In his other works, Hippocrates also described the various kinds of attacks, including convulsions and spells preceded by premonitory signs. He differentiated between 'idiopathic' and 'symptomatic' seizures and went on to describe the effects of various factors such as age, temperament, menstruation and seasonal changes on seizures. Many of these early writings still hold true today. Epilepsy is now recognized as a condition characterized by a tendency for recurrent seizures (defined as two or more spells) unprovoked by any immediate insult. In contrast, a seizure is defined as a paroxysmal disorder of the central nervous system associated with abnormal neuronal discharges.

It is estimated that approximately 1.5 million individuals have active epilepsy in the United States (Hauser & Hersdorffer 1990). From 70 000 to 128 000 new cases of epilepsy are reported each year. With the introduction of anticonvulsant medication, many patients with epilepsy have achieved better seizure control. Furthermore, the development of epilepsy surgery within the last decade has provided an alternative therapy for those individuals in whom seizures are intractable to medical treatment. As a consequence, the natural history of epilepsy has been altered significantly. Compared with the low remission rate of less than 30% in the early 1900s (Habermaas 1901; Turner 1907; Volland 1908), the overall prognosis of epilepsy has improved significantly one century later, with cure rates ranging from 50% to 80%.

The epilepsies are a heterogeneous group of symptom complexes, most of them empirically determined, whose only common denominator, as stated above, is the recurrence of seizures caused by abnormal neuronal discharge. Accordingly, the natural course of one type of epilepsy differs from the next. For instance, absence seizures and Benign Focal Epilepsy of Childhood usually have an excellent prognosis, with remission of the disease by the mid to late teens. In contrast, the seizure complexes constituting the Lennox–Gastaut syndrome are known to be indolent, persistent, and refractory to most or all medical therapy. Given this heterogeneity, treatment of the epilepsies must be tailored specifically to the epilepsy and seizure type, and outcome is to a large degree determined by the specific diagnosis.

Classification of epileptic seizures and the epilepsies

Before we can begin a discussion on the outcome of epilepsy, a review of the classification of seizures and epilepsy syndrome is in order. In 1970, the first attempt to classify epileptic seizures based on their clinical characteristics was proposed in the International Classification of Epileptic Seizures (Gastaut 1970). The criteria used to characterize each seizure type included the clinical semiology, ictal and interictal electrographic (EEG) pattern, age of onset, aetiology and anatomical substrate. It was the first classification system to impress upon the medical community the difference between partial and generalized seizures. This was a tentative proposal and a revision was published in 1981 by the Commission on Classification and Terminology of the International League Against Epilepsy (ILAE) (Table 22.1). The criteria utilized in the 1970 classification were judged to have been excessive in including age of onset, aetiology and anatomical substrate. In some respects, they were overextended into the classification of epileptic syndromes. For that reason, the criteria for seizure classification were now restricted to empirical data regarding the clinical seizure itself and the accompanying ictal EEG only. The Commission subdivided partial seizures into different types according to preservation or lack of consciousness. It made provisions for the progression of the epileptic seizures, and allowed for overlaps of symptomatology of simple and complex partial seizures. Furthermore, it eliminated confusing terms such as 'compound form', 'akinetic' seizures and 'infantile spasms'.

This classification of *seizures* is extremely useful in the diagnosis and treatment of patients. However, it is restricted in providing information about prognosis and long-term therapeutic decisions. A more useful approach is to use seizure type and other information to classify patients into meaningful patterns representing epileptic syndromes or diseases. For this, clinical semiology, interictal and ictal EEG patterns, as well as age of onset, aetiology, anatomical and physiological substrates, neurological and psychiatric findings, and imaging studies would be important. Such thinking was the basis for the Classification of the Epilepsies (Commission on Classification and Terminology of the ILAE 1970, 1985). The committee thus divided *epilepsy* into two main categories: localized and non-localized. Each category was further divided into 'idiopathic' (no known aetiology) and 'symptomatic' (known or suspected CNS disease) (Table 22.2).

Medical outcome

In studying outcome of medical therapy, three areas are commonly addressed: risk of recurrence after a first unprovoked seizure, remission from seizures and relapse after drug withdrawal. Investigations into these areas have been difficult to analyse and interpret. There are often too many variables confounding the data analysis. For example, looking at the clinical history alone, we find heterogeneous patient populations, epilepsy types, medication history and length of follow-up. Studies also emphasize different factors. The greatest difficulty is in patient ascertainment. Studies that depend on hospital or institution-based referrals acquire a disproportionately high number of patients with chronic epilepsy who tend to be refractory to medical treatment. Thus, data from these studies tend to reflect a worse prognosis. The method of recruiting patients also affects the statistical results. Retrospective studies by means of chart review run the risk of acquiring incomplete information. In the case of seizure recurrence following a first unprovoked seizure, hospital charts may indicate that the patient had more than one seizure at the time of consultation. Thus, the patient population may be skewed towards a more complicated group with poor prognosis. On the other hand, chart review of patients in remission may miss those who have had a relapse since the last visit. In this case, outcome would appear more favourable than expected. Studies of seizure recurrence that rely on EEG records as a means of identifying patients in the community may neglect a considerable number of epileptic individuals because the physician or patient did not see the need for an EEG. Prospective studies are perhaps nearer to the ideal and have better control over the variables. However, identifying all persons in the community with the problem of interest is difficult and often incomplete.

Another problem with most medical outcome studies involves the heterogeneity of epilepsy as a whole. Unlike the ILAE classification, most outcome studies do not examine one type of epilepsy at a time. Rather, idiopathic and symptomatic, generalized and partial seizures are all considered simultaneously. This lumping is sometimes facilitated by consideration of epilepsy of all ages within a population. We know that children make up a large percentage of epileptics. They also have a considerable number of epilepsy syndromes with benign course. Thus, it is easy to see how predominance of one seizure type within a series may affect the overall prognosis of epilepsy as reported in general.

Medication history is another confounding factor in analysis of epilepsy prognosis. In the case of the first unprovoked seizure, some patients are followed on no treatment, while others have medication initiated. In studies of remission rate, some patients are entered into the study on no medication, some on monotherapy and some on polytherapy. Remission is not achieved when medication fails, but we are uncertain as to what is meant by 'failed medical therapy'. Most studies do not define medication history so we rarely know whether appropriate anticonvulsant medication was used in the proper way. Inappropriate medication selection can also *exacerbate* some seizures. Monotherapy came into fashion about a decade ago. Prior to that, if a patient failed one drug he was more likely tried on an additional drug rather than switched to a different monotherapy regimen. Lastly, drug compliance is a confounding factor. Unfortunately, it is difficult to detect and to control.

Table 22.1. *Clinical and electroencephalographic classification of epileptic seizures*

I. Partial (focal, local) seizures
A. Simple partial seizures
(consciousness not impaired)
    1. With motor signs
        (a) Focal motor without march
        (b) Focal motor with march (Jacksonian)
        (c) Versive
        (d) Postural
        (e) Phonatory (vocalization or arrest of speech)
    2. With somatosensory or special-sensory (simple hallucinations, e.g. tingling, light flashes, buzzing)
        (a) Somatosensory
        (b) Visual
        (c) Auditory
        (d) Olfactory
        (e) Gustatory
        (f) Vertiginous
    3. With automatic symptoms or signs (including epigastric sensation, pallor, sweating, flushing, piloerection and pupillary dilatation)
    4. With psychic symptoms (disturbance of higher cerebral function). These symptoms rarely occur without impairment of consciousness and are much more commonly experienced as complex partial seizures
        (a) Dysphasic
        (b) Dysmnesic (e.g. dejà-vu)
        (c) Cognitive (e.g. dreamy states, distortions of time sense)
        (d) Affective (fear, anger, etc.)
        (e) Illusions (e.g. macropsia)
        (f) Structured hallucinations (e.g. music, scenes)
B. Complex partial seizures
(with impairment of consciousness; may sometimes begin with simple symptomatology)
    1. Simple partial onset followed by impairment of consciousness
        (a) With simple partial features (A.1–A.4) followed by impaired consciousness
        (b) With automatisms
    2. With impairment of consciousness at onset
        (a) With impairment of consciousness only
        (b) With automatisms
C. Partial seizures evolving to secondarily generalized seizures
(This may be generalized tonic-clonic, tonic, or clonic)
    1. Simple partial seizures
        (a) Evolving to generalized seizures
    2. Complex partial seizures
        (b) Evolving to generalized seizures
    3. Simple partial seizures evolving to complex partial seizures evolving to generalized seizures

II. Generalized seizures (convulsive or non-convulsive)
A. 1. Absence seizures
        (a) Impairment of consciousness only
        (b) With mild clonic components
        (c) With atonic components

Table 22.1 (*cont.*)

(d) With tonic components
(e) With automatisms
(f) With automatic components
(b through f may be used alone or in combination)
2. Atypical absence
   May have:
   (a) Changes in tone that are more pronounced than in A.1
   (b) Onset and/or cessation that is not abrupt
B. Myoclonic seizures
   Myoclonic jerks (single or multiple)
C. Clonic seizures
D. Tonic seizures
E. Tonic-clonic seizures
F. Atonic seizures (astatic)
   (Combinations of the above may occur, e.g. B and F, B and D)

III. Unclassified epileptic seizures
   Includes all seizures that cannot be classified because of inadequate or incomplete data
   and some that defy classification in hitherto described categories. This includes some
   neonatal seizures, e.g. rhythmic eye movements, chewing and swimming movements

Prognosis of a first unprovoked seizure

Early studies by Blom *et al.* (1978) reported a recurrence rate of 56% in 76 children within 3 years of the index seizure. Their patient population included both chronic and acute symptomatic seizures, as well as idiopathic seizures. The inclusion of acute symptomatic seizures questions the validity of some of the 'unprovoked' seizures in this series. Johnson *et al.* (1972) followed 77 men in the navy with a first idiopathic seizure who were not treated. Sixty-four per cent of the men had another seizure within 3 years, and 77% of the recurrences were within the first year after the index seizure. Unfortunately, 18% of these men were also diagnosed with psychogenic seizures. Thus, the nature of epileptogenic seizure in this series is questionable.

Studies from the early 1980s to the present have all taken a different approach to their data. Individuals or specific sets of parameters were examined for predictive value on outcome. They included idiopathic versus symptomatic classification, type of presenting seizure (generalized versus partial; status epilepticus, or multiple seizures within a 24 hour period versus isolated seizure), EEG patterns, gender, abnormal neurological examination and age of seizure onset.

The overall risk of recurrence at 1 year varied from 16% to 36% among the different studies. The risk of recurrence is greatest within the first year of the index seizure and decreases considerably with increasing time beyond this point. The risk of having another seizure following a second seizure increases to 79% (Camfield *et al.* 1985). A history of remote symptomatic seizures is associated with a higher risk of recurrence than for idiopathic seizures (Sillanpaa 1993; Berg *et al.* 1996). Hauser *et al.* (1982) report a

Table 22.2. *International classification of epilepsies and epileptic syndromes*

I. Localization-related (focal, local, partial) epilepsies and syndromes
A. Idiopathic with age-related onset
  1. Benign childhood epilepsy with centrotemporal spike
  2. Childhood epilepsy with occipital paroxysms
B. Symptomatic
  1. Frontal lobe epilepsies
    (a) Supplementary motor
    (b) Cingulate
    (c) Anterior (polar) frontal region
    (d) Orbito-frontal
    (e) Dorsolateral
  2. Epilepsies of the motor cortex
  3. Temporal lobe epilepsies
    (a) Hippocampal (mesiobasal, limbic, or primary rhinencephalic psychomotor) epilepsy
    (b) Amygdalar (anterior polar-amygdalar)
    (c) Opercular (insular)
  4. Parietal lobe epilepsies
  5. Occipital lobe epilepsy

II. Generalized epilepsies and syndromes
A. Idiopathic, with age-related onset, listed in order of age
  1. Benign neonatal familial convulsions
  2. Benign neonatal convulsions
  3. Benign myoclonic epilepsy in infancy
  4. Childhood absence epilepsy (pyknolepsy)
  5. Juvenile absence epilepsy
  6. Juvenile myoclonic epilepsy (impulsive petit mal)
  7. Epilepsy with grand mal seizures (GTCS) on awakening
    Other generalized idiopathic epilepsies, if they do not belong to one of the above syndromes, can still be classified as generalized idiopathic epilepsies
B. Idiopathic and/or symptomatic, in order of age of appearance
  1. West syndrome (infantile spasms, Blitz–Nick–Salaam Krämpfe)
  2. Lennox–Gastaut syndrome
  3. Epilepsy with myoclonic-astatic seizures
  4. Epilepsy with myoclonic absences
C. Symptomatic
  1. Non-specific aetiology
    (a) Early myoclonic encephalopathy
  2. Specific syndromes.
    (a) Malformations
      (1) Aicardi syndrome
      (2) Lissencephaly – pachygyria
      (3) Neurophakomatoses (tuberous sclerosis, Sturge–Weber syndrome)
    (b) Proven or suspected inborn error of metabolism
      (1) Neonate
        Nonketotic hyperglycinaemia
        D-glyceric acidaemia
      (2) Infant
        Phenylketonuria
        Phenylketonuria variant (biopterins deficiency)

Table 22.1 (*cont.*)

Tay–Sachs disease
Sandhoff disease
Santuavori–Haltia–Hagberg disease
Pyridoxine dependency

(3) Child
      Jansky–Bielschowski disease
      Huntington's disease, infantile form
(4) Child and adolescent
      Gaucher disease, juvenile form
      Spielmeyer–Vogt–Sjogren disease
      Lafora disease
      Progressive myoclonic epilepsy (Lundborg type)
      Ramsay–Hunt syndrome
      Sialidosis
  (5) Adult
      Kuff's disease

III. Epilepsies and syndromes undetermined as to whether they are focal or generalized

A. With both generalized and focal seizures
    1. Neonatal seizures
    2. Severe myoclonic epilepsy in infancy
    3. Epilepsy with continuous spike-waves during slow wave sleep
    4. Acquired epileptic aphasia (Landau–Kleffer syndrome)
B. With unequivocal generalized or focal features
    All cases with GTCS where clinical and EEG findings do not permit classification as clearly generalized or localization-related, such as in many cases of sleep grand mal

IV. Special syndromes

A. Situation-related seizures (Gelegenheitsanfälle)
    1. Febrile convulsions
    2. Seizures related to other identifiable situations such as stress, hormonal changes, drugs, alcohol or sleep deprivation
B. Isolated, apparently unprovoked epileptic events
C. Epilepsies characterized by specific modes of seizure precipitation
D. Chronic progressive epilepsia partialis continua of childhood

---

recurrence risk of 31% for the symptomatic seizure group, and 20% for the idiopathic seizure group ($P = 0.004$). A later follow-up study found similar results (Annegers *et al.* 1986). The cumulative risk of recurrence of the idiopathic seizure group was 26% and 45% at 1 year and 5 years respectively, while it nearly doubled for the symptomatic seizure group (56% by 1 year and 77% by 5 years). Shinnar *et al.* (1990), in a prospective study of 283 children, reported similar results, with the remote symptomatic seizure group having a greater risk of recurrence (55%) than the idiopathic seizure group (32%). Another prospective study by Hauser *et al.* (1990) included 208 patients of variable age groups. These authors also found the risk of recurrence to vary significantly between the idiopathic and remote symptomatic seizure groups. In the former, the risks were 10%, 24% and 29% at 1, 3 and 5 years respectively. This was contrasted with 26%, 41% and

48% at 1, 3 and 5 years for the symptomatic seizure group.

The significance of seizure type at the time of presentation varies from study to study. Hauser *et al.* (1982, 1990) found that status epilepticus occurred more frequently within the symptomatic seizure group (20%) than the idiopathic seizure group (7%, $P < 0.01$). There was a significantly higher risk of recurrence in the symptomatic seizure group when the index seizure was status epilepticus. Camfield *et al.* (1985) found complex partial seizures to have a higher recurrence risk (78.9%) than generalized tonic clonic seizures (44%). This study concurs with the reports by Annegers *et al.* (1986), in which generalized seizures were associated with a lower risk of recurrence for both the idiopathic and symptomatic seizure groups. Shinnar *et al.* (1990) found that partial seizures only increased the risk of recurrence for the symptomatic seizure group. Furthermore, a previous history of febrile seizures was significantly associated with increased risk of recurrence (86% in comparison with 50%, $P < 0.05$) for the symptomatic seizure group. Hauser *et al.* (1990) also found a remote history of acute symptomatic seizure, particularly febrile seizure, to have significant influence on recurrence in both subgroups. The variability among the studies may in part be attributed to patient selection and sample size influencing statistical analysis.

EEG abnormality has some predictive value for seizure recurrence, but the specific EEG patterns vary among the different studies. Epileptiform discharges found on EEG after a first unprovoked seizure have been associated with a recurrence risk of 83% within 2 years in adults (Van Donselaar *et al.* 1992) and 58% in children (Berg & Shinnar 1991). Hauser *et al.* (1982, 1990) found that generalized spike-wave complexes on EEG were significantly associated with recurrence among the idiopathic seizure group. Camfield *et al.* (1985), on the other hand, found only focal epileptiform discharges to be a significant factor; there is no indication whether this applies to the symptomatic or idiopathic seizure group. Annegers *et al.* (1986) reported an abnormal EEG of any type to be associated with an increased risk of recurrence in the idiopathic seizure group. Shinnar *et al.* (1990) found an abnormal EEG to occur more frequently within the symptomatic seizure group than the idiopathic seizure group. The abnormal EEG, however, did not have predictive value in the symptomatic seizure group. On the other hand, it was found to be the most important predictor of outcome ($P < 0.001$) for the idiopathic group, although a specific EEG pattern was not identified. It is of note that a normal EEG does not necessarily rule out seizure recurrence completely. Recurrence risk as high as 12% after a first unprovoked seizure has been reported in patients with a normal EEG (Van Donselaar *et al.* 1992).

Whether treatment with an antiepileptic drug after a first unprovoked seizure has any effect on long-term outcome has always been a controversial issue. Approximately 70% of patients with epilepsy go into remission, and at least half of these will eventually be able to discontinue their antiepileptic drug (Annegers *et al.* 1979; Cockerell *et al.* 1995). Results from the British National General Practice Study of Epilepsy found that the number of pretreatment seizures does not have a substantial impact on the probability of outcome (Cockerell *et al.* 1995). Further support for this comes from population-based studies from developing countries where antiepileptic drugs are not readily available. Long-term seizure outcome studies from Ecuador and Nigeria showed high remission rates even though most patients did not receive any treatment (Osuntokun *et al.* 1987; Placencia *et al.* 1992). Recent well-controlled epidemiological studies have shown that half or fewer of the patients with first unprovoked seizures have a second seizure (Berg & Shinnar 1991). The First Seizure Trial Group (1993) performed a randomized study to address seizure outcome between treated and untreated patients after a first unprovoked seizure. Treated patients had only about half the risk of a second seizure compared with the untreated group. However, with longer follow-up there was no difference between the two groups in terms of probability of achieving remission (Musicco *et al.* 1994). What has become clear is that antiepileptic drugs may help prevent a second seizure from occurring but do not alter the overall natural course of the epileptic syndrome. Factors such as the type of epileptic syndrome, underlying aetiology, age of seizure onset and pre-existing abnormal neurological examination play a more important role in predicting outcome, and should be considered in helping a physician decide on whether to initiate treatment or not.

In summary, the most consistent factor influencing the prognosis of a first unprovoked seizure is the presence of symptomatic versus idiopathic seizures. The other factors discussed are so variable in their expression as to be of questionable or undefined significance. The reasons for this were discussed previously and relate to patient selection, data acquisition and data analysis.

Remission of epilepsy

The only documentation of the natural history of untreated seizure was by Gowers (1881), who wrote 'the spontaneous cessation of the disease is an event too rare to be reasonably anticipated in any given case'. With the introduction of bromide treatment in 1857, Gowers noted a significant improvement in seizure outcome. Bromide was not an effective anticonvulsant by today's standards. At the turn of the century, the remission rate remained poor, ranging from 3% to 30% (Habermass 1901; Turner 1907; Volland 1908). With the introduction of more effective medications (phenobarbital in 1912, diphenylhydantoin in 1938, and other anticonvulsant medications including carbamazepine and valproic acid over the next three decades), one would expect remission from seizures to be significantly improved. However, in a comprehensive review of the literature on the prognosis of epilepsy, Rodin (1968) found that approximately two-thirds of epileptics develop a chronic form of the disease and cannot be helped by standard medications. Rodin's study represented a retrospective cross-sectional study of referral hospitals and institutions. As a consequence, chronic or uncontrolled epilepsy patients were overrepresented, while newly diagnosed cases and epilepsy in remission were underrepresented.

Studies reported within the last 15 years present a more favourable outcome. Despite differences in the definition of remission, varying between 1 and 5 years seizure-free, complete remission ranges from 50% to 70%. The Group for the Study of Prognosis of Epilepsy in Japan (1981) reported a 3 year remission rate of 58.3%. Elwes *et al.* (1984) reported the actuarial percentage of patients attaining a 1 year seizure-free period to be 40% by 1 year, 73% by 2 years, 84% by 3 years, 88% by 4 years, 84% by 5 years and 92% by 8 years. Similar percentages were seen among the 2 year seizure-free group. Outcome became more favourable with longer follow-up. Loiseau *et al.* (1987) reported remission rates in adolescents to be 33.5% at 5 year follow-up, 46% at 10 years, 54.4% at 15 years and 57.8% at 20 years, with a trend towards better outcome with longer follow-up. Annegers *et al.* (1979) used more stringent criteria for remission (5 years seizure-free). The estimated probability of achieving remission within 10 years after diagnosis was 65%, and within 20 years was 76%. Remission rates stabilized after 20 years. All studies found that a longer duration required to achieve seizure control was associated with a lower likelihood of seizure remission.

Generalized idiopathic seizures are one of the most important prognostic indicators of remission. The probability of remission by 20 years was equal for both idiopathic and symptomatic seizures (70–75%) in Annegers' study (1979). However, when symptomatic seizures were related to perinatal injury, this figure dropped to 46%. Among the idiopathic seizure group, generalized seizures had a higher remission rate (85% for generalized tonic clonic and 80% for absence) than partial seizures (65% for complex partial seizures). The Japan Study Group (1981) also found the idiopathic seizure group to have better outcome than the symptomatic seizure group. With respect to specific seizure types, absence seizures, generalized tonic clonic seizures, simple partial seizures, secondarily generalized tonic clonic seizures and complex partial seizures all had comparable remission rates of 68%, 69%, 50%, 60% and 61%, respectively. When partial seizures were associated with generalized tonic clonic seizures, the remission rate dropped substantially to 30% for complex partial seizures and 42% for simple partial seizures. Lennox–Gastaut syndrome and infantile spasms had the worst prognosis, with remission rates of 37% and 51%, respectively. The mean annual incidence rate of relapse was determined to be 1.6% (Annegers *et al.* 1979). The probability of relapse by 20 years was 6% for absence seizures, 21% for generalized tonic clonic seizures and 32% for complex partial seizures.

Conflicting results have been reported with regard to the age of seizure onset as a predictor of seizure remission. Earlier studies have reported better outcome in younger patients (Annegers *et al.* 1979; Japan Study Group 1981). The probability of remission by 10 years after diagnosis is 75% for seizure onset after age 1 and before 10 years, 68% for those 10–19 years old at seizure onset, and 63% for those 20–59 years old (Annegers *et al.* 1979). The difference is even more impressive when one considers remission in terms of those who are seizure free off medication: 51% probability of remission for seizure onset before 10 years old, 40% for those 10–19 years old, and 28% for those 20–59 years old. Conversely, the probability of relapse increases with older age of seizure onset. The relapse rate by 20 years is 13% for those with seizure onset before 9 years old, 22% for those 10–19 years old, and 32% for those older than 20 years. In a recent case–control study, Berg *et al.* (1996) found that early age of seizure onset was a consistent predictor of intractability on both univariate and multivariable analyses. The predictive value of age was not limited to onset before 1 year of age. Conversely, Camfield *et al.* (1993) found that older age at onset was a significant predictor of remission. Other factors which had significant predictive value to intractability included a history of status epilepticus before the diagnosis of epilepsy, poor short-term outcome with treatment, and high initial seizure frequency (Silanpaa 1993; Berg *et al.* 1996).

Factors which appear to have no prognostic value include gender, race, family history, time between diagnosis and initiation of therapy, and EEG abnormality. Abnormal neurological examination is of uncertain significance.

Relapse following discontinuation of anticonvulsant therapy

Many patients become seizure free on anticonvulsant therapy. Since the long-term effect of medication on remission is not known, and the cumulative side effects of medication can be significant, some studies have been undertaken specifically to examine the outcome following medication withdrawal. The overall relapse rate ranges from 20% to 36.5% (Emerson *et al.* 1981; Thurston *et al.* 1982; Todt 1984; Shinnar *et al.* 1985; Bouma *et al.* 1987; Callaghan *et al.* 1988; Arts *et al.* 1988). Children have lower relapse rates of 12–36.3% (Emerson *et al.* 1981; Thurston *et al.* 1982; Todt 1984; Shinnar *et al.* 1985; Bouma *et al.* 1987; Arts *et al.* 1988; Matricardi *et al.* 1989) in comparison with adults, with rates of 26–63% (Juul-Jensen 1964; Overweg *et al.* 1987). The discrepancy may be attributed to more benign epilepsy syndromes occurring in childhood, and more epilepsies symptomatic of cerebrovascular diseases and brain tumours in adults.

Most relapses occur within the first year from the start of withdrawal. In fact, 50–80% of relapses occur *during* medication withdrawal (Emerson *et al.* 1981; Todt 1984; Shinnar *et al.* 1985; Matricardi *et al.* 1989). This observation poses a question with regard to the true nature of these seizure recurrences: are they true relapses or the result of withdrawal effect from medication? Most studies taper their medication over a 2–4 month period. Although this schedule is appropriate for some anticonvulsant medication, it may be too rapid for others, such as the highly dependent drugs like barbiturates and benzodiazepines; these cause withdrawal seizures. Few studies account for this effect. When this factor is taken into account and patients with seizures during the tapering period are excluded from the study, the relapse rate is reduced to as low as 12% (Matricardi *et al.* 1989).

In interpreting cross-sectional studies on medication withdrawal, one realizes the variability in the definition of remission in seizures. Some studies require a seizure-free period of at least 2 years, while others require 4 years before considering drug withdrawal. The significance of 2 years versus 4 years is not known and serves as another confounding factor in data analysis. Two studies attempted to address this question, but do not agree on the number of years of remission maintained on medication before discontinuation. Todt (1984) reports a significant increase in risk of relapse if medications are withdrawn in less than 3 years of being seizure free. Matricardi (1989) reports a minimum of 4 years for better outcome. Braathen *et al.* (1996) reported outcome in uncomplicated childhood epilepsy treated with antiepileptic drug for 1 versus 3 years following remission. The overall remission rate was significantly higher (71%) in the group treated for 3 years than in the group treated for 1 year (53%). The difference in remission rate only reached statistical significance for the group with complex partial seizures.

A number of studies have tried to identify factors that may have predictive value for outcome, with inconsistent results. EEG findings at the time of medication withdrawal have been promoted by many investigators as having good predictive value for outcome. Emerson *et al.* (1981) found that patients whose EEG demonstrated spikes and sharp waves had a relapse rate of 57%, in comparison with only 4% in those with normal EEG ($P < 0.001$). Todt (1984) found several EEG characteristics predictive of outcome. Paroxysmal changes were associated with a higher incidence of seizure recurrence. EEGs which showed normal background or demonstrated resolution of paroxysmal activity at the time of remission correlated with low relapse rate ($P < 0.05$). Matricardi *et al.* (1989) found similar results, with the presence of focal activity, generalized spike and wave, or polyspike on EEG prior to drug discontinuation associated with a high risk of relapse. However, not all authors agree on the significance of EEG findings (Thurston *et al.* 1982; Bouma *et al.* 1987). Overweg *et al.* (1987) reported no difference in outcome with respect to EEG patterns when all other factors were held constant. In a different approach, Arts *et al.* (1988) did not consider medication withdrawal unless the seizure-free patient had a normalized EEG. Patients were maintained on medication for 2–5 years prior to drug withdrawal. Interestingly, relapse rate was constant among the different time points, at 20–26%.

Some factors hold a more consistent relationship with prognosis. Mental retardation and abnormal neurological examination are consistently associated with poor outcome. The relapse rate among this group is approximately 50% (Thurston *et al.* 1982; Todt 1984).

Outcome of the different seizure types has been difficult to define. Oller-Daurella & Oller (1987), found a higher rate of relapse among the symptomatic seizure group (37.9%) than the idiopathic seizure group (19.6%). Relapse rate for generalized tonic clonic seizures varies from 14% to 37% (Thurston *et al.* 1982; Callaghan *et al.* 1988). Similarly, typical absence seizures have been found to have a relapse rate from as low as 0 (Arts *et al.* 1988) to as high as 41% (Matricardi *et al.* 1989). Remission is difficult to predict accurately in most patients with childhood absence epilepsy at the time of diagnosis. In a population-based study, Wirrell *et al.* (1996) found certain factors predictive of poor outcome. These included cognitive impairment at diagnosis, absence status prior to or during treatment with an antiepileptic drug, development of generalized tonic clonic seizures or myoclonic seizures during treatment, abnormal background on the initial EEG, and family history of generalized seizures in first-degree relatives. Patients with these findings were more likely to go on to develop juvenile myoclonic epilepsy, requiring a lifetime treatment with antiepileptic medications. Complex partial seizures alone carry a better prognosis, with relapse rate of 16%. However, outcome changes dramatically when secondary generalization is added (relapse rate 54%). Thurston *et al.* (1982) and Todt (1984) found a relapse rate of 45% with a febrile seizure history compared with 12% in those with no such history.

Factors which were found not to have predictive values included gender, race and family history. The significance of the age of onset of seizure history was conflicting among the different centres. Emerson *et al.* (1981) found relapse rate to be high in children aged less than 2 years (17%), but low in those older than 7 years (6%, $P < 0.02$). Shinnar *et al.* (1985) and Bouma *et al.* (1987), however, reported low relapse rates among children aged less than 2–3 years. Most other studies do not find any significance in age of onset at all. The discrepancy can be due to a number of factors. First, some studies only include children, while others include patients of all age groups. Furthermore, among the children, studies have different criteria, with some excluding certain seizure types, such as neonatal seizures, absence seizures, Lennox–Gastaut syndrome, infantile spasms and benign focal epilepsy of childhood. The duration of seizure history has been found by some to have predictive value. However, the critical discriminating year between good and bad outcome has been highly variable among studies, ranging anywhere from 2 to 7 years.

The Quality Standards Subcommittee of the American Academy of Neurology (1996) recently published their recommendations for discontinuing antiepileptic drugs in seizure-free patients. Their recommendations were based on a review of the medical literature from 1967 to 1991 relating to the issue of remission and relapse, seizure prognosis and discontinuance of antiepileptic drugs. Among the 53 articles cited during this time period, they identified nine factors observed among these different studies which related to the probability of successful antiepileptic withdrawal. These included sex, age of seizure onset, seizure type, aetiology, neurological examination and IQ, duration of seizure freedom on antiepileptic drugs, treatment regimen, age at relapse, and normalization of the EEG. Only 17 of the 53 studies addressed all nine factors. An analysis of the studies yielded a weighted mean relapse rate of 31.2% for children and 39.4% for adults. The longer the duration of seizure control with antiepileptic drugs, the better the prognosis. Patients meeting the following profile had the greatest chance of successful drug withdrawal: seizure free for 2–5 years on antiepileptic drugs (mean 3.5 years), single type of partial or generalized seizures, normal neurological examination and IQ, and normalized EEG with treatment. Children meeting the above profile had at least a 69% chance and adults a 61% chance of successful withdrawal.

Conclusion

Approximately 50–80% of epileptics achieve a seizure-free state with medical therapy. Results from different centres are variable and difficult to interpret. This is mostly related to differences in definitions and criteria employed. Patient selection remains the biggest variable, with most studies basing their outcome on patients referred to tertiary centres. Responsiveness to medication, judged by remission, is also not well defined. Should 1 year, 2 years or 5 years seizure-free be defined as remission? When should medications be discontinued? Ideally, a multicentre prospective population-based study is required to address these issues. Finally, outcome studies should be designed for individual epileptic syndromes in order to define medical responsiveness of specific syndromes. Such information will be invaluable as we consider patient eligibility for epilepsy surgery.

Surgical outcome

Medically intractable complex partial seizures represent 20% of incident epilepsy. Approximately 10–25% of those patients with partial epilepsy may be amenable to surgery for control of their seizures. Surgery is also performed to manage intractable epilepsy without definite foci, and refractory epilepsy with hemiplegia. Studies of post-surgical seizure control are difficult to compare because of differing inclusion criteria, surgical techniques, definition of outcomes, and duration of follow-up among the many epilepsy centres. Inclusion criteria are poorly specified. In most studies, patients are required to have medically refractory seizures despite adequate blood levels. Few studies, however, report blood levels. Whether a patient has failed all standard anticonvulsant medications, both as monotherapy and in combination with other drugs, is not known. EEG evidence of a localized epileptogenic focus amenable to resection is necessary. However, varying recording methods are used to identify the foci. Surgical outcome can be analysed in terms of seizure control, in which complete cure can be considered as cessation of seizures and auras. Unfortunately, most centres have provisions for 'good' and 'worthwhile' outcome, specifying 70–80% reduction of the patient's presurgical seizure frequency. Finally, conclusions with regard to outcome have been drawn from data collected from follow-up as short as 6 months to as long as 10 years or more.

Before we can address surgical results, we have to recognize that different categories of epilepsy surgery exist for different conditions. Focal cortical resection, hemispherectomy and corpus callosotomy are the most common procedures. These approaches must be considered separately since they have different purposes and outcome. The first two aim to stop seizures by removing the brain that is responsible; they are thus only appropriate for symptomatic localization-related epilepsies. Corpus callosotomy is not intended to suppress seizure activity completely, but only to alleviate the intensity and severity of seizures.

Focal cortical resections

Sir Victor Horsley became a pioneer in epilepsy surgery when he performed a craniotomy and corticectomy on three patients with epilepsy in 1886. Over the next 50–60 years, surgery as a treatment for epilepsy continued to be explored, mostly by Penfield and his colleagues. Penfield's early procedures were limited to resection of structural abnormalities, with cure rates of 25–43% (Penfield & Erickson 1941; Penfield & Steelman 1947; Penfield & Paine 1955). Today, partial lobectomies are performed widely for the treatment of medically intractable epilepsy, with reported cure rates as high as 80%.

Temporal lobectomy

Temporal lobectomy represents the largest subgroup of cortical resection in the treatment of complex partial seizures. For the most part, this is due to the frequency of the disease localized to this area. Furthermore, methods for localization of the seizure-generating area to the temporal lobe are better refined than for other neocortical areas. Standard preoperative evaluations performed at most major epilepsy centres include video-EEG telemetry, neuropsychological testing, intracarotid sodium amytal (WADA) test, and neuroimaging studies. All these tests are designed to help localize the seizure focus.

Surgical techniques Temporal lobectomy for the treatment of non-lesional epilepsy was first performed in the early 1950s by Penfield (Penfield & Jasper 1954). He was able to significantly reduce seizure frequency or stop seizures altogether in 40–75% of his patients. Outcome was significantly better in patients with lesions than those without. Over the years, successful outcome has improved to as high as 80–90% in some series, thanks to the development of new EEG recording techniques and imaging studies.

Discrepancies in surgical outcome among the different epilepsy centres reflect to some degree differences in surgical approaches. Three approaches are now commonly employed: anterior temporal lobectomy with amygdalohippocampectomy, amygdalohippocampectomy only, and anterior temporal lobectomy without hippocampectomy. These differing techniques were controversial in the 1950s and continue to be so in the 1990s. Each epilepsy centre has adopted one method or another. It is not clear that outcome differs substantially, but the variability makes comparison studies extremely difficult.

Epilepsy centres which perform anterior medial temporal lobectomies with amygdalohippocampectomy have reported complete remission rates of 60–80% (Cahan *et al.* 1984; Spencer *et al.* 1984a; King *et al.* 1986). Similar results, however, are reported by centres employing other techniques. In Wieser's series (1988), of 52 patients with non-lesional temporal lobe epilepsy who underwent a selective amygdalohippocampectomy, 61% were seizure free, 6% had 'rare' seizures and 16% had worthwhile improvement. Overall, 83% of patients benefited from the surgery. At the second International Palm Desert Conference on epilepsy surgery in 1993, outcomes of the different temporal lobectomy approaches were polled from epilepsy centres around the world. Outcomes for anterior medial temporal lobe resection and selective amygdalohippocampectomy were quite comparable, approximately 68% of patients being seizure free, 22–24% being improved and 9% unchanged. To date, there is only one epilepsy centre which has attempted to compare outcome between the two approaches (Arruda *et al.* 1996). They found no significant difference in seizure control between selective amygdalohippocampectomy and anterior medial temporal lobectomy. Rather, outcome was more dependent on difference in degree of hippocampal atrophy as seen on head MRI-volumetrics. Patients with unilateral hippocampal atrophy had the best outcome, followed by those with bilateral hippocampal atrophy. Patients with no apparent atrophy had the worst outcome.

Goldring *et al.* (1992) contended that the amygdala did not contribute to epileptogenesis in temporal lobe epilepsy and, thus, elected not to remove the amygdala. Of 70 patients who underwent this procedure, 79% benefited from surgery: 33% were seizure free, 27% had one or several seizures and 18.6% had more than 90% seizure reduction. The extent of hippocampal resection has also been debated. In Hermann's study (1989), standard anterior medial temporal lobectomy with resection of variable amounts of hippocampus resulted in 73% of patients being seizure free, and an additional 24% significantly improved. Wyler *et al.* (1995) randomized 70 patients with non-lesional unilateral medial temporal lobe epilepsy into two surgical groups: 34 patients had a partial hippocampectomy with posterior resection up to the anterior edge of the cerebral peduncle, and 36 patients had a total hippocampectomy with posterior resection to the level of the superior colliculus. All patients had a 4.5 cm anterior temporal neocortical resection. Follow-up at 1 year showed that 69% of the patients with a complete hippocampectomy were seizure free compared with only 38% of the patients with partial hippocampectomy. Although the follow-up interval was short, the results demonstrate that the surgical procedure of choice in patients with clear evidence of non-lesional medial temporal lobe epilepsy is a total hippocampectomy.

In all these series, postoperative seizure outcome was better when the electrographically demonstrated area of initial seizure onset was included in the resection. Furthermore, good outcome was highly correlated with specific pathology.

EEG telemetry Specific criteria for patient selection vary. Although selection is based on medical intractability and localization by means of EEG, neuropsychology and/or neuroimaging studies, methodology of EEG recording differs dramatically. In the 1950s to 1970s, most seizure foci were identified by scalp-recorded interictal epileptiform activities. Ictal EEGs were rarely recorded as part of the evaluation. The extent of resection was further determined by intraoperative electrical stimulation and electrocorticography. Patients with bilateral interictal EEG epileptiform discharges were usually dismissed as not being candidates for surgery. This was based on many studies showing only 25% worthwhile outcome in this group of patients (Penfield & Flanigin 1950; Bailey & Gibbs 1951; Bloom *et al.* 1959/1960; Van Buren *et al.* 1975). With the increasing popularity of intracranial depth electrode recording in the 1980s, a resectable seizure focus which could not previously be localized by scalp EEG recording was now more often identified. Seventy per cent of patients with bitemporal interictal epileptiform discharges on scalp EEG recording who had been excluded from surgical therapy showed localization of seizure discharges to a discrete region on intracranial recording (So *et al.* 1989a; Hirsch *et al.* 1991b). However, centres which utilize intracranial electrode recording usually deal with the more complicated seizure population, which may predispose to a worse outcome. This point is well exemplified by the UCLA experience in epilepsy surgery (Cahan *et al.* 1984). Despite very rigid criteria to qualify patients for surgery following an intracranial study, only 62% of their intracranial patients became seizure free, in contrast to 75% of patients localized by scalp EEG only. Similarly, 73% of patients who underwent intracranial EEG recording and 100% with scalp EEG monitoring achieved total remission in the series of King *et al.* (1986).

So *et al.* (1989b) addressed the issue of bitemporal epileptiform abnormalities detected on intracranial studies. Only 29% of their patients achieved complete remission. This may in fact be due to the less stringent criteria by which they offered surgery to these patients, including many with multifocal disease. In addition, the hippocampus was inconsistently resected. Hirsch *et al.* (1991b) addressed the same issue, but used more stringent criteria and included hippocampal resection. They offered surgery to 12 patients with bitemporal disease proven by intracranial EEG recording. Eighty-two per cent of these patients are now seizure free.

Despite the numerous variables and inconsistency in the evaluation and surgical techniques among the many epilepsy centres, temporal lobectomy is still able to provide good seizure control for 60–80% of individuals who were previously medically intractable. Similarly, although intracranial depth EEG recording may capture a population of patients with more severe intractable epilepsy, it can be regarded as a continuum of the surgical evaluation in that it makes it possible to offer surgery to the additional 50% of patients who otherwise would not have had their seizure foci localized by scalp EEG monitoring alone; this group has similar 60–80% worthwhile results.

Neuroimaging studies Recent advances in structural and functional neuroimaging techniques have made a significant contribution to the preoperative evaluation of patients with suspected mesial temporal lobe epilepsy and predicting outcome. Evidence of hippocampal sclerosis on qualitative MRI in patients with mesial temporal lobe epilepsy correlates significantly with seizure relief after temporal lobectomy (Bronen 1992; Chan *et al.* 1993). The two most consistent MR features for diagnosing hippocampal sclerosis are volume loss and hyperintense signal changes on T2-weighted sequences of the ipsilateral hippocampus. A decrease in the size of the hippocampus has shown correlation with the degree of neuronal cell loss, a history of childhood febrile seizures, age of seizure onset, verbal memory performance, epileptiform EEG abnormalities and postoperative seizure control (Bronen 1992; Jack 1993, 1994; Jackson 1994). In patients with concordant EEG and MR findings, a satisfactory postoperative outcome was reported in 97% of cases in one centre (Jack *et al.* 1992). When hippocampal atrophy alone was identified by MRI without an identified EEG focus, there was an 86% positive predictive value for excellent postoperative seizure control based on MRI results (Kuzniecky *et al.* 1993). If no MR abnormality was observed in a surgical candidate, the postoperative success rate for seizure control dropped to only 44% (Jack *et al.* 1992; Kuzniecky *et al.* 1993).

Interictal cerebral glucose metabolism imaged with FDG-positron emission tomography (PET) has been found to be helpful in localizing the seizure focus in patients with mesial temporal lobe epilepsy. There is a 60–90% incidence of hypometabolism in the affected temporal lobe in medically refractory mesial temporal lobe epilepsy (Henry *et al.* 1993). Often both the lateral and mesial temporal lobe demonstrate hypometabolism. Patients with non-refractory temporal lobe epilepsy are more likely to demonstrate normal PET findings than those with medically refractory disease.

Single photon emission tomography (SPECT) using HMPAO evaluates focal alteration of cerebral blood flow (CBF). Interictal SPECT has not been consistently reliable in localizing the seizure focus in patients with temporal lobe epilepsy, demonstrating hypoperfusion in the affected temporal lobe in only 50% of cases (Rowe *et al.* 1990, 1991b). Ictal SPECT, on the other hand, has consistently demonstrated a characteristic pattern of unilateral global temporal hyperperfusion with relative decreased perfusion in other cortical areas, both ipsilaterally and contralaterally (Berkovic *et al.* 1993). During a seizure, CBF is markedly increased at and around the site of ictal onset, and this pattern may persist for injections given up to 30 seconds after seizure termination. Later postictal injections demonstrate the 'postictal switch' (Rowe *et al.* 1989, 1991a). Injections done at 1–5 minutes after termination of the seizure show the initial hyperperfused area to have shrunken in size to a characteristic small crescent in the mesial and anterior parts of the temporal lobe, with hypoperfusion in the remaining temporal lobe. The scan returns to the interictal state again within 20 minutes after termination of the seizure. In cases of bilateral independent temporal ictal onsets, ictal SPECT studies show images congruent with the EEG localization. Needless to say, timing is critical in obtaining a diagnostic ictal and postical SPECT scan. Furthermore, knowledge of the sequence of seizure activity at the time of injection is important for proper interpretation of the results.

Extratemporal resection

Surgical outcome from extratemporal resection has been disappointing in most centres. This is attributed primarily to poor localization of the seizure focus in the absence of an abnormal lesion identified by imaging studies. Localization often requires intracranial EEG recordings. Careful planning is required for electrode placement in the vicinity of the seizure focus. Even then, recording of the seizure onset is not always achieved. Furthermore, neuropsychological testing is not very specific for extratemporal disease, and functional imaging studies, such as PET and SPECT, have been inconsistent in demonstrating neocortical abnormalities. Finally, once a seizure focus is identified, the extent of its resection may be limited by adjacent functional cortex.

The Montreal Neurological Institute has the most extensive experience in neocortical resections, totalling 381 non-lesional patients from 1929 to 1975 (Rasmussen 1963,

1975a–c). Cure rates were 23%, 25% and 31% for frontal, occipital and parietal lobectomies, respectively. Other centres report similar results. Hajek and Weiser (1988) reported only 20% of patients with frontal lobectomy to be seizure free. The Cleveland Clinic was a pioneer in subdural grids in the 1970s and used this method extensively to localize neocortical seizure foci. Despite this, only 17% of patients were seizure free, and an additional 14% became seizure free after prolonged follow-up (Van Ness 1991). Interestingly, all the patients with complete cure had structural lesions on preoperative MRI and CT scans, providing further evidence for the difficulty in localizing non-lesional neocortical seizure foci. Of six patients who underwent extratemporal lobec tomies in the UCLA series, none were cured of their seizures (Sutherling *et al.* 1990). Similarly, only one of five patients with frontal or frontoparietal lobectomies in the Yale series had significant seizure reduction (Williamson and Spencer 1986). In another study, Spencer *et al.* (1990) reported their experience in four patients with neocortical temporal seizures localized by intracranial electrodes. All these patients continued to have seizures following an anteromedial temporal lobectomy and hippocampectomy. This observation provides additional support for the difficulties in localizing extrahip-pocampal seizure foci, even within the temporal lobe.

Studies which have found good outcome with neocortical resections have included a disproportionately higher number of patients with lesions. Bonis (1980) reported good outcome in 73.3% of 294 patients. Good seizure control was seen in 57% of frontal lobectomies, 60% of central resections, 70.9% of parietal lobectomies and 86.5% of temporal lobectomies. However, 91% of these patients had a structural lesion.

Long-term seizure outcome

The outcome data on epilepsy surgery discussed above are limited and do not provide the information on long-term outcome that is critical in counselling patients and adjusting antiepileptic medication after surgery. Data regarding the likelihood of continuing to be seizure free after a period of remission are sparse. Rougier *et al.* (1992) found that the probability of being seizure free for 1 year was 66% at 1 year, 61% at 2 years and 62% at 5 years. The probability of remaining seizure free was fairly optimistic: 83% between the first and second year, 87% between the second and third year and 96% between the third and fourth year. Elwes *et al.* (1991) also found a favourable longitudinal outcome. In this series, the probability of 1 year of remission after epilepsy surgery was 50% at 1 year, 70% at 2 years and 77% at 7 years. The probability of remaining seizure free was 90% after 1 year, and 94% after 2 consecutive years of being seizure free.

In 1995, Berkovic and colleagues published an actuarial analysis of epilepsy surgery outcome, according to pathological substrates. The probability of becoming seizure free for 2 years determined at 5 years follow-up was 62% in patients with mesial temporal sclerosis (MTS), 80% in patients with cortical tissue lesions and 36% in the normal tissue group. Freedom from seizures for 5 continuous years occurred in 50% of patients with MTS, 69% of patients with cortical tissue lesions and 21% of patients with normal tissue. This more sobering estimate suggests a decline in seizure outcome in the MTS group over time – a group that has traditionally been considered to be among the best for persistent relief of seizures after epilepsy surgery. In fact, Berkovic *et al.* (1995) found that all relapses after 30 months occurred in the MTS group. We recently reported our own long-term outcome based on pathological substrates (Spencer 1996). In this series, we only included patients who had at least 2 years of postoperative follow-up, and had pathological findings of either glioma, MTS, vascular malformation or developmental lesion. Continued seizure control was seen most often in patients with gliomas (75%), followed by patients with MTS (67%). Similar to Berkovic's findings, relapse was extremely rare in patients with gliomas or normal tissue, and relatively low in patients with vascular lesions (10%). However, relapse rate reached 15% in patients with MTS, and 25% in patients with developmental lesions. The findings in these two studies suggest that patients with MTS and developmental lesions are at risk of having recurrent seizures after epilepsy surgery. Therefore, it may be prudent to continue these patients on antiepileptic drugs, regardless of the duration of remission after surgery. Possible causes for seizure relapse in these patients include multifocal involvement in the case of developmental lesions, and dual pathology and bilateral hippocampal sclerosis in patients with MTS. We have also studied factors which may be predictive of successful seizure control in focal corticectomies (Spencer *et al.* 1993). In the temporal lobe group, evidence of MTS in the resected tissue, a known cause of the epilepsy, and absence of secondary generalization were predictive of good outcome. The only predictor in the extratemporal group was a known cause of epilepsy.

Psychosocial outcome

Most studies addressing the outcome of epilepsy surgery have focused primarily on seizure control. Psychosocial issues have been addressed, but not as extensively. Even then, most of these studies looked at changes in cognitive function, and only a few addressed quality of life. Comparison of different psychosocial studies is difficult, since most of these contain small numbers of patients, precluding meaningful multivariable analysis and analysis by subgroup. The few studies that have accumulated large numbers of patients did so over a prolonged period of time. Since epilepsy surgery is an evolving field, techniques, patient selection, and evaluation are continuously changing, yielding a heterogeneous patient population in such long-term analyses.

Neuropsychological tests Since temporal lobectomies are by far the most common resection done in epilepsy surgery, most psychosocial data have been reflective of this group of patients. Cognitive function can be evaluated in this group in terms of memory and learning function. Early experience in the contribution of the temporal lobes to memory is well exemplified by Scoville's celebrated patient HM (Scoville and Milner 1957) who underwent bilateral temporal lobectomy for intractable seizures and acquired severe and debilitating memory loss. The results of HM's surgery were devastating, but taught an important lesson about memory function in the temporal lobes. Now, preoperative neuropsychological evaluations are carefully performed to establish the level of memory function in the contralateral hemisphere, lest removal of one temporal lobe produce another HM.

In patients with dominant temporal lobe epilepsy, preoperative neuropsychological testing usually shows impaired language function and worse verbal memory in comparison with visuospatial memory and pattern recognition. Patients with good seizure control following dominant temporal lobectomy may have worsening of immediate and delayed verbal memory and verbal learning (Cavazzuti *et al.* 1980; Novelly *et al.* 1984; Ojemann & Dodrill 1985; Ivnik *et al.* 1987). These patients are less efficient on language dependent cognitive tasks, particularly those that involve complex learning and memory. The extent of verbal memory and verbal learning deterioration after surgery is inversely related to the magnitude of the deficit preoperatively (Cavazzuti *et al.* 1980). Ojemann & Dodrill (1985) found that the degree of postoperative memory deficit was more related to the extent of lateral temporal resection than medial resection; they noted that preoperative verbal memory performance was more reflective of the extent of medial temporal lobe pathology, whereas postoperative memory deficits were dependent on the extent of lateral resection. Visuospatial memory, on the other hand, improves significantly with dominant temporal lobectomy (Cavazzuti *et al.* 1980; Novelly *et al.* 1984).

Patients with non-dominant temporal lobe epilepsy have worse visuospatial function and memory in comparison with verbal memory and language function preoperatively. After surgery, there is improvement in verbal memory (Cavazzuti *et al.* 1980; Novelly *et al.* 1984; Ivnik *et al.* 1987). In contrast to the ipsilateral memory deficit sometimes seen after dominant temporal lobectomy, either no change or only a slight decline in non-verbal abilities is the rule (Novelly *et al.* 1984; Ivnik *et al.* 1987). In fact, Novelly *et al.* (1984) found a significant improvement in verbal and performance IQs in patients with non-dominant temporal lobectomies, in contrast to no improvement in IQs among patients with dominant temporal lobectomies.

In contrast to the findings in patients who have well-controlled seizures following surgery, patients who have recurrent seizures are found to have no improvement in any aspect of memory function. Instead, Novelly *et al.* (1984) noticed a global decline in most of their patients. Other factors predictive of poor postoperative cognitive function include absence of specific pathology in the resected specimen and continued abnormal EEG (Lieb *et al.* 1982).

Quality of life and employment Very few studies have addressed the quality of life in patients with epilepsy surgery, or epilepsy at all. Factors such as employment, functional independence, social interaction and sexuality are as important as seizure control and cognitive function. Studies looking at employment and social adjustment suffer the same biases discussed previously under the medical management, namely selection bias from a tertiary centre versus the general population. Furthermore, questionnaires to employers face the prejudice against epileptics being highly functional individuals. Because of the stigma of epilepsy, such disorders may also not be reported to employers. In general, epileptics have higher unemployment rates than the general population. A twofold difference was seen in unemployment in one Rochester study, where 7.6% of epileptics with IQs above 70 were unemployed in comparison with 3.6% of the general population (Hauser & Hesdorffer 1990). The overall level of occupation attained by epileptics is usually lower than that of the general population, with an underrepresentation of managerial and professional occupations. There is no difference between the two groups in utilizing health care services, absenteeism and proneness to accidents. Neurological factors predictive of employment are centred around the history of seizures themselves. The mere presence or absence of seizures influences employment; particularly frequent generalized tonic clonic seizures tend to decrease the likelihood of employment. Successful employment, however, is more related to intelligence and motivation, rather than neurological variables. Furthermore, the amount of time employed since entering the work force is positively correlated with current employment.

Employment increases following successful control with surgery. Crandall (1975) found that the percentage of patients able to maintain employment or successfully manage families and home responsibilities increased from 32% preoperatively to 66% postoperatively. In a series of 32 patients with temporal lobectomies, Augustine et al. (1984) found the number of patients fully employed to increase from 43% to 71% postoperatively. Furthermore, the number of underemployed decreased from eight patients to zero. Seizure control was found to be an important predictor of post-operative employment. The mean seizure frequency was significantly better for the employed group. Changes in employment took place primarily during the first year after surgery. Most of these patients were previously underemployed. Similar to the findings in other studies (Hauser & Hesdorffer 1990; Guldvog et al. 1991), current employment was highly correlated with presurgical employment history. Unemployed welfare patients continued to receive welfare postoperatively.

Other non-neurological factors also influence employment. Both psychiatric and social situations affected employment irrespective of seizure control. There was a significantly higher number of moderate to severe psychiatric disorders such as personality disorder, suicidal depression, schizophrenia and paranoia among the unemployed group. In contrast, most patients in the employed group either had no psychiatric history or mild disorders such as anxiety, adjustment or mild affective disorder. Similarly, significantly more patients in the unemployed group had a criminal record, for example, drug abuse.

Sperling et al. (1995) also found improved employment following temporal lobectomy in 86 patients. The unemployment rate declined from 25% before surgery to 11% after surgery ($P < 0.05$). Underemployment also tended to diminish. They found a strong correlation between postoperative seizure control and occupational status. Patients who were seizure free demonstrated a high rate of improvement in employment status (49%) after surgery, as did patients who had few seizures postoperatively (39%). In contrast, patients with persistent seizures rarely improved (6%) and more often deteriorated (17%) ($P < 0.005$). The authors also examined other variables which may contribute to postoperative occupational outcome. They found that length of postoperative follow-up, educational level, full-scale IQ, and global memory and global psychopathology scores had no bearing on occupational outcome. Age at surgery was the only variable that significantly differed between patients who remained unemployed (mean age at surgery 42.4 ± 10.9 years) and those who became employed (mean age at surgery 31.0 ± 8.0 years; $P < 0.05$). The authors also found that it took up to 6 years in several patients before any noticeable vocational improvement could be seen. This longer time period may account for the lower employment rate reported in other studies which had a shorter follow-up period.

To date, there has been one study which compared psychosocial outcome between postoperative patients and matched control patients with medically treated epilepsy not fully controlled by medications (Guldvog et al. 1991). In a retrospective cohort study of patients in the Danish Epilepsy Registry, Guldvog ascertained outcomes with respect to survival, seizure control, neurological deficits and social outcomes such as employment, receipt of disability insurance and onset of new psychiatric conditions. Two hundred and one patients surgically treated and 185 patients medically treated were entered into the study. Self-reported change in working ability indicated improvement in over half of the surgical group compared with a quarter of the non-surgical group. However, there was no actual change in work or educational situations. In general, patients in the surgical group were more likely to become employed or stay employed and were less likely to require disability pensions compared with the non-surgical group. Similar to other studies, a long-standing history of pretreatment employment was correlated with current employment. With respect to marital status and fertility, there was no statistical difference between the two groups. Similarly, there was no difference between the two groups for social dependency.

Despite the variability in different study designs, there is an overall trend toward surgical treatment being effective in controlling seizures and having positive effects on psychosocial factors. When seizure foci are well localized to a resectable area, surgery in these patients will not only provide good seizure control, but may also improve psychosocial functions. There remains the need to develop rehabilitative programmes for patients who are not highly functional preoperatively. Such programmes would involve vocational training, as well as helping patients adjust to social situations and independent living.

Hemispherectomy

Hemispherectomy was first introduced by Dandy (1928) and Lhermitte (1928) in an attempt to treat brain tumours. Twenty-five years later, Krynauw (1950) applied it to the treatment of epilepsy in 12 children with infantile hemiplegia. Early results were successful in controlling seizures. However, approximately two of three patients presented 3–25 years later with increased intracranial pressure. This lethal complication of superficial cerebral haemosiderosis was the result of repeated bleeding into the sub-arachnoid space. As a consequence, hemispherectomies were abandoned. In 1983, Rasmussen proposed a modified procedure: a 'functional hemispherectomy'. About one-quarter to one-third of the hemisphere, usually the frontal and occipital lobes, were left behind with intact circulation. Superficial cerebral haemosiderosis has not been seen as a late complication with this method. However, only 45% of patients achieved seizure control, in comparison with 59% of patients after complete hemis-pherectomy. In 1988, Tinuper *et al.* reported the results of a modification of the functional hemispherectomy. In addition to the standard procedure described previ-ously by Rasmussen, a corpus callosotomy was also performed. Using this modified technique, 71% of their patients obtained complete seizure remission. Early complica-tions included hydrocephalus in rare cases which was responsive to shunting. To date, there have been no long-term complications reported.

Inclusion criteria for functional hemispherectomy are quite different from those of temporal lobectomy. Patients are often severely debilitated from their seizures and hemiparesis. EEG findings in some patients may be localized to one lobe, often the temporal lobe, but often these patients have diffuse but unilateral EEG abnormality. Localization is very difficult, however. Their seizures are focal in onset, but may generalize rapidly. Very frequent focal attacks may occur, even continuously, contralat-eral to the hemispheric defect. Many have drop attacks, from either tonic or atonic seizures, resulting in frequent falls and injuries. The hemiparesis is most prominent in the upper extremity. The patient has minimal or no fine motor skills in the hand. However, the arm can be used for gross motor activity. Ambulation, although asym-metric, is possible.

The pathologies responsible for such a clinical picture are diverse and include perinatal injury, cerebral infarction, superior longitudinal sinus thrombosis, meningi-tis, acute encephalitis and head trauma. Patients with Sturge–Weber syndrome presen-ting with hemiparesis and seizures have benefited from this procedure, with complete cessation of seizure activity. Hemimegalencephaly, a neuronal migration disorder, can cause mental retardation, hemiparesis and intractable epilepsy of varying degree. The continued mental deterioration in this condition is suspected to be related to the frequent seizure activity. Finally, Rasmussen's encephalitis is a chronic viral encephali-tis which presents with intractable epilepsy and progressive hemiparesis and/or hemianopia. Since the ultimate outcome is hemiplegia with or without surgery, it has been recommended that a functional hemispherectomy be performed early in order to preserve cognitive function (Rasmussen & Andermann 1991).

Approximately 75% of patients undergoing functional hemispherectomy become seizure free. Among those with poor outcome, the single most important predictor of failure is bilateral independent ictal and interictal EEG findings on preoperative evalu-ation. This pattern may indicate diffuse cerebral pathology. Low IQ is not a contraindi-cation to the surgery. Even among patients with persistent seizures, the intensity and frequency of seizure activity improve significantly postoperatively. There is no change in the degree of hemiparesis. Some patients may acquire a hemianopia demonstrated on examination, but this is usually not functionally disabling. With respect to psychosocial outcome, Rasmussen (1983) found improvement in behaviour in all 41 of his patients. The changes were always within 1–2 months of surgery. Thirty-six of 41 patients had either no change or improvement in IQ testing. Following surgery, many patients were able to attend regular schools or attend special classes in regular schools. A number of patients were able to obtain regular jobs.

Corpus callosotomy

There remains a population of medically intractable epileptics who cannot be helped by focal resection or hemispherectomy. It is often this group of patients who require some form of surgical intervention, since their seizures are frequently generalized, rendering the patient physically debilitated. Corpus callosotomy has become increasingly popular over the last few decades for this group of patients. Its intent is not to suppress seizures altogether, but to stop generalization of seizure activity, thereby preventing falls and injuries.

Corpus callosotomy was first applied to human epileptics by Van Wagenen and Harren in 1940. Their approach involved sectioning of the entire corpus callosum, hippocampal commissure, anterior commissure and one fornix. Early experiences with corpus callosotomy, however, were associated with an unacceptably high morbidity rate, which included ventriculitis, hydrocephalus and meningitis. For these reasons, the procedure was not very popular until the late 1970s, when Donald Wilson and his colleagues at Dartmouth University revised the procedure. They initially proposed a 'frontal commissurotomy' which involved sectioning of the rostral one-half of the corpus callosum, anterior commissure and one fornix (Wilson *et al.* 1977). Later, they changed the procedure to what is today called a 'central commissurotomy'. This involves section of the corpus callosum and hippocampal commissure only (Wilson *et al.* 1982). Seizure control in either of the two revised procedures was similar to a complete commissurotomy; however, complications were significantly reduced. The final modification was to perform a two-stage operation in which sectioning of part of the corpus callosum was done first, followed by completion of the callosotomy a few months later (Harbaugh *et al.* 1983). The two-stage approach was found to dramatically reduce the duration and severity of postoperative disconnection syndrome, characterized by abulia, incontinence, apraxia of the non-dominant hand and visual agnosia in the non-dominant field (Ross *et al.* 1984).

Comparing the outcome of corpus callosotomy at different centres is extremely difficult. The primary problem is related to the heterogeneous patient population. Patients who have been considered for this surgery include those with symptomatic generalized epilepsy of variable types, multifocal diseases and poorly localized focal epilepsy. Given the diversity of patients, baseline cognitive function is also highly variable. Most series are not large enough to allow multivariable analysis of subgroups.

To complicate data analysis further, the surgical procedure is not standardized. Central commissurotomy is the standard technique performed today. However, some centres advocate complete commissurotomies to be done as either a one- or two-stage procedure. Other centres contend that a partial anterior corpus callosotomy is adequate for seizure control. Finally, definition of surgical outcome is more difficult in this population since there are so many different seizure types involved. Many patients have mixed seizure types. For example, in one series, 26 of 80 patients had mixed seizure types; 7 of these had more than four different types of seizures (Fuiks *et al.* 1991). Should 'good' outcome be defined as significant reduction of seizure frequency? The quantitative approach does not take into account the possibility that reduction of one seizure type may be associated with increased frequency of a different type. Perhaps more appropriate for this population is to define outcome according to the purpose of the procedure, namely effectiveness of the surgery in reducing injury. Unfortunately, not all centres include this variable in their outcome definition.

In general, corpus callosotomy decreases the incidence of generalized seizures in 50–70% of patients, and in particular atonic, tonic and generalized tonic clonic seizures. On the other hand, patients develop different seizure patterns postoperatively. These may appear to be generalized seizures, but a partial onset in the form of either an aura or simple partial symptomatology enables the patient to secure him- or herself, or to slowly slump to the floor, avoiding injury. Other patients develop hemibody involvement only. Although most patients continue to have seizures postoperatively, the partial manifestations minimize injury significantly (Harbaugh *et al.* 1983; Gates *et al.* 1984, 1987; Purves *et al.* 1988; Spencer 1988; Spencer *et al.* 1988; Oguni *et al.* 1991). Some patients complain of being more frightened with these partial seizures due to the more prolonged duration of awareness for episodes that had previously resulted in prompt loss of consciousness (Gates *et al.* 1987; Spencer *et al.* 1988).

The preferred extent of corpus callosotomy remains controversial. Centres which perform partial callosotomy find no significant difference in outcome with respect to postoperative generalized seizure frequency between partial and complete corpus callosotomy. However, some of these centres do not offer additional surgery to patients who do poorly after partial section (Purves *et al.* 1988; Oguni *et al.* 1991). Centres which offer complete corpus callosotomy do it inconsistently. For instance, the extent of section was documented in only 15 of 24 patients in Gates' series (1987). Of the 15, only six were found to have complete callosal section. Gates *et al.* found no difference in seizure outcome in their series, yet they did not account for the remaining nine patients who did not have verification of the extent of corpus callosotomy. Similarly, Fuiks *et al.* (1991) performed a second surgery to complete the callosotomy in only 10 of 17 patients who had no improvement after the first surgery. Furthermore, their classification of seizure outcome was according to absolute numbers of postoperative seizures. Thus, a patient with complete callosotomy may have benefited from fewer generalized seizures and fewer falls but more partial seizures. As a consequence, his or her overall outcome following complete corpus callosotomy is similar to that following partial corpus callosotomy, since the absolute number of seizures remained the same.

At our institution we perform a two-stage procedure. This method minimizes the severity of disconnection syndrome discussed previously. Furthermore, it provides an opportunity to examine the response of generalized seizures after partial callosotomy. Patients who are not helped by the first surgery are then offered a second surgery to complete the section. We found that 80% of patients with complete corpus callosotomy have cessation of their generalized seizures and falls, in comparison with 50% of patients with partial and anterior corpus callosotomy (Spencer 1988). This finding indicates that completion of corpus callosotomy may have some benefit in selected patients.

Corpus callosotomy, partial or complete, is also inconsistently effective in controlling partial seizures. Patients who benefit the most are those with a lateralized seizure focus on EEG, structural abnormality involving one hemisphere, or hemiparesis (Luessenhop et al. 1970; Herbaugh et al. 1983; Geoffroy et al. 1983; Spencer et al. 1988; Oguni et al. 1991). These patients may have complete resolution of their partial seizures postoperatively. However, Spencer et al. (1984b) reported five patients who developed more intense focal seizures postoperatively. Characteristic features included violent bilateral or unilateral tonic and/or clonic activity, feelings of fear during the motor activity, prolonged postictal hemiparesis and retention of consciousness. The onset of these seizures ranged from 3 months to several years postoperatively. Interestingly, all these patients had bilateral independent EEG foci on preoperative evaluation and more localized bifrontal EEG abnormality postoperatively. This phenomenon may be explained by the cutting of inhibitory fibres from the contralateral hemisphere.

Several factors have been found to be predictive of outcome following corpus callosotomy. Patients with low intelligence, specifically IQ less than 40, are more likely to have persistent generalized seizures following surgery. Patients who acquired focal deficits relatively early in life have a better outcome (Spencer 1988; Oguni et al. 1991). Preoperative EEGs which demonstrate secondary bisynchrony or lateralized EEG discharges are associated with good outcome. On the other hand, patients who have multifocal independent discharges are found to have recurrent generalized seizures postoperatively. Age at seizure onset, duration of epilepsy and age at surgery do not consistently show positive correlation with outcome (Fuiks et al. 1991; Oguni et al. 1991).

Long-term follow-up after corpus callosotomy shows no significant effect on intelligence and memory. Language function is intact in most patients except in those with crossed dominance for language and handedness. In this particular group there may be persistent dysfunction of verbal output for both speech and writing. Verbal receptive and reasoning abilities are affected but not to the same extent (Sass et al. 1990). On formal testing, these patients display variable degrees of dysgraphia and dyslexia. Apraxia and right–left antagonism is variably seen in post-callosotomy patients.

The effect of corpus callosotomy on behaviour is poorly studied. Early reports by

Wilson *et al.* (1977, 1978, 1982) demonstrate a significant improvement in behaviour and psychosis following surgery. It should be noted, however, that most of Wilson's patients gave a history suggestive of more localized partial seizures. Due to the limited tools available for preoperative evaluation at the time, these patients were offered corpus callosotomy. Thus, their patient population may have included a disproportionate number of higher functioning individuals. Spencer *et al.* (1988) more recently found that patients who have preoperative aggressive behavioural disorders display more pronounced aggression postoperatively. Unfortunately, there have been no other studies of this issue.

Corpus callosotomy in a selected group of patients is beneficial. Patients who have frequent generalized seizures with associated falls and injuries benefit the most.

Conclusion

We have come a long way from the days of Gowers, when the natural history of epilepsy was dismal. Today, approximately 50–80% of patients with epilepsy achieve a seizure-free state with medical treatment. Patients with generalized idiopathic epilepsy have consistently responded to medical treatment. On the other hand, some 20% of patients with partial seizures are medically intractable. Of this group, approximately 15% may be helped by surgery, with 60–80% of these patients achieving good seizure control with cortical resection.

There remains a small percentage of patients who cannot be helped by either of these therapies. With the introduction of new anticonvulsant drugs on the horizon, there is a glimmer of hope for these people. Future directions in the treatment of epilepsy will probably involve both novel medical and surgical approaches. As research in the areas of molecular genetics and neurophysiology continues, it is to be hoped that it will shed new light on the basic mechanisms of the different epileptic syndromes and provide clues for designing creative therapy, perhaps combining medical and surgical intervention.

References

Annegers, J. F., Hauser, W. A. & Elveback, L. R. (1979). Remission of seizures and relapse in patients with epilepsy. *Epilepsia* **20**, 729–37.

Annegers, J. F., Shirts, S. B., Hauser, W. A. & Kurland, L. T. (1986). Risk of recurrence after an initial unprovoked seizure. *Epilepsia* **27**, 43–50.

Arruda, F., Cendes, F., Andermann, F. *et al.* (1996). Mesial atrophy and outcome after amygdalohippocampectomy or temporal lobe removal. *Ann. Neurol.* **40**, 446–50.

Arts, W. F. M., Visser, L. H., Loonen, M. C. B. *et al.* (1988). Follow-up of 146 children with epilepsy after withdrawal of antiepileptic therapy. *Epilepsia* **29**, 244–50.

Augustine, E. A., Novelly, R. A., Mattson, R. H. *et al.* (1984). Occupational adjustment following neurosurgical treatment of epilepsy. *Ann. Neurol.* **15**, 68–72.

Bailey, P. & Gibbs, F. A. (1951). The surgical treatment of psychomotor epilepsy. *JAMA* **145**, 365–70.

Berg, A. T., Levy, S. R., Novotny, E. J. & Shinnar, S. (1996). Predictors of intractable epilepsy in childhood: a case–control study. *Epilepsia* **37**, 24–30.

Berg, A. T. & Shinnar, S. (1991). The risk of seizure recurrence following a first unprovoked seizure: a quantitative review. *Neurology* **41**, 965–72.

Berkovic, S. F., Newton, M. R., Chiron, C. & Dulac, O. (1993). Single photon emission tomography. In *Surgical Treatment of the Epilepsies*, 2nd edn, ed. J. Engel Jr, pp. 233–43. New York: Raven Press.

Berkovic, S. F., McIntosh, A. M., Kalnins, R. M. *et al.* (1995). Preoperative MRI predicts outcome of temporal lobectomy: an actuarial analysis. *Neurology* **45**, 1358–63.

Blom, S., Heijbel, J. & Berfors, P. G. (1978). Incidence of epilepsy in children: a follow-up study three years after the first seizure. *Epilepsia* **19**, 343–50.

Bloom, D., Jasper, H. & Rasmussen, T. (1959/1960). Surgical therapy in patients with temporal lobe seizures and bilateral EEG abnormality. *Epilepsia* **1**, 351–65.

Bonis, A. (1980). Long-term results of cortical excisions based on stereotactic investigation in severe drug resistant epilepsies. *Acta Neurochurg.* **30**(Suppl.), 55–66.

Bouma, P. A. D., Peters, A. C. D., Arts, R. J. H. *et al.* (1978). Discontinuation of antiepileptic therapy: a prospective study in children. *J. Neurol. Neurosurg. Psychiatry* **50**, 1579–83.

Braathen, G., Andersson, T., Gylje, H. *et al.* (1966). Comparison between one and three years of treatment in uncomplicated childhood epilepsy: a prospective study. I. Outcome in different seizure types. *Epilepsia* **37**, 822–32.

Bronen, R. A. (1992). Epilepsy: the role of MR imaging. *AJR* **159**, 1165–74.

Cahan, L. D., Sutherling, W., McCullough, M. A. *et al.* (1984). Review of the 20-year UCLA experience with surgery for epilepsy. *Cleve. Clin. Q.* **51**, 313–18.

Callaghan, N., Garrett, A. & Goggin, T. (1988). Withdrawal of anticonvulsant drugs in patients free of seizures for two years. *N. Engl. J. Med.* **318**, 942–6.

Camfield, P. R., Camfield, C. S., Dooley, J. M. *et al.* (1985). Epilepsy after a first unprovoked seizure in childhood. *Neurology* **35**, 1657–60.

Camfield, C., Camfield, P., Gordon, K. *et al.* (1993). Outcome of childhood epilepsy: a population-based study with a simple scoring system for those treated with medication. *J. Pediatr.* **122**, 861–8.

Cavazzuti, V., Winston, K., Baker, R. & Welch, K. (1980). Psychological changes following surgery for tumours in the temporal lobe. *J. Neurosurg.* **53**, 618–26.

Chan, S., Silver, A. J., Hilal, S. K. *et al.* (1993). Identification of mesial temporal sclerosis using STIR MRI. *Epilepsia* **34** (Suppl. 6), 142.

Cockerell, O. C., Johnson, A. L., Sander, J. W. A. S. *et al.* (1995). Remission of epilepsy: results from the National General Practice Study of Epilepsy. *Lancet* **346**, 140–4.

Commission on Classification and Terminology of the International League Against Epilepsy (1981). Proposal for revised clinical and electroencephalographic classification of epileptic seizures. *Epilepsia* **22**, 489–501.

Commission on Classification and Terminology of the International League Against Epilepsy (1985). Proposal for classification of epilepsies and epileptic syndromes. *Epilepsia* **26**, 268–78.

Crandall, P. H. (1975). Postoperative management and criteria for evaluation. In *Neurosurgical Management of the Epilepsies*, vol. 8, eds. D. P. Purpura, J. K. Penry & R. D. Walter, pp. 265–280. New York: Raven Press.

Dandy, W. E. (1928). Removal of right cerebral hemisphere for certain tumors with hemiplegia. *JAMA* **90**, 823–5.

Elwes, R. D., Dunn, G., Binnie, C. D. & Polkey, C. E. (1991). Outcome following resective surgery for temporal lobe epilepsy: a prospective follow-up study of 102 consective cases. *J. Neurol. Neurosurg. Psychiatry* **54**, 949–52.

Elwes, R. D. C., Johnson, A. L., Shorvon, S. D. & Reynolds, E. H. (1984). The prognosis for seizure control in newly diagnosed epilepsy. *N. Engl. J. Med.* **311**, 944–7.

Emerson, R., D'Souza, B. J., Vining, E. P. *et al.* (1981). Stopping medication in children with epilepsy. Predictors of outcome. *N. Engl. J. Med.* **304**, 1125–9.

First Seizure Trial Group (1993). Randomized clinical trial on the efficacy of antiepileptic drugs in reducing the risk of relapse after a first unprovoked tonic-clonic seizure. *Neurology* **43**, 478–83.

Fuiks, K. S., Wyler, A. R., Hermann, B. P. & Somes, G. (1991). Seizure outcome from anterior and complete corpus callosotomy. *J. Neurosurg.* **74**, 573–8.

Gastaut, H. (1970). Clinical and electroencephalographic classification of epileptic seizures. *Epilepsia* **11**, 114–19.

Gates, J. R., Leppik, I. E., Yap, J. & Gumnit, R. J. (1984). Corpus callosotomy: clinical and electroencephalographic effects. *Epilepsia* **25**, 308–16.

Gates, J. R., Rosenfeld, W. E., Maxwell, R. E. & Lyons, R. E. (1987). Response to multiple seizure types to corpus callosum section. *Epilsepsia* **28**, 28–34.

Geoffroy, G., Lassonde, M., Delisle, F. & Decarie, M. (1983). Corpus callosotomy for control of intractable epilepsy in children. *Neurology* **33**, 891–7.

Goldring, S., Edwards, I., Harding, G. W. & Bernardo, K. L. (1992). Results of anterior temporal lobectomy that spares the amygdala in patients with complex partial seizures. *J. Neurosurg.* **77**, 185–93.

Gowers, W. R. (1881). *Epilepsy and Other Chronic Convulsive Diseases*. London: Churchill.

The Group for the Study of Prognosis of Epilepsy in Japan (1981). Natural history and prognosis of epilepsy: report of a multi-institutional study in Japan. *Epilepsia* **22**, 35–53.

Guldvog, B., Loyning, Y., Hauglie-Hanssen, E. *et al.* (1991). Surgical versus medical treatment for epilepsy. II. Outcome related to social areas. *Epilepsia* **32**, 477–86.

Habermas, S. (1901). Ueber die prognose der epilepsie. *Z. Psychiatr.* **58**, 243–53.

Hajek, M. & Weiser, H. G. (1988). Extratemporal, mainly frontal, epilepsies: surgical results. *J. Epilepsy* **1**, 103–19.

Harbaugh, R. E., Wilson, D. H., Reeves, A. G. & Gazzaniga, M. S. (1983). Forebrain commissurotomy for epilepsy. Review of 20 consecutive cases. *Acta Neurochirurg.* **68**, 263–75.

Hauser, W. A., Anderson, V. E., Loewenson, R. B. & McRoberts, S. M. (1982). Seizure recurrence after a first unprovoked seizure. *N. Engl. J. Med.* **307**, 522–8.

Hauser, W. A. & Hesdorffer, D. C. (1990). *Epilepsy: Frequency, Causes and Consequences*. New York: Epilepsy Foundation of America.

Hauser, W. A., Rich, S. S., Annegers, J. F. & Anderson, V. E. (1990). Seizure recurrence after a first unprovoked seizure: an extended follow-up. *Neurology* **40**, 1163–70.

Henry, T. R., Chugani, H. T., Abou-Khalil, B. W. *et al.* (1993). Positron emission tomography. In *Surgical Treatment of the Epilepsies*, 2nd edn, ed. J. Engel Jr., pp. 211–232. New York: Raven Press.

Hermann, B. P., Wyler, A. R., Ackerman, B. & Rosenthal, T. (1989). Short-term psychological outcome of anterior temporal lobectomy. *J. Neurosurg.* **71**, 327–34.

Hirsch, L. J., Spencer, S. S., Williamson, P. D. *et al.* (1991*a*). Comparison of bitemporal and unitemporal epilepsy defined by depth electroencephalography. *Ann. Neurol.* **30**, 340–6.

Hirsch, L. J., Spencer, S. S., Spencer, D. D. *et al.* (1991*b*). Temporal lobectomy in patients with bitemporal epilepsy defined by depth electroencephalography. *Ann. Neurol.* **30**, 347–56.

Ivnik, R. J., Sharbrough, F. W. & Laws E. R. (1987). Effects of anterior temporal lobectomy on cognitive function. *J. Clin. Psychol.* **43**, 128–37.

Jack, C. R. (1993). Epilepsy surgery and imaging. *Radiology* **189**, 635–46.

Jack, C. R. (1994). MRI-based hippocampal measurements in epilepsy. *Epilepsia* **35** (Suppl. 6), S21–9.

Jack, C. R., Sharbrough, F. W. & Cascino, G. D. (1992). MRI-based hippocampal volumetry: correlations with outcome after temporal lobectomy. *Ann. Neurol.* **31**, 138–46.

Jackson, G. D. (1994). New techniques in magnetic resonance and epilepsy. *Epilepsia* **35** (Suppl. 6), S2–13.

Johnson, L. C., DeBolt, W. L., Long, M. T. *et al.* (1972). Diagnostic factors in adult males following initial seizures: a three-year follow-up. *Arch. Neurol.* **27**, 193–7.

Juul-Jensen, P. (1964). Frequency of recurrence after discontinuance of anti-convulsant therapy in patients with epileptic seizures. *Epilepsia* **5**, 352–63.

King, D. W., Flanigin, H. F., Gallagher, B. B. *et al.* (1986). Temporal lobectomy for partial complex seizures: evaluation, results, and 1-year follow-up. *Neurology* **36**, 334–9.

Krynauw, R. A. (1950). Infantile hemiplegia treated by removing one cerebral hemisphere. *J. Neurol. Neurosurg. Psychiatry* **13**, 243–67.

Kuzniecky, R., Burgard, S. *et al.* (1993). Predictive value of magnetic resonance imaging in temporal lobe epilepsy surgery. *Arch. Neurol.* **50**, 65–9.

Lhermitte, J. (1928). L'ablation complete de l'hemisphere droit dans les case de tumeur cerebrale localisee compliquee d'hemiplegie: la decebration suprathalamique unilaterale chez l'homme. *Encephale* **23**, 314–23.

Lieb, J. P., Rausch, R., Engel, J., Brown, W. J. & Crandall, P. H. (1982). Changes in intelligence following temporal lobectomy: relationship to EEG activity, seizure relief, and pathology. *Epilepsia* **23**, 1–13.

Loiseau, P., Pestre, M. & Dartigues, J. F. (1987). Symptomatology and prognosis in adolescent epilepsies (a study of 1033 cases). *Epilepsy Res.* **1**, 290–6.

Luessenhop, A. J., de la Cruz, T. C. & Fenichel, G. M. (1970). Surgical disconnection of the cerebral hemispheres for intractable seizures. Results in infancy and childhood. *JAMA* **213**, 1630–6.

Matricardi, M., Brinciotti, M. & Benedetti, P. (1989). Outcome after discontinuation of antiepileptic drug therapy in children with epilepsy. *Epilepsia* **30**, 582–9.

Merlis, J. K. (1970). Proposal for an international classification of the epilepsies. *Epilepsia* **11**, 114–19.

Musicco, M., Beghi, E., Solari, A., the First Seizure Trial Group (1994). Effect of antiepileptic treatment initiated after the first unprovoked seizure on the long-term prognosis of epilepsy. *Neurology* **44** (Suppl. 2), A337–8.

Novelly, R. A., Augustine, E. A., Mattson, R. H. *et al.* (1984). Selective memory improvement and impairment in temporal lobectomy for epilepsy. *Ann. Neurol.* **15**, 64–7.

Oguni, H., Olivier, A., Andermann, F. & Comair, J. (1991). Anterior callosotomy in the treatment of medically intractable epilepsies: a study of 43 patients with a mean follow-up of 39 months. *Ann. Neurol.* **30**, 357–64.

Ojemann, G. A. & Dodrill, C. B. (1985). Verbal memory deficits after left temporal lobectomy for epilepsy. Mechanism and intraoperative prediction. *J. Neurosurg.* **62**, 101–7.

Oller-Daurella, L. & Oller, F.-V. L. (1987). Suppression of antiepileptic treatment. *Eur. Neurol.* **27**, 106–13.

Osuntokun, B. O., Adeuja, A. O. G., Nottidge, V. A. *et al.* (1987). Prevalence of the epilepsies in Nigerian Africans: a community-based study. *Epilepsia* **28**, 272–9.

Overweg, J., Binnie, C. D., Oosting, J. & Rowan, A. J. (1987). Clinical and EEG prediction of seizure recurrence following antiepileptic drug withdrawal. *Epilepsy Res.* **1**, 272–83.

Penfield, W. & Erickson, T. C. (1941). *Epilepsy and Cerebral Localization.* Springfield, Illinois: Thomas.

Penfield, W. & Flanigin, H. (1950). Surgical therapy of temporal lobe seizures. *Arch. Neurol. Psychiatry* **64**, 491–500.

Penfield, W. & Jasper, H. (1954). *Epilepsy and the Functional Anatomy of the Human Brain.* Boston: Little, Brown.

Penfield, W. & Paine, K. (1955). Results of surgical therapy for focal epileptic seizures. *Can. Med. Assoc. J.* **73**, 515–31.

Penfield, W. & Steelman, H. (1947). The treatment of focal epilepsy by cortical excision. *Ann. Surgery* **126**, 740–62.

Placencia, M., Shorvon, S. D., Paredes, V. *et al.* (1992). Epileptic seizures in an Andean region of Ecuador: incidence and prevalence of regional variation. *Brain* **115**, 771–82.

Purves, S. J., Wada, J. A., Woodhurst, W. B. *et al.* (1988). Results of anterior corpus callosum section in 24 patients with medically intractable seizures. *Neurology* **38**, 1194–201.

Quality Standards Subcommittee of the American Academy of Neurology (1996). Practice parameter: a guideline for discontinuing antiepileptic drugs in seizure-free patients-summary statement. *Neurology* **47**, 600–2.

Rasmussen, T. (1963). Surgical therapy of frontal lobe epilepsy. *Epilepsia* **4**, 181–98.

Rasmussen, T. (1975*a*). Cortical resection in the treatment of focal epilepsy. In *Advances in Neurology*, vol. 8, eds. D. P. Purpura, J. K. Penry, & R. D. Walter, pp. 139–54. New York: Raven Press.

Rasmussen, T. (1975*b*). Surgery of frontal lobe epilepsy. In *Advances in Neurology*, vol. 8, eds. D. P. Purpura, J. K. Penry & R. D. Walter, pp. 197–205. New York: Raven Press.

Rasmussen, T. (1975*c*). Surgery for epilepsy arising in regions other than the temporal and frontal lobes. In *Advances in Neurology*, vol. 8, eds. D. P. Purpura, J. K. Penry & R. D. Walter, pp. 207–226. New York: Raven Press.

Rasmussen, T. (1983). Hemispherectomy for seizures revisited. *Can. J. Neurol. Sci.* **10**, 71–8.

Rasmussen, T. & Andermann, F. (1991). Rasmussen's syndrome: symptomatology of the symdrome of chronic encephalitis and seizures. In *Epilepsy Surgery*, ed. H. Luders, pp. 173–82. New York: Raven Press.

Rodin, E. A. (1968). *The Prognosis of Patients with Epilepsy.* Springfield, Illinois: Thomas.

Ross, M. K., Reeves, A. G. & Roberts, D. W. (1984). Post-commissurotomy mutism. *Ann. Neurol.* **16**, 114.

Rowe, C. C., Berkovic, S. F., Austin, M. C. *et al.* (1990). Interictal and postictal blood flow in temporal lobe epilepsy. In *Focal Epilepsy: Clinical Use of Emission Tomography*, eds. M. Baldy-Moulinier, N. A. Lassen, J. Engel Jr, pp. 143–150. London: Libbey.

Rowe, C. C., Berkovic, S. F., Austin, M. C. *et al.* (1991*a*). Patterns of postictal cerebral blood flow in temporal lobe epilepsy: qualitative and quantitative analysis. *Neurology* **41**, 1096–103.

Rowe, C. C., Berkovic, S. F., Austin, M. C. *et al.* (1991*b*). Visual and quantitative analysis of interictal SPECT with Tc-99m HMPAO in temporal lobe epilepsy. *J. Nucl. Med.* **32**, 1688–94.

Rowe, C. C., Berkovic, S. F., Sia, S. T. B. *et al.* (1989). Localization of epileptic foci with postictal single photon emission computed tomography. *Ann. Neurol.* **25**, 660–8.

Sass, K. J., Novelly, R. A., Spencer, D. D. & Spencer, S. S. (1990). Postcallosotomy language impairments in patients with crossed cerebral dominance. *J. Neurosurg.* **72**, 85–90.

Scoville, W. B. & Milner, B. (1957). Loss of recent memory after bilateral hippocampal lesion. *J. Neurol. Neurosurg. Psychiatry* **20**, 11–21.

Shinnar, S. & Berg, A. T. (1996). Does antiepileptic drug therapy prevent the development of chronic epilepsy? *Epilepsia* **37**, 701–8.

Shinnar, S., Berg, A. T., Moshe, S. L. (1990). Risk of seizure recurrence following a first unprovoked seizure in childhood: a prospective study. *Pediatrics* **85**, 1076–85.

Shinnar, S., Vining, E. P. G., Mellitis, E. D. *et al.* (1985). Discontinuing antiepileptic medication in children with epilepsy after two years without seizures. A prospective study. *N. Engl. J. Med.* **313**, 976–80.

Sillanpaa, M. (1993). Remission of seizures and prediction of intractability in long-term follow-up. *Epilepsia* **34**, 930–6.

So, N., Gloor, P., Quesney, F. *et al.* (1989*a*). Depth electrode investigations in patients with bitemporal epileptiform abnormalities. *Ann. Neurol.* **25**, 423–31.

So, N., Olivier, A., Andermann, F. *et al.* (1989*b*). Results of surgical treatment in patients with bitemporal epileptiform abnormalities. *Ann. Neurol.* **25**, 432–9.

Spencer, D. D., Spencer, S. S., Williamson, P. D. *et al.* (1984*a*). Access to the posterior medial temporal lobe structures in the surgical treatment of temporal lobe epilepsy. *Neurosurgery* **15**, 667–71.

Spencer, S. S. (1988). Corpus callosotomy in the treatment of intractable seizures. In *Recent Advances in Epilepsy*, ed. T. A. Pedley & B. S. Meldrom, pp. 181–204. New York: Churchill Livingstone.

Spencer, S. S. (1996). Long-term outcome after epilepsy surgery. *Epilepsia* **37**, 807–13.

Spencer, S. S., Berg, A. T. & Spencer, D. D. (1993). Predictors of remission of one year after resective epilepsy surgery. *Epilepsia* **34** (Suppl. 6), 27.

Spencer, S. S., Spencer, D. D., Glaser, G. H. *et al.* (1984*b*). More intense focal seizure types after callosal section: the role of inhibition. *Ann. Neurol.* **16**, 686–93.

Spencer, S. S., Spencer, D. D., Williamson, P. D. & Mattson, R. H. (1990). Combined depth and subdural electrode investigation in uncontrolled epilepsy. *Neurology* **40**, 74–9.

Spencer, S. S., Spencer, D. D., Williamson, P. D. *et al.* (1988). Corpus callosotomy for epilepsy. I. Seizure effects. *Neurology* **38**, 19–24.

Sperling, M. R., Saykin, A. J., Roberts, F. D. *et al.* (1995). Occupational outcome after temporal lobectomy for refractory epilepsy. *Neurology* **45**, 970–7.

Sutherling, W. W., Risinger, M. W., Crandall, P. H. *et al.* (1990). Focal functional anatomy of dorsolateral frontocentral seizures. *Neurology* **40**, 87–98.

Thurston, J. H., Thurston, D. L., Hixon, B. B. & Keller, A. J. (1982). Prognosis in childhood epilepsy: additional follow-up of 148 children 15 to 23 years after withdrawal of anticonvulsant therapy. *N. Engl. J. Med.* **306**, 831–6.

Tinuper, P., Andermann, F., Villemure, J.-G., Rasmussen, T. B. & Quesney, L. F. (1988). Functional hemispherectomy for treatment of epilepsy associated with hemiplegia: rationale, indications, results, and comparison with callosotomy. *Ann. Neurol.* **24**, 27–34.

Todt, H. (1984). The late prognosis of epilepsy in childhood: results of a prospective follow-up study. *Epilepsia* **25**, 137–44.

Turner, W. A. (1907). *Epilepsy: a Study of the Idiopathic Disease*. London: Macmillan.

Van Buren, J. M., Ajmone Marsan, C. & Mutsuga, N. (1975). Temporal lobe seizures with additional foci treated by resection. *J. Neurosurg.* **43**, 596–607.

Van Donselaar, C. A., Schemischeimer, R. J., Geerts, A. T. & Derlerck, A. C. (1992). Value of electroencephalogram in adult patients with untreated idiopathic first seizures. *Arch. Neurol.* **49**, 231–7.

Van Ness, P. C. (1991). Surgical outcome for neocortical (extrahippocampal) focal epilepsy. In *Epilepsy Surgery*, ed. H. O. Luders, pp. 613–24. New York: Raven Press.

Van Wagenen, W. P. & Harren, R. Y. (1940). Surgical division of commissural pathways in the corpus callosum. *Acta Neurol. Psychiatr.* **44**, 740–59.

Volland, H. (1908). Statistische untersuchungen ueber geheilte epileptiker. *Z. Psychiatr.* **65**, 18–27.

Wieser, H. G. (1988). Selective amygdalo-hippocampectomy for temporal lobe epilepsy. *Epilepsia* **29** (Suppl. 2), S100–13.

Williamson, P. D. & Spencer, S. S. (1986). Clinical and EEG features of complex partial seizures of frontal lobe origin. *Epilepsia* **27** (Suppl 2), S46–63.

Wilson, D. H., Reeves, A. G., Gazzaniga, M. & Culver, C. (1977). Cerebral commissurotomy for control of intractable seizures. *Neurology* **27**, 708–15.

Wilson, D. H., Reeves, A. G. & Gazzaniga, M. (1978). Division of the corpus callosum for uncontrollable epilepsy. *Neurology* **28**, 649–53.

Wilson, D. H., Reeves, A. G. & Gazzaniga, M.S. (1982). Central commissurotomy for intractable generalized epilepsy: series two. *Neurology* **32**, 687–97.

Wirrell, E. C., Camfield, C. S., Camfield, P. R. *et al.* (1996). Long-term prognosis of typical childhood absence epilepsy: remission or progression to juvenile myoclonic epilepsy. *Neurology* **47**, 912–18.

Wyler, A. R., Hermann, B. P. & Somes, G. (1995). Extent of medial temporal resection on outcome from anterior temporal lobectomy: a randomized prospective study. *Neurosurgery* **37**, 982–91.

23 Post-traumatic syndrome, 'myalgic encephalomyelitis' and headaches

J. M. S. PEARCE

Post-traumatic syndrome

The clinical problem

In our opinion, the subjective posttraumatic syndrome, characterised by ..., is organic and is dependent on a disturbance in intracranial equilibrium due directly to the blow on the head, We suggest the term postconcussion syndrome for this symptom complex. *Strauss and Savitsky 1934*

or

The most consistent clinical feature is the subject's unshakable conviction of unfitness for work, a conviction quite unrelated to overt disability, even if his symptomatology is taken at face value. *Miller 1961*

Survivors of severe head injury commonly suffer neurological symptoms, cognitive (Pearce 1994), personality and behavioural changes which are easily related to focal or diffuse brain damage. Their symptoms improve in the first year, but if present at 1–2 years tend to persist indefinitely.

The more difficult problem is in determining the clinical features and outcome of minor head injuries. These patients have complaints and disabilities which are extraordinarily variable, often seeming disproportionate to the injury sustained. They are commonly attributed to the post-traumatic syndrome. Since it has no defining or consistent clinical signs nor biochemical, radiological or pathological accompaniments, it is not a diagnostic entity (Pearce 1994).

A term of convenience, it denotes a variable collection of symptoms that succeed head (and other) injuries. The well-known features are shown in Table 23.1. In most circumstances a knock on the head causes local bruising and abrasions no different from those resulting from a kick on the shin; local pain subsides within days, without sequelae. The emotional vulnerability of the head and the common recourse to medicolegal compensation complicate both symptoms and mechanisms. By contrast, many victims of severe head injury (for prognosis see Table 23.5), wake from coma without headache. Similarly, the headache of patients after uncomplicated craniotomy

441

Table 23.1. *Post-traumatic syndrome[a]*

I. Headaches	71%
II. Fatigue	55.5%
III. Dizziness (usually not vertigo),	50.3%
IV. Sleep disturbance	43.9%
V. Forgetfulness,	39.4%
VI. Depression	36.1%
VII. Anxiety	32.9%
VIII. Thinking	29.7%
IX. Poor concentration	29.7%
X. Intolerance of noise	22.6%

[a] Selected data from Three Centre Study (Levin 1989).

Table 23.2. *Crude outcome after head injury*

	Outcome		
Initial severity	Good or mild disability	Severe disability or vegetative	Dead
Mild 1324 patients	99%	1%	< 1%
Moderate 168 patients	86%	14%	< 1%
Severe 79 patients	22%	39%	39%

Data from 1571 patients aged < 65 years at time of head injury (Pentland *et al.* 1986)

seldom lasts more than 3 to 10 days. Those with minor injury, often without loss of consciousness provide the greatest number of complaints.

Diffuse axonal injury (DAI), implied by Symonds (1962), results from the shearing forces between different parts of the brain that stretch, distort or rupture parenchymal axons and may cause neuronal damage or death. It may be caused by angular acceleration of the head, and can arise without increased intracranial pressure or hypoxia. There is a spectrum of graded severity beginning with axonal swelling and retraction balls in parasagittal white matter. Every patient with DAI loses consciousness after injury, and up to one half have a lucid interval (Blumberg *et al.* 1989). Thus, without substantial impairment of consciousness, DAI is not an acceptable explanation for cognitive changes. Teasdale (1987) states: 'When there is a gap of some weeks between the injury and the onset of "postconcussional" symptoms, it is likely that psychological [*sic*] factors are prominent'. Severe and prolonged disability is not a problem unless early organic damage has been underrated (Pentland *et al.* 1986) (Table 23.2).

Definition

The crucial importance of strict definition (Pearce *et al.* 1987) is emphasized by the vague and often inconsistent subjective complaints of plaintiffs. We seek reliable hallmarks to allow the clinician to verify both the presence and severity of the condi-

Table 23.3. *Criteria of severity of head injury*[a]

	Mild	Moderate	Severe
GCS	13–15	9–12	3–8
PTA	0–1 hour	1–24 hours	> 24 hours

GCS, Glasgow Coma Scale; PTA, post-traumatic amnesia.
[a] Dikmen *et al.* (1986); Levin (1989); Evans (1992); Dikmen & Levin (1993).

tion. Many 'experts' are culpable of breaking the obvious rule: that a post-concussional syndrome is excluded if there is no concussion, i.e. brief loss of consciousness.

A major problem in studying outcome is the variability of criteria employed – exemplified by Table 23.6. Social factors, premorbid intelligence, work patterns (Stambrook *et al.* 1990), and motivation – which are often unspecified – also profoundly influence outcome. Consensus criteria defining severity are shown in Table 23.3.

Outcome: assessment of symptoms and disability

Methodological issues include classification of head injury severity, biases in selection of patients with mild head injury, and use of controls to account for morbidity owing to other injuries, preexisting disease, and emotional responses to, and circumstances surrounding the accident (Dikmen & Levin 1993). Whereas other sequelae of injury tend to improve from the time of trauma, symptoms of the post-traumatic syndrome tend to persist for years, or even worsen, so that many a clinician's good prognostication has proved false.

> To inquire ... whether the symptoms under consideration are functional or organic, psychogenic or physiogenic, is fruitless, for they must always be both ... It is questionable whether the effects of concussion, however slight, are ever completely reversible. (Symonds 1962)

Nonetheless, many patients who have sustained minor head injuries exhibit such symptoms but no neurological signs and have normal brain images. It is indeed remarkable that the plethora of symptoms is often greater than those reported after severe head injuries. Their genuine nature has been supported by claims of cognitive deficits present in the mildly injured with brief post-traumatic amnesia (PTA). However, there is clear evidence that the majority of such patients leave hospital within a few days, have no organic signs, recover quickly (Miller 1961), and return to work without further complaints. For example, Lowdon and Cockin (Lowdon *et al.* 1989) studied 114 adults with a minor head injury from the accident department. Follow-up showed that 90% of patients suffered symptoms lasting an average of 2 weeks. The patients who were discharged had symptoms that lasted a *shorter* time than those briefly detained. After injury during contact sports, many victims continue the game, or return to physical activities within days without ill effect.

Neuropsychological deficits

Some patients with minor injury complain of impaired memory, concentration, poor capacity for learning, lack of initiative and mental agility (Levin 1989). The literature abounds with claimed deficits of cognitive function that seek to explain such symptoms (Rimel *et al.* 1981). It is misleading to regard abnormality in tests of cognition as the equivalent of patients' complaints. Dikmen *et al.* (1986) have shown mild but 'probably clinically non-significant difficulties' at 1 month after minor head injury. They claimed that Rimel's results were flawed by faulty selection, e.g. previous head injuries in 31%, and by other (orthopaedic) injuries which contributed to psychosocial problems.

Tests of neuropsychological impairment

Investigators have shown impaired reaction times (Van Zomeven & Deelman 1987), faulty attention and speed of information processing (e.g. Paced Auditory Serial Addition Test/PASAT) and also inconsistency in performance (Stuss *et al.* 1989). Leininger *et al.* (1990) have shown defects of reasoning, information processing and verbal learning, independent of neurological status *immediately* after injury. Critics allege that some of these abnormalities are due, not to brain injury, but to concomitant analgesic and sedative drugs, or to depression. Serial tests show recovery in 1–3 months in most patients (Lowdon *et al.* 1989). Deliberate slowness and errors in performing tests are common in medicolegal practice, but hard to prove. Bias and expectation of the psychologist tester can confound the results.

Anxiety states, phobias, loss of self-esteem, resentment, and depression are genuine accompanying features in some cases, and serve to induce or to aggravate headache and other complaints. A diagnosis of post-traumatic neurosis or depression may be attributable to injury and should be based on the same constellation of clinical symptoms as in the non-injured subject.

'Post-traumatic stress disorder' represents a fashionable vogue for scales but it is no more than an arbitrary clinical convenience, without an established clinicopathological substrate. In a study of road traffic accidents (Mayou *et al.* 1993), psychiatric complications and 'post-traumatic stress disorder' were identified respectively in 18% and 7% at 3 months, and in 12% and 5% at 1 year; in two-thirds the 'intrusive thoughts' were present but 'not frightening'. Phobic travel anxiety was a problem in 21% at 3 months and in 18% at 1 year.

In 2493 participants examined in a general-population survey of psychiatric disorders (Helzer *et al.* 1987) the prevalence of post-traumatic stress disorder was high only in those wounded in warfare (Table 23.4). The authors conclude 'Although some symptoms of post-traumatic stress disorder occurred commonly in the general population, the full syndrome as defined by the DSM 111R, was common only among veterans wounded in Vietnam'. This argues against the validity of the widespread use of this label in those subjected to minor injuries.

Table 23.4. *Prevalence of post-traumatic stress disorder (PTSD)[a]*

	Total population 2493 subjects	Unwounded civilians exposed to attack & Vietnam veterans	Wounded Vietnam veterans
Prevalence of PTSD	1%	3.5%	20%

[a] Helzer *et al.* (1987).

Resentment figures prominently (Symonds 1962; Kelly 1975) in deciding protracted complaints: resentment against an inconsiderate employer, or against the other driver for unkind comments, or for drunken or runaway driving. 'That b ... d has ruined my life' is a familiar protest. Psychogenic symptoms are not always straightforward. The man so exhausted that he cannot return to a nine-to-five job as a bank clerk but who can jog for 5 or 10 miles 'in an attempt to get myself fit and build up my strength' is one extreme; the uncomplaining, haggard face painted with sadness and despair in a depressed woman, is the other.

A long history of *anxiety symptoms, phobias, depression* and of numerous minor somatic complaints is revealing. The average number of symptoms 1 year after injury was 7.3 for claimants as compared with 4.5 ($P < 0.1$) in a matched group with no claim. (McKinlay *et al.* 1983). Assessment of motivation has been described (Binder 1990). It is surprising how many plaintiffs ascribe every ailment, however remote, to their injuries.

Malingering or deliberate exaggeration in other cases is motivated by a quest for financial gain and attention which may confound analysis and invalidate outcome studies. Malingering may be more common than is palatable for physicians to credit, but as a diagnosis it is sustainable only when the patient is 'caught out'. Insurance companies now often produce such evidence on video films. Some subjects give the strong impression of a well-rehearsed and even tutored performance.

Binder (1990) comments:

> The possibility of malingering should be considered whenever an opportunity for financial gain exists or when the subjective complaints outweigh the objective findings.... Observations of untruthfulness, test abnormalities more severe than predicted by knowledge of the injury ... provided useful diagnostic data. Performance on a forced-choice technique that is significantly worse than chance is presumed to result from the deliberate production of wrong answers.

Prognosis

Stambrook *et al.* (1990) reported that survival from significant closed head injury is frequently associated with cognitive defects, physical impairment, personality change, interpersonal difficulty and, some degree of social dependence and a poor post-injury vocational status. However, these depend on demonstrable brain damage not evident in most minor injuries.

Early headaches, fatigue, dizziness, loss of recent memory, (Table 23.6) distractibility

Table 23.5. *The outcome of severe closed head injury in 746 patients rated 3–8 on the Glasgow Coma Scale (GCS)[a]*

Total 746 patients GCS 3–8	Mortality at 6 months = 36%
GCS 3	76%
GCS 6–8	18%
Surgical lesions	31%
Acute subdural haematoma	50%

[a] Marshall *et al.* (1991).

Table 23.6. *Percentage of patients with symptoms after mild head injury collated from different series[a]*

	1 week	1 month	3 months	1 year	4 years
Headache	36,71	31,56,90	47,78	8,18,35	24
Memory disturbance	—	19	8	4	19
Dizziness	19,53	12,22,35	22	5,14,26	18
Irritability	—	19,25	—	5	19
			20 at 6 months		
Psychological complaints[a]	—	—	51,84	15,33	15

—, No data; [a] personality change: irritability, anxiety and depression
[a] Data modified from Evans (1992)

Table 23.7. *Estimated return to work related to post-traumatic amnesia (PTA)*

Duration of PTA	Return to work
< 1 hour	1 month
< 1 day	2 months
< 1 week	4 months
> 1 week	± 1 year

Data from Lishman (1968)

and lack of initiative are organic symptoms of concussive minor injuries (*vide supra*) which disappear in 1 to 3 months in most young victims. Symptoms present after this time are of mixed aetiology but predominantly psychogenic. The period taken to return to work (Table 23.7) is closely related to age, personality and motivation. In mild head injury as defined, most patients can safely return to light work within a few days or weeks, and to full duties (depending on the nature of the job) within 2 months.

The speed and quality of recovery (Gordon *et al.* 1995) depend on many factors most of which are adverse: age over 45 (Vollmer *et al.* 1991); pre-injury personality, psychiatric history and resilience; motivation; type of job; insecure medical reassurance; alcoholism; previous head injury; multiple injuries or anoxia; coercion from union officials and legal advisers; resentment (Mayou *et al.* 1993) and delay in settlement. Complaints

Table 23.8. *Summary of studies on prognosis in severe head injury*

Author	Patients (n)	Features	Follow-up	GOS 4–5	Deaths
Miller 1961	100	PTA avg 13d	11 years	77/92 working	8
Heiden et al., 1983	213	GCS <8	1 year	35%	55%
Stambrook et al. 1990	131 males	Severe	?	55%	?
Costeff et al. 1990	31 children	Coma >7d	5–11 years	30%	1
Groswasser & Sabon 1990	72	Coma >30 d	?	50% independent+ 20% partly dependent	7% (in 1st year)
Marshall et al. 1991	746	GCS < 8	6 months	?	76% with GCS 3. 18% with GCS 6–8
Tennant et al. 1995	190 mixed HI	In Hosp. 33d	7 years	77%	7.4%
Fearnside et al. 1993	181	GCS < 8	2 years	88%	?
Gordon et al. 1995	1264	GCS < 9	21	55%	24%
Ashwal et al. 1994	847	Children PVS	Survival curves	0	<18 years = 3.2–5.2 years; >19 = 9.9 years
Dubroja et al. 1995	19	GCS > 8 PVS	5 years	30% mod disability	7 PVS

HI, head injury; GCS, Glasgow coma scale; GOS, Glasgow outcome scale; PVS, persistent vegetative state.

often improve when the patient returns to work, but do not invariably disappear (Van Zomeven & Deelman 1987) after settlement (Table 23.6). Sadly, more suggestible or easily manipulated plaintiffs in time come to believe the sick role they have chosen to adopt; they may remain tragically, but unnecessarily, crippled for life. A summary of outcome data shown in Table 23.8.

'Myalgic encephalomyelitis' (ME) and the chronic fatigue syndrome (CFS)

This is another fashionable 'new disease'. It has so far made little impact in the courts, but figures prominently and commonly in all realms of clinical practice (Wesseley 1991; Landay et al. 1991) in the UK and elsewhere.

Definition (Levine et al. 1992)

(1) Severe persistent fatigue following an acute illness appearing in an individual with no previous physical or psychological symptoms; (2) presenting signs and symptoms of an acute infection; (3) severe and persistent headache and/or myalgias; and (4) abrupt change in cognitive function or the appearance of a new mood disorder.

Chronic fatigue syndrome (CFS) is a disabling illness of uncertain but probably protean aetiology. It is characterized by a chronic, sustained or fluctuating sense of debilitating fatigue without any other known underlying medical conditions. It is associated with both somatic and neuropsychological symptoms. Most patients with the chronic fatigue syndrome have sleep disorders, which are likely to contribute to daytime fatigue. Both physical and laboratory findings are usually unremarkable. Athletes, both amateur and professional seem unusually prone. Perhaps because of their self-image of invulnerability and physical perfection, when dented by physical or psychological impediments they are subject to a catastrophic breakdown of the whole organism. It is mainly a disorder of the young, age 15 to 40, both sexes are affected.

Search for aetiological markers

CFS patients have mild memory impairment, but only on tasks requiring conceptually driven encoding and retrieval processes. There are no associations between the nature of the precipitating illness, self-ratings of fatigue, physical findings, or laboratory findings, objective memory performance or, self-report of memory functioning (Grafman et al. 1993).

Skeletal muscle bioenergetics and control of intracellular pH have been investigated in 46 patients (Barnes et al. 1993) with CFS by phosphorus magnetic resonance spectroscopy. The results have been compared with those from healthy controls and with mitochondrial cytopathies affecting skeletal muscle. No consistent abnormalities of glycolysis, mitochondrial metabolism or pH regulation were identified in the group when taken as a whole. These findings do not support the hypothesis that any specific metabolic abnormality underlies fatigue in this syndrome although abnormalities may be present in a minority of patients.

Only minor morphological changes were detected in 9 of 20 patients of one series. The non-specific morphological changes in muscle tissue and the lack of class 1 MHC expression do not support the viral aetiology of muscle fatigue in CFS (Grau et al. 1992)

Diagnostic criteria

Diagnostic criteria in current use do not allow isolation of a homogeneous subgroup. An infectious or immunological cause has not been shown conclusively (Cathebras et al. 1993), although a persistent enterovirus or herpesvirus type 6 infection or chronic immune activation (Landay et al. 1991) possibly play a role in some cases. Patients present with psychiatric morbidity, essentially depressive, and in 50% of the cases the mental disorders precede CFS (Grafman et al. 1993). Grau et al. (1992) regard the syndrome as 'a social construction reproducing or renovating the neurasthenia of the late 19th century'.

Regional cerebral blood flow (rCBF) was assessed in 60 clinically defined CFS patients and 14 normal control (NC) subjects, using ^{99m}Tc- hexamethyl propyleneamine oxime single photon emission computed tomography (SPECT). Compared with the NC group, the CFS group showed significantly lower cortical/cerebellar rCBF ratios, throughout multiple brain regions. The findings were, however, not diagnostic (Ichise *et al.* 1992) and may be epiphenomena. PET studies have shown variable changes in cerebral metabolism that do not equate with symptoms and are currently regarded as non-diagnostic.

But many patients exhibit no acute or subacute viral illness recognizable at the onset. The label, ME, endangers alleged victims, since its acceptance as a disease entity can mislead physicians who may overlook more treatable organic diseases such as hyper thyroidism, mycobacterial, and a variety of neoplastic and inflammatory diseases. Patients often suggest the diagnosis to doctors. In this context, Woods and Goldberg (1991) discuss attribution, stigma, collusion between doctor and patient and abnormal illness behaviour. They indict 'special vulnerability factors in these patients' personalities' before the viral [sic] illness.

Identical symptoms have been well known and previously attributed to chronic psychoneurosis, stress syndromes, hypochondriacal states, allergies, and post-viral depression. This trendy new diagnosis and the establishment of a vogue can induce iatrogenic 'illness behaviour'. Diagnostic bewilderment and therapeutic impotence can be inferred from the plethora of terms used (Editorial 1996). The invention of yet another diagnostic label, as if it were a disease, does not serve us well.

Treatment and outcome

Antidepressant drugs are the most successful therapy even in those without obvious depression, but are not universally effective. In contrast with the reported clinical improvement with high doses of essential fatty acids, the clinical condition was not improved after 3 months of L-carnitine therapy (Barnes *et al.* 1993).

There is little doubt that the severity of disability can be marked, with frequent periods of absence from work, profound apparent restriction of physical effort in work and in leisure activities. Many patients lose their jobs because of their poor work records. Such problems are, however, variable and often intermittent. We can best measure disability by absence from work and by assessing limitations of physical activities. More sophisticated scales do not exist, and both measurable and objective abnormalities are almost invariably absent. Good data for prognosis are scanty. Many studies have shown a good prognosis but recovery can be delayed for months or years. After 3 years of follow-up, almost all subjects in one report (Levine *et al.* 1992) could return to pre-illness activity. Personal resilience and motivation are paramount.

Headache

Representative of many studies, one thousand 25–64-year-old men and women, who lived in the western part of Copenhagen County were randomly drawn from the

National Registry (Rasmussen *et al.* 1991). The lifetime prevalences of headache (including anybody with any form of headache), migraine, and tension-type headache were 93%, 8% and 69%, respectively in men and 99%, 25% and 88%, respectively in women. The point prevalence of headache was 11% in men and 22% in women. Prevalence of migraine in the previous year was 6% in men and 15% in women and the corresponding prevalences of tension-type headache were 63% and 86%. Differences according to sex were significant with a male: female ratio of 1:3 in migraine, and 4:5 in tension-type headache. The prevalence of tension-type headache decreased with increasing age, whereas migraine showed no correlation with age within the studied age interval.

Tension headache

Diagnostic issues

Definition is shown in the Appendix. Difficulties in providing reliable criteria for tension headache as opposed to common migraine bedevil epidemiological studies, assessment of outcome, and, therapeutic trials. The common coexistence of tension headache – as clinically defined – with migraine compounds the problems. Studies from Asia, South America and Africa have shown a smaller prevalence for all types of headache as compared with North America and Western Europe. Since different diagnostic criteria, different cultural stoicism, use of words and diagnostic criteria confound definition, such studies are not easily interpreted.

Acute episodic tension headache is the most common of human complaints, constituting 70% of referrals to a 'Headache Clinic'. It is often a short-lived complaint with an obvious preceding cause: overwork, lack of sleep or an emotional crisis. This is benign, and is often referred to, by patients, as 'my normal headaches'. Tension headaches outnumber migraine by 5:1. In most series 75% of sufferers are women.

Current systems classify the most common recurring headaches as either migraine or tension-type. Some suggest that these two headache patterns are but different expressions of the same pathophysiological process, having overlapping symptomatic presentations with certain features emphasized to a greater or lesser extent. The same therapies have been shown to be effective for patients in either headache group (Marcus 1992). An alternative continuum classification model has been suggested since there is an undoubted overlap between common migraine and tension headache, though their common coexistence has added to the confusion.

By contrast, Solomon and Lipton (1991) propose criteria derived from a study comparing the features of 100 patients with migraine without aura and 100 patients with chronic daily ('tension') headache. The author's criteria for the diagnosis of migraine without aura were highly sensitive and adequately discriminated the two groups.

There are also differences in laboratory data. Electromyographic (EMG) studies have shown muscle contraction in both headache types (Phillips 1978; Pikoff 1984) and the expected increase of EMG activity with increased headache severity and reduction with biofeedback techniques (Schoenen *et al.* 1991) have not been found. Thus, muscle contraction is not specific to tension headache and as a marker or diagnostic criterion is valueless. Platelet [³II]imipramine binding was measured and a significant reduction was found in migraine compared with controls but not in tension headache (Jarman *et al.* 1991). A significant reduction in peripheral blood mononuclear cell beta-endorphin concentrations was observed in migraine patients with and without aura, but not in tension-type headache patients (Leone *et al.* 1992). Adult and childhood migraineurs without aura have an increased amplitude of the Contingent Negative Variation (CNV) between attacks (Besken *et al.* 1993). Similarly, vascular phenomena, well described in migraine, contrast with transcranial Doppler ultrasound (TCD) of blood flow velocities in chronic tension headache which show no significant differences from controls.

We must conclude that there are no consistent or objective criteria that separate common migraine from tension headache. However, clinical evidence shows that the two syndromes are often distinct, though they overlap and commonly coexist.

Acute tension headache is experienced transiently, at some time, by over 80% of people. More rarely it presents as an emergency and may simulate subarachnoid bleeding. The emotional basis is usually obvious and recovery ensues quickly.

Chronic tension headache (chronic daily headache) is more common than the acute syndrome. Pain is diffusely felt all over the head, often located on the vertex, or may start in the forehead or in the neck. Primary tension headache is psychogenic; its mechanisms are not wholly understood (Pearce 1984). Most patients continue to work.

Treatment and outcome

There is almost no information about prognosis in standard headache monographs and papers. In patients presenting with a short history, social and psychological factors (family deaths, a friend with a brain tumour, etc.) may be identified, and sometimes reversed; these patients have an excellent prognosis. Others have symptoms for years without evident deterioration of general health. Symptoms are worse when the patient is tired or under pressure of work, or domestic stresses (Ende & Holm 1992). Most sufferers have insight; many are emotional and anxious with fears of brain tumours, hypertension or 'clots in the brain'. Analgesic abuse may aggravate the situation; with persuasion, it can be reversed with dramatic benefit. Short-lived improvement may succeed a new doctor, a new therapeutic approach or a change in life style.

The late development of chronic daily headache in a patient with previous episodic migraine is common and is misleadingly called 'transformed migraine' (Saper 1986). It is accompanied by tension, depression, insomnia and analgesic abuse, each of which should be identified and treated, as soon as possible.

To cure such headaches after many years is a daunting and often unsuccessful task (Kunkel 1989). Sensitive patients with fragile personalities may be unable to cope with life's stresses and unconsciously use headaches to escape responsibilities with which they cannot cope. Sedatives, tranquillizers and tension-relieving drugs are of limited value unless the psychological issues are adequately handled. Glib reassurance will not eradicate headache if fundamental psychological problems are unresolved. When the history is short and if a cause is exposed, explanation and reassurance may suffice. Latent depression presenting as tension headache is easily overlooked. Full doses of tricyclic antidepressants (Pearce 1987) or fluoxetine are needed. The prognosis for depression is often good. However, when daily pain has persisted for years, the prognosis for headache is poor; but supportive psychotherapy, short courses of benzodiazepines or amitriptyline may be helpful. Treatment offers partial but worthwhile relief that enables most patients to continue their work.

Migraine

Migraine with and without aura correspond to classical and common migraine; the International Headache Society (IHS) definitions are not wholly satisfactory, but are given in the Appendix.

Incidence A study from Olmsted County, Minnesota (Strang *et al.* 1992) confirms the overall incidence of about 10% in the population. These workers determined the incidence of migraine in a defined population. From 6400 patient records 629 residents fulfilled the International Headache Society's (1988) criteria for migraine between 1979 and 1981. The overall age-adjusted incidence was 137 and 294 per 100 000 person years for males and females, respectively. The highest incidence was in females aged 20 to 24 years (689 per 100 000 person years), whereas in boys, aged 10 to 14 years the incidence was 246 per 100 000 person years.

Prevalence Based on a study (Rasmussen 1992) of 1000 persons using the IHS criteria, the overall lifetime prevalence of classic migraine was 5% with a male to female ratio of 1 : 2. The overall lifetime prevalence of common migraine was 8%, with a male to female ratio of 1 : 7. Women were more likely to have common than classic migraine. Neither classic nor common varieties correlated with age, but in both types the most conspicuous precipitating factors were stress and mental tension.

Consultations The rate of consultation is of concern for those planning medical resources. Among subjects with classic and common migraine, 50% and 62%, respectively, consult their general practitioner because of migraine at some time in their lives. Patients frequently attend for medical help, and lose much time from work that is often unrecorded. In a random sample (Rasmussen *et al.* 1992) of 740 subjects, aged 25 to 64 years living in Copenhagen County, 119 had migraine and 578 had tension headache (1 : 5). Among subjects with migraine 56% had consulted their general practitioner in the previous year for migraine; of subjects with tension headache 16% had had consultations. Specialists had been consulted by 16% of migraine sufferers and by 4% of subjects with tension-type headache. Less than 3% of all patients studied had required hospital admissions and laboratory investigations for headache. Half the migraine sufferers and 83% of subjects with tension-type headache in the previous year had taken drug therapy. Thus migraine and tension headaches are potent sources of demand for medical attention and for the consumption of drugs.

Table 23.9. *Migraine: outcome*

Author; No. patients	Age (years)	Follow-up (years)	Headaches ceased	Headaches improved	Headaches unchanged or worse
(Bille 1984) 67	13–21	6	51%	34%	15%
(Hinriches & Keith 1965) 58	mean 21	9–14	33%	47%	20%
(Hockaday 1978) 102	< 20	8–25	26%	48%	17%
(Whitty & Hockaday 1968) 92	25–64	15–20	29%	48%	23%

Work loss In the preceding year, in the Danish study, 43% of employed migraine sufferers and 12% of employed subjects with tension-type headache had lost working time. The total loss of workdays per year due to migraine was estimated at 270 days per 1000 persons per year; for tension headache the corresponding figure was 820/1000. Women consult a doctor more often than men, but there is no sex difference in absenteeism.

Outcome

Migraine starts in childhood before the age of 10 in about one-third, and before the age of 30 in over 80% of sufferers. Exacerbations both of severity of attacks and frequency accompany stress, insecurity, conflict, menstruation, and oestrogenic contraceptives. Hypertension and the menopause may provoke transient worsening, whereas pregnancy sees a remission, usually in the second and third trimesters in 75% women. Headaches are commonly increased by the advent of tension headache.

Outcome studies are sparse. In children (Table 23.9) between 20 and 40% have a substantial or lasting remission. However when Bille (1984) followed up his children's series he found that 60% were having some attacks at the age of 30, showing that late adult recurrence is common. In adults data are even fewer.

Whitty and Hockaday's study (1968) is shown in the Table 23.9, but though outdated, is the only published examination of this kind. They found the menopause in 40 patients left four with cessation or improvement, 18 with no change, and six were worse. Attacks changed in content in 22 of 62 patients: five lost the aura, four had aurae but lost their headaches, two noted the emergence of cluster headache, and two lost cluster headache but continued classical migraine. Both loss of vomiting and loss of aura appeared to be associated with advancing age. 'No consistent change was noted with the development either of raised blood pressure or cervical spondylosis.' Further long-term studies are needed, but there is little to suggest that any drug therapy alters the natural history of either classical or common migraine, though suppression and control of symptoms are attainable in the majority.

Cluster headache

It is traditional to classify cluster headache (synonym: periodic migrainous neuralgia, Harris's syndrome, Horton's syndrome) into episodic and chronic types. The classifical temporal features of the *episodic type* are: pain of agonizing severity with attacks lasting for 30 to 120 minutes, occurring usually once or twice every day for about 4 weeks to 4 months (Pearce 1992). Total remission is then the rule, until the next cluster ensues months or a year or two later (Pearce 1994).

In *chronic cluster headache*, constituting about 10% of all cases, the clinical features of each attack (Pearce 1994) are identical to those of episodic cluster headache. The difference is that the remissions that characterize the episodic form fail to occur. The term chronic cluster is thus a misnomer (Pearce 1987, 1992). Those patients with no remission, but suffering daily attacks from the outset, are labelled 'Primary Chronic'; those who start with episodic clusters but in a later attack have chronic persisting symptoms are labelled 'Secondary Chronic'. Chronic paroxysmal hemicrania, described by Sjaastad and Dale (1976; Pearce & Pearce 1986) is a rare variant with distinctive features.

Studies of the natural history and outcome of cluster headache are sparse. A common difficulty is retrieving patients some of who have an episodic disorder, or who, in implacable cases, have despaired of therapeutic help and are therefore reluctant to receive further medical attention. But do episodic and chronic cluster headaches behave similarly?

Episodic cluster headache

Kudrow (1982) reported patients who were initially lost to follow-up for a period of 3 to 8 years. Of the 149 'drop-out patients', 75 (50.3%) reported no change in headache. Eleven (7.4%) had experienced a shift in headache type, that is, from chronic to episodic or from episodic to chronic, equally. Fifty-one (34.2%) had experienced a prolonged remission, and 12 (8.1%) had died. The major determinants of 'drop-out' status included remissions longer than usual remission duration, and death (42.3%). Remission and mortality rates increased with duration of cluster disorder. Patients in Kudrow's paper however are specifically selected from 'drop-out patients', and one would anticipate such default if the subject was in remission, or obviously, if dead.

Another study (Sacquegna *et al.* 1987) in 72 patients with episodic clusters disclosed 62 cases (86%) with a 'regular frequency' of clusters per year. Most patients suffered from one or two bouts per year. A prolonged remission (> 1 year) did not change the frequency pattern of clusters per year. Fifty patients (69%) had a fixed pattern both of frequency and duration of bouts. Thirty-seven patients (51%) had a regular frequency of bouts per year, a fixed duration of bouts and a fixed frequency of attacks a day. The authors conclude that the natural history of most cluster headache patients is characterized by a regular pattern.

Krabbe reported (1991) follow-up of 226 patients and 13 dead traced from 290 cases; symptoms varied from 2 to 58 years. Twenty-seven had terminated their headaches for

Table 23.10. *Outcome in episodic cluster headache*

Author	No. patients	Follow-up (years)	Remission
Krabbe (1991)	239	2–58	27 (11%) 1–9 years
Pearce (1993)	123	10–25	12 (11%) > 4 years
Kudrow (1982)	149	?	51 (34%) 'drop-outs'
Saquegna *et al.* (1987)	72	?	< 14% remit; 86% continue

Table 23.11. *Episodic cluster headache: outcome (personal series)*

	At onset	Follow-up[a]
No. patients	123	101
Male:Female	117:6	96:5
Age (mean)	36.7	54.2
Clusters/years	1.4	0.9
Duration cluster (weeks)	10.8	10.2
Clusters/day	1.3	1.4
Duration attack (minutes)	72	68
Changed to chronic	—	4 (3.96%)
Remission > 4 years	—	12 (11.88%)
Pattern unchanged	—	85 (84.2%)

[a] Over 10–25 years, mean 13.9 years.

1 to 9 years, but for most patients cluster headache is a life-long disease (Table 23.10).

In a personal series (Pearce 1993) the data on patients seen with episodic cluster headache are summarized in Table 23.11. The number of clusters per year decreased slightly over the period, but the duration of each cluster remain at about 10 weeks. Within each 24 hours, the number of clusters was unchanged, and the duration of pain stayed constant at 70 minutes. In four patients, the episodic changed to a chronic cluster pattern.

Only a small but significant number (11.88%) experienced a prolonged and spontaneous remission (arbitrarily taken as at least 4 years). This occurred mainly in patients who have previously experienced their usual remissions of 1 year or longer. For the majority (84.2%) the pattern of episodic cluster headache continued, with very similar symptoms and similar numbers and duration of headaches within each cluster. In three patients the headache switched to the other side in some clusters; these 'contralateral' attacks were milder in severity in each case, and often reverted to the original side in subsequent clusters.

Chronic cluster headache

Boiardi and colleagues (1983) in a follow-up study (3.2 years), of 56 patients with chronic cluster headache who had had no remissions for at least a year, reported treatment with lithium carbonate, methysergide and prednisone singly and in combination. The course of chronic cluster headache was variable: some improved with lithium, but many persisted despite treatment.

Table 23.12. *Chronic Cluster Headache: outcome*

Author	No. patients	Mean follow-up (years)	Outcome
Boiardi *et al.* (1983)	56	3.2	'Variable'
Watson & Evans (1987)	46	4	33% free, 26% satisfied, but 52% had surgery
Pearce (1993)	9	13.9	57% continue,
		10–25	28% – > episodic,
			15% – > remit

Watson and Evans (1987) in a review of chronic cluster headache described data on extended follow-up of 46 patients (median 4 years). Treatment was generally difficult and often 'trial and error' in nature. Lithium carbonate, methysergide, corticosteroids and indomethacin were of limited usefulness as prophylactic agents. Long-term follow-up revealed that 33% of patients were free of headache and 26% were categorized as satisfactory by patients and examiner. But 14 (52%) of these had undergone a surgical procedure, and we learn little of the true natural history. In my own series the number of chronic cluster headache patients is small, constituting 9 of 132 of the whole series (Table 23.12). This differs from the findings of Kudrow and others, and may reflect more stringent criteria for diagnosis. Of nine such patients, seven were available for review and four of these had maintained their continual pattern of cluster headaches without remission. Two patients ceased to have a chronic pattern and developed episodic clusters with the usual remissions lasting 3 to 22 months. Two patients had unexplained total remissions of 3 and 12 months, respectively, without episodic cluster, and then reverted to the chronic pattern. However for four of the seven patients followed, the chronic pattern was unchanged.

Treatment

Rational therapy should consider the limited knowledge of pathogenesis. Based on orbital phlebography and signs of inflammation in episodic and chronic cluster headache it has been suggested that episodic cluster headache is due to 'temporary sympathicoplegia' caused by venous vasculitis in the cavernous sinus; and, chronic cluster headache may be a permanent post-inflammatory sympathicoplegia in the middle fossa (Hannevz 1991). Sumatriptan and oxygen inhalation are useful in 70%–80% of attacks providing relief within 10–20 minutes. Ergotamine suppositories, inhaler or injection will abort a similar proportion of attacks if taken 30–60 minutes *before the anticipated attack*. Methysergide is valuable on a regular prophylactic basis 3–6 mg/d, but courses should not exceed 4 months. Verapamil 80–160 mg tds is a useful, safer, but probably less efficacious alternative. Indomethacin is relatively specific for chronic paroxysmal hemicrania. And, lithium is effective in 60–70% of patients with chronic cluster headache, but requires plasma level monitoring.

The various drug therapies (for details see Rasmussen *et al.* 1991) used whilst the patients were in a headache cluster, resulted in good symptomatic control in 81 (80%) patients of episodic cluster, and in four patients (57%) with chronic cluster headaches

(Leone *et al.* 1992). However, attempts by patients to stop treatment in an active phase were invariably followed by a brisk return of symptoms within 24 to 72 hours.

Appendix. Definitions of the International Headache Society (IHS) (Olesen 1988)

Tension headache

2.1. Episodic: recurrent attacks of a tight, pressing sensation in the head, usually bilateral. The episodes are usually precipitated by physical or mental stress and a subvariety is associated with excessive muscle contraction and muscle tenderness.

2.2. Chronic: Chronic tension-type headache recurs 15 or more days in a month, commonly every day. It has the same heavy or tight quality as the episodic variety and may or may not be associated with overactivity of the jaw and facial muscles.

Migraine without aura

A. At least 5 attacks fulfilling B–D
B. Headaches attacks lasting 4–72 hours
C. Headache has at least two of the following characteristics
    1. Unilateral location
    2. Pulsating quality
    3. Moderate or severe (inhibits daily activities)
    4. Aggravation by walking stairs or similar physical activity
D. During headache at least one of
    1. Nausea and/or vomiting
    2. Photophobia or phonophobia
E. At least one of 3 clauses: excluding any or related major head trauma or intracranial pathology

Migraine with aura

A. At least 2 attacks fulfilling B
B. At least 3 of the following
    1. One or more fully reversible aura symptoms indicating focal cerebral cortical and/or brain stem dysfunction
    2. At least one aura symptom develops gradually over more than 4 minutes or, 2 or more symptoms occur in succession
    3. No aura symptoms last more than 60 minutes. If more than one aura symptom, accepted duration is proportionately increased
    4. Headache follows the aura with a free interval of less than 60 minutes. It may be simultaneous with aura
C. At least one of 3 clauses in B: excluding any or related major head trauma or intracranial pathology

References

Ashwal, S., Eyman, R. K. & Call, T. L. (1994). Life expectancy of children in a persistent vegetative state. *Pediatr. Neurol.* **10**, 27–33.

Barnes, P. R. J., Taylor, D. J., Kemp, G. J. & Radda, G. K. (1993). Skeletal muscle bioenergetics in the chronic fatigue syndrome. *J. Neurol. Neurosurg. Psychiatry* **56**, 679–83.

Besken, E., Pothmann, R. & Sartory, G. (1993). Contingent negative variation in childhood migraine. *Cephalalgia* **13**, 42–3.

Bille, B. (1984). Migraine in childhood and its prognosis. *Cephalalgia* 1, 71–5.

Binder, L. M. (1990). Malingering following minor head trauma. *Clin. Neuropsychol.* 4, 25–36.

Blumberg, P. C., Jones, N. R. & North, J. B. (1989). Diffuse axonal injury in head trauma. *J. Neurol. Neurosurg. Psychiatry* 52, 838–41.

Boiardi, A., Bussone, G., Merati, B. *et al.* (1983). Course of chronic cluster Headache. *Ital. J. Neurol. Sci.* 4, 75–8.

Cathebras, P., Bouchou, K., Charmion, S. *et al.* (1993). Syndrome de fatigue chronique: une revue critique. *Rev. Med. Interne* 14, 233–42.

Costeff, H., Groswasser, Z. & Goldstein, R. (1990). Long-term follow-up review of 31 children with severe closed head trauma. *J. Neurosurg.* 73, 684–7.

Dikmen, S. S. & Levin, H. S. (1993). Methodological issues in the study of mild head injury *J. Head Trauma. Rehabil.* 8, 30–7.

Dikmen, S., McLean, A. & Temkin, N. (1986). Neuropsychological and psychosocial consequences of minor head injury. *J. Neurol. Neurosurg. Psychiatry* 49, 1227–32.

Dubroja, I., Valent, S., Miklie, P. & Kesak, D. (1995). Outcome of posttraumatic unawareness persisting for more than a month. *J. Neurol. Neurosurg. Psychiatry* 58, 465–6.

Editorial (1996). Frustrating survey of chronic fatigue. *Lancet* 348 (October 12).

Ehde, D. M. & Holm, J. E. (1992). Stress and headache: comparisons of migraine, tension, and headache-free subjects. *Headache Q.* 3, 54–60.

Evans, R. W. (1992). *Neurologic Clinics 1992*; November 10, 815–49. Philadelphia: Saunders.

Fearnside, M. R., Cook, R. J., McDougall, P. & Lewis, W. A. (1993). The Westmead Head Injury Project. Physical and social outcomes following serious head injury. *Br. J. Neurosurg.* 7, 643–50.

Gordon, E., van Holse, H. & Rudehill, A. (1995). Outcome of head injury in 2298 patients treated in a single clinic during a 21 year period. *J. Neurosurg. Anesthesiol.* 4, 235–47.

Grafman, J., Schwartz, V., Dale, J. K. *et al.* (1993). Analysis of neuropsychological functioning in patients with chronic fatigue syndrome. *J. Neurol. Neurosurg. Psychiatry* 56, 684–9.

Grau, J. M., Casademont, J., Pedrol, E. *et al.* (1992). Chronic fatigue syndrome: studies on skeletal muscle *Clin. Neuropathol.* 11, 329–32.

Groswasser, Z. & Sazbon, L. (1990). Outcome in 134 patients with prolonged posttraumatic unawareness. Part 2: Functional outcome of 72 patients recovering consciousness *J. Neurosurg.* 72, 81–4.

Hannerz, J. (1991). Orbital phlebography and signs of inflammation in episodic and chronic cluster headache. *Headache* 31, 540–2.

Heiden, J. S., Small, R., Caton, W., *et al.* (1983). Severe head injury. Clinical assessment and outcome. *Phys. Ther.* 63, 1946–51.

Helzer, J. E., Robins, L. N. & McEvoy, L. (1987). Post-traumatic stress disorder in the general population: findings of the epidemiologic catchment area survey. *N. Engl. J. Med.* 317, 1630–4.

Hinrichs, W. L. & Keith, H. M. (1965). Migraine in childhood: follow-up report. *Mayo Clin. Proc.* 40, 593–6.

Hockaday, J. M. (1978). Late outcome of childhood onset migraine and factors affecting outcome. In *Current Concepts in Migraine Research*, ed. R. Greene, pp. 41–8. New York: Raven Press.

Ichise, M., Salit, I. E., Abbey, S. E. *et al.* (1992). Assessment of regional cerebral perfusion by (99)Tc(m)-HMPAO SPECT in chronic fatigue syndrome. *Nucl. Med. Comm.* 13, 767–72.

International Headache Society (1988). Classification. Diagnostic criteria. *Cephalalgia* 8 (Suppl. 7), 19–45.

Jarman, J., Davies, P. T. G., Fernandez, M., Glover, V., Steiner, T. J., Rose, F. C. & Sandler, M.

(1991). Platelet Himipramine binding in migraine and tension headache in relation to depression. *J. Psychiatr. Res.* **25**, 205–11.

Kelly, R. (1975). The post-traumatic syndrome: an iatrogenic disease. *Forensic Sci.* **6**, 17–24.

Krabbe, A. (1991). The prognosis of cluster headache. A long-term observation of 226 cluster headache patients. *Cephalalgia* **11** (Suppl. 11), 250–1.

Kudrow, L. (1982). Naural history of cluster Headache, part 1, outcome of drop-out patients. *Headache* **22**, 203–6.

Kunkel, R. S. (1989). Muscle contraction (tension) headache. *Clin. J. Pain* **5**, 39–44.

Landay, A. L., Jessop, C., Lennette, E. T. & Levy, J. A. (1991). Chronic fatigue syndrome: clinical condition associated with immune activation. *Lancet* **338**, 707–12.

Leininger, B. E., Gramling, S. E., Farrell, E. D. *et al.* (1990). Neuropsychological deficits in patients with minor head injury after concussion and mild concussion. *J. Neurol. Neurosurg. Psychiatry* **53**, 293–6.

Leone, M., Sacerdote, P., D'Amico, D., Paneraei, A. E. & Bussone, G. (1992). Beta-endorphin concentrations in the peripheral blood mononuclear cells of migraine and tension-type headache patients. *Cephalalgia* **12**, 155–7.

Levin, H. S. (1989). Neurobehavioural outcome of mild to moderate head injury. In: *Mild to Moderate Head Injury*, eds. J. Hoff, T. Anderson, T. Cole, pp. 153–87. Boston: Blackwell.

Levine, P. H., Jacobson, S., Pocinki, A. G. *et al.* (1992). Clinical, epidemiologic, and virologic studies in four clusters of the chronic fatigue syndrome. *Arch. Intern. Med.* **152**, 1611–16.

Lishman, W. A. (1968). Brain damage in relation to psychiatric disability after head injury. *Br. J. Psychiatry* **114**, 373–410.

Lowdon, I. M. R., Briggs, M. & Cockin, J. (1989). Post-concussional symptoms following minor head injury. *Injury* **20**, 193–4.

Marcus, D. A. (1992). Migraine and tension-type headaches: the questionable validity of current classification systems. *Clin. J. Pain* **8**, 28–36.

Marshall, L. F., Gautille, T., Klauber, M. R. *et al.* (1991). The outcome of severe closed head injury. *J. Neurosurg.* **75**(Suppl.), S28–36.

Mayou, R., Bryant, B. & Duthie, R. (1993). Psychiatric consequences of road traffic accidents. *Br. Med. J.* **307**, 647–51.

McKinlay, W. W., Brooks, D. M. & Bond, M. R. (1983). Post-concussional symptoms, financial compensation and outcome after severe blunt head injury. *J. Neurol. Neurosurg. Psychiatry* **46**, 1084–91.

Miller, H. (1961). Accident neurosis. *BMJ* I, 919–25, 992–8.

Olesen, J. (1988). Classification and diagnostic criteria for headache disorders, cranial neuralgias and facial pain. *Cephalalgia* **8** (Suppl. 7), 9–96.

Pearce, J. M. S. (1984). Tension headaches: clinical features and mechanisms. In *The Neurobiology of Pain*, eds. A. V. Holden and W. Winlow, pp. 235–43. Manchester: Manchester University Press.

Pearce, J. M. S. (1992). Cluster headache and its variants. Festchrift for Lord Walton. *Postgrad. Med. J.* **68**, 517–21.

Pearce, J. M. S. (1993). Natural history of cluster headache. *Headache* **33**, 253–7.

Pearce, J. M. S. (1987). Headache. In *Oxford Textbook of Medicine*, 2nd edn, vol. 2, sect. 21, pp. 28–33. D. J. Weatherall, J. G. G. Ledingham & D. A. Warrell. Oxford: Oxford University Press.

Pearce, J. M. S. (1994). Headache. In: *Oxford Textbook of Medicine*, 3rd edn, eds. D. J. Weatherall, J. G. G. Ledingham & D. A. Warrell. Oxford: Oxford University Press.

Pearce, J. M. S. (1994). The post-traumatic syndrome and whiplash injury. In *Recent Advances in*

Clinical Neurology, vol. 8, ed. C. Jennard. Edinburgh: Churchill Livingstone.

Pearce, J. M. S. & Pearce, S. H. S. (1986). Benign paroxysmal cranial neuralgia' or 'cephalgia fugax'. *BMJ* **292**, 1015–16.

Pentland, B., Jones, P. A. & Miller, J. D. (1986). Head injury in the elderly. Age Aging **15**, 193–202.

Phillips, C. (1978). Tension headache: theoretical problems. *Behavi. Res. Ther.* **16**, 249–61.

Pikoff, H. (1984). Is the muscular model of headache still viable? *Headache* **24**, 186–98.

Rasmussen, B. K. (1992). Migraine with aura and migraine without aura: An epidemiological study. *Cephalalgia* **12**, 221–8.

Rasmussen, B. K., Jensen, R., Schroll, M. *et al.* (1991). Epidemiology of headache in a general population: a prevalence study. *J. Clin. Epidemiol.* **44**, 1147–57.

Rasmussen, B. K., Jensen, R. & Olesen, J. (1992). Impact of headache on sickness absence and utilisation of medical services: a Danish population study. *J. Epidemiol. Commun. Health* **46**, 443–6.

Rimel, R., Giordani, M., Barth, J. *et al.* (1981). Disability caused by minor head injury. *Neurosurgery* **9**, 221–8.

Sacquegna, T., De Carolis, P., Agati, R. *et al.* (1987). The natural history of episodic cluster Headache. *Headache* **27**, 370–1.

Saper, J. R. (1986). Changing perspectives on chronic headache. *Clin. Pain* **2**, 19–28.

Schoenen, J., Gerard, P., De Pasqua, V. & Juprelle, M. (1991). EMG in pericranial muscles during postural variation and mental activity in volunteers and patients with chronic tension headache. *Headache* **31**, 321–4.

Sjaastad, O. & Dale, J. (1976). A new (?) headache entity 'Chronic paroxysmal hemicrania'. *Acta Neurol. Scand.* **54**, 140–59.

Solomon, S. & Lipton, R. B. (1991). Criteria for the diagnosis of migraine in clinical practice. *Headache* **31**, 384–7.

Stambrook, M., Moore, A. D., Peters, L. C. *et al.* (1990). Effects of mild, moderate and severe closed head injury on long-term vocational status. *Brain Inj.* **4**, 183–90.

Stang, P. E., Yanagihara, T., Swanson, J. W. *et al.* (1992). Incidence of migraine headache: a population-based study in Olmsted County, Minnesota. *Neurology* **42**, 1657—62.

Stuss, D. T., Stethem, L. L., Hugenholtz, H. *et al.* (1989). Reaction time after head injury. *J. Neurol. Neurosurg. Psychiatry* **52**, 742–8.

Symonds, C. P. (1962). Concussion and its sequelae. *Lancet* **1**, 1–3.

Teasdale, G. M. (1987). Head injuries. In *Oxford Textbook of Medicine*, 2nd edn, vol. 2, sect. 21, eds. D. J. Weatherall, J. G. G. Ledingham & D. A. Warrell. Oxford: Oxford University Press.

Tennant, A., Macdermott, N. & Neary, (1995). The long-term outcome of head injury. *Brain Inj.*, **9**, 595–605.

Van Zomeren, A. H. & Deelman, D. G. (1987). Long-term recovery of visual time after closed head injury. *J. Neurol. Neurosurg. Psychiatry* **41**, 452–7.

Vollmer, D. G., Torner, J. C., Jane, J. A. *et al.* (1991). Age and outcome following traumatic coma: why do older patients fare worse? *J. Neurosurg.* **75** (Suppl.), S37–49.

Watson, C. P. N. & Evans, R. J. (1987). Chronic cluster headache: a review of 60 patients. *Headache* **27**, 158–65.

Wesseley, S. (1991). Chronic fatigue syndrome. *J. Neurol. Neurosurg. Psychiatry* **54**, 669–72.

Whitty, C. W. M. & Hockaday, J. M. (1968). Migraine: a follow-up study of 92 patients. *BMJ* **1**, 735–6.

Woods, T. O. & Goldberg, D. P. (1991). Psychiatric perspectives: an overview. *Br. Med. Bull.* **47**, 908–18.

24 Outcome in coma

N. E. F. CARTLIDGE

Historical introduction

From the time of mankind's earliest writings there are records of abnormalities of consciousness, and in many of these there is reference to outcome. Some of the most vivid descriptions are reviewed in an excellent book by Courville (1955).

The Edwin Smith Papyrus can be regarded as the first known medical textbook, being an incomplete copy of a work probably written during the period 2500–3000 BC (Breasted 1930). It contains a series of case histories and case 22 describes an individual who suffered a head injury and who was 'unable to speak'. The outcome in this patient can be guessed from the conclusion that is written 'an ailment not to be treated'.

Within the Hippocratic writings can be found many references to disorders of consciousness and outcome. For example, within the Hippocratic *Aphorisms* there is reference to coma as evidenced by the comment 'in cases of concussion of the brain produced by any cause the patients of necessity lose their speech'. Hippocrates clearly recognized the importance of being able to predict outcome with the sentence 'It seems to be highly desirable that a physican should pay much attention to prognosis'. The poor outcome of coma is referred to in a number of case descriptions such as case one in book one of *Epidemics*: 'The patient on the fifth day of the fever developed delirium, lost his voice, [presumably lapsed into coma] and then died' (Chadwick & Mann 1950).

In more modern times a major step forward in our understanding of the pathophysiology of coma occurred with the recognition of the close relationship between coma and sleep and the subsequent recognition of the importance of the brain in maintaining normal consciousness (Sigerist 1967). In 1853, Carpenter recognized the importance of links between subcortical structures and the cortex but it was the development of the electroencephalogram (EEG) which led to the concept of a subcortical pacemaker (Berger 1929) subsequently recognized to be the ascending reticular activating system (the reticular formation) by Moruzzi & Magoun (1963). This structure was recognized to extend from the brainstem and to have diffuse projections to the cerebral cortex.

These studies thus gave the framework for an understanding of normal consciousness and hence its disorders such as coma. Normal consciousness depends on a close interaction between the brainstem reticular formation and its connections with the cerebral cortex. Disorders of consciousness can thus either result from abnormalities of the cerebral cortex, or the reticular formation, or both, and of these the most important is coma.

Definition of coma

The patient who appears to be asleep and is at the same time incapable of sensing or responding to external stimuli or inner needs is in a state of coma. A simple and understandable definition of coma is that of unarousable unresponsiveness. This implies not only a defect in arousal but also one of awareness of self and environment. A more practical definition may be obtained using the Glasgow Coma Scale (Table 24.1). Coma is defined as a certain pattern of behavioural responses at the lower end of the scale. In precise terms, coma may be defined as the lower two responses of eye-opening, the lower two verbal responses and the lower three motor responses. At best, such patients do not open their eyes to a voice or spontaneously, do not localize a painful stimulus and utter recognizable words. The depth of coma may vary from a patient showing total absence of responses to the best responses as noted above.

The clinical picture of coma needs to be differentiated from two similar conditions, the vegetative state and the locked-in syndrome.

Vegetative state

This was the term suggested by Jennett & Plum (1972) to describe patients who recover the arousal component of consciousness but not, as far as can be determined, awareness. The commonest causes are head injury and hypoxic/ischaemic damage to the brain following cardiac arrest, although in one study from Japan, stroke was said to have caused one fifth of the cases. Such patients emerge from coma, as evidenced by eye opening, yet remain unresponsive and unaware.

Locked-in syndrome

The ventral pontine or locked-in syndrome describes a condition of total paralysis below the level of the third nerve nuclei. Such patients can open their eyes and elevate and depress their eyes. However, horizontal eye movements are lost and no other voluntary movement is possible. The diagnosis of this locked-in state depends on the recognition that the patient can open his eyes voluntarily rather than spontaneously as in the vegetative state (Feldman 1971).

Pathophysiology of coma

In order to fully understand the significance of outcome in coma a clear understanding of the specific pathophysiological mechanisms is necessary.

Table 24.1. *The Glasgow Coma Scale*

A. Eye opening
1. Nil
2. Pain
3. Verbal
4. Spontaneous

B. Motor response
1. Nil
2. Abnormal extension
3. Abnormal flexion
4. Weak flexion
5. Localization
6. Obeys command

C. Verbal
1. Nil
2. Incomprehensible
3. Inappropriate
4. Confused
5. Orientated fully

Coma due to cerebral hemisphere lesion

To produce coma cerebral hemisphere disturbances must be diffuse and extensive. These may be structural such as diffuse anoxic damage, or metabolic such as hepatic dysfunction or hypoglycaemia.

Coma due to lesions of the reticular formation

Discrete brainstem lesions can readily damage the reticular formation. Lesions caudal to the lower pons do not produce coma but rostral to this level bilateral lesions, even if quite small, may impair consciousness.

Brainstem infarction or haemorrhage often causes coma though this is rare with brainstem gliomas or brainstem plaques of demyelination. Massive demyelination as seen in central pontine myelinolysis may impair consciousness. Drug coma results largely from depression of the reticular formation though many drugs have additional effects on the cerebral cortex.

Coma from unilateral hemisphere or supratentorial lesions

It is axiomatic that a localized unilateral supratentorial lesion will not in itself produce coma though it is common clinical experience that, for example, a patient with a unilateral cerebral haemorrhage is almost invariably unconscious. Whilst a unilateral hemisphere lesion may compromise consciousness by direct infiltration of ascending projections from the reticular formation, a more common mechanism is downward shift of the cerebral hemisphere with brainstem distortion and dysfunction; the syndrome of rostrocaudal herniation (Grinker 1945).

There are many other factors which may contribute to either initial loss of consciousness after a head injury or prolonged coma including cerebral hypoxia, intracranial haemorrhage and secondary ischaemic brain damage (Miller 1993).

Clinical approach to coma

From the clinical point of view, three groups of comatose patients can be recognized.

Drug coma

Drug coma usually results from self-poisoning, either deliberate or accidental (Cartlidge 1981). The mechanism of action of drugs on consciousness depends in part on the pharmacology of the drug and in part on its dose. Opiates, barbiturates and benzodiazepines are thought to cause coma by their action on the brainstem reticular formation (Przybyla & Wang 1968), though the former two undoubtedly have more widespread effects upon the cerebrum (Larrabee & Posternak 1952).

Head injury

Controversy continues as to the precise mechanism by which the brain is injured by a direct blow to the head, though it is generally agreed that, at the moment of impact, there is a sharp rise in intracranial pressure (Gurdjian et al. 1955) and rapid movement of the brain within the skull. A more detailed account of the mechanics of brain injuries may be found elsewhere (Ripperger 1975). Ommaya showed that immobilization of the neck by means of a collar was an effective means of preventing concussion in the monkey, and therefore an important determinant of loss of consciousness at the time of a head injury is movement of the head on the cervical spine and hence brain on spinal cord (Ommaya et al. 1964). This implies involvement of the reticular formation and its cortical connections.

Medical coma

Transient loss of consciousness is not uncommon in the context of many medical illnesses but prolonged coma lasting for more than 6 hours is relatively uncommon. The international collaborative study of coma examined 500 patients in coma for more than 6 hours and the list of causes includes a wide variety of general medical conditions (Table 24.2) (Levy et al. 1981).

Table 24.2. *'Medical' causes of coma*

	UK	USA	Total
1. Hypoxia-ischaemia			
Respiratory arrest	5	17	22
Cardiac arrest	26	129	155
Hypotension	13	20	33
Total	44(20%)	166(60%)	210(42%)
2. Cerebrovascular			
Occlusive	40	10	56
Parenchymal haermorrhage	39	33	72
Subarachnoid haemorrhage	29	9	38
Other	4	11	15
Total	118(52%)	63(23%)	181(36%)
3. Hepatic	34(15%)	17(6%)	51(10%)
4. Other	29(13%)	29(11%)	58(12%)
Total	225	275	500

Hypoxic ischaemic coma

This form of coma in which the brain is deprived of its supply of oxygen most commonly follows cardiac arrest, though it may result from any disorder of oxygen supply to the brain, including respiratory arrest, cardiac dysrhythymia, or hypotension, and may be seen following problems in the course of medical anaesthesia. Rarer causes relate to carbon monoxide poisoning, suffocation and strangulation, drowning and air embolism. Coma that follows cardiopulmonary bypass operations is also thought likely to be due to hypoxic ischaemia (Shaw *et al.* 1989).

Cerebrovascular disease

There may be sudden loss of consciousness following a subarachnoid haemorrhage when blood escapes into the meninges and results in a sudden rise in intracranial pressure affecting the intracranial circulation. Vasospasm accompanying this phenomenon may result in diffuse ischaemia or infarction, and communicating hydrocephalus or localized collections of blood, such as haematoma, may complicate the picture.

The more common ischaemic stroke arising from occlusion of blood vessels within the cerebrum causes coma either by producing brainshift due to swelling at the site of infarction or from a discrete brainstem infarct involving the ascending reticular-activating substance. Massive intracerebral haemorrhage may result in coma due to swelling of brain tissue and consequent herniation.

Hepatic coma

The most common form of coma due to disorders of metabolism is that seen in hepatic disease. The pathophysiology is generally believed to be due to a toxic agent interfering with brain function, and an increase in blood and brain ammonia level has been identified though the level does not invariably explain the findings (Plum & Hindfelt 1976). A neurotransmitter disorder has been suggested and the discovery of increased levels of the amine octopamine supports this theory (Fischer & Baldessarini 1976). The response in some patients to the administration of L-dopa (Lunzer *et al.* 1974) would be compatible with the concept of a neurotransmitter defect, but the response to such treatment is not consistent or reproducible.

Miscellaneous causes of coma

These are relatively uncommon.

Metabolic disorders

These include uraemia and acid-base and electrolyte disorders which are most commonly seen in renal failure, and disorders of glucose metabolism as seen in patients with diabetes.

Infections

Meningitis and encephalitis are two other causes of coma due to diffuse bihemispheric disease. Coma may initially result from ischaemia to the cortical tissues following vasoconstriction and deterioration will result if there is cerebral oedema or hydrocephalus and secondary herniation through the tentorium, or when there is direct invasion of the cerebral cortex by the infecting organism extending down the Virchow–Robin spaces (Levin *et al.* 1978).

Acute viral encephalitis is the most common of the encephalitids to cause coma. This is due to disruption of cortical neuronal activity due to the infecting virus or the development of cerebral oedema resulting in herniation.

Mass lesions

Supra-and infratentorial mass lesions may cause coma by pressure on the ascending reticular activating substance.

Differential diagnosis

The differential diagnosis of coma includes the locked-in syndrome and the persistent vegetative state (see above). A variety of psychiatric disorders, most particularly those associated with catatonia may be confused with coma though such patients usually have spontaneous eye-opening and are obviously aware, a factor which can be demon-

Table 24.3. *The Paediatric Coma Scale*

Age	Eyes open	Motor response		Verbal response		Total
0–6 months	4	Flexion	3	Cries	2	9
6–12 months	4	Localizes	4	Vocalizes	3	11
1–2 years	4	Localizes	4	Words	4	12
2–5 years	4	Obeys	5	Words	4	13
Over 5 years	4	Obeys	5	Orientated	5	14

strated by the preservation of a menace response to visual stimuli. Feigning of coma as a pseudocoma is quite rare and readily diagnosed from true coma by the preservation of a normal oculovestibular response.

Coma in children

Coma in children in general has a similar pattern of causes to that of adults (Johnston & Mellits 1980). The definition of coma, however, in young children cannot be so precise as in adults and requires the use of a modified paediatric coma scale (Table 24.3) (Simpson & Reilly 1982).

Outcome in coma

Coma is thus the result of a wide variety of specific causes with an even wider variety of differing pathophysiological mechanisms. Not surprisingly outcome shows considerable variation.

Definitions of outcome

Many attempts have been made to produce outcome scales for coma and of these the Glasgow Outcome Scale is unquestionably the simplest (Jennett & Bond 1975). This was devised for brain damage in general and has been used successfully in the many international collaborative studies of head injury and non-traumatic coma. The scale can be varied from the fully expanded scale to a shortened version (Jennett *et al.* 1981) (Table 24.4).

Outcome in coma depends predominantly on three factors: (1) the cause of the coma; (2) clinical signs; and (3) investigations. Of these the most important determinant of outcome is the cause of the coma and the three main groups of coma, as outlined above, will be considered in relation to outcome with a note on the influence of physical signs and investigations.

Table 24.4. *Variations on the Glasgow Coma Scale*

Extended		Original		Contracted scales			
Dead		Dead	Dead		Dead or vegetative	Dead or vegetative	Dead
Vegetative		Vegetative					
Degree of disability			Dependent				
	5	Severely disabled		Severely disabled			
	4						Survivor
	3	Moderately disabled				Conscious	
	2		Independent	Independent			
	1	Good recovery					
	0						
Total categories	8	5	3			2	

Drug-induced coma

Uncomplicated coma due to drug overdose is not associated with structural brain damage and the prognosis in most instances is good. Death in drug-induced coma is usually a result of the complications of anoxia, pneumonia or cardiac arrhythmia.

Head injury coma

The increased interest in head injury research of the past few years with the resulting improvement in management of patients after head injury has resulted in a 15%–20% reduction in mortality for patients in coma after head injury (Miller 1993). Studies of outcome in head injury are beset with problems that include determination of study population, length of follow-up, definition of outcome and appropriate methodology. Brookes (1989) provided a very useful critique of head injury outcome studies to which potential researchers should refer. Some of the most important studies were initiated from the Glasgow School of Neurosurgery and are summarized in the many publications from Glasgow (see Jennett & Teasdale 1981). These studies have defined prognostic features based on depth of coma and other neurological signs which enable patients to be allocated into either those who are likely to have a good outcome and those who are likely to have a bad outcome.

The important factors determining outcome in head injury coma are the age of the

Table 24.5. *Outcome in head injury coma*

Indicant (best state in first 24 hours)	n	Outcome	
		Dead/PVS	Moderate disability/good recovery
Age (years)			
0–19	199	37%	56%
20–59	310	53%	39%
60+	91	88%	5%
Eye movements			
Intact	239	31%	59%
Impaired	96	64%	27%
Absent	98	95%	4%
Pupils			
Reacting	449	42%	50%
Not reacting	125	95%	5%
Motor response:			
Obeys/localizes	80	34%	57%
Withdrawal/flexor	126	63%	37%
Extensor/nil	103	83%	10%
Ranking by coma scale:			
1 (most responsive)	32	6%	91%
2	124	27%	59%
3	215	54%	28%
4 (least responsive)	173	80%	13%

PVS, persistent vegetative state.

patient, the depth of coma, the length of coma, and certain patterns of physical signs (Table 24.5) (Jennett *et al.* 1979).

Recovery after prolonged coma

Prolonged coma after head injury is accepted as a poor prognostic indicator. Sazbon & Groswasser (1990) published a retrospective study of 134 patients in a condition described as prolonged unawareness which, in effect, meant that the patients were comatose for over 1 month after head injury. They evaluated various parameters in a search for those that were able to predict non-recovery of consciousness. They found six features that were present during the first week after trauma which predicted non-recovery: *fever of central origin, diffuse body sweating, disturbances of anti-diuretic hormone secretion, abnormal motor reactivity* (unresponsiveness, decerebrate or decorticate posturing), *respiratory disturbance* and *diffuse non-neurological injuries.* A further two later factors (after the first week of injury), *late epilepsy* and *communicating hydrocephalus*, were also significant in predicting non-recovery. Of particular interest, in part two of their paper they reported that 72 out of the 134 patients (54%) recovered consciousness after coma of at least 1 month's duration. Eventually, about half of these individuals became independent in activities of daily living. Eleven per cent were able to resume open employment; 49% were engaged in some sort of sheltered employment. Overall around 70% of these patients were able to enjoy a reasonable quality of life.

There is still no evidence of any effective mechanism to accelerate recovery from persistent coma. Interestingly, two papers regarding coma arousal programmes using intense sensory stimulation have produced conflicting results. Pierce *et al.* (1990) showed no significant improvements, where as Mitchell *et al.* (1990) showed the period of coma to be shortened significantly.

Investigations and prediction of outcome

Increasingly studies are emerging in which there have been attempts to correlate a variety of investigative procedures with outcome. Jaggi *et al.* (1990) attempted to correlate outcome with early measurement of cerebral blood flow and metabolism. They found that cerebral blood flow correlated with the degree of functional recovery; lower blood flows were seen in patients with severe residual disability. They also found that the cerebral metabolic rate of oxygen combined with the better known outcome predictors (age, initial score on the Glasgow Coma Scale, and intracranial hypertension) enabled an accuracy of 82% prediction of survival or non-recovery.

Hans *et al.* (1989) combined a similar range of known outcome predictors with measurement of the cerebrospinal fluid-extrapolated creatine kinase BB isoenzyme activity and achieved a total prediction efficiency of 91% on the Glasgow Outcome Scale. The creatine kinase BB isoenzyme was felt to be a marker of the degree of initial brain damage.

Colquhoun and Burrows (1989) described the prognostic significance of the appearance of the basal cisterns and third ventricle on computed tomography (CT) scanning. Compression or obliteration of either the third ventricle and/or the basal cisterns were found to be useful predictors of the extent of primary brain damage; the authors proposed that detection of these signs with CT should lead to an early attempt to reduce intracranial pressure and thus, hopefully, improve eventual outcome. The study of evoked potentials in head injury did not provide equal prediction of prognosis. Lindsay *et al.* (1990) found that brainstem auditory and central somatosensory evoked potentials correlated with the clinical indices of brain damage, but they did not add to prediction accuracy. However, the authors did make the reasonable point that such measures do add useful prognostic information in paralysed or sedated patients.

Combining the results of investigations with the clinical features of the patient in coma has been undertaken in an attempt to improve the accuracy of prediction of outcome in head injury coma (Gibson & Stephenson 1989). These authors proposed a 20-point scale based on age, level of consciousness, pupil reactions, intracranial press-

Table 24.6. *Cause of medical coma and outcome*

	Best 1-year recovery				
	No recovery (%)	Vegetative state (%)	Severe disability (%)	Moderate disability (%)	Good recovery (%)
All patients (*n* = 500)	61	12	11	4	12
Subarachnoid haemorrhage (*n* = 38)	74	5	8	10	3
Other cerebrovascular disease (*n* = 143)	74	5	13	3	5
Hypoxia-ischaemia (*n* = 210)	58	20	10	2	10
Hepatic encephalopathy (*n* = 51)	49	2	14	8	27
Miscellaneous (*n* = 58)	45	9	12	3	31

ure, CT findings, blood pressure, and other injuries. They claimed that their scale predicts death with 100% accuracy. The scale clearly holds promise but as with any predictive system it is often impossible to assess the level of consciousness in an acutely rescusitated head injury patient because of the intubation and muscle relaxants which have been administered.

Summary

Serious physical, psychological and social sequelae occur in people who have been in coma subsequent to a head injury. Outcome is worse in patients in deep coma, prolonged coma, and when certain so-called adverse physical signs are present. Investigations in the early stages after coma have only limited value in predicting outcome.

Medical coma

Medical coma comprises a wide variety of different clinical conditions. Outcome depends to a significant extent on the cause as demonstrated in the international cooperative study of 500 patients in medical coma for more than 6 hours (Table 24.6). Outcome is better in patients in metabolic coma than in patients in coma after stroke.

Clinical signs and outcome

Many retrospective studies have attempted to define physical signs seen in the comatose patient that might be of predictive value. The majority of these studies, being retrospective, provided inaccurate clinical information.

The papers by Jorgensen (Jorgensen & Malchow-Moller 1981) were a landmark in the early clinical assessment in patients in coma after cardiac arrest. For example, Jorgen-

Table 24.7. *Outcome in medical coma related to signs noted at the time of admission*

Sign	Cohort	Best outcome at 1 year (%)		
		Death/ vegetative	Moderate/ severe disability	Disability/ Good recovery
Two of the following absent: Corneal reflex Pupillary reflex Oculovestibular reflex	120	97	2	1
Better than above but no motor response	83	80	8	12
Better than above but motor poorer than withdrawal	135	69	14	17
Better than above but no vocalization	106	58	19	23
Better than above plus vocalization	56	46	13	41

sen showed that the recovery of the pupillary light reflex within 12 minutes after cardiac arrest is compatible with neurological survival whereas the absence of a pupillary light reflex after 28 minutes indicates that neurological recovery is unlikely. This was the first prospective study of clinical signs in coma after cardiac arrest.

The international collaborative study provided further clinical data based on a prospective study. The level of coma as measured on the Glasgow Coma Scale is predictive of outcome, patients with higher levels having better outcomes, and the duration of the coma also correlates with outcome. None of these features are sufficiently specific or selective to help in establishing the prognosis in an individual patient. Some clinical signs are significantly associated with a poor prognosis: in the total cohort of 500 patients corneal reflexes were absent 24 hours after the onset of coma in 90 patients and this sign was incompatible with survival (Table 24.7). In a more uniform group who had suffered anoxic injury there were 210 patients: 52 of these had no pupillary reflex at 24 hours, all of whom died. By the third day 70 were left with a motor response poorer than withdrawal and all died. By the seventh day the absence of roving eye movements was seen in 16 patients all of whom died. The confidence intervals for all of these individual criteria were 0.95 and yet, statistically, even with such a large prospective study it remains possible that up to 5% of individual patients with such clearly defined abnormal signs could actually make a good or moderate recovery.

The possibility of using combinations of different clinical signs to improve accuracy of prognosis was analysed by Levy *et al.* (1981) but although this improved the accuracy of prediction of good prognosis in those patients who had or regained some clinical signs early in the course of the disease it could not eliminate the small possibility that some patients lacking important responses early in the course of coma might ultimately make a good recovery. More recent studies from Longstreth *et al.* (1983) utilizing a combination of clinical and laboratory features (motor response, pupillary light response, spontaneous eye movements and blood glucose) to manufacture an 'awakening' score have a false-positive rate in the poor outcome category of 16 of our 98 patients (16%). This study was based on patients surviving out-of-hospital cardiac arrest and the timing of the assessments with relation to the resuscitation is variable and difficult to evaluate. A large retrospective study performed by Mullie *et al.* (1988) using the Glasgow Coma Scale alone to predict outcome made a false-positive prediction of 1 in 51 patients (2%). In both of these studies the confidence intervals would suggest that the possibility of error would lie between 5% and 20% making these indicants unacceptable for purposes of deciding to withdraw therapy in the course of coma.

A large prospective study (Hamel *et al.* 1995) of 395 patients in non-traumatic coma has produced further information concerning estimation of prognosis. Five clinical variables available on the third day of coma were useful in predicting a bad prognosis. For example, 97% of patients who had abnormal brainstem responses, absent verbal responses, absent withdrawal to pain, a creatinine level greater than 1.5 mg/dcl and age of 70 years or more were dead within 2 months.

Investigations and outcome

Increasingly, attempts have been made to assess the value of investigations performed in the early stages of coma as predictors of outcome.

Electrophysiology

The possibility of neurophysiological, imaging or chemical investigations providing more definitive indicants for prognosis has been increasingly studied during the past 20 years. Five grades of EEG abnormality in coma are internationally accepted: alpha rhythm, dominant theta, diffuse dominant delta, burst suppression and isoelectric. At 48 hours these grades provide prediction with an accuracy of about 88% (Edgren *et al.* 1987). The evaluation of compressed spectral arrays (CSA) of EEG is still being undertaken though it seems that the accuracy is unlikely to improve upon that provided by clinical assessment. CSA is a useful method for monitoring patients in coma and variation in pattern of response may indicate a potential for neurological recovery.

Evoked potential studies have also failed to demonstrate greater accuracy than that possible with clinical methods. In general brainstem evoked responses (BSER) are of use in identifying brain death and somatosensory evoked potential are of greater value in prediction of outcome. It is suggested that the bilateral loss of cortical SSEP is of value in the early prediction of a poor outcome from coma but currently available results involve small numbers of patients and are not uniform (Walser *et al.* 1986). There is also the technical problem of difficulties arising in the peripheral nerves and roots which might cause false-positive errors. It is unlikely that these methods will achieve better accuracy than clinical evaluation.

Imaging

Imaging techniques including computed tomography, magnetic resonance imaging and single photon emission spectroscopy, together with other methods measuring blood flow are extremely useful in determining the diagnosis of coma and in identifying brain death but their value in prediction is not better than clinical signs. Even the use of cerebral metabolic rate for oxygen (CMRO) appears only to allow correct prediction in approximately 82% of patients (Jaggi *et al.* 1990). Although invasive studies are still being reported, particularly in paediatric coma, there is no evidence that their accuracy is an improvement over clinical signs. Most of the statistics relating to clinical signs have been derived from adult populations and may not necessarily be applied in a paediatric population.

Biochemistry

Biochemical studies, either of cerebral metabolic rate for oxygen or of the concentration of chemicals of cerebrospinal fluid believed to be indicative of tissue damage such as brain-type creatine kinase and neuron-specific enolase, have been correlated with outcome. The sensitivity obtained is only of the order of 74% though the specificity is said to be as high as 100% (Roine *et al.* 1989). Problems will be likely to occur in conditions such as bronchogenic neoplasm and neuroblastomas where the enzyme levels may be falsely elevated.

Summary

Outcome in medical coma is related to the cause of the coma independent of the physical signs, depth of coma or length of coma. Certain clinical signs, particularly those of brainstem responses, motor and verbal responses are the most useful and best-validated clinical predictors. Even these useful clinical predictors are not sufficient to avoid a 5% risk of a positive error. Investigations seem only to have limited value in predicting outcome in medical coma.

Conclusion

Patients in coma have a disturbance of the normal functional interaction between the brainstem reticular formation and the cerebral cortex. Biochemical disturbances of the brain affecting either the cortex as in hepatic coma, or the brainstem reticular formation as in drug coma are potentially recoverable. Structural damage to the brain affecting either the brainstem reticular formation or the cortex is associated with a much worse prognosis, the outcome depending on the extent and type of the damage. In those patients who have suffered structural brain damage the pattern of neurological signs demonstrable in the early stages of coma may enable prediction of outcome whatever the precise cause of the damage.

References

Berger, H. (1929). Über das Elektrenkephalogramm des Menschen *Arch. Psychiatr. Nervenkr.* **87**, 527–70.

Breasted, J. H. (1930). *The Edwin Smith Surgical Papyrus.* Chicago: University of Chicago Press.

Brookes, N. (1989). Defining outcome. *Brain Injury* **3**, 325–9.

Carpenter, W. B. (1853). *Principles of Human Physiology.* Philadelphia: Blanchard and Lea.

Cartlidge, N. E. F. (1981). Drug-induced coma. *Adv. Drug React. Bull.* **88**, 320–3.

Chadwick, J. & Mann, W. N. (1950). *Hippocratic Writings.* Oxford: Blackwell Scientific Publications.

Colquhoun, I. R. & Burrows, E. H. (1989). The prognostic significance of the third ventricle and basal cisterns in severe closed head injury. *Clin. Radiol.* **40**, 13–16.

Courville, C. B. (1955). *Commotio-Cerebri.* Los Angeles: San Lucas Press.

Edgren, E., Hedstrend, U., Nordin, M. *et al.* (1987). Prediction of outcome after cardiac arrest. *Crit. Care Med.* **15**, 820–5.

Feldman, M. H. (1971). Physiological observations in a chronic case of locked-in syndrome. *Neurology* **21**, 459–78.

Fischer, J. E. & Baldessarini, R. J. (1976). Pathogenesis and therapy of hepatic coma. In *Progress in Liver Disease*, eds F. Schaeffner & H. Popper. New York: Bruyn and Smith.

Gibson, M. & Stephenson G. C. (1989). Aggressive management of severe closed head trauma: time for reappraisal. *Lancet* **II**, 369–71.

Grinker, I. M. (1945). Transtentorial herniation of the brain-stem: a characteristic clinico-pathologic syndrome: pathogenesis of haemorrhages in the brain-stem. *Arch. Neurol. Psychiatry* **53**, 289–98.

Gurdjian, E. S., Webster, J. E. & Lissner, H. R. (1955). Observations on the mechanism of brain concussion, contusion and laceration. *Surg. Gynecol. Obstet.* **101**, 680–92.

Hamel, M. B., Goldman, L., Teno, J., Lynn, J., Davis, R. B., Harrell, F. E., Connors, A. F., Califf, R., Kussin, P., Bellamy, P., Vidallet, H. & Phillips, R. S. (1995). Identification of comatose patients at high risk for death or severe disability. *JAMA* **273**, 1842–8.

Hans, P., Albert, A., Franssen, C. & Born, J. (1989). Improved outcome prediction based on CSF extrapolated creatinine kinase BB-isoenzyme activity and other risk factors in severe head injury. *J. Neurosurg.* **71**, 54–8.

Jaggi, J. L., Obrist, W. D., Gennarelli, T. A., Langfitt, T. W. (1990). Relationship of early cerebral blood flow and metabolism to outcome in acute head injury. *J. Neurosurg.* **72**, 176–82.

Jennett, B. & Bond, M. (1975). Assessment of outcome after severe brain damage. *Lancet* **i**, 480.

Jennett, W. B. & Plum, F. (1972). The persistent vegetative state: a syndrome in search of a name. *Lancet* **I**, 734–7.

Jennett, B. & Teasdale, G. (1981). *Management of Head Injuries.* Philadelphia: Davis.

Jennett, B., Teasdale, G., Braakman, R., Minderhoud, J. & Knill-Jones, R. (1979). Predicting outcome in individual patients after severe head injury. *Lancet* **II**, 1031–4.

Jennett, B., Snoek, J., Bond, M. R. & Brooks, N. (1981). Disability after severe head injury: observations on the use of the Glasgow Outcome Scale. *J. Neurol. Neurosurg. Psychiatry* **44**, 285–93.

Johnston, R. B. & Mellits, E. (1980). Pediatric coma: prognosis and outcome. *Develop. Med. Child. Neurol.* **22**, 3–12.

Jorgensen, E. O. & Malchow-Moller, A. (1981). Natural history of global and critical brain ischaemia. *Resuscitation* **9**, 133–91.

Larrabee, M. G. & Posternak, J. M. (1952). Selective action of anaesthetics on synapses and axons in mammalian sympathetic ganglia. *J. Neurol. Physiol.* **15**, 91–114.

Levin, S., Harris, A. A. & Sokalskei, S. J. (1978). Bacterial meningitis. In *Infections of the Nervous System*, part I, *Handbook of Clinical Neurology*, vol. 33, eds. P. J. Vinken & G. W. Bruyn, pp. 1–19. New York: Elsevier/North Holland.

Levy, D. E., Bates, D., Corona, J. J. *et al.* (1981). Prognosis in non-traumatic coma. *Ann. Intern. Med.* **94**, 293–301.

Lindsay, K., Pasoglu, A., Hirst, D., Allardyce, G., Kennedy, I. & Teasdale, G. (1990). Somatosensory and auditory brain stem conduction after head injury: a comparison with clinical features in prediction of outcome. *Neurosurgery* **26**, 278–85.

Longstreth, W. T., Diehr, P. & Inuit, S. (1983). Prediction of awakening after out-of-hospital cardiac arrest. *N. Engl. J. Med.* **308**, 1378–82.

Lunzer, M., James, I. M., Weinman, J. *et al.* (1974). Treatment of chronic hepatic encephalopathy with levodopa. *Gut* **15**, 555–61.

Miller, J. D. (1993). Head injury. *J. Neurol. Neurosurg. Psychiatry* **56**, 440–7.

Mitchell, S., Bradley, V., Welch, J. L., Britton, P. G. (1990). Coma arousal procedure: a therapeutic intervention in the treatment of head injury. *Brain Inj.* **4**, 273–9.

Moruzzi, G. & Magoun, H. W. (1963). Brain stem reticular formation and activation of the EEG. *Electroenceph. Clin. Neurophysiol.* **1**, 455–73.

Mullie, A., Buylaert, W., Michem, N. *et al.* (1988). Predictive value of Glasgow Coma Score for awakening after out of hospital cardiac arrest. *Lancet* **1**, 137–40.

Ommaya, A. K., Rockoff, S. D. & Baldwin, M. (1964). Experimental concussion. *J. Neurosurg.* **21**, 249–63.

Pierce, J. P., Lyle, D. M., Quine, S., Evans, N. J., Morris, J. & Fearnside, M. R. (1990). The effectiveness of coma arousal intervention. *Brain Inj.* **4**, 191–7.

Plum, F. & Hindfelt, B. (1976). The neurological complications of liver disease. In *Metabolic and Deficiency Disease of the Nervous System*, part I, *Handbook of Clinical Neurology*, vol. 27, eds. P. J. Vinken, G. W. Bruyn & H. L. Clowans, pp. 349–77. New York: Elsevier/North Holland.

Przybyla, A. C. & Wang, S. C. (1968). Mechanisms of action of the benzo-diazepines. *J. Pharmacol. Exp. Ther.* **163**, 349–47.

Ripperger, E. A. (1975). The mechanics of brain injuries. In *Injuries of the Brain and Skull*, part I, *Handbook of Clinical Neurology*, vol. 23, eds P. J. Vinken & G. W. Bruyn. Amsterdam: North Holland.

Roine, R. O., Somer, H., Kaste, M. *et al.* (1989). Neurological outcome after out-of-hospital cardiac arrest: prediction by cerebrospinal fluid enzyme analysis. *Arch. Neurol.* **46**, 753–6.

Sazbon, S. & Groswasser, Z. (1990). Outcome in 134 patients with prolonged post-traumatic unawareness, part 1, parameters determining late recovery of consciousness. *Neurosurgery* **72**, 75–80.

Sigerist, H. E. (1967). *A History of Medicine 1.* New York: Oxford University Press.

Shaw, P. J., Bates, D., Cartlidge, N. E. F., French, J. M., Heaviside, D., Julian, D. G. & Shaw, D. A.

(1989). An analysis of factors predisposing to neurology injury in patients undergoing coronary bypass operations. *Q. J. Med.* **267**, 633–46.

Simpson, D. & Reilly, P. (1982). The Paediatric Coma Scale. *Lancet* II, 450–2.

Walser, H., Murat, E. & Janzer, R. (1986). Somatosensory evoked potentials in comatose patients: correlations with outcome and neuropathological findings. *J. Neurol.* **233**, 34–40.

25 Syringomyelia

BERNARD WILLIAMS*

Syringomyelia is the presence of longitudinally disposed cavities in the grey matter of the spinal cord. It is thus not a disease but a condition almost always associated with other lesions. If hydrocephalus, posterior fossa arachnoid pouches or spina bifida are present in a patient with syringomyelia they indicate a disturbance of cerebrospinal fluid (CSF) physiology. Sometimes the associated lesions are clearly causing the syringomyelia, such as intrinsic spinal cord or posterior fossa tumours. In these cases the prognosis is that of the tumour.

Syringomyelia is a surgical disorder, the outcome is thus related to the appropriateness of the surgery and the skill and experience of the surgeon. The following notes follow the author's classification of syringomyelia (Williams 1991).

Hindbrain-related syringomyelia

Chiari malformation, tonsillar prolapse and cerebellar ectopia are all terms which can be replaced by 'hindbrain herniation'. This is the commonest associated lesion and the clinical picture is often dominated by the effects of the hindbrain hernia rather than the associated syringomyelia. The commonest form of syringobulbia is bulbar symptomatology related to hindbrain herniation (Morgan & Williams 1992; Williams 1993). If left alone the progression of syringobulbia is commonly fatal within 20 years or so. The pessimism of earlier authors was because it was quickly fatal cases which came to post mortem examination (Tomesco-Sisesti 1924; Schliep 1968) and thereby to a diagnosis. Such patients dominate the essentially pathological descriptions prior to the surgical era of syringomyelia management which commenced after the work of Gardner (Gardner 1973; Gardner et al. 1977). Benign hindbrain impaction, if treated by adequate decompression before the onset of permanent structural damage such as syringomyelia or fourth ventricular clefts has an excellent prognosis (Morgan & Williams 1992; Shannan et al. 1981; Susuki et al. 1985).

If the patient comes to surgery late, and if the cord is damaged by prolonged

---

* Mr Williams died on 9 August 1995: he left this chapter in its present incomplete form. I thought it best to publish it without alteration, in his memory. *M.S. (Editor)*

478

distension and the formation of a thick gliotic lining to the cavity, then the most effective surgery, as judged by magnetic resonance imaging (MRI) criteria, is not good enough to prevent slow deterioration. This may be due to the progression of gliosis affecting the blood supply of the cord. The natural processes of ageing may affect such a cord adversely. It is a natural assumption that the flattening of the cord produced by surgical treatment improves the prognosis but there is no proof. Correlation between flattening of the cord and clinical improvement is poor, and the assumption that deflating the syrinx makes the prognosis better depends on such traditionally suspect assumptions as 'Well it must be better, mustn't it?'

The hindbrain symptoms including headache and all lower cranial nerve dysfunction from the oculomotor nerve downwards correlate well with the MRI appearances. Careful surgery with resection of the tonsils and leaving the dura open with no grafts produces good clinical results (Dyste *et al.* 1989; Morgan & Williams 1992; Williams 1981, 1993). Clinical results of the symptoms presumed to be coming from the cord are often helped less than the MRI appearances.

Patients with meningeal fibrosis are sometimes described as having 'arachnoiditis'. Active inflammation is seldom present at the time that they present with syringomyelia. At the foramen magnum meningeal fibrosis is sometimes uncorrectable without the risks of vascular damage; for example, by attempting to dissect the cerebello-medullary fissure. Shunting of the CSF from the ventricles or the spinal subarachnoid space may help (Vengsarkar *et al.* 1991).

Spinal meningeal fibrosis

The second commonest cause of syringomyelia in the author's practice is spinal meningeal fibrosis. Patients may be divided into two, those with localized fibrosis, for example due to a fractured spine or to Pott's disease, and those with diffuse fibrosis such as that due to epidural abscess, meningitis or the injection of toxic chemicals such as antibacterial agents, or myodil (Pantopaque). The prognosis for the last group is grim and relentless advance leading to death may not be preventable. Post-traumatic syringomyelia, detected pathologically, was found in about 20% of the patients with traumatic cord lesions reported by Squier and Lehr (1994). This incidence is rather higher than reported from clinical data.

The treatment of the localized variety is the establishment of a free pathway for CSF past the obstruction. After operation the dura should be left widely open.

Drainage of syrinx cavities is often recommended in both hindbrain- and non-hindbrain-related syringomyelia (Shannon *et al.* 1981; Suzuki *et al.* 1985; Tator *et al.* 1982), but in the author's view is seldom required (Williams 1992). If the CSF pathways are restored to normal pressure and as nearly as possible normal anatomy, then the prognosis largely depends upon the damage which has been done before surgery was instituted.

Acknowledgement

This work has been partly financed by Anne's Neurological Trust, a self-help Group and fund-raising charity.

References

Dyste, G., Menezes, A. H. & Van Gilder, J. C. (1989). Symptomatic Chiari malformations: an analysis of presentation, management and long-term outcome. *J. Neurosurg.* **71**, 159–68.

Gardner, W. J. (1973). *The Dysraphic States*. Amsterdam: Excerpta Medica.

Gardner, W. J., Bell, H. S., Poolos, P. N., Dohn, D. F. & Steinberg, M. (1977). Terminal ventriculostomy for syringomyelia. *J. Neurosurg.* **46**, 609–17.

Jonesco-Sisesti, N. (1924). Syringobulbia: a contribution to the pathophysiology of the brainstem. Paris: Masson. (Translation and updating by R. T. Ross (1986). New York: Praeger.)

Morgan, D. W. & Williams, B. (1992). Syringobulbia, a surgical appraisal. *J. Neurol. Neurosurg. Psychiatry* **55**, 1132–41.

Schliep, G. (1978). Syringomyelia and syringobulbia. In *Handbook of Clinical Neurology*, vol. 32. *Congenital Malformations of the Brain and Spinal Cord*, eds. P. J. Vinken & G. W. Bruyn, pp. 255–327. Amsterdam: North Holland.

Shannon, N., Symon, L., Logue, V., Cull, D., Kang, J. & Kendall, B. E. (1981). Clinical features, investigation and treatment of post-traumatic syringomyelia. *J. Neurol. Neurosurg. Psychiatry* **44**, 35–42.

Squier, M., Lehr, P. (1994). Post-traumatic syringomyelia. *J. Neurol. Neurosurg. Psychiatry* **57**, 1095–8.

Suzuki, M., Davis, C., Symon, L. & Gentili, G. (1985). Syringoperitoneal shunt for treatment of cord cavitation. *J. Neurol. Neurosurg. Psychiatry* **48**, 620–7.

Tator, C. H., Meguro, K., Rowed, D. W. (1982). Favourable results with syringosubarachnoid shunts for treatment of syringomyelia. *J. Neurosurg.* **56**, 517–23.

Vengsarkar, U. S., Panchal, V. G., Tripathi, P. D., Patkar, S. V., Agarwal, A., Doshi, P. K. & Kamat, M. M. (1991). Percutaneous thecoperitoneal shunt for syringomyelia. *J. Neurosurg.* **74**, 827–31.

Williams, B. (1991). 'Malformations'. In *Clinical Neurology*, vol. 2, eds. M. Swash & J. Oxbury, pp. 1533–82. Edinburgh: Churchill Livingstone.

Williams, B. (1992). Post-traumatic syringomyelia (cystic myelopathy). In *Handbook of Clinical Neurology*, vol. 17, *Spinal Cord Trauma*, eds. P. J. Vinken & G. W. Bruyn, pp. 375–98. Amsterdam: North Holland.

Williams, B. (1981). Simultaneous cerebral and spinal fluid pressure recordings. 2. Cerebrospinal dissociation with lesions at the foramen magnum. *Acta Neurochir.* **59**, 123–42.

Williams, B. (1993). Surgery for hindbrain related syringomyelia. In *Advances and Technical Standards in Neurosurgery*, vol. 20, ed. L. Symon, pp. 107–164. New York: Springer.

26 Neurosurgical treatment of pain syndromes

R. R. TASKER

Introduction

The problem of chronic pain, one of the most economically important issues in medicine, encompasses a vast array of disease states and neurosurgical procedures to treat it. This chapter reviews outcomes of surgery for chronic pain. Neurosurgical operations in regular use will be briefly reviewed, giving a brief summary of status for the relief of a particular disease state and then, in the form of tables, published, and where available, personal data on success rate and incidence of complications. The decision to review outcomes of particular procedures will be influenced by the author's experience and perception of overall contemporary significance. For example, the use of infusion pumps to administer morphine in pain patients is a medical procedure that will not be reviewed here.

Measurement of outcome

In stressing the importance of attempting to provide a database for outcomes, this volume has hit the nail on the head, a very sensitive and wobbly head at that in the case of these functional procedures. Outcomes in the therapy of head injury can be assessed by measurements of activities of everyday living; that in tumour surgery by the Karnovsky Scale and survival statistics. But semi-quantitative outcome assessment in pain disorders is not readily achieved. Chronic pain patients usually suffer from underlying disease states responsible for their pain in the first place and these influence outcome significantly. Moreover these disease processes are usually unpredictably progressive and as time goes on may induce new problems and different pain syndromes not envisaged at the time of original pain surgery. For example, cancer may in time induce neuropathic in addition to nociceptive pain (Tasker 1987), while degenerative disc disease and its consequences in patients with low back pain, hemiplegia in stroke-induced pain, amputation in phantom pain play as large a role as the pain in the patient's outcome. And how does one deal with the often associated psychogenic problems? For chronic pain suffered for a long time appears to warp psychological well-being. And what of the 'placebo' effect (Wall 1992)? Improving pain status (complete relief is virtually impossible) simply makes life more comfortable, an immeasurable entity.

Even when these features are taken into account, how can one compare published results from different centres? Do reported differences reflect the skills and techniques of the authors, length of follow-up, the sample selection from and the constitution of the original patient population upon which results are being reported, the methods for assessment of results (questionnaire? impartial semi-quantitative measurement?) How does one measure pain in the first place? Gybels (1991) has critically addressed this problem in pain patients as well as in his book with Sweet (Gybels & Sweet 1989). After pain surgery, complete relief never happens and eventual recurrence is the rule (Tasker 1993). The best that can be done is to try to report the incidence of significant relief of pain over a reasonable period of follow-up, say 50% or more over 6–12 months. But it is rare to find such outcome consensus in publications on the subject. Does an '85% successful result' after dorsal column stimulation for pain mean that 85% of all patients accepted for treatment did well (how well? for how long?); or that 85% of patients who could be traced did well; or 85% of patients who passed some initial selection process such as trial stimulation; or does it mean that 85% of patients in whom everything went well with no interfering complications or technical problems did well? These issues are often not specified.

One aim of this chapter is to compare the courses of patients that have been operated upon with those not surgically treated. Such comparisons are routine in, say, reviewing glioma surgery but there is no comparable relevant information of which I am aware applicable to patients with pain. Patients with chronic pain have the life expectancy of their underlying disease, cancer patients with pain die of cancer and pain surgery doesn't make any difference except to add complications. Though in pain associated with degenerative disc disease pain surgery might increase activities of everyday living which are capable of semi-quantitative assessment, such information is rarely provided.

The reader will have to be content, therefore, with a review of published series of a variety of well-known surgical procedures which are difficult to compare with one another. It can only be hoped that in future more attention will be paid to developing and following outcome databases as advocated by Gybels (Gybels 1991).

Surgery for intractable pain

Though the number of neurosurgical procedures advocated for the relief of intractable pain is legion, only a few appear to be in sufficiently regular use to be adequately assessed in the literature for the purpose of this chapter and these are listed in Table 26.1.

Though general difficulties in assessing surgical results have been discussed in the Introduction, some specific problems concerning pain surgery require further elaboration. Chronic pain syndromes have a number of differing pathophysiologies. Clearly a particular surgical procedure is designed to correct a particular pathophysiology. If it is used in a patient with a pain problem not caused by that particular pathophysiology, it

Table 26.1. *Neurosurgical procedures in regular use to relieve chronic pain*

Facet 'rhizotomy'
Percutaneous cordotomy
Dorsal column stimulation
Stereotactic mesencephalic tractotomy
Medial thalamotomy
Deep brain stimulation

can hardly succeed. However, pain mechanisms are complex and poorly understood. Not only may the individual surgeon make diagnostic errors resulting in a poor choice of surgical technique, but also he may be unaware of scientific information that bears on his choice of operation. And the pathophysiology of all too many pain syndromes remains unknown to science so that expert use of all available technology may result in the treatment being ineffective. On the other hand, the mechanisms by which some surgical operations such as dorsal column stimulation modify pain are unknown, still further compromising their intelligent application.

Quite apart from choice of operation, destructive pain surgery, even when perfectly tailored to the patient's needs, may be confounded by the astounding responses of the nervous system to the surgically induced injury. Regeneration may reconstitute severed pain pathways; iatrogenic neuropathic pain may replace the original pain after neurectomy, rhizotomy, cordotomy and mesencephalic tractotomy; somatotopographic reorganization, capable of bypassing the iatrogenic lesion may lead to recurrence of the original pain. None of these procedures can be adequately dealt with.

Facet rhizotomy

In 1971 Rees (1971) advocated a new operation for the relief of chronic back pain in which, through a stab wound, he sought to locate and cut with a scalpel the nerves of Luschka that supplied sensation to the facet joints. Some questions have since been raised as to whether his procedure could, in fact, cut these nerves so that it has been replaced with percutaneous radiofrequency (RF) facet rhizotomy (Shealy 1975).

Patient selection

Not really a rhizotomy, this procedure aims to denervate the facets, under the assumption that certain types of back pain localized to the paravertebral area, particularly if aggravated by extension, arise chiefly in the facet joints which are almost exclusively innervated by the medial branches of the dorsal rami from the segment above the joint, with contributions from the next more cephalad level as well as from communicating branches from the sympathetic trunk (Auleroche 1983; Bogduk *et al.* 1982; Groen *et al.* 1990; Stolker *et al.* 1984). Unfortunately it is unclear whether a typical 'facet pain syndrome' can be recognized clinically, and there may be additional innervation to facet joints to that arising in the segmental posterior rami. In selecting patients for RF facet rhizotomy most surgeons require that, in addition to an appropriate clinical picture, the pain be relieved temporarily by a local anaesthetic test block. The latter is done in a variety of ways and the criteria for successful block are not standard. In most cases, up to 2 ml of 2% lidocaine, with or without steroids, is injected into the implicated facet joints, a successful result being deemed 50% or more pain reduction (Boas 1982). Such blocks often lead to unbelievably long periods of relief of pain, even of pain elements located in parts of the body that could not possibly arise in facet joints. Moreover, this method of testing does not duplicate RF denervation, the use of steroids is an uncontrollable variant, while 2 ml of local anaesthetic is likely to spill over into other structures. Thus the test is a poor predictor of the eventual outcome of facet 'rhizotomy'. It would seem that test blocks with smaller, say 0.5 ml volumes, of a long-acting local anaesthetic agent, such as 0.5% marcaine, applied at the expected site of the nerve rather than into the joint, might be a better predictor, but there are no data to confirm this to be the case (Marks *et al.* 1992; Nash 1990; Marks 1989). Even so, in the author's experience, less than half the patients undergoing RF facet blocks after successful local blocks derive significant relief and Dunsker *et al.* (1977) reported a 40% figure. Thus a diverse population of patients are treated by percutaneous RF facet 'rhizotomy' (Fox & Rizzoli 1973; Pedersen *et al.* 1956).

Technique

The facet nerves are usually interrupted under intravenous sedation on the side(s) and at the levels of the pain as well as one segment above its cephalic limit, using image intensification. A guide needle is introduced to the expected site of the facet nerves as revealed by X-ray and a suitable electrode passed through it to the site when the guide needle is partly withdrawn to bare the electrode tip. Some authors rely only on X-ray localization but physiological corrobation of electrode placement is usually achieved by electrical stimulation. Many surgeons seek reproduction of the patient's pain with 60–100 Hz stimulation to confirm adequate positioning of their electrode, after which a radiofrequency lesion is made with a 1 to 2-mm diameter electrode with about a 5-mm bare tip capable of temperature monitoring. Current and temperature are gradually increased allowing maximal duration of maximal current flow before current 'falloff' occurs. The latter is caused by boiling at the electrode tip, the insulating gases formed precluding further lesion enlargement at that particular site. Boiling too soon results in an ineffectively small lesion. Some authors make duplicate lesions at each level to increase the chance of success or attempt to interrupt superior and inferior branches of the posterior ramus separately.

This protocol seems illogical; first the procedure is very uncomfortable and the necessary intravenous sedation interferes with patient cooperation. Moreover, stimulation of the nervous system rarely produces pain, but usually causes paraesthesiae (Tasker *et al.* 1982*a*). Thus the significance of stimulation-induced pain is open to question. It seems more effective to perform the procedure under general anaesthetic relying on inducing contractions in paravertebral muscles but not in muscles supplied by anterior rami as the physiological guide to appropriate electrode position. Responses to stimulation at or below 1.0 volt suggest that the electrode is close enough to the nerve to make an effective lesion. Such muscle contractions should not persist during brief curarization; otherwise they could arise from direct stimulation of muscle.

Complications

Whatever the technique used, complications are usually minimal. Nevertheless ischemic cord damage has been described after the procedure in the lower thoracic area (Koning *et al.* 1991; Sluijter *et al.* 1991). One to two per cent of patients report unexplainable postoperative aggravation of their pain and, occasionally, heating of the corresponding anterior ramus may induce patchy sensory loss in its distribution. Most important is the fact that facet 'rhizotomies' at or cephalad to L2 induce sensory loss from unavoidable concomitant damage to the cutaneous branches of the dorsal rami, often with transient neuropathic pain. These sensory branches are prominent in the case of C2/3 in which they consitute the occipital nerves and in the upper lumbar area where they form the cluneal nerves. They are absent, however, in the lower lumbar area and small elsewhere, innervating patches of paravertebral skin.

Table 26.2 reviews reported results. Most authors feel that the procedure is less successful in patients who have had previous spinal surgery, presumably because of disturbed anatomy. And certainly fusion masses may prevent percutaneous access to the nerves. Finally, since the lesion is a post-ganglionic one, nerve regeneration is to be expected with recurrence of pain in a year or so.

Comment

Facet rhizotomy is of considerable socioeconomic importance. Low back pain is increasingly common, and its spiralling costs worldwide are making it one of the most expensive issues in the health care budgets of developed countries. For example, in Sweden in 1990 (Uden 1994) low back pain cost 1.4 billion Swedish crowns for medical costs, 21.1 billion for disability and pension payments totalling 22.5 billion crowns or 3.6 billion Canadian dollars. The pressures to treat low back pain are therefore mounting, including the pressure to carry out facet rhizotomy. With the uncertainties of patient selection and choice of technique alluded to above and the wide variation in results, it is an economically significant matter to make a proper study of this procedure in order to be able to assign it to its appropriate role.

Percutaneous cordotomy

Percutaneous RF cordotomy, the modern adaptation (Sweet *et al.* 1960; Mullan *et al.* 1963; Rosomoff *et al.* 1965; Gildenberg *et al.* 1969; Taren *et al.* 1969; Taren 1971; Onofrio 1971; Tasker & Organ 1973; Hitchcock & Tsukamoto 1973; Tasker *et al.* 1973; Kanpolat *et al.* 1989) of Spiller and Martin's historic open procedure (Spiller & Martin 1912) is one of

Table 26.2. *Published results of 'Facet Rhizotomy'*

Significant pain relief (% of patients)			Reference
Previous spinal surgery			
Yes	No	?	
41 (27 if fused)	79		Shealey 1975
59	89		Oudenhoven 1974
		50–80 lit review	Stolker *et al.* 1993
		22 personal	Stolker *et al.* 1993
	67	42	Burton 1976
	67		McCulloch 1976
	20		Dunsker *et al.* 1977
		50–60	Tasker 1985, 1988*a*
		60	Johnson 1974
		60	Boas 1982
		50 (25 after 1 year)	Mehta & Sluijter 1979
26	61	40	Lora & Long 1976
	62	20	McCulloch & Organ 1977
		58	Sluijter 1981
54	68	60	Savitz 1991
50	75	69	Silvers 1990

the most successful and useful procedures for the relief of nociceptive pain, particularly that caused by cancer, and is the author's choice of surgical procedure whenever simpler therapy fails (Tasker 1994). Whereas arguments are still presented for performing cordotomy by open techniques, in this author's opinion there are few situations where the procedure should not be performed percutaneously; in children or un-cooperative patients it can be done under general anaesthesia. (Tasker 1976, 1977, 1982*a*, 1984; Poletti 1988; Probst 1990; Isumi *et al.* 1992).

Patient selection

Success and complication rates depend so heavily upon patient selection that it is most difficult to compare data from different centres. The procedure can succeed only if patients are selected whose pain is associated with transmission in pain pathways in the cord. The most obvious example is pain resulting from continual stimulation of nociceptors in a long bone by cancer resulting in signal transmission in spino-reticulothalamic paths, known as nociceptive pain. However, the commonest pain syndrome that leads to cordotomy results from direct stimulation of the lumbosacral plexus by cancer, where nociceptors may not be involved, also a nociceptive syndrome. But cancer is not the only disease process capable of inducing nociceptive pain; non-malignant skeletal disease can do the same thing. Furthermore, pain syndromes other than nociceptive syndromes also appear to be dependent upon transmission in pain pathways. Clinical experience (Tasker *et al.* 1992) suggests that intermittent,

Table 26.3. *Differential effect of surgical procedures on different elements of central pain of spinal cord origin*

	Patients significantly relieved (%)	
Pain element	Destructive surgery[a]	Chronic stimulation[b]
Steady, causalgic dysaesthetic, aching	26	36
Intermittent shooting	89	0
Allodynia and hyperpathia	84	16

[a] Cordotomy, cordectomy, DREZ.
[b] Dorsal column, deep brain stimulation producing paraesthesiae in pain area.

neuralgic, lancinating pain, possibly caused by ectopic impulse generation at an injury site, and evoked pain (allodynia and hyperpathia) associated with central pain of cord origin are dependent upon spinothalamic transmission because they are alleviated by cordotomy as shown in Table 26.3. Laboratory work has shown that evoked pain caused by peripheral neuropathic lesions is also dependent upon spinothalamic tract transmission (Woolfe 1992) and the same may be true of central pain caused by brain lesions (Parrent *et al.* 1992). However, the commonest element in all neuropathic syndromes the constant dysaesthetic, causalgic or aching element, does not behave as if it is dependent upon transmission in pain pathways and usually does not respond to cordotomy (Tasker & Dostrovsky 1989) as is shown by our experience with cordotomy before we appreciated this fact (Table 26.4). Such constant pain responds best to chronic stimulation that induces paraesthesiae in the patient's area of pain.

These observations are contrary to the gradually developed feeling that cordotomy (and other manipulations of spinoreticulothalamic transmission) is effective for cancer but not 'benign' pain. Further, in patients with cancer, pain is most often caused by plexus compression, a nociceptive pain syndrome. However, this compression eventually damages the plexus and can add neuropathic pain to the original nociceptive type whose steady component does not respond to cordotomy (Tasker 1987, 1994). These factors complicate proper selection of patients and assessment of published experience with cordotomy.

Pain return after cordotomy

Quite apart from issues such as these, pain may still recur in the postoperative period for reasons other than inappropriate execution of the procedure (Tasker 1994): spread of disease to involve new areas, appearance of 'mirror pain', progression of cancer to induce neuropathic pain not present at the time of surgery, recurrence of neuropathic pain not recognized preoperatively, but temporarily relieved by cordotomy, and development of postcordotomy dysaesthesia.

Of these, 'mirror' pain has received some degree of recent attention leading to the conclusion that it results from opening up of existing dormant circuits in the cord

(Nathan 1956; Ventafridda *et al.* 1982; Nagaro *et al.* 1993*b*, Ischia *et al.* 1984*a*, *b*, 1985; Nagaro *et al.* 1987; Bowsher 1988; Ischia & Ischia 1988). Recent observations by Nagaro *et al.* (1993*b*) suggest that mirror pain is triggered by afferents from the painful region towards which the cordotomy was directed.

Technique

Percutaneous cordotomy can be done by the high lateral (Sweet *et al.* 1960; Mullan *et al.* 1963; Rosomoff *et al.* 1965; Gildenberg *et al.* 1969; Taren *et al.* 1969; Taren 1971; Onofrio 1971; Tasker & Organ 1973; Hitchcock & Tsukamoto 1973; Tasker *et al.* 1973; Kanpolat *et al.* 1989) high dorsal and low anterior cervical approaches (Crue *et al.* 1968; Hitchcock 1969; Lin *et al.* 1960) of which the author prefers the first (Tasker 1982*a*, 1994). Under intravenous sedation and image intensification a lumbar puncture (LP) needle is introduced into the subarachnoid space in the middle of the C1/C2 interspace and an air/positive contrast myelogram carried out to delineate the dentate ligament. A sharpened electrode insulated with Teflon tubing except for its 2-mm bare tip is then inserted through the LP needle to impale the cord (monitored by impedance) just at or anterior to the dentate ligament; 2-Hz stimulation producing contraction of ipsilateral neck muscles and 100-Hz stimulation inducing a contralateral sensation of warmth or cold complete the localization whereupon an RF lesion is made.

Results

Tables 26.4–26.6 display the author's and published incidence of pain relief and complications after unilateral and bilateral cordotomy. The methods by which different authors state their results vary and are sometimes complex so that the author apologizes for any errors incurred in converting them to these standard tables.

Complications

In the case of bilateral procedures the overall success rate is, as expected, the square of that for one side only. The complication rates follow the same algorithm except for two problems: respiratory complications and their associated mortality, and bladder decompensation, since they arise only if the related cord pathways are interrupted bilaterally. In fact, respiratory complications are the usual cause of operative mortality after percutaneous cordotomy other than that caused by progression of advanced cancer, so that mortality figures reflect the aggressiveness of the surgeon in attempting to treat cancer pain in higher-risk patients. They therefore deserve special comment. As contrasted with voluntary respiration in response to the command 'take a breath', mediated by the corticospinal tract, unconscious respiration is mediated by the strictly ipsilaterally distributed reticulospinal pathways (Nathan 1963; Belmusto *et al.* 1963; Belmusto *et al.* 1965; Hitchcock & Leece 1967; Mullan & Hosobuchi 1968; Tenicela *et al.* 1968; Rosomoff *et al.* 1969; Fox 1969). With bilateral normal lungs and reticulospinal innervation, this pathway is expendable on one side. But if the lung or phrenic nerve on one side has been damaged by, say, cancer in Pancoast syndrome, cordotomy designed

Table 26.4. *Results of percutaneous cordotomy in nociceptive and neuropathic pain*

Type of pain	Relief of the pain for which cordotomy done (%)			
	At discharge from hospital		At latest follow-up	
	Complete	Partial	Complete	Partial
Nociceptive (n = 179)	90	6	70	12
Neuropathic (n = 15)	69	8	29	43
Mixed neuropathic-nociceptive (neuropathic element, n = 40)	72	8	53	16
Mixed neuropathic-nociceptive (nociceptive element, n = 40)	79	13	73	18

Table 26.5. *Published success after unilateral percutaneous cordotomy*

Pain relief (% of patients)		References
Complete	Significant	
63		O'Connell 1969
75	96	Lorenz 1976
77	89	Grote & Roosen 1976[a]
75	83	Scröttner 1978[a]
79	—	Meglio & Cioni 1981
—	68	Kühner 1981
75	—	Lipton 1981
—	81	Ventafridda *et al.* 1982
71	82.3	Tasker 1982*a*
—	75	Siegfried *et al.* 1984
—	80	Lipton 1984
—	71	Ischia *et al.* 1984*a*
64	87	Lahuerta *et al.* 1985
76	92.5	Ischia *et al.* 1985
—	89	Farcot *et al.* 1988
74.5	87.8	Tasker 1988*b*
90, immediately		Rosomoff *et al.* 1990
84, 3 months		
61, 1 year		
43, 1–5 years		
37, 5–10 years		
64	82	Amano *et al.* 1991
	59–96	Tasker 1993 (literature review)
72	84	Tasker 1994*b*
	81.1	Ischia *et al.* 1984*b*
	38	Ventafridda *et al.* (literature review) 1982
	84 after 3 months	Rosomoff *et al.* 1990
	60 after 1 year	

[a] Mostly cancer pain and unilateral cordotomy.

Table 26.6. *Published success after bilateral percutaneous cordotomy*

Relief (% of patients)		Reference
Complete	Significant	
58	77	Rosomoff 1969
—	71.4	Tasker 1982*a*
47	59.5	Ischia *et al.* 1984*a*
76	95	Amano *et al.* 1991
	47	Tasker 1993 (literature review)

to relieve the associated pain and performed on the opposite side may sever the only remaining reticulospinal tract since the latter lies close to the spinothalamic fibres serving the cervical dermatomes in the spinal cord. Similarly, if percutaneous cordotomy has been done on one side, the reticulospinal tract may have been severed by that cordotomy exposing the patient to risk with second-sided cordotomy. The result in either case is failure of automatic respiration during sleep or distraction as in reading, often loosely referred to as 'Ondine's curse'.

One other factor controlling outcome in cordotomy is post-cordotomy dysaesthesiae. This is a central pain syndrome just like that seen after traumatic spinal cord injury, affecting unpredictably about 5% of cordotomy patients.

Comment

Percutaneous cordotomy is a very precise procedure that is highly effective for the treatment of nociceptive pain with reasonably predictable results within the above-discussed limitations. Even so, the surgically induced level of analgesia fades over years and pain recurs, sometimes capable of being relieved a second time by repeating the procedure. The mechanism of this phenomenon is unknown, spinothalamic tract regeneration never having been demonstrated in the spinal cord. The chief complications to be feared are the respiratory ones which can be avoided, and bladder decompensation and post-cordotomy dysaesthesiae that cannot.

Mesencephalic tractotomy

Indications

Whenever possible, percutaneous cordotomy should be used to treat nociceptive pain, particularly that caused by cancer. When cordotomy is contraindicated and simpler therapy is unavailable, a stereotactic procedure for the interruption of cranial pain pathways is one option, mesencephalic tractotomy and medial thalamotomy being most often employed. Frank *et al.* (1987) have compared these two operations concluding that mesencephalic tractotomy offers the better chance of pain relief (84% compared with 58% for medial thalamotomy) but at the cost of greater risk: 1.8% mortality and 10% morbidity compared with 70% transient confusion for medial thalamotomy.

Technique

Mesencephalic tractotomy which can be viewed as a cranial extension of cordotomy is performed stereotactically. Using a suitable frame, the frame xyz coordinates of the anterior (AC) and posterior (PC) commissures are calculated using the same technique as for stereotactic biopsy. With reference to a suitable atlas, (Schaltenbrand & Bailey 1959; Schaltenbrand & Wahren 1977) the probable coordinates of the spinothalamic tract are extrapolated. This is facilitated in our practice by the use of a set of sagittal diagrams generated by digitization with a personal computer from an atlas with their AC/PC lines stretched or shrunk so as to match those of the patient and ruled in stereotactic coordinates. The location of the spinothalamic tract 7–9 mm from midline is then confirmed physiologically by electrical stimulation. It is easiest to first locate the larger medial lemniscus (ML) located 10–12 mm from the midline, to which the spinothalamic tract lies dorsomedial. As the electrode is advanced in 1 to 2-mm steps from 10-mm above to up to 10 mm beyond the expected location of ML, the patient feels a sequence of contralateral somatotopographically organized paraesthesiae outlining ML. As the stimulating trajectories are moved medially and dorsally in 2-mm steps the spinothalamic tract will be traversed, heralded by a change in the effects induced by stimulation from contralateral paraesthesiae to warm, cold, painful or burning. An RF lesion is then made with a 1.1-mm electrode with a 3-mm bare tip so centred that the generated lesion will interrupt both the spinothalamic tract and the medially adjacent reticulothalamic tract (which cannot be identified easily physiologically) extending all the way to periaqueductal grey. The lesion produces contralateral dissociated sensory loss particularly in the upper quarter of the body.

Results and complications

As already stated, cancer can cause neuropathic pain particularly when it involves the brachial plexus whose steady component responds as poorly to tractotomy as it does to cordotomy. Bosch (1991) has recently reiterated this point. Failure to identify the presence of such neuropathic pain in a reported series of cancer patients makes the results difficult to evaluate.

Nevertheless mesencephalic tractotomy has also been used to treat neuropathic pain. Particularly, Schieff & Nashold (1990) have used it to treat stroke-induced central pain. Our experience, however, is that the operation is selectively effective for evoked and neuralgic elements and unsuccessful for steady pain. Since surgeons often report results in mixed series of patients with nociceptive and neuropathic pain, published data may be difficult to interpret.

There have been a number of general reviews in addition to the data cited (Nashold 1982; Pagni 1974).

Medial thalamotomy

The other regularly employed procedure for the relief of chronic pain when cordotomy is contraindicated is medial thalamotomy, a safer but less effective alternative to mesencephalic tractotomy (Frank *et al.* 1987). The rationale for its use arises out of the concept of two diencephalic pain pathways: a paucisynaptic somatotopographically organized rapidly conducting spinothalamic tract relaying to cortex via lateral thalamus, and a multisynaptic non-somatotopographically organized more slowly conducting pathway relaying through medial thalamus. Mesencephalic tractotomy may interrupt both while it is the latter to which medial thalamotomy is directed.

The original attempts to interrupt pain pathways in the thalamus were directed at the primary somatosensory pathway in the Ventrocaudal nucleus (Vc) (Monnier & Fischer 1951; Hécaen *et al.* 1949) and there has been some return to this region with more recent interest in Hassler's parvocellular portion of Vc (Vcpc) (Hassler 1972; Halliday & Logue 1981; Hitchcock & Teixeira 1981) thought to be the relay for spinothalamic tract. However, apart from this limited experience with Vcpc it was found that lesions made in medial thalamus were more effective than those in Vc and they never induced the dysesthesiae so common after Vc lesions (Ervin & Mark 1960; Mark *et al.* 1961, 1963; Mark & Ervin 1965; Mark & Tsutsumi 1974; Mark *et al.* 1960).

Technique

The procedure is performed stereotactically in the same manner as mesencephalic tractotomy except that the medial thalamic structures cannot be recognized physiologically; their stimulation usually evokes no conscious response just as lesioning them produces no clinically detectable sensory loss. The medial thalamus therefore must be localized by extrapolation. The easiest way to do this is, first, to locate and corroborate physiologically the position of the tactile relay nucleus in Vc by either stimulating to produce somatotopographically organized paraesthesiae or recording the receptive fields of tactile neurons in the contralateral body; medial thalamus is then located by extrapolation using a brain atlas. An RF lesion is then made in it as in mesencephalic tractotomy.

A major problem with medial thalamotomy, other than the inability to verify physiologically that a probe lies within the structure, or that an appropriate lesion has been made in it afterwards since no clinically detectable effect is induced, is the lack of consensus about the optimal lesion site, different surgeons choosing parafascicular, centre median, submedial, or centrolateral nuclei or else the internal thalamic lamina.

Results and complications

Though mesencephalic tractotomy and thalamotomy may be looked upon as cranial extensions of cordotomy, they are more complex procedures to perform whose results are less predictable and satisfactory than those of cordotomy. And of course, they are not the only options if cordotomy is contraindicated; particularly morphine infusion in the CSF being a viable alternative.

Their application differs from that of cordotomy in that both procedures have been more extensively used to treat neuropathic pain than cordotomy has, though their efficacy in this condition, whose main component is a steady causalgic dysaesthetic element, appears little better. Our experience with these procedures in evoked and intermittent neuralgic pain associated with neuropathic pain syndromes is similar to that with cordotomy in central cord pain though much more limited (Tasker *et al.* 1992): they selectively suppress these features of the pain better than they do the steady pain for which dorsal column stimulation (DCS) or deep brain stimulation (DBS) are best.

Dorsal column stimulation (DCS)

One of the original tenets of the Melzack–Wall Gate Theory of pain (Melzack & Wall 1965) was the notion that nociceptive pain could be suppressed by electrical stimulation of large afferent nerve fibres. Put into practice clinically using nerve stimulation (Wallesweet 1967), the new technique proved promising and was extended to dorsal cord (DCS) (Shealy *et al.* 1970) and lateral thalamic stimulation (deep brain stimulation, DBS) (Hosobuchi *et al.* 1974; Mazars *et al.* 1974). However, as experience broadened, it became plain that chronic stimulation was more effective for the relief of neuropathic than nociceptive pain (Tasker 1991) when paraesthesiae were induced in the patient's area of pain.

The two major problems with treating pain with chronic stimulation are that it is unclear by what mechanism pain is relieved and why stimulation is effective in only about half the apparently appropriate patients; of two patients with identical pain syndromes, technically successful stimulation will relieve one but not the other. For thus far it has not been possible to predict the 'winners' though our preliminary results (Tasker & Dostrovsky 1989) suggested that the latter had nervous systems susceptible to modulation by electrical stimulation in that such stimulation suppressed the late events of the somatosensory evoked potentials. Moreover, as has been mentioned above, chronic stimulation appears to be much more effective for the treatment of the steady, often causalgic or dysaesthetic, element of cord central pain than for the evoked (allodynia, hyperpathia) or neuralgic elements.

The procedure is usually done, first, by carrying out a trial of DCS in likely candidates, though some surgeons proceed directly to a permanent stimulation system. Under intravenous sedation and image intensification an epidural mono- or multipolar electrode is introduced percutaneously into the spinal epidural space at the appropriate level to achieve stimulation of the dorsal columns supplying the painful part. Or else a flat multipolar electrode is introduced at laminotomy. The patient then test stimulates for several days and a permanent system is inserted in those achieving 50% or more pain relief without unpleasant side effects. The permanent system usually consists of a multipolar electrode activated either by RF coupling or a totally implantable battery-

powered stimulator. Some surgeons use separate electrodes for testing and for permanent installation while others simply internalize the test electrode if adequate pain
relief occurs. Thus there is considerable variation in the complexity of equipment used
by different surgeons. It has been suggested that stimulation is more successful when
multipolar programmable electrodes are used since multiple choices of pole selection
are available to achieve optimal effects and in the event of electrode migration,
otherwise reoperation would be necessary. This is an important matter since electrode
migration is such a common complication of DCS.

It is difficult to assess results with DCS. Authors vary in the manner in which they
quote them. There seems to this reviewer no other way than to quote the percentage of
all patients undergoing trial stimulation who achieve significant, i.e. > 50% pain relief
over the longer term.

Most published results concern patients with neuropathic pain syndromes. However, in North America, chronic intractable back and leg pain associated with lumbar
degenerative disc disease is the commonest indication. One would have predicted that
the low back element of such pain would not, while the neuropathic leg pain in
radicular distribution should, respond to DCS. Published results by no means support
this notion though they do show that nociceptive pain caused by cancer does not
usually respond.

Deep brain stimulation (DBS)

DCS, especially using the percutaneous technique, is the most convenient, simplest
and safest manner of treating the constant element of neuropathic pain and should be
used whenever feasible because of its simplicity and low risk. Except for percutaneous
stimulation of the trigeminal nerve, peripheral nerve stimulation is more formidable
and difficult to control in this author's opinion; and this certainly applies to DBS.

Indications

The indications for DBS are, essentially, patients in whom DCS is indicated but not
technically possible, as in central pain caused by stroke and certain highly selected
cases of nociceptive pain. The former group of indications includes patients with the
appropriate part of the epidural space rendered inaccessible by previous surgery,
patients with complete or nearly complete cord lesions and some with phantom pain
or pain from massive root or nerve lesions in whom the appropriate dorsal column
fibres have died back to the dorsal column nuclei. In central pain caused by stroke, DCS
has not been effective in this author's hands even if it induces paraesthesiae in the
painful part of the body. In patients with complete or post-ganglionic trigeminal
lesions in whom trigeminal stimulation is ineffective in producing facial paraesthesiae,
DBS is the only alternative. If DCS produces paraesthesiae in the patient's area of pain
but fails to relieve the pain, DBS is usually also unsuccessful.

Based on the work of Reynolds (Reynolds 1969; Mayer & Price 1976), Richardson &

Akil (1977a,b) pioneered the use of DBS of the periventricular grey (PVG) for pain relief, presumably activating the descending serotoninergic path from nucleus raphe magnus that blocks access of nociceptive impulses into the spinothalamic tract in the cord. On basic principles one would predict that such stimulation would be effective for those types of pain that were dependent upon transmission in spinoreticulothalamic tract.

Thus, a dichotomy was proposed: DBS in the lemniscal system to produce paraesthesiae in the area of pain for the constant dysaesthetic causalgic element of neuropathic pain and PVG stimulation for nociceptive pain (and, according to our experience, allodynia, hyperpathia and the neuralgic elements of neuropathic pain (Tasker *et al.* 1992; Parrent *et al.* 1992). This concept led to Hosobuchi's use of the morphine screening test. In cancer pain where it may be difficult to rationalize the expense of a permanent DBS system, Meyerson and his associates (Meyerson *et al.* 1978) have shown that transcutaneous PVG stimulation can be carried on safely in the long term.

Neat as it seems, there is no consensus on this concept of a DBS dichotomy, many surgeons finding that either type of stimulation may be effective in either class of pain syndrome (Richardson & Akil 1977a,b, 1982; Hosobuchi *et al.* 1977; Gybels 1990; Ray & Burton 1980; Richardson 1982a,b; Amano *et al.* 1982; Boivie & Meyerson 1982; Young *et al.* 1985; Tsubokawa *et al.* 1985, 1986; Young & Brechner 1987; Young & Chambi 1985; Levy *et al.* 1987; Hosobuchi 1988; Meyerson 1988; Barbaro 1988 and suggesting that multiple descending inhibitory paths exist).

Young *et al.* (1993) however, showed significant rises in ventricular endorphin and met-encephalin during PVG but not lateral thalamic stimulation, tending to support the dichotomy. Moreover, the changes they saw in endorphins correlated with the patient's pain reduction characterized on a visual analogue scale.

Finally, though Richardson & Akil (1977a,b) originally reported that, though stimulation in both PVG and periaqueductal grey (PAG) could relieve pain, stimulation in PAG was too unpleasant to be exploited for pain relief. Not all observers have confirmed this fact; some use PAG stimulation preferentially (Young & Brechner 1987; Young & Chambi 1985; Young *et al.* 1985).

These issues not only cloud the matter of patient selection for DBS at the two sites but also the evaluation of results. Many authors do not, or do not feel it is important to, distinguish results in patients with neuropathic or nociceptive pain in their reported series, and may present data derived from mixed groups of patients with DBS that produces paraesthesiae and that in PVG-PAG or both. Whether because electrodes are rarely implanted there in these patients, or because of pathophysiological reasons, paraesthesiae-inducing DBS is rarely successful in patients with cancer pain.

Finally, the commonest indicator for DBS in North America is 'failed back' pain syndrome which may consist of a mixture of nociceptive and neuropathic pain syndromes for which stimulation at either the medial or lateral site or both may be appropriate.

Technique

The procedure is performed stereotactically as for mesencephalic tractotomy. The coordinates of AC and PC are determined with CT or MR and the locations of stimulation sites selected with reference to an atlas and the positions of AC and PC. Many surgeons choose a site in medial parafascicular nucleus for their PVG stimulation site, commonly 2–5 mm rostral to PC on the AC/PC line 2 mm lateral to the third ventricular wall. Though sometimes its position can be confirmed physiologically this is not consistently the case so that purely anatomical localization is most often used.

A site to produce localized paraesthesiae is usually located in Vc, for wider body areas in medial lemniscus. These sites are first selected on anatomical grounds as for PVG and then confirmed physiologically as described in medial thalamotomy. When an appropriate site (or sites) is located, a suitable chronic stimulating electrode with multiple poles is advanced to the site, locked in place and attached to a percutaneous extension. The latter is tunnelled under the scalp to a suitable locus where it is brought out through the skin for a period of trial stimulation. When successful trial stimulation is completed, the percutaneous lead is discarded and the electrode attached to either a battery-powered totally programmable or a radiofrequency-coupled stimulating device, otherwise electrodes are removed.

Results and complications

Paraesthesiae-producing DBS and that in PVG-PAG have been reviewed. It seems clear that the former is ineffective in the nociceptive pain of cancer. Few data have accumulated with PVG-PAG stimulation in undoubted neuropathic pain syndromes, most surgeons appearing to have used paraesthesiae-inducing DBS for this, extending the doctrine of DCS cephalad. Since the largest single group of patients treated with the technique – the 'failed back group' suffers from pain of mixed types, in which either type of DBS may be effective, this may be the reason that no consensus has been reached in the use of the two techniques. Even in central pain syndromes caused by stroke, we have found PVG stimulation preferentially useful for allodynia, hyperpathia and neuralgic pain, paraesthesiae-producing DBS often being unpleasant in the presence of evoked pain.

References

Amano, K., Tanikawa, T., Kawamura, H. *et al.* (1986*a*). Endorphin and pain relief: further observations on electrical stimulation of the periaqueductal gray matter during rostral mesencephalic reticulotomy for pain relief. *Appl. Neurophysiol.* **45**, 123.

Amano, K., Kawamura, H., Tanikawa, T. *et al.* (1986*b*). Long-term follow-up study of rostral mesencephalic reticulotomy for pain relief: report of 34 cases. *Appl. Neurophysiol.* **49**, 105.

Amano, K., Kawamura, H., Tanikawa, T., Kawabatake, H., Iseki, H., Iwataw, Y. & Taira, T. (1991). Bilateral versus unilateral percutaneous high cervical cordotomy as a surgical method of pain relief. *Acta Neurochir.* **52** (Suppl.), 143–5.

Askenasy, H. M. & Levinger, M. (1968). Stereoencephalotomy for relief of pain. *Harefuah* 74, 85–9.

Auleroche, P. (1983). Innervation of the zygoapophyseal joints of the lumbar spine. *Anat. Clin.* 5, 17–28.

Barbaro, N. M. (1988). Studies of PAG/PVG stimulation for pain relief in humans. In *Progress in Brain Research*, vol. 77, eds. H. L. Fields & J. M. Besson, pp. 165–73. Amsterdam: Elsevier.

Belmusto, L., Brown, E. & Owens, G. (1963). Clinical observations on respiratory and vasomotor disturbances as related to cervical cordotomies. *J. Neurosurg.* 20, 225–32.

Belmusto, L., Woldring, S. & Owens, G. (1965). Localization and patterns of potentials of the respiratory pathways in the cervical spinal cord in the dog. *J. Neurosurg.* 22, 277–83.

Bettag, W. & Yoshida, I. (1967). Über stereotaktische Schmerzoperationen. *Acta Neurochirurg.* 8, 299–317.

Boas, R. A. (1982). Facet joint injections. In *Chronic Low Back Pain*, eds. M. Stanton-Hicks & R. Boas, pp. 199–211. New York: Raven Press.

Bogduk, N., Wilson, A. S. & Tynan, W. (1982). The human dorsal rami. *J. Anat.* 134, 383–97.

Boivie, J. & Meyerson, B. A. (1982). A correlative anatomic and clinical study of pain suppressed by deep brain stimulation. *Pain* 13, 113.

Bosch, D. A. (1991). Stereotactic rostral mesencephalotomy in cancer pain and deafferentation pain: a series of 40 cases with follow-up results. *J. Neurosurg.* 75, 747–51.

Bowsher, D. (1988). Contralateral mirror-image pain following anterolateral cordotomy. *Pain* 33, 63–5.

Bulacio, E. N., Pozzetti, A. & Barros, M. (1972). Dolor crónico Effectos de lesiones en nucleos centro-medianus y parafascicularis. *Buenos Aires Medet.* 32, 363–72.

Burton, C. V. (1976). Percutaneous radiofrequency facet denervation. *Appl. Neurophysiol.* 39, 80–6.

Cooper, I. S. (1972). Clinical and physiologic implications of the thalamic surgery for disorders of sensory communication. Thalamic surgery for intractable pain. *J. Neurol. Sci.* 2, 493–519.

Crue, B. L., Todd, E. M. & Carregal, E. J. A. (1968). Posterior approach for high cervical percutaneous radiofrequency cordotomy. *Confin. Neurol.* 30, 41–52.

Demierre, B. & Siegfried, J. (1983). Traitement neurochirurgicale de la neuralgie postherpetiform. *Med. Hyg.* 41, 1960.

de Montreuil, C. B., Lajat, Y., Resche, F. *et al.* (1983). Apport de la neurochirurgie stereotaxique dans le traitement des algies des cancers cervico-faciaux. *Ann. Otolaryngol. Chir. Cervicofac.* 100, 181.

Dunsker, S. B., Wood, M., Lotspeich, E. S. & Maysfield, E. E. (1977). Percutaneous electrocoagulation of lumbar articular nerves. In *Pain Management*, ed. J. F. Lee, pp. 123–127. Baltimore: Williams and Wilkins.

Ervin, F. R. & Mark, V. H. (1960). Stereotactic thalamotomy in the human. II. Physiologic observations on the human thalamus. *Arch. Neurol.* 3, 368–80.

Fairman, D. (1967). Unilateral thalamic tractotomy for the relief of bilateral pain in malignant tumours. *Confin. Neurol.* 29, 146–58.

Fairman, D. (1972). Hypothalamotomy as a new perspective for alleviation of intractable pain and regression of metastatic malignant tumours. In *Present Limits of Neurosurgery*, eds. I. Fusek & Z. Kune, pp. 525–8. Prague: Avicenum.

Fairman, D. & Llavallol, M. A. (1973). Thalamic tractotomy for the alleviation of intractable pain in cancer. *Cancer* 31, 700–7.

Farcot, J.-M., Mercky, F., Tritschler, J.-L. & Schaeffer, F. (1988). Cordotomies cervicales percutanées dans les douleurs cancéreuses thoraciques primitives ou secondaires (à propos de 19 cas). *Agressologie* **29**, 87–9.

Frank, F., Tognetti, F., Gaist, G. *et al.* (1982). Stereotaxic rostral mesencephalotomy in treatment of malignant faciothoracobrachial pain syndromes. *J. Neurosurg.* **56**, 807.

Frank, F., Fabrizi, A. P. & Gaist, G. (1989). Stereotaxic mesencephalic tractotomy in the treatment of chronic cancer pain. *Acta Neurochir. (Wien)* **99**, 38–40.

Frank, F., Fabrizi, A. P., Gaist, G. *et al.* (1987). Stereotaxic lesions in the treatment of chronic pain syndromes: mesencephalotomy versus multiple thalamotomies in the treatment of chronic cancer pain syndromes. *Appl. Neurophysiol.* **50**, 314.

Forster, D. M. C., Leksell, L., Meyerson, B. A. & Steiner, L. (1979). Gamma thalamotomy in intractable pain. In *Pain: Basic Principles – Pharmacology –Therapy*, eds. R. Janzen *et al.*, pp. 194–198. Stuttgart: Thieme.

Fox, J. L. (1969). Localization of the respiratory pathway in the upper cervical spinal cord following percutaneous cordotomy. *Neurology* **19**, 1115–18.

Fox, J. L. & Rizzoli, H. V. (1973). Identification of radiological coordinates for the posterior articular nerve of Luschka in the lumbar spine. *Surg. Neurol.* **1**, 343–6.

Gildenberg, P. L., Zanes, C., Flitter, M. A., Lin, R. M. & Lautsch, E. V. (1969). Impedance monitoring device for detection of penetration of the spinal cord in anterior percutaneous cervical cordotomy. Technical note. *J. Neurosurg.* **30**, 87–92.

Gioia, D. F., Wallace, P. B., Fuste, F. J. *et al.* (1967). A stereotaxic method of surgery for the relief of intractable pain. *Int. Surg.* **48**, 409.

Green, J. R., Kanshepolsky, J. & Turkian, B. (1974). Incidence and significance of central nervous system infections in neurosurgical patients. *Adv. Neurol.* **6**, 223.

Groen, G. J., Baljet, B., Drukker, J. (1990). Nerves and nerve plexuses of the human vertebral column. *Am. J. Anat.* **188**, 282–96.

Grote, W., Roosen, C. W. (1976). Die percutane Chordotomie. *Langebecks Archiv. fur. Chirurgie.* **342**, 101–8.

Gybels, J. (1977). Electrical stimulation of the brain for pain control in humans. *Verh. Dtsch. Ges. Inn. Med.* **86**, 1553.

Gybels, J. M. (1991). Indications for the use of neurosurgical techniques in pain control. In *Proceedings of the VIth World Congress on Pain*, eds. M. R. Bond, J. E. Charlton & C. J. Woolf, pp. 475–82. Amsterdam: Elsevier.

Gybels, J. & Kuipers, R. (1990). Deep brain stimulation in the treatment of chronic pain in man: where and why? *Neurophysiol. Clin.* **20**, 389–98.

Gybels, J. M. & Sweet, W. H. (1989). *Stereotactic Mesencephalotomy: Neurosurgical Treatment of Persistent Pain*, pp. 210–19. Basel: Karger.

Halliday, A. M. & Logue, V. (1981). Painful sensations evoked by electrical stimulation in the thalamus. In *Neurophysiology Studied in Man*, ed. G. G. Somjen, pp. 221–30. Amsterdam: Excerpta Medica.

Hassler, R. (1972). The division of pain conduction into systems of pain sensation and pain awareness. In *Pain: Basic Principles – Pharmacology –Therapy*, eds. R. Janzen *et al.*, pp. 98–112. Stuttgart: Thieme.

Hassler, R. & Riechert, T. (1959). Klinische und anatomische Befunde bei stereotaktischen Schmerzoperationen im Thalamus. *Arch. Psychiatr. Nervenkrankh.* **200**, 93–122.

Heimburger, R. F., Campbell, R. L., Kalsbeck, J. E., Mealey, J. Jr. & Goodill, C. L. (1966). Positive contrast roentgenography using water soluble media. *J. Neurol. Neurosurg. Psychiatry* **29**, 281–90.

Hécaen, H., Talairach, J., David, M. & Dell, M. B. (1949). Coagulations limitées du thalamus dans les algies du syndrome thalamique. *Rev. Neurol. (Paris)* **81**, 917–31.

Hitchcock, E. R. (1969). An apparatus for stereotactic spinal surgery. A preliminary report. *J. Neurosurg.* **31**, 386–92.

Hitchcock, E. R. & Leece, B. (1967). Somatotopic representation of the respiratory pathways in the cervical cord of man. *J. Neurosurg.* **27**, 320–9.

Hitchcock, E. R. & Teixeira, M. J. A. (1981). A comparison of results from center-median and basal thalamotomies for pain. *Surg. Neurol.* **15**, 341–51.

Hitchcock, E. R. & Tsukamoto, Y. (1973). Distal and proximal sensory responses during stereotactic spinal tractotomy in man. *Ann. Clin. Res.* **5**, 68–73.

Hood, T. W. & Yap, J. C. (1981). A survey of infections in stereotactic surgery. *Appl. Neurophysiol.* **44**, 314–19.

Hosobuchi, Y. (1988). Analgesia induced by brain stimulation with chronically implanted electrodes. In *Operative Neurosurgical Techniques, Indications, Methods and Results*, 2nd edn., eds. H. H. Schmidek & W. H. Sweet, pp. 1089–1095. New York: Grune and Stratton.

Hosobuchi, Y. (1986). Subcortical electrical stimulation for control of intractable pain in humans. *J. Neurosurg.* **64**, 543–53.

Hosobuchi, Y., Adams, J. E. & Linchitz, R. (1977). Pain relief by electrical stimulation of the central gray matter in humans and its reversal by naloxone. *Science* **179**, 181.

Hosobuchi, Y., Adams, J. E. & Fields, H. L. (1974). Chronic thalamic and internal capsule stimulation for the control of facial anesthesia dolorosa and the dysesthesia of thalamic syndrome. In *Advances in Neurology*, vol. 4, ed. J. J. Bonica, pp. 783–7. New York: Raven Press.

Ischia, S. & Ischia, A. (1988). A mechanism of new pain following cordotomy (letter). *Pain* **32**, 383–4.

Ischia, S., Ischia, A., Luzzani, A., Toscano, D. & Steele, A. (1985). Results up to death in the treatment of persistent cervico-thoracic (Pancoast) and thoracic malignant pain by unilateral percutaneous cervical cordotomy. *Pain* **21**, 339–55.

Ischia, S., Luzzani, A., Ischia, A. & Maffezzoli, G. (1984a). Bilateral percutaneous cervical cordotomy immediate and long-term results in 36 patients with neoplastic disease. *J. Neurol. Neurosurg. Psychiatry* **47**, 141–7.

Ischia, S., Luzzani, A., Ischia, A., Magon, E. & Toscano, D. (1984b). Subarachnoid neurolytic block (L5–S1) and unilateral percutaneous cervical cordotomy in the treatment of pain secondary to pelvic malignant disease. *Pain* **20**, 139–49.

Ischia, S., Luzzani, A., Ischia, A. & Pacini, L. (1984c). Role of unilateral percutaneous cervical cordotomy in the treatment of neoplastic vertebral pain. *Pain* **19**, 123–31.

Izumi, J., Hirose, Y. & Yazaki, T. (1992). Percutaneous trigeminal rhizotomy and percutaneous cordotomy under general anesthesia. *Stereotact. Funct. Neurosurg.* **59**, 62–8.

Jannetta, P. J., Gildenberg, P. L., Loeser, J. D., Sweet, W. H. & Ojemann, G. A. (1990). Operations on the brain and brainstem for chronic pain. In *The Management of Pain*, 2nd edn, ed. J. J. Bonica, pp. 2082–103. Philadelphia: Lea and Febiger.

Johnson, I. (1974). Radiofrequency percutaneous facet rhizotomy. *J. Neurosurg. Nurs.* **6**, 92–6.

Kanpolat, Y., Deda, H., Akyar, S. & Bilgic, S. (1989). CT-guided percutaneous cordotomy. *Acta Neurochir. Suppl.* **46**, 67–8.

Koning, H. M., Koster, H. G. & Niemeijer, R. P. (1991). Ischaemic spinal cord lesion following percutaneous radiofrequency spinal rhizotomy. *Pain* **45**, 161–6.

Koulousakas, A. & Nittner, K. (1982). Bilateral C1–C2 cordotomies. Can complications be avoided? *Appl. Neurophysiol.* **45**, 500–3.

Kudo, T., Yoshii, N. & Shimizu, S. (1968). Stereotaxic surgery for pain relief. *J. Exp. Med.* **96**, 219–34.

Kühner, A. (1981). La cordotomie percutanée. Sa place actuelle dans la chirurgie de la douleur. *Anesth. Analg.* **38**, 357–9.

Kumar, K., Wyant, S. M. & Nath, R. (1990). Deep brain stimulation for control of intractable pain in humans, present and future: a ten-year follow-up. *Neurosurgery* **26**, 774–82.

Lahuerta, T., Lipton, S. & Wells, J. C. D. (1985). Percutaneous cervical cordotomy: results and complications in a recent series of 100 patients. *Ann. R. Coll. Surg. Engl.* **67**, 41–4.

Leksell, L., Meyerson, B. A. & Forster, D. M. C. (1972). Radiosurgical thalamotomy for intractable pain. *Confin. Neurol.* **34**, 264.

Lenz, F. A., Dostrovsky, J. O., Kwan, H. C., Tasker, R. R., Yamashiro, K. & Murphy, J. T. (1988*a*). Methods for microstimulation and recording of single neurons and evoked potentials in the human central nervous system. *J. Neurosurg.* **68**, 630–4.

Lenz, F. A., Dostrovsky, J. O., Tasker, R. R., Yamashiro, K., Kwan, H. C. & Murphy, J. T. (1988*b*). Single-unit analyses in the human ventral thalamic nuclear group: somatosensory responses. *J. Neurophysiol.* **59**, 299–316.

Levy, R. M., Lamb, S. & Adams, J. E. (1987). Treatment of chronic pain by deep brain stimulation: long-term follow-up and review of the literature. *Neurosurgery* **21**, 885.

Lin, R. M., Gildenberg, P. L. & Polakoff, P. P. (1960). An anterior approach to percutaneous lower cervical cordotomy. *J. Neurosurg.* **25**, 553–60.

Lipton, S. (1978). Percutaneous cervical cordotomy and the injection of the pituitary with alcohol. *Anaesthesia* **33**, 953–7.

Lipton, S. (1981). Percutaneous cervical cordotomy. *Acta Anaesthesiol. Belg.* **32**, 81–5, with additional personal communication.

Lipton, S. (1984). Percutaneous cordotomy. In *Textbook of Pain*, eds. P. D. Wall & R. Melzack, pp. 632–8. Edinburgh: Churchill Livingstone.

Lora, J. & Long, D. (1976). So-called facet denervation in the management of intractable back pain. *Spine* **1**, 121–6.

Lorenz, R. (1976). Methods of percutaneous spinothalamic tract section In, *Advances and Technical Standards in Neurosurgery*, vol. 3, ed. H. Krayenbühl, pp. 123–145. Vienna: Springer.

Mark, V. H. & Ervin, F. R. (1965). Role of thalamotomy in treatment of chronic severe pain. *Postgrad. Med.* **35**, 563–71.

Mark, V. H. & Tsutsumi, H. (1974). The suppression of pain by intrathalamic lidocaine. In *Advances in Neurology*, vol. 4, ed. J. J. Bonica, pp. 715–21. New York: Raven Press.

Mark, V. H., Ervin, F. R., Hackett, T. P. (1960). Clinical aspects of stereotactic thalamotomy in the human. I. The treatment of chronic severe pain. *Arch. Neurol.* **3**, 351–67.

Mark, V. H., Ervin, F. R. & Yakovlev, P. I. (1961). Correlation of pain relief, sensory loss, and anatomical lesion sites in pain patients treated by stereotactic thalamotomy. *Trans. Am. Neurol. Assoc.* **86**, 86–90.

Mark, V. H., Ervin, F. R. & Yakovlev, P. (1963). Stereotactic thalamotomy. III. The verification of anatomical lesion sites in the human thalamus. *Arch. Neurol.* **8**, 78–88.

Marks, P. V. (1993). Stereotactic surgery for post-traumatic cerebellar syndrome: an analysis of seven cases. *Stereotact. Funct. Neurosurg.* **60**, 157–67.

Marks, R. (1989). Distribution of pain provoked from lumbar facet joints and related structures during diagnostic spinal infiltration. *Pain* **39**, 37–40.

Marks, R. C., Houston, T. & Thulbourne, T. (1992). Facet joint injection and facet nerve block: a randomized comparison in 86 patients with chronic low back pain. *Pain* **49**, 325–8.

Mayer, D. J. & Price, P. D. (1976). Central nervous system mechanisms of analgesia. *Pain* 2, 379–404.

Mazars, G. L., Merienne, L. & Ciolocca, C. (1974). Treatment of certain types of pain by implantable thalamic stimulators. *Neurochirurgie* 29, 117–24.

Mazars, G., Pansini, A., Chiarelli, J. (1960*a*). Coagulation du faisceau spino-thalamique et du faisceau quinto-thalamique par stéréotaxie: Indications: résultats. *Acta Neurochir.* 8, 324.

Mazars, G., Roge, R. & Pansini, A. (1960*b*). Stereotactic coagulation of the spinothalamic tract for intractable trigeminal pain (abstract). *J. Neurol. Neurosurg. Psychiatry* 23, 352.

McCulloch, J. A. (1976). Percutaneous radiofrequency lumbar rhizolysis (rhizotomy). *Appl. Neurophysiol.* 39, 87–96.

McCulloch, J. A. & Organ, L. W. (1977). Percutaneous radiofrequency lumbar rhizolysis. *Can. Med. Assoc. J.* 116, 300–11.

Meglio, M., Cioni, B. (1981). The role of percutaneous cordotomy in the treatment of chronic cancer pain. *Acta Neurochir.* 59, 111–21.

Mehta, M. & Sluijter, M. E. (1979). The treatment of chronic back pain. *Anesthesia* 34, 768–75.

Melzack, R. & Wall, P. D. (1965). Pain mechanisms: a new theory. *Science* 150, 971–9.

Meyerson, B. A. (1980). Aspects on the present state of intracerebral stimulation for pain. In *Brain Stimulation and Neuronal Plasticity*, ed. T. Tsubokawa, p. 33. Tokyo: Neuron.

Meyerson, B. A. (1988). Problems and controversies in PVG stimulation and sensory thalamic stimulation as treatment for pain. In *Progress in Brain Research* 77, eds. H. L. Fields & J. M. Besson, pp. 175–88. Amsterdam: Elsevier.

Meyerson, B. A., Boëthius, J. & Carlsson, A. M. (1978). Percutaneous central gray stimulation for cancer pain. *Appl. Neurophysiol.* 41, 57–65.

Monnier, M., Fischer, R. (1951). Localisation, stimulation et coagulation du thalamus chez l'homme. *J. Physiol.* 43, 818.

Mullan, S. & Hosobuchi, Y. (1968). Respiratory hazards of high cervical percutaneous cordotomy. *J. Neurosurg.* 28, 291–7.

Mullan, S., Harper, P. V., Hekmatpanah, J., Torres, H. & Dobbin, G. (1963). Percutaneous interruption of the spinal pain tract by means of a strontium 90 needle. *J. Neurosurg.* 20, 931–9.

Mundinger, F. (1974). Stereotaktische Operationen gegen anderweitig unbehandelbar schwere Schmerz-zustände. *Z. Allgemeinmed.* 50, 860–4.

Nagaro, T., Kimura, S. & Arai, T. (1987). A mechanism of new pain following cordotomy; reference of sensation. *Pain* 30, 89–91.

Nagaro, T., Amakawa, K., Arai, T. & Ochi, G. (1993*a*). Ipsilateral referral of pain following cordotomy. *Pain* 275–6.

Nagaro, T., Amakawa, K., Kimura, S. & Arai, T. (1993*b*). Reference of pain following percutaneous cervical cordotomy. *Pain* 53, 205–11.

Nash, T. P. (1990). Facet joints. Intra-articular steroids or nerve block. *Pain Clin.* 3, 77–82.

Nashold, B. S. Jr (1982). Brainstem stereotaxic procedures. In Stereotaxy of the Human Brain. Anatomical Physiological and Clinical Applications, eds. G. Schaltenbrand & A. E. Walker, pp. 475–83. Stuttgart: Thieme.

Nathan, P. W. (1956). Reference of sensation at the spinal level. *J. Neurol. Neurosurg. Psychiatry* 19, 88–100.

Nathan, P. W. (1963). The descending respiratory pathway in man. *J. Neurol. Neurosurg. Psychiatry* 26, 487–99.

Niizuma, H., Kwak, R., Saso, S. *et al.* (1980). Follow-up results of center median thalatomy for central pain. *Appl. Neurophysiol.* 43, 336.

O'Connell, J. E. A. (1969). Anterolateral chordotomy for intractable pain in carcinoma of the rectum. *Proc. R. Soc. Med.* **62**, 31–3, 1223–5.

Onofrio, B. M. (1971). Cervical spinal cord and dentate delineation in percutaneous radiofrequency cordotomy at the level of the first to second cervical vertebrae. *Surg. Gynecol. Obstet.* **133**, 30–4.

Orthner, H. & von Koeder, F. (1966). Further clinical and anatomical experiences with stereotactic operations for relief of pain. *Confin. Neurol.* **27**, 418–30.

Oudenhoven, R. C. (1974). Articular rhizotomy. *Surg. Neurol.* **2**, 275–8.

Pagni, C. A. (1974). Place of stereotactic technique in surgery for pain. In *Advances in Neurology*, vol. 4, ed. J. J. Bonica, pp. 699–706. New York: Raven Press.

Palma, A., Hozer, J., Cuadra, O. & Palma, J. (1988). Lateral percutaneous spinothalamic tractotomy. *Acta Neurochir.* **93**, 100–3.

Papadakis, N. & Mark, V. H. (1980). Intermittent decortication and progressive hyperthermia, hypertension and tachycardia following methylglucamine iothalamate ventriculogram. *Appl. Neurophysiol.* **43**, 59–66.

Parrent, A., Lozano, A., Tasker, R. R. & Dostrovsky, J. (1992). Periventricular gray stimulation suppresses allodynia and hyperpathia in man. *Stereotact. Funct. Neurosurg.* **59**, 82.

Pedersen, H. E., Blunck, C. F. J. & Gardner, E. (1956). The anatomy of lumbosacral posterior rami and meningeal branches of spinal nerves (sinu-vertebral nerves) with an experimental study of their functions. *J. Bone Joint Surg.* **38A**, 377.

Poletti, C. E. (1988). Open cordotomy medullary tractomy. In *Operative Neurosurgical Techniques: Indications, Methods and Results*, 2nd edn, eds. H. H. Schmidek & W. H. Sweet, pp. 1155–68. Orlando: Grune and Stratton.

Probst, C. L. (1990). Microsurgical cordotomy in 20 patients with epi/intradural fibrosis following operation for lumbar disc herniation. *Acta Neurochir.* **107**, 30–6.

Ray, C. D. & Burton, C. V. (1980). Deep brain stimulation for severe chronic pain. *Acta Neurochirurgica* **30** (Suppl.), 289–93.

Rees, W. E. S. (1971). Multiple bilateral subcutaneous rhizolysis of segmental nerves in the treatment of the inter-vertebral disc syndrome. *Ann. Gen. Pract.* **26**, 126–7.

Reynolds, D. V. (1969). Surgery in the rat during electrical analgesia induced by frontal brain stimulation. *Science* **164**, 444–5.

Richardson, D. E. (1974a). Recent advances in the neurosurgical control of pain. *South. Med. J.* **60**, 1082–6.

Richardson, D. E. (1974b). Thalamotomy for control of chronic pain. *Acta Neurochirurgica* **21** (Suppl.), 77–88.

Richardson, D. E. (1982a). Long-term follow-up of deep brain stimulation for relief of chronic pain in the human. In *Modern Neurology*, ed. M. Brock, pp. 449–53. Berlin: Springer-Verlag.

Richardson, D. E. (1982b). Analgesia produced by stimulation of various sites in the human beta-endorphin system. *Appl. Neurophysiol.* **45**, 116.

Richardson, D. E. & Akil, H. (1977a). Pain reduction by electrical brain stimulation in man. I. Acute administration in periacqueductal and periventricular sites. *J. Neurosurg.* **47**, 178–83.

Richardson, D. E. & Akil, H. (1977b). Long-term results of periventricular gray self-stimulation. *Neurosurgery* **1**, 200.

Richardson, D. E. & Akil, H. (1982). Pain reduction by electrical brain stimulation in man. II. Chronic self-administraion in periventricular gray matter. *J. Neurosurg.* **47**, 184.

Rosomoff, H. L. (1969). Bilateral percutaneous radiofrequency cordotomy. *J. Neurosurg.* **31**, 41–6.

Rosomoff, H. L., Carroll, E., Brown, J. & Sheptak, P. (1965). Percutaneous radiofrequency cervical cordotomy; technique. *J. Neurosurg.* **23**, 639–44.

Rosomoff, H. L., Krieger, A. J. & Kuperman, A. S. (1969). Effects of percutaneous cervical cordotomy on pulmonary function. *J. Neurosurg.* **31**, 620–7.

Rosomoff, H. L., Papo, I., Loeser, J. D. & Bonica, J. J. (1990). Neurosurgical operations on the spinal cord. In *The Management of Pain*, 2nd edn, ed. J. J. Bonica, pp. 2067–81. Philadelphia: Lea & Febiger.

Sano, K. (1977). Intralaminar thalamotomy (thalamolaminotomy) and posterior hypothalamotomy in the treatment of intractable pain. In *Progress in Neurological Surgery*, vol. 8, eds. J. Krayenbühl, P. E. Maspes & W. H. Sweet, pp. 50–103. Basel: Karger.

Sano, K. (1979). Stereotaxic thalamolaminotomy and posteromedial hypothalamotomy for the relief of intractable pain. In *Advances in Pain Research and Therapy*, vol. 2, eds. J. J. Bonica & V. Ventafridda, pp. 475–85. New York: Raven Press.

Sano, K., Yoshioka, M., Ogashiwa, M. *et al.* (1966). Thalamolaminotomy: a new operation for relief of intractable pain. *Confin. Neurol.* **27**, 63–6.

Sano, K., Yoshioka, M., Sekino, H. *et al.* (1970). Functional organization of the internal medullary lamina in man. *Confin. Neurol.* **32**, 374–80.

Savitz, M. H. (1991). Percutaneous radiofrequency rhizotomy of the lumbar facets: ten years' experience. *Mt Sinai J. Med.* **58**, 177–8.

Schaltenbrand, G. & Bailey, P. (1959). *Introduction to Stereotaxis with an Atlas of the Human Brain.* Stuttgart: Thieme.

Schaltenbrand, G., Wahren, W. (1977). *Atlas for Stereotaxy of the Human Brain*, 2nd edn, Stuttgart: Thieme.

Schröttner, O. (1978). Die perkutane zervikale anterolaterale Chordotomie. *Wien. Klin. Wochenschr.* **90**, 372–4.

Shealy, C. N. (1975). Percutaneous radiofrequency denervation of spinal facets. *J. Neurosurg.* **43**, 448–51.

Shealy, C. N., Mortimer, J. T. & Hagfors, N. R. (1970). Dorsal column electroanalgesia. *J. Neurosurg.* **32**, 560–4.

Shieff, C. & Nashold, B. S. Jr (1990). Stereotactic mesencephalotomy. In *Neurosurgery Clinics of North America*, ed. W. A. Friedman, pp. 825–59. Philadelphia: Saunders.

Siegfried, J. (1991). Therapeutic neurostimulation. *Acta Neurochir.* **52** (Suppl.), 112–17.

Siegfried, J., Kühner, A. & Sturm, V. (1984). Neurosurgical treatment of cancer pain. Recent results. *Cancer Res.* **89**, 148–55.

Silvers, H. R. (1990). Lumbar percutaneous facet rhizotomy. *Spine* **15**, 36–40.

Sluijter, M. E. (1981). Percutaneous facet denervation and partial posterior rhizotomy. *Acta Anaesthesiol. Belg.* **1**, 63–79.

Sluijter, M. E., Dingemans, W. A., Barendse, G. A. & Van Kleef, M. (1991). Comment on ischaemic spinal cord lesion following percutaneous radiofrequency spinal rhizotomy. *Pain* **47**, 241–2.

Spiegel, E. A. & Wycis, H. T. (1953). Mesencephalotomy in treatment of "intractable" facial pain. *AMA Arch. Neurol. Psychiatry* **69**, 1.

Spiegel, E. A. & Wycis, H. T. (1962). *Stereoencephalotomy: II. Clinical and Physiological Applications.* New York: Grune and Stratton.

Spiegel, E. A. & Wycis, H. T. (1962). *Stereoencephalotomy*, part II, *Clinical and Physiological Applications.* Monographs in Biology and Medicine, New York: Grune & Stratton.

Spiller, W. G. & Martin, E. (1912). The treatment of persistent pain of organic origin in the lower part of the body by division of the anterolateral column of the spinal cord. *JAMA* **58**, 1489–90.

Steiner, L., Forster, D., Leksell, L. *et al.* (1972). Gammathalamotomy in intractable pain. *Acta Neurochir.* **52**, 173–84.

Stolker, R. J., Vervest, A. C. M. & Groen, G. J. (1994). The management of chronic spinal pain by blockades: a review. *Pain* **58**, 1–20.

Sugita, K., Musuga, N., Takaoka, Y. & Doi, T. (1972). Results of stereotaxic thalamotomy for pain. *Confin. Neurol.* **34**, 265–74.

Sweet, W. H., Mark, V. H. & Hamlin, H. (1960). Radiofrequency lesions in the central nervous system of man and cat: including case reports of eight bulbar pain-tract interruptions. *J. Neurosurg.* **17**, 213–25.

Taren, J. A. (1971). Physiologic corroboration in stereotactic high cervical cordotomy. *Confin. Neurol.* **33**, 285–90.

Taren, J. A., Davis, R. & Crosby, E. C. (1969). Target physiologic corroboration in stereotactic cervical cordotomy. *J. Neurosurg.* **30**, 569–84.

Tasker, R. R. (1965). Simple localization for stereoencephalotomy using the 'portable' central beam of the image intensifier. *Confin. Neurol.* **26**, 209.

Tasker, R. R. (1976). The merits of percutaneous cordotomy over the open operation. In *Current Controversies in Neurosurgery*, ed. T. P. Morley, pp. 496–501. Philadelphia: Saunders.

Tasker, R. R. (1977). Open cordotomy. In *Progress in Neurological Surgery. Pain, Its Neurosurgical Management*, Part 11, vol. 8, eds. H. Krayenbühl, P. E. Maspes & W. H. Sweet, pp. 1–4. Basel: Karger.

Tasker, R. R. (1982*a*). Percutaneous cordotomy: the lateral high cervical technique. In *Operative Neurosurgical Techniques. Indications, Methods and Results*, eds. H. H. Schmidek & W. H. Sweet, pp. 1137–53. New York: Grune and Stratton.

Tasker, R. R. (1982*b*). Thalamic stereotaxic procedures. In *Stereotaxy of the Human Brain*, eds. G. Schaltenbrand & A. E. Walker, pp. 484–97. Stuttgart: Thieme.

Tasker, R. R. (1984). Stereotaxic surgery. In *Textbook of Pain*, eds. P. D. Wall & R. Melzack, p. 639. Edinburgh: Churchill Livingstone.

Tasker, R. R. (1985). Surgical approaches to the primary afferent and the spinal cord. In *Advances in Pain Research and Therapy*, vol. 9, eds. H. L. Fields, R. Dubner & F. Cervero, pp. 299–324. New York: Raven Press.

Tasker, R. R. (1987). The problem of deafferentation pain in the management of the patient with cancer. *J. Pall. Care* **2**, 8–12.

Tasker, R. R. (1988*a*). Neurostimulation and percutaneous neural destructive techniques. In *Neural Blockade in Clinical Anesthesia and Management of Pain*, eds. M. J. Cousins & P. O. Bridenbaugh, pp. 1085–117. Philadelphia: Lippincott.

Tasker, R. R. (1988*b*). Percutaneous cordotomy: the lateral high cervical technique. In *Neurosurgical Techniques Indications, Methods and Results*, 2nd edn, pp. 1191–205. Orlando: Grune and Stratton.

Tasker, R. R. (1990*a*). Percutaneous cordotomy. In *Neurological Surgery*, 3rd edn, *A Comprehensive Reference Guide to the Diagnosis and Management of Neurosurgical Problems*, ed. J. R. Youmans, pp. 4045–58. Philadelphia: Saunders.

Tasker, R. R. (1990*b*). Management of nociceptive, deafferentation and central pain by surgical intervention. In *Pain Syndromes in Neurology*, ed. H. L. Fields, pp. 143–200. London: Butterworth.

Tasker, R. R. (1991). Deafferentation pain syndromes. Introduction. In *Advances in Pain Research and Therapy*, vol. 19, *Deafferentation Pain Syndromes: Pathophysiology and Treatment*, eds. B. S. Nashold & J. Ovelmen-Levitt, pp. 241–57. New York: Raven Press.

Tasker, R. R. (1993). Ablative central nervous system lesions for control of cancer pain. In *Management of Cancer-Related Pain*, ed. E. Arbit, pp. 231–55. Mt Kisco, N.Y.: Futura.

Tasker, R. R. (1994b). The recurrence of pain after neurosurgical procedures. *Quality of Life Res.* **3**, 543–9.

Tasker, R. R. (1994c). Percutaneous cordotomy. In *Operative Neurosurgical Techniques*, eds. H. H. Schmidek & W. H. Sweet, 3rd edn, 1595–611. Philadelphia: Saunders.

Tasker, R. R. (1994d). Stereotactic surgery. In *Textbook of Pain*, 3rd edn, eds. P. D. Wall & R. Melzack. Edinburgh: Churchill Livingstone.

Tasker, R. R. & Dostrovsky, J. O. (1989). Deafferentation and central pain. In *Textbook of Pain*, 2nd edn, eds. P. D. Wall & R. Melzack, pp. 154–80. Edinburgh: Churchill Livingstone.

Tasker, R. R. & Organ, L. W. (1973). Percutaneous cordotomy. Physiological identification of target site. *Confin. Neurol.* **35**, 110–17.

Tasker, R. R., Organ L. W., Hawrylyshyn P. A., (1982a). *The Thalamus and Midbrain of Man. A Physiological Atlas Using Electrical Stimulation*. Springfield: Thomas.

Tasker, R. R., De Carvalho, G. T. C. & Dolan, E. J. (1992). Intractable pain of spinal cord origin: clinical features and implications for surgery. *J. Neurosurg.* **77**, 373–8.

Tasker, R. R., Organ, L. W. & Smith, K. C. (1973). Physiological guidelines for the localization of lesions by percutaneous cordotomy. *Acta Neurochir.* **21** (Suppl.), 111–17.

Tenicela, R., Rosomoff, H. L., Feist, J. *et al.* (1968). Pulmonary function following percutaneous cervical cordotomy. *Anesthesiology* **29**, 7–16.

Tsubokawa, T., Katayama, Y., Yamamoto, T. & Hirayama, T. (1985). Deafferentation pain and stimulation of the thalamic sensory relay nucleus: clinical and experimental study. *Appl. Neurophysiol.* **48**, 166–71.

Tsubokawa, T., Hirayama, T., Yamamoto, T. *et al.* (1986). Differential effects between thalamic sensory relay nucleus and peri-aqueductal gray stimulation on neural activity within the normal and deafferented trigeminal medullary dorsal horn. In *Brain Stimulation and Neuronal Plasticity*, ed. T. Tsubokawa, p. 65. Tokyo: Neuron.

Uden, A. (1994). Specific disease in 532 cases of back pain. In *Quality of Life Res.* **3**, 533–4.

Urabe, M., Tsubokawa, T. (1965). Stereotaxic thalamotomy for the relief of intractable pain. *Tohoku J. Exp. Med.* **85**, 286–300.

Ventafridda, V., De Conno, F., Fochi, C. (1982). Cervical percutaneous cordotomy. In *Advances in Pain Research and Therapy*, vol. 4, *Management of Superior Sulcus Syndrome (Pancoast Syndrome)*, eds. J. J. Bonica, Ventafridda & C. A. Pagni, pp. 185–98. New York: Raven Press.

von Roeder, F. & Orthner, H. (1961). Erfabrungen mit stereotaktischen Eingriffen III Mitteilung. *Confin. Neurol.* **21**, 51–97.

Voris, H. C. & Whisler, W. W. (1978). Results of stereotaxic surgery for intractable pain. *Confin. Neurol.* **37**, 86.

Wall, P. D. (1992). The placebo effect: an unpopular topic. *Pain* **51**, 1–3.

Wall, P. D. & Sweet, W. H. (1967). Temporary abolition of pain in man. *Science* **155**, 108–9.

Ward, A. A. Jr, McCulloch, W. S. & Magoun, H. W. (1948). Production of an alternating tremor at rest in monkeys. *J. Neurophysiol.* **11**, 317–30.

Whisler, W. W. & Voris, H. C. (1978). Mesencephalotomy for intractable pain due to malignant disease. *Appl. Neurophysiol.* **47**, 52.

Woolf, C. J. (1992). Excitability changes in central neurons following peripheral damage; role of central sensitization in the pathogenesis of pain. In *Hyperalgesia and Allodynia*, ed. W. Willis, pp. 221–43. New York: Raven Press.

Wycis, H. T. & Spiefel, E. A. (1962). Long-range results in the treatment of intractable pain by stereotaxic midbrain surgery. *J. Neurosurg.* **19**, 101.

Young, R. F. (1989). Brain stimulation. In *Textbook of Pain*, 2nd edn, eds. P. D. Wall & R. Melzack, pp. 925–9. Edinburgh: Churchill Livingstone.

Young, R. F. (1990). Brain stimulation. In *Stereotactic Neurosurgery*, ed. W. Friedman. *Neurosurg. Clin. North Am.* **1**, 865–79.

Young, R. F. & Brechner, T. (1987). Electrical stimulation of the brain for relief of intractable pain due to cancer. *Cancer* **57**, 1266.

Young, R. F. & Chambi, V. I. (1985). Pain relief by electrical stimulation of the periaqueductal and periventricular gray matter. *J. Neurosurg.* **66**, 364.

Young, R. F., Bach, F. W., Van Norman, A. S. & Yakih, T. L. (1993). Release of β-endorphin and methionine enkephalin into cerebrospinal fluid during deep brain stimulation for chronic pain. Effects of stimulation locus and site of sampling. *J. Neurosurg.* **79**, 816–25.

Young, R. F., Kroening, R., Fulton, W., Fedlman, R. A. & Chambi, I. (1985). Electrical stimulation of the brain in treatment of chronic pain. Experience over 5 years. *J. Neurosurg.* **62**, 389–96.

27 Neurosurgical treatment of pain: trigeminal neuralgia

KIM J. BURCHIEL AND KEVIN R. MOORE

Introduction

In this chapter we will focus on a chronic pain problem which is unique. Trigeminal neuralgia stands apart from other pain syndromes in two important areas. First, the diagnosis can be made quickly and relatively simply by interview, and second we have many excellent medical and surgical treatments for this disorder. Since this volume is intended for a general audience, we will not dwell on the technical aspects of the various surgical procedures. These are well covered in numerous other texts. Instead we will highlight the indications for treatment, the choice of medical and surgical options, the results and potential morbidity of treatment, with an overall discussion of each surgical procedure.

History

Facial pain has been noted and described since antiquity. Aretaeus described the condition as 'Cephalaea' in the first century A.D., and discussions of the disorder known as 'trigeminal neuralgia' have been described from thirteenth to seventeenth centuries in English literature (Burchiel 1987a). John Locke first described the condition in the medical literature in 1677. Although Nicholas Andre first apparently recognized trigeminal neuralgia as a definite clinical entity, John Fothergill's classical description in 1776 is often noted as the first clinical treatise on the subject (Burchiel 1987a). Although often the term trigeminal neuralgia is used loosely to describe facial pain in the distribution of the trigeminal nerve, it actually relates to a distinct clinical sub-population of facial pain patients with very characteristic signs and symptoms. This distinction is of more than academic interest since idiopathic trigeminal neuralgia is a very treatable disease, while most of the other facial pain syndromes can be considerable treatment dilemmas. We will concentrate on the entity of 'essential' trigeminal neuralgia and its effective management in this chapter, but will also address invasive procedures for management of atypical or malignant facial pain.

Signs and symptoms

Trigeminal neuralgia is typically described as a fleeting, lancinating pain occurring in the sensory distribution of the trigeminal nerve. This story is strikingly reproducible and unmistakable. The pain characteristically lasts seconds to minutes and is almost always unilateral. Curiously, the disease course is not static and is notable for pain-free intervals that may last months to year. The division most commonly affected is the maxillary distribution at 35%, with mandibular (29%) and ophthalmic (4%) less commonly affected. V_2 and V_3 simultaneously occur at 19% and all three together 1% (Katusic *et al.* 1990). The pain is described as paroxysmal and electrical in nature. Attacks are usually brought on by such triggering stimuli as talking, eating, oral hygiene, or even cool temperatures or wind on the face. Light tactile stimulation is often all that is needed to provoke a volley of paroxysms, and this can be so profound that sufferers will neglect grooming on the affected side secondary to elicited pain. Patients may not wash their face, brush teeth, eat on that side, or may even pool their secretions for fear of swallowing. Age distribution is usually older individuals in their 60s and above but ranges from the second to the tenth decade. There is a slight preponderance of females over males (5.9 compared with 3.4 per 100 000 population, respectively) with an age and sex adjusted incidence of 4.7 per 100 000 population (Katusic *et al.* 1990). Relationships to hypertension, multiple sclerosis, hemifacial spasm, and familial occurrences have all been reported. Season of onset, side of face, etc. are not statistically significant, although the right side is slightly more commonly affected (Jannetta 1980; Katusic *et al.* 1990).

Medical therapy

Approximately 70% of trigeminal neuralgia patients are well controlled non-operatively. Perhaps the quintessential drug used is carbamazepine (Tegretol) started at 100 mg p.o. b.i.d. then increased by 100–200 mg a day every 2 to 3 days to a final effective dose in the range of up to 600–1000 mg. Not only will most patients respond to this regimen, but this is also a powerful and reliable modality in the diagnosis of trigeminal neuralgia. That is, if a patient with facial pain responds to carbamazepine, the diagnosis of trigeminal neuralgia is assured. Unfortunately, use of the drug is limited by development of hypersensitivity reactions or side effects such as drowsiness, decreased mental acuity, subjective dizziness and ataxia (particularly in older patients), dose-related mild leukopenia, or a very rare non-dose-dependent idiosyncratic bone marrow suppression (aplastic anaemia) which can occur early in treatment. For these reasons a baseline white blood cell (WBC) count is obtained and repeat studies are done at 3–4 week intervals. In patients who cannot tolerate carbamazepine other options include baclofen (Lioresal) or phenytoin (Dilantin). Baclofen can be a good choice in patients who get effective relief from carbamazepine but cannot tolerate its side effects, and it is usually started at 5 mg t.i.d. and increased by 5–10 mg every 2–3 days to a maximum dose of 80 mg per day. It is usually not effective in patients who do not derive benefit from carbamazepine. Phenytoin is rarely of use when carbamazepine or baclofen have failed, but may be helpful in combination with one of the other medications.

Although most patients are well controlled initially by medical management, many of these will become non-responders as drug therapy becomes ineffective and break-through pain begins. In fact, probably the majority of patients will eventually fail medical management if followed carefully over a period of years. Fortunately, many of these patients subsequently derive excellent relief from surgical modalities.

Surgical treatment

Most patients are initially treated with conservative medical modalities and often do not present to the surgeon until they have maximized medical management without adequate relief. Like medical management, at least initially surgical management is very rewarding.

There have been many procedures developed over the years for management of trigeminal neuralgia, and a logical classification is division into two groups; minor procedures involving local or brief general anaesthesia and short hospital stay or ambulatory surgery, and major procedures requiring general anaesthesia and several days of hospitalization. It is worth noting that no one technique is completely satisfactory, as evidenced by the number of surgical strategies available.

Minor versus major procedures

There are three main minor procedures; percutaneous retrogasserian glycerol rhizolysis (PRGR), percutaneous radiofrequency trigeminal gangliolysis (PRTG) and percutaneous trigeminal ganglion compression (PTGC). The choice of procedure depends on the experience and preference of the surgeon. All are effective with relative advantages and disadvantages to each. PTGC is technically simple, causes only mild sensory loss and has an acceptable recurrence rate. However, it is impossible to restrict the lesion to a single division. PRGR causes mild to no sensory loss, but is technically more difficult to perform. The failure rate also seems to be higher in most operators' hands, as is the relapse rate over 5 years. PRTG affords immediate pain relief in a very high percentage of patients with a low recurrence rate but produces a considerable sensory loss. It is also effective for trigeminal neuralgia associated with multiple sclerosis or tumour. It is easier to perform for V_3 than V_2 because of the potential overlap with V_1.

One of the primary criticisms of the minor procedures is that they do not address the underlying pathology and remove the cause of the pain. On the other hand, they are effective procedures with relatively minimal morbidity and almost non-existent mortality, an important consideration for a non-lethal condition such as trigeminal neuralgia.

The primary major procedures are microvascular decompression (MVD) and partial sensory rhizotomy (PSR). Although microvascular decompression is the only surgical modality directly addressing the presumed aetiology of trigeminal neuralgia and probably provides the longest-lasting pain relief, it has several significant drawbacks; it is a major surgical procedure with a reported mortality of 1%, non-negligible postoperative complications, and transient or permanent cranial nerve deficits (Fraoili *et al.* 1989). Several have questioned the use of a procedure with defined morbidity and mortality for benign disease, and propose the use of the percutaneous procedures for most surgical management of trigeminal neuralgia (Morley 1985; Adams 1989).

The ultimate choice between major and minor procedures in patients refractory to medical management should be made between the patient and physician. Older patients are often biased toward minor procedures because of considerations such as life expectancy, other health concerns, longer hospital stay, increased recovery time, and avoidance of a craniotomy. On the other hand, in a young healthy patient the longer duration of effective pain relief offered by microvascular decompression may offset these considerations.

Minor procedures

Percutaneous injection of alcohol into the peripheral trigeminal nerve or its ganglion (ethanol block) and peri/intraganglionic injection of alcohol (alcohol gangliolysis) are procedures that are rarely performed and will not be discussed further. Peripheral neurectomy is no longer a state of the art procedure, but it can be employed to provide simple effective pain relief for very sick elderly patients who would not tolerate surgery and in whom pain will almost certainly return within a few years requiring re-lesioning. It also will not be discussed further.

State of the art minor procedures are: percutaneous retrogasserian glycerol rhizolysis (PRGR), percutaneous radiofrequency trigeminal gangliolysis (PRTG), and percutaneous trigeminal ganglion compression (PTGC). These offer the substantial benefits of outpatient surgery with minimal anaesthetic risk and morbidity/mortality, and utilize local or brief general anaesthetics rather than general endotracheal anaesthesia. In addition to effective short-acting general anaesthesia, methylhexital (Brevital) and propofol (Diprivan) also provide a welcome amnestic effect. It is important to note that these agents provide no analgesia, however, and their use requires supplementation with analgesic agents. The surgical indication for these procedures is medically intractable trigeminal neuralgia. These techniques are particularly well suited for elderly or ill patients who do not desire or would be poor candidates for major operative procedures. However, the lesions seldom last more than a few years, necessitating repeat procedures.

Percutaneous retrogasserian glycerol rhizolysis

Percutaneous retrogasserian glycerol rhizolysis (PRGR) derives from Hakanson's (Hakanson 1981) serendipitous discovery that glycerol injected into the cistern of

Meckel's cave in patients with trigeminal neuralgia produces lasting pain relief with minimal sensory loss (Hakanson 1978). Current evidence suggests that glycerol may preferentially exert its effects on small myelinated or unmyelinated fibres of the nerve, and particularly on the damaged large myelinated fibres, which have been implicated in the genesis of trigeminal neuralgia (Burchiel 1987a). PRGR is less dependent on patient input than PRTG, in which one needs a semi-awake patient to produce a tailored sensory deficit, and thus permits one to be more generous with local anaesthetic and intravenous sedation. It can be difficult to perform, and although it offers a lower reliability for pain relief than either PTGC or PRTG, its relative lack of complications and lower rate of sensory dysaesthesias compared with the other denervative procedures lead many to employ it as their first choice in previously untreated patients with trigeminal neuralgia.

Results

About one half of patients will be pain-free within 24 hours after injection, while the remainder may continue to have typical pain that disappears over a period of days to weeks. Effective pain relief is achieved within 48 hours in 72% to 96% of patients (Burchiel 1987a; 1988; Fraoili et al. 1989; Fujimaki et al. 1990; Sahami et al. 1990; Zhang et al. 1990). Technical failure is reported as high as 15% (Burchiel 1988). Recurrence rate is difficult to evaluate because of the heterogeneity of the follow-up reported, but at one year is 27% and ranges from 18.5% to 72% over follow-up from 3 to 72 months (Saini 1987; Burchiel 1988; Fraoili et al. 1989; Fujimaki et al. 1990; Sahni et al. 1990). Median time to recurrence is 16 to 36 months (Fujimaki et al. 1990; North et al. 1990; Sahni et al. 1990). Patients having previous procedures recur sooner than those not having previous procedures (Saini 1987; Fujimaki et al. 1990; North et al. 1990; Zhang et al. 1990). It is worth noting that many recurrences are initially amenable to medical treatment and do not require surgical re-lesioning until later in their course.

Complications

The complications of PRGR are the same as those for the other percutaneous procedures, namely paraesthesias, dysaesthesias, anaesthesia dolorosa, corneal hypaesthesia or anaesthesia, diminished corneal reflex, neuroparalytic keratitis, masticatory muscle weakness, herpes labialis, or haematoma at needle entry site. The minor complications seem to be dependent on the experience of the operator.

The most dreaded complications are anaesthesia dolorosa and keratitis. Anaesthesia dolorosa, intractable facial pain refractory to all medical and surgical procedures, occurs from 0% to 2% (Burchiel 1988; De La Porte et al. 1990; Fujimaki et al. 1990; Sahni et al. 1990; Zhang et al. 1990), but has been reported as high as 5% (Saini 1987). Keratitis has been reported rarely (Saini 1987; Fraoili et al. 1989).

Discussion

Most authors agree on the following clinical indicators of successful lesion: brisk CSF flow following cisternal puncture, distinct cisternogram findings demonstrating typical

anatomic localization, rapid egress of the radiocontrast, and ipsilateral facial dysaesthesias following glycerol injection.

The following prognostic factors are believed to predict a good outcome: classic
presentation ('essential' trigeminal neuralgia), female sex, prior successful medical
therapy (especially carbamazepine), short duration of symptoms, and young age
(North *et al.* 1990). Factors which have been shown to be *not* significant include: the
division involved, side of face affected, presence of a discrete trigger zone, previous
radiofrequency lesion or microvascular decompression, degree and duration of success of prior procedures, and response to phenytoin or baclofen (North *et al.* 1990).

In attempting to analyse the myriad disparate data in the literature, a careful eye
must be trained on a few technical considerations. First, 'good' result is poorly defined
and varies significantly among researchers. Second, the duration of follow-up reported
varies widely, as does the patient population; many include patients with multiple
sclerosis, tumours, and post-herpetic pain as well as 'essential' trigeminal neuralgia.
Lastly, as in all procedures there is a learning curve, and the best results and fewest
complications occur as established groups gain more experience. Patients are better
served by surgeons who do these procedures frequently and deftly. The primary
attractiveness of this procedure has been its reputation as one that avoids sensory loss
and dysaesthesias, but the literature clearly disputes that assumption. In fact, one
group reports that it now favours microvascular decompression for this reason
(Fujimaki *et al.* 1990). Nevertheless, in experienced hands it is still a safe, effective
procedure with minimal side effects that lends itself well as an initial surgical procedure.

Percutaneous radiofrequency trigeminal gangliolysis

Initially described by Sweet and Wepsic (1974) percutaneous radiofrequency trigeminal
gangliolysis (PRTG) has beome one of the most widely used minor surgical modalities
for trigeminal neuralgia. It is the procedure of choice for multiple sclerosis and is very
good for tumour-related pain. It is very effective for V_3 distribution pain, but less so for
V_2 and V_1. It is difficult to make an isolated V_1 lesion without corneal anaesthesia, and
thus glycerol rhizolysis may be a better choice. Advantages include high immediate
pain relief, low relapse rate, effectiveness in symptomatic trigeminal neuralgia, avoidance of craniotomy, ease of repeating lesion if needed, minimal morbidity and mortality, and less expense than with microvascular decompression. Disadvantages include
prominent hypaesthesia and a steeper learning curve than PRGR or PTGC.

Results

Trigeminal neuralgia confined to V_1 has the least favourable outcome, and V_3 the best
(Burchiel 1987*a*; Piquer *et al.* 1987): 78%–100% of patients have immediate pain relief
with a 6%–7% technical failure rate (Burchiel 1987*a*). Initial response is variably defined
but ranges from 82% to 99.2% (Fraoili *et al.* 1989; Reglio & Cioni 1989; Broggi *et al.* 1990;

Moraci *et al.* 1992). Immediate failures result in 1%–17% of patients, but average time to recurrence has been reported as 18.5 months (Meglio & Cioni 1989). One year recurrence ranges from 4% to 32% (Burchiel *et al.* 1981; Burchiel 1987*a*; Piquer *et al.* 1987; Fraoili *et al.* 1989) and 3 year from less than 10% up to 66% (Burchiel *et al.* 1981; Piquer *et al.* 1987; Fraoili *et al.* 1989; Meglio & Cioni 1989; Broggi *et al.* 1990). At 4 to 5 years 39%–85% will remain in remission (Burchiel 1987*a*). Temperature of the probe has no effect on early pain relief, but is directly related to rate of recurrence (Moraci *et al.* 1992).

Complications

Mortality from PRTG is essentially unheard of. Reduction or loss of facial sensation occurs in direct proportion to lesion temperature in up to 80% of patients (Moraci *et al.* 1992). Postoperative paraesthesias occur in 20% and dysaesthesias from 5.2% to 24.2% (Burchiel *et al.* 1981; Mealio and Cioni 1989; Moraci *et al.* 1992). Anaesthesia dolorosa occurs less commonly at 0.3% to 4% (Burchiel *et al.* 1981; Piquer *et al.* 1987; Fraoili *et al.* 1989; Broggi *et al.* 1990; Moraci *et al.* 1992). Unwanted V_1 hypaesthesia is reported at 17.3% to 19.7% (Piquer *et al.* 1987; Fraoili *et al.* 1989; Broggi *et al.* 1990) with V_1 anaesthesia less commonly at 3% (Burchiel *et al.* 1981; Fraoili *et al.* 1989) and frank keratitis 0.5% to 3.0% (Burchiel *et al.* 1981; Piquer *et al.* 1987; Fraoili *et al.* 1989; Broggi *et al.* 1990; Moraci *et al.* 1992). Patients with substantial analgesia or anaesthesia have half the rate of recurrence at 4.5 years follow-up compared with those with only hypalgesia (13% versus 26%); at 9 years the recurrence rate for patients with hypaesthesia compared with analgesia is 41% versus 7.5% (Broggi *et al.* 1990). In comparison, patients with partial or no permanent sensory deficit have a recurrence rate of 60% (Piquer *et al.* 1987). Herpes labialis, diminution of hearing, and oculomotor palsy all occur in about 1% or less (Burchiel *et al.* 1981; Piquer *et al.* 1987; Broggi *et al.* 1990; Moraci *et al.* 1992). Minor masticatory weakness is reported in up to 10.5% of patients (Meglio & Cioni 1989; Fraoili *et al.* 1989; Broggi *et al.* 1990) and generally involves the ipsilateral masseter muscle.

Inadvertent intracranial placement of the electrode with lesion formation can result in unsuspected intracranial (temporal lobe) lesions. Haemorrhagic lesions resulting from intracranial penetration through unsuspected skull defects or supernumerary foramina as well as unusual extratrigeminal complications such as cranial nerve injuries (II, III, VI, VII, VIII, and XII), subarachnoid haemorrhage, carotico-cavernous fistulas, or internal carotid artery injuries at the foramen lacerum anteriorly or at the intrapetrous level through a rare osseous defect have all been described (Puca *et al.* 1992). Careful fluoroscopic surveillance is essential to avoid these pitfalls.

Discussion

PRTG is an efficacious therapeutic modality for trigeminal neuralgia, particularly V_3 and less so V_2 since there may be contiguous denervation of V_1 with attendant side effects. It can provide immediate pain relief and dense hypaesthesia or anaesthesia to heat, touch, and partial deep sensation, and good results are obtained in patients having previous PRGR, PTGC, or even previous PRTG lesions (Fraoili *et al.* 1989).

Patients with trigeminal neuralgia confined to V_1 have a less favourable outcome than the other divisions (Piquer *et al.* 1987; Fraoili *et al.* 1989). It is difficult to perform isolated V_1 lesions without producing a diminished-to-absent corneal reflex, and it is more advisable to perform a PRGR or PTGC in these patients. In patients with postoperative corneal sensory deficits, 31.4% had lesions preoperatively and 14.4% did not (Broggi *et al.* 1990). PRTG is the procedure of choice over microvascular decompression for multiple sclerosis patients, but seems to be less successful in atypical trigeminal neuralgia patients (20%) (Fraoili *et al.* 1989).

Variance in reported success and recurrence rates may depend on the definition of recurrence and whether one strictly adheres to retrogasserian placement of the needle (with CSF flow), thus achieving ganglion and root lesions instead of ganglion and nerve lesions (Burchiel *et al.* 1981). Overall recurrence rate is correlated to the degree of postoperative sensory deficit (Broggi *et al.* 1990), patients with marked sensory deficits had a diminished rate of recurrence (Piquer *et al.* 1987).

PRTG's lower recurrence rate compared with the other minor procedures comes at the price of increased undesirable sequelae such as dysaesthesias, keratitis, corneal anaesthesia, and anaesthesia dolorosa. Unfortunately, these are directly related to the amount of sensory deficit produced (Burchiel *et al.* 1981; Broggi *et al.* 1990). Thus, degree of anaesthesia produced and consequent pain relief obtained must be balanced against the risk of unwanted side effects.

Percutaneous trigeminal ganglion (micro) compression

Percutaneous trigeminal ganglion (micro)compression (PTGC) was first introduced in 1978 and published by Mullan & Lichtor in 1983. This procedure evolved from an adaptation of the technique of trigeminal compression through temporal craniotomy espoused by Shelden *et al.* (1955). This procedure is useful in patients who are infirm or elderly, young patients not wishing a major procedure, or in patients who had undergone destructive procedures previously but did not have major dysaesthesias (Brown & Preul 1989). It is thought that the beneficial effects are due to the balloon-induced ischaemic and mechanical damage to rootlet and ganglion cells (Belber & Rak 1987). PTGC's primary advantages are its slight permanent sensory deficit, its technical ease, moderate relapse rate in skilled hands, quickness, and that patient cooperation is not needed (Fraoili *et al.* 1989). On the other hand, one cannot confine lesions to one division only, it requires at least light general anaesthesia, it is characterized by hypertension and bradycardia (Fraoili *et al.* 1989), and the larger needle than that used with PRGR or PRTG may be more difficult to insert through the foramen ovale (Lobato *et al.* 1990).

Results

The rate of immediate pain relief is quoted from 89.9% to 100% (Belber & Rak 1987; Meglio *et al.* 1987; Brown & Preul 1989; Fraoili *et al.* 1989; Meglio & Cioni 1989; Lobato *et al.* 1990; Mullan & Lichtor 1990). Mullan & Lichtor currently have the longest reported series at 10 years follow-up. They report 80% technical success at 60 months and 70% at 120 months. Average recurrence time is reported as 4.2 to 6.5 months (Meglio *et al.* 1987; Meglio & Cioni 1989). Total recurrence is widely variable, from 55% to 77.4% at 36 months (Meglio *et al.* 1987; Meglio & Cioni 1989) to 30% at 120 months (Mullan & Lichtor 1990) and these relapses are often easily managed with carbamazepine, even if they were not prior to PTGC. The majority of recurrences are within 48 months, but also continue steadily for up to 9 years (Mullan & Lichtor 1990). The 13% 5-year reoperative rate is better than after PRTG (21%–28%) or microvascular decompression (17%–26%). Despite this apparent success, 15% of patients with life expectancy greater than 10 years will require more invasive intracranial surgery of some sort. The length of compression time is controversial; earlier studies have stressed longer times to achieve some degree of permanent ganglion damage (Belver & Rak 1987; Meglio *et al.* 1987; Meglio & Cioni 1989) but currently one minute is thought to provide equivalent recurrence rates to longer times (Fraoili *et al.* 1989; Lobato *et al.* 1990; Mullan & Lichtor 1990). Sensory deficit is related to duration of compression (Belber & Rak 1987; Fraoili *et al.* 1989; Lobato *et al.* 1990) and is directly proportional to duration of pain relief (Fraoili *et al.* 1989; Lobato *et al.* 1990; Moraci *et al.* 1992). In fact, a lack of post-procedure hypaesthesia probably implies for relatively short-term pain relief.

Complications

A mild degree of V_3 hypaesthesia is the rule, and most patients become accustomed to it. Mortality is distinctly uncommon. Keratitis or loss of corneal reflex is rare because the needle enters the middle fossa through the foramen ovale adjacent to the inferolateral V_3 fibres, missing the superomedial V_1 fibres (Brown & Preul 1989). Reported complications include ipsilateral masticatory muscle weakness, hypaesthesia, dysaesthesias, anaesthesia dolorosa, balloon failure, herpetic eruptions, abducens nerve palsy (3%–5%), cheek haematoma, aseptic meningitis (5%), and transient otalgia (5%) (Brown & Preul 1989; Lobato *et al.* 1990). Significant masseter weakness has been reported from 1% to 100% initially (Belber & Rak 1987; Meglio *et al.* 1987; Brown & Preul 1989; Fraoili *et al.* 1989; Meglio & Cioni 1989; Lobato *et al.* 1990; Mullan & Lichtor 1990), with a 3% permanent incidence (Fraoili *et al.* 1989). It seems clear that nearly 100% of patients will have at least some ipsilateral masseter weakness that generally disappears in about 3 months but can last up to a year (Belber & Rak 1987; Lobato *et al.* 1990). Dysaesthesias have been noted in 6.7% to 8.5% (Meglio *et al.* 1987; Meglio & Cioni 1989; Fraoili *et al.* 1989) with only one incident of anaesthesia dolorosa (Fraoili *et al.* 1989). Aseptic meningitis is infrequently encountered, and one case of pneumococcal meningitis has been reported secondary to penetration of the oral mucosa during cannulation of the foramen ovale (Lobato *et al.* 1990). Hypertension requiring sodium nitroprusside and bradycardia are well-characterized perioperative phenomena (Lobato *et al.* 1990). There is some debate whether the bradycardia is significant; some routinely use external pacers and atropine for heart rate less than 45 beats per minute (Brown & Preul

1989), others give atropine intramusculary preoperatively and intravenously perioperatively for bradycardic episodes during cannulation (Belber & Rak 1987), while still others do not routinely treat these generally self-limited episodes, but instead use them to indicate whether they are in the foramen and later that they have achieved an adequate compression (Mullan & Lichtor 1990).

Discussion

Unlike the other percutaneous procedures, patient cooperation is not needed for PTGC. On the other hand, it requires at least light general anaesthesia, it is not possible to confine lesions to one division only, and the 14-gauge needle may be more difficult to cannulate througfh the foramen ovale than the 19-gauge needle used with PRGR or PRTG (Lobabo *et al.* 1990). Also, some may consider the characteristic intraoperative hypertension and bradycardia a disadvantage (Fraoili *et al.* 1989). However, the relative ease of this procedure compared with other percutaneous procedures makes it a more attractive choice for the surgeon who does not treat large numbers of trigeminal neuralgia patients.

Major procedures

Microvascular decompression

Patients with essential trigeminal neuralgia who are young or in whom the additional risk of a craniotomy is outweighed by the benefits of a high probability of long-term palliation of pain with minimal to no sensory loss are good candidates for microvascular decompression (MVD). It effectively addresses what may be the aetiologic basis for trigeminal neuralgia with minimal occurrence of the feared complications keratitis or anaesthesia dolorosa.

Dandy (1932; 1934) and Gardner & Miklos (1959) provided the framework for what Jannetta (1967; 1980) later developed into the technique of microvascular decompression. They proposed that the principle of neurovascular compression was aetiologic in trigeminal neuralgia; frequently an artery or vein or less often an arteriovenous malformation (AVM) or tumour compresses the trigeminal nerve at its junction with the pons (the root entry zone or REZ), and surgical decompression provides remarkable alleviation of pain. Currently it is the most widely applied major procedure for idiopathic trigeminal neuralgia.

Results

The variety of disease processes manifesting as trigeminal neuralgia and consequent multitude of prior procedures leaves most patients in these series with pre-existing lesions so interpretation of outcome is difficult. Patients who are dysaesthetic preoperatively are likely to remain so postoperatively. Facial pain may continue for a few days postoperatively, then gradually subside and disappear, particularly when the nerve has been manipulated very little during decompression (Janetta 1980).

The concept of neurovascular compression is critical for understanding microvascular decompression. Neurovascular compression is found in 70 to 90% or more of microvascular decompressions with more surgeon's experience resulting in less incidence of negative findings at operation (Piatt & Wilkins 1984; Hamlyn & King 1992; Klun 1992). Findings at the REZ are 59% to 76% arterial, 5% to 14% venous, 23% mixed arteriovenous, 3.6% tumour, 2% venous angioma, occasional osseous contact, and 0.25% each aneurysm, AVM, or no pathology (Jannetta 1980; Hamlyn & King 1992). Arterial compression usually involves the SCA but may also include AICA, PICA, VA, or BA (Jannetta 1980; Piatt & Wilkins 1984; Zorman & Wilson 1984; Sweet 1985; Hamlyn & King 1992). In a more recent article on microsurgical anatomy (Matsushima *et al.* 1989), the lateral mesencephalic segment of the SCA near its bifurcation often (70% of cases) compressed the trigeminal nerve at multiple points on the nerve's medial surface. Arterial contact at the REZ has a significantly better prognosis than venous or no contact (73% versus 51% cure respectively) after microvascular decompression; major recurrence rate is 17% for arterial compression, 75% for venous compression, and 60% for both venous and arterial (Hamlyn & King 1992). In addition, patients with anatomical arterial distortion of the trigeminal nerve or wedging into the pontine 'crevice' did better than those with other types of arterial contact (83% versus 62%) (Piatt & Wilkins 1984). Anatomical studies of the REZ of asymptomatic cadavers have been inconclusive regarding the incidence of vascular compression in the general population without trigeminal neuralgia (Hardy & Rhobon 1978; Adams 1989; Hamlyn & King 1992). The relationship between intentional intraoperative neural trauma and pain relief is not clearly related to the degree of trauma, as commonly accepted. Venous and bony incursion cause more severe nerve compression, but have a much higher recurrence rate after microvascular decompression than arterial compression (Burchiel *et al.* 1988). In one study 79% of patients pain-free after operation had neurovascular compression, but only 55% of major recurrences had arterial neurovascular compression initially (Burchiel *et al.* 1988). Another group reports that over a 5-year period they achieved 78% satisfactory results and 22% poor outcome in patients with arterial contact versus 54% satisfactory and 46% poor outcome or recurrence in patients with no arterial contact (Piatt & Wilkins 1984). Multiple sclerosis-related trigeminal neuralgia seldom benefits from microvascular decompression due to internal plaques and compression (Klun 1992).

The largest experience and best results have been reported by Jannetta. In this chapter, satisfactory outcome includes patients totally pain-free and those with mild pain or pain-free with lower doses of medication added. If one includes all patients improved, including those who have satisfactory pain control with adjunctive medical therapy, over 96% long-term pain-free results can be obtained (Jannetta 1980). In patients with unilateral trigeminal neuralgia, the rate of immediate pain relief is 70% to greater than 96% (Jannetta 1980; Klun 1992). At 48 months, 72% still have excellent results (Piatt & Wilkins 1984). At 60 months the recurrence rate is about 6%, compared with 50% recurrence following partial sensory rhizotomy (Burchiel *et al.* 1988; Klun 1992); 83% have satisfactory results (pain-free with or without treatment or with mild pain), 12% are pain-free initially but recur after 1 month, and 5% have outright poor outcome (Bederson & Wilson 1989). At 100 months 58% are pain-free, 12% have had minor recurrences, and 30% have had major recurrences (Burchiel *et al.* 1988). Minor recurrence is defined as minor resumption of neuralgic pain (transient, infrequent or mild) that is amenable to medical adjunctive treatment, and major recurrence is defined as resumption of previous trigeminal neuralgic pain intractable to medical regimens (Burchiel *et al.* 1988). The average time to recurrence seems to be about 2 years, at which time 12% have recurred. The rate thereafter is about 2% recurrence per year, divided into 3.5% for major recurrences and 1.5% for minor recurrences annually (Burchiel *et al.* 1988; Bederson & Wilson 1989). In contrast to previous shorter duration follow-up studies (Piatt & Wilkins 1984), long-term follow-up now suggests that there seems to be no point at which patients can be considered cured; microvascular decompression only seems to arrest trigeminal neuralgia with gradual fallout due to recurrences (Burchiel *et al.* 1988). Most patients having recurrent pain undergo re-exploration; although the incidence of neurovascular compression discovered at time of surgery is extremely variable (Tytus 1982; Bederson & Wilson 1989). Those patients without evidence of compression generally undergo partial sensory rhizotomy with 85% satisfactory results (Bederson & Wilson 1989).

Negative prognostic indicators include a less advanced degree of neurovascular compression (Szapiro *et al.* 1985; Bederson & Wilson 1989; Klun 1992), venous compression (Klun 1992), longer duration of symptoms (Klun 1992), sensory deficit of more than two divisions (Szapiro *et al.* 1985), prior surgery (Szapiro *et al.* 1985; Burchiel *et al.* 1988), or the presence of a constant pain component in addition to paroxysmal pain (Szapiro *et al.* 1985). Paroxysmal pain only has about a 95% cure rate while paroxysmal plus permanent has only 58% cure over 60 months (Sweet 1985). Relationship between outcome and age or sex is less clear (Szapiro *et al.* 1985; Bederson & Wilson 1989; Hatsushima *et al.* 1989). Men are more likely to have root distortion than women and thus seem to have a better outcome (Bederson & Wilson 1989). Degree of neurovascular compression does not seem to correlate with sensory deficit (Sweet 1985; Bederson & Wilson 1989). Shorter duration of symptoms gives better outcome (Bederson & Wilson 1989) in some studies but not others (Klun 1992). Duration seems only important for prognosis if neurovascular compression is present; there is no relation between duration of symptoms and outcome if neurovascular compression is not present at operation (Bederson & Wilson 1989). Patients with previous proximal ablative procedures (PRTG, PRGR, subtemporal retrogression rhizotomy) do significantly poorer and are more likely to have major recurrences than those with no previous operations, microvascular decompression, or a peripheral procedure (32% versus 2%) (Szapiro *et al.* 1985; Burchiel *et al.* 1988; Bederson & Wilson 1989). Also, previous PRTG increases incidence of trigeminal nerve injuries after microvascular decompression (Matsushima *et al.* 1989).

Bilateral trigeminal neuralgia is uncommon (1%–6% in most series); these patients have a lower rate of pain relief or cure than those with unilateral disease. The right side is generally affected before the left (77% versus 20%), with 3% simultaneously bilaterally. Pain on the contralateral side generally develops an average of 9 years later, with a range up to 20 years. Compared with unilateral trigeminal neuralgia, there is a higher incidence of 'familial trigeminal neuralgia' and increased cranial nerve dysfunction. Women are also more frequently in the poor outcome group with bilateral trigeminal neuralgia. Following bilateral microvascular decompression, nearly 100% of patients have satisfactory immediate results; 100% of patients at 12 months and 92% at 60 months have satisfactory control. However, only 5% are well controlled off medication or with medication only. In patients with separate incidence of unilateral trigeminal neuralgia, immediately satisfactory results are obtained in 89% of treated sides. At 12 months, 82% of patients obtain satisfactory results with 13% poorly controlled by adjunctive medical therapy. At 60 months, the percentage with satisfactory results decreases to 66% with 22% not well controlled. By 120 months the number with satisfactory results is 60% with 22% not well controlled. As many as 25% of patients may never achieve a satisfactory result (Pollack *et al.* 1988).

Complications

Large series quote a 10% to 19% total incidence of complications (Piatt & Wilkins 1984; Pollack *et al.* 1988; Bederson & Wilson 1989). Operative mortality runs from 0% to 1.4% (Jannetta 1980; Piatt & Wilkins 1984; Pollack *et al.* 1988; Bederson & Wilson 1989; Meglio *et al.* 1990; Zhang *et al.* 1990; Hamlyn & King 1992; Klun 1992). Herpes labialis has been described from 0% to greater than 50% incidence and is related to the degree of intraoperative nerve manipulation. Transient cranial nerve deficits occur with a 4% incidence lasting 6 weeks to 6 months (78% facial, 22% vestibulocochlear nerve) (Bederson & Wilson 1989). Overall incidence of permanent cranial nerve deficits runs from 5.6% to 10% (Jannetta 1980; Piatt & Wilkins 1984). With more experience and the utilization of intraoperative brainstem auditory evoked response (BAER) monitoring these complications should be decreasing (Piatt & Wilkins 1984; Sweet 1985; Klun 1992). Trigeminal nerve lesions are naturally more prevalent in partial sensory rhizotomy patients, while facial and vestibulocochlear lesions are more prevalent in those undergoing microvascular decompression (Piatt & Wilkins 1984; Bederson & Wilson 1989). Incidence of sensory loss in microvascular decompression is less than for partial sensory rhizotomy (25% versus 100%) (Burchiel *et al.* 1988). Hypaesthesia is rare (6% to 14%) (Sweet 1985; Pollack *et al.* 1988), as are paraesthesias (8%) (Piatt & Wilkins 1984) and dysaesthesias (0% to 2.4%) (Piatt & Wilkins 1984; Bederson & Wilson 1989; Hamlyn & King 1992; Klun 1992). Corneal hypaesthesia occurs in around 1.7% (Sweet 1985) with frank anaesthesia in 0% to 0.5% (Bederson & Wilson 1989; Klun 1992). Transient diplopia secondary to abducens nerve involvement is also infrequently encountered in 0.8% to 2.7% (Zorman & Wilson 1986; Klun 1992). Facial paresis, both transient and permanent, is well recognized with an incidence of 0.4% to 2.8% (Piatt & Wilkins 1984; Sweet 1985; Zorman & Wilson 1986; Pollack *et al.* 1988; Bederson & Wilson 1989.

Perhaps one of the most serious under-recognized sequelae of microvascular decompression is hearing loss, which can be quite profound (Piatt & Wilkins 1984). The rate of minor hearing loss is generally quoted as 0% to 6%, with major permanent hearing loss in up to 8% (Piatt & Wilkins 1984; Zarman & Wilson 1984; Sweet 1985; Fritz *et al.* 1988; Pollack *et al.* 1988; Bederson & Wilson 1989; Schwartz & Gennarelli 1990; Hamlyn & King 1992; Klun 1992; Sindou *et al.* 1992). Deafness is usually noted immediately postoperatively and generally resolves within 6 months (Schwartz & Gennarelli 1990). Probably the rate of objective hearing loss found during formal testing is much higher than the subjective reports in the literature. One prospective study of postoperative hearing loss reveals a 23.8% incidence of impairment on detailed testing (Fritz *et al.* 1988). Irreversible deficit of the vestibulocochlear nerve can occur secondary to excessive traction or manipulation of the acoustico-facial bundle or its vascular supply or heat from nearby electrocoagulation (Piatt & Wilkins 1984; Sindou *et al.* 1992). Intraoperative entry of blood and CSF into the mastoid air cells with middle ear effusion on the operative side results in a conductive hearing loss and may be prevented with careful waxing of bone and air cells. Detailed audiological testing of these patients demonstrates a flattened tympanogram with diminution of speech comprehension and tone decay of 15–20 dB (Fritz *et al.* 1988). Those patients with normal impedance and normal tympanogram have a retrocochlear lesion. Contralateral hearing loss is due to pressure on the cochlear nerve in the brain stem (crossed reflex) while ipsilateral hearing loss is secondary to retractor compression of the vestibulocochlear nerve in the internal acoustic canal.

CSF leak has been described as occurring 0% to 2.8% (Piatt & Wilkins 1984; Pollack *et al.* 1988; Bederson & Wilson 1989; Zhang *et al.* 1990; Klun 1992). CSF rhinorrhea, due to translation of CSF through the Eustachian tubes, occurs 0.5% to 1% of the time (Jannetta 1980; Piatt & Wilkins 1984). Meningitis is also fairly frequent; aseptic is quoted at 3% to 4.4% (Piatt & Wilkins 1984; Zorman & Wilson 1984; Bederson & Wilson 1989) and bacterial ranges from 0.4% to 2.4% (Jannetta 1980; Bederson & Wilson 1989; Zhang *et al.* 1990; Hamlyn & King 1992) although as high as 14.3% has been reported (Tsubaki *et al.* 1989). Rounding out the litany of sequelae are more general postoperative complications such as pulmonary embolus, epidural haematoma, chronic subdural haematoma, pneumonia, infarction, intracerebral haemorrhage and deep venous thrombosis.

Discussion

Microvascular decompression does not appear to 'cure' trigeminal neuralgia; the procedure only seems to arrest the disorder for a prolonged period with gradual fallout due to recurrence. Gross recurrence rate has been reported at 2% per year (Bederson & Wilson 1989) or even higher (3.5% per year for major recurrences and 1.5% for minor references) (Burchicl *et al.* 1988). Minor recurrence is defined as transient, infrequent, or mild resumption of neuralgic pain and is often amenable to adjunctive medical treatment, while major recurrence is defined as resumption of previous trigeminal neuralgia pain intractable to medical regimens. If enough intrinsic damage to the system has already occurred, there remains a progressive erosion in the number of pain-free patients over time. Thus, the earlier that essential trigeminal neuralgia is addressed the better the potential outcome. Symptoms persisting for more than 8 years have a worse prognosis than more recent onset, and probably represent the formation of permanent non-reversible intrinsic lesions secondary to constant pressure on the REZ that are not addressed by microvascular decompression. It is not always clear why pain recurs; some ideas espoused are that multiple vessels are common and may not be appreciated at first operation, and that veins which have been coagulated and divided may recanalize causing recurrence of symptoms (Janetta 1980). Patients are usually maintained on their preoperative anticonvulsants, if any, and medication is withdrawn slowly after discharge home. Early recurrence of pain can frequently be treated effectively by resumption of previously ineffective doses of medications.

In the older literature, microvascular decompression has been associated with a significant incidence of morbidity as well as mortality. Some authors have even condemned microvascular decompression as a therapeutic option for trigeminal neuralgia because the high incidence of complications and the approximately 1% mortality seem untenable for a benign disease with no associated mortality (Morley 1985). There is also not complete agreement that trigeminal neuralgia is explained entirely by neurovascular compression or that microvascular decompression is the best modality to treat the aetiology of trigeminal neuralgia, with both ardent supporters (Jannetta 1967; 1980) as well as detractors (Morley 1985; Adams 1989).

Detailed preoperative imaging of the root entry zones is critical to rule out a tumour, AVM or multiple sclerosis before attempting microvascular decompression. Cryptic angiomas have also been mentioned as a rare cause of trigeminal neuralgia (Tsubaki *et al.* 1989). Although generally the neurovascular compression is at the REZ, there are cases where the nerve is actually transfixed by veins or, much rarer, arteries (Tashiro *et al.* 1991). These probably fare better with a modification of partial sensory rhizotomy rather than microvascular decompression. MRI is probably the most useful screening tool for tumours and AVMs, and also provides the additional advantage of imaging the trigeminal REZ for evidence of vascular compression or multiple sclerosis plaques. MRA (magnetic resonance angiography) is a non-invasive modality which may be of value for defining vascular relationships at the level of the REZ.

There are still many questions about microvascular decompression that need to be answered. Uncommonly, neurovascular compression is seen at REZ of asymptomatic cranial nerves, yet trigeminal neuralgia pain can present with subtle or absent evidence of neurovascular compression (Jannetta 1980). The incidence of hearing loss seems unacceptably high and needs to be addressed; probably the prime offenders are conduction problems due to less than meticulous avoidance of entering the mastoid air cells, and nerve deficit due to excessive exposure or retraction. Modification in technique and use of intraoperative electrophysiological monitoring can lower the incidence of these complications (Sindou *et al.* 1992). Although inconsistencies exist, neurovascular compression still seems to be the best explanation for many cases of trigeminal neuralgia, and microvascular decompression still has by far the highest percentage cure rate.

Partial sensory rhizotomy

Trigeminal root section by the subtemporal extradural approach (Frazier approach) has long been employed in the treatment of trigeminal neuralgia. As newer procedures have been developed, the literature has contained fewer accounts of the outcome of subtemporal rhizotomy. A posterior fossa approach can be used following attempted microvascular decompression in the event that no vascular compression of the nerve is identified. This is called partial sensory rhizotomy (PSR). Currently, the most common indication for PSR is as an alternative to microvascular decompression when no convincing neurovascular impingement is noted, as has been reported in from 14% to 21% of cases in which the original intent was to perform a microvascular decompression (Burchiel *et al.* 1981; Piatt & Wilkins 1984; Burchiel 1987*b*).

Results

Unfortunately, most recent studies tend to combine their PSR and microvascular decompression statistics rather than report them individually. Compared with microvascular decompression, PSR has fewer good results, and generally major recurrences are more frequent than minor (Burchiel *et al.* 1988). Initial results are quite good, ranging from 86% to 100% immediate pain relief (Hussein *et al.* 1982; Klun 1992) tapering to about 50% pain-free at 5 years (Klun 1992). Patients having a poor result varies from 4% to 25% depending on the time interval studied. Rate of recurrence is widely variable in the literature and ranges from 4% to 63% of patients depending on follow-up interval and surgeon (Jannetta 1980; Hussein *et al.* 1982; Piatt & Wilkins 1984; Burchiel *et al.* 1988; Zhang *et al.* 1990; Klun 1992). Most recurrences seem to occur in the first year postoperatively (Hussein *et al.* 1982; Zhang *et al.* 1990; Klun 1992). The rate of recurrence and initial results seem to be clearly related to the aggressiveness of the sectioning, with quick recurrence generally due to an overly cautious resection.

Complications

Mortality is similar to that of microvascular decompression (0.8% to 1.6%). Initial sensory loss is up to 100% (Burchiel *et al.* 1988), although the eventual degree of sensory loss is variable and generally much less than expected (Hussein *et al.* 1982). Persistent paraesthesias are reported as frequently as 36%, while persistent dysaestheiae run from 0% to 8% (Hussein *et al.* 1982; Piatt & Wilkins 1984; Klun 1992). Anaesthesia dolorosa occurs in from 0% to 2.3% (Bederson & Wilson 1989; Klun 1992). In studies looking at both microvascular decompression and partial sensory rhizotomy, the majority of dysaesthesiae and anaesthesia dolorosa occurs with partial sensory rhizotomy (Bederson & Wilson 1989). Corneal anaesthesia occurs with 0% to 4.6% incidence (Bederson & Wilson 1989; Klun 1992) and the corneal reflex is impaired in a further 32% (Hussein *et al.* 1982). Keratitis has not been reported when the approach is made through the posterior fossa, but is seen in up to 15% of cases approached subtemporally (Zorman & Wilson 1984; Zhang *et al.* 1990).

Inadvertent cranial nerve injuries occurred as often as 10% (Piatt & Wilkins 1984). In general, partial sensory rhizotomy seems to be associated more with injuries to the trigeminal nerve, while microvascular decompression more with facial and vestibulocochlear nerve. Transient abducens (4%) and facial nerve (8%) palsies have been noted (Hussein *et al.* 1982) with PSR, but permanent lesions are uncommon; trochlear, abducens, and facial nerve palsies, and persistent hearing loss occur at 0.8%, 0.8%, 0% to 1.6%, and 0% to 3.2%, respectively (Hussein *et al.* 1982; Zorman & Wilson 1984; Bederson & Wilson 1989).

Other complications include CSF leak (0% to 4%) (Burchiel *et al.* 1988; Klun 1992), aseptic meningitis (94%) (Zorman & Wilson 1984), and hydrocephalus (2–3%) (Bederson & Wilson 1989). Epidural haematoma, chronic subdural haematoma, infections, and thromboembolic events such as deep venous thrombosis and pulmonary embolus are all seen, but are generally rare (Piatt & Wilkins 1984; Zorman & Wilson 1984; Bederson & Wilson 1989). The incidence of annoying labial herpes outbreak occurs from 50% to 100% (Hussein *et al.* 1982; Klun 1992).

Discussion

Partial sensory rhizotomy is an effective modality when no neurovascular compression is noted at operation. However, it often produces a significant, variable sensory deficit, and a greater incidence of dysaesthesias, and recurrence that makes microvascular decompression more attractive as an initial procedure.

Most surgeons report similar results for partial sensory rhizotomy and microvascular decompression, although unfortunately many studies tend to combine partial sensory rhizotomy results with their microvascular decompression statistics rather than report them individually. Of the two, however, only microvascular decompression corrects the presumed pathology at the point of origin (REZ) and relieves facial pain while preserving facial sensation. Compared with microvascular decompression, partial sensory rhizotomy has fewer good results and many more major recurrences. Rate of recurrence and initial results seem to be related to aggressiveness of the sectioning. Remarkably, due to the intrinsic somatotopy of the trigeminal nerve with V_1 located superiorly, rhizotomy usually spares the ophthalmic division and touch sensation on the majority of the face. The degree of sensory loss is often suprisingly small, even in patients having near total rhizotomy. It is possible to produce a dissociated sensory loss of pinprick and light touch by sectioning the posterior portion of the root (less effective when V_1 is involved), seeming to suggest an anatomical separation of fibres subserving light touch and pinprick in the posterior nerve root (Hussein *et al.* 1982).

There is relatively little evidence favouring Frazier's approach over the posterior fossa approach when the goal is performing a rhizotomy; both have similar efficacy, morbidity, and mortality. Keratitis is much more frequent with the subtemporal approach than the posterior fossa approach, but likewise hearing loss is not seen much in the subtemporal approach but is unfortunately all too common with the posterior fossa approach. Probably the only general indication for rhizotomy today is when a microvascular decompression is attempted but no extrinsic neurovascular compression is noted. However, in those patients with vascular contact but no distortion of the trigeminal REZ, some have advocated both partial sensory rhizotomy and microvascular decompression (Bederson & Wilson 1989).

Trigeminal tractotomy

Destruction of the descending spinal tract of the trigeminal nerve in the dorsal medulla (Sjoqvist procedure (1938)) produces analgesia and thermoanalgesia in the distrubtion of the ipsilateral nerve with preservation of tactile sensation. This can be performed as either an open (Hosobuchi & Rutkin 1971; Zorman & Wilson 1984; Burchiel 1987b) or percutaneous stereotaxic (Nashold & Crue 1982; Schvarcz 1989) procedure and can be done bilaterally. Although occasionally used in recalcitrant idiopathic trigeminal neuralgia, this is primarily a procedure for treatment of intractable pain associated with malignant disease of the head and neck, and can be combined with other procedures such as nucleotomy and rhizotomy for improved results. The open medullary tractotomy is generally ineffective in cases of deafferentation pain, although the literature presents mixed success in treating post-herpetic neuralgia (Burchiel 1987b; Schvarcz 1989). Stereotactic trigeminal nucleotomy of the second order neurons at the oral pole of nucleus caudalis has been found to be quite effective in such patients with deafferentation pain (Schvarcz 1989). Unlike essential trigeminal neuralgia, the dysaesthetic pain in deafferentation is directly proportional to the extent of sensory deficit.

Results

Recent series with physiological monitoring are small. The success rate for trigeminal neuralgia depends inversely on the duration of pain. Virtually all patients have dense analgesia in the corresponding region of the face. The rate of relief in trigeminal neuralgia patients is about 58% pain-free and 42% with partial relief. Follow-up at 6 years shows 58% pain-free and 42% partially improved (Plangger *et al.* 1987). Between 50% and 85% of patients with intractable pain associated with malignant disease of the head and neck can achieve satisfactory relief (Burchiel 1987b; Schvarcz 1989). Long-term follow-up is often problematic in cancer patients due to the nature of their primary disease, and reports in the literature are scarce. Typically, success rate tends to dwindle in proportion to disease. There also appears to be some benefit for post-traumatic and post-herpetic deafferentation pain (Plangger *et al.* 1987), but there is no consensus (Schvarcz 1989). Stereotatic trigeminal nucleotomy of the second order neurons at the oral pole of nucleus caudalis is more effective than tractotomy itself and provides satisfactory pain relief in 76% of patients with deafferentation pain due to post-herpetic neuralgia or from anaesthesia dolorosa (Schvarez 1989).

Complications

Many of the reported complications stem from poor anatomical localization of the descending tract and the difficulty in correctly placing lesions within the medulla. The descending tract extends from the area of the second dorsal cervical nerve root medially to the line of emergence of the filaments of the spinal accessory nerve. At the level of the obex, this tract becomes ventrolateral to the restiform body, and its identification becomes problematic. It is preferable to perform the tractotomy after localization by evoked potentials recorded from the brain stem during continuous peripheral trigeminal stimulation.

Keratitis, hemiparesis, facial palsy, masticatory paresis, and anaesthesia dolorosa are all exceedingly rare (Plangger *et al.* 1987). Ipsilateral limb ataxia has been described in 10% and contralateral limb sensory loss in 14% of patients (Hosobuchi & Rutkin 1971). These occur secondary to lesion extension into the adjacent restiform body and spinothalamic tract respectively and are more common in large ophthalmic distribution lesions (Schvarcz 1989). Proprioceptive loss in the ipsilateral arm and leg occasionally occurs secondary to aggressive lesioning far dorsally in attempts to render the mandibular and oropharyngeal areas anaesthetic. Although all of these lesions are usually transient, they can persist. Mortality is minimal with careful physiological monitoring.

Discussion

The indications for tractotomy today are few for several reasons. First, improved delivery of adjunctive regimens such as chemotherapy and radiation therapy decreases the number of advanced stage cancer patients needing invasive pain procedures. Also improved (and less invasive) analgesic delivery systems such as intrathecal morphine infusion pumps have been shown to be effective in malignant head and neck pain (Andersen *et al.* 1991). In benign pain, all other modalities should be considered first before tractotomy is contemplated.

Tractotomy lesions are surprisingly tolerable but produce dense analgesia and thermoanalgesia with preservation of light touch, corneal reflex, and a modicum of thermal sensibility. The afferent impulses for tongue, facial, and other reflexes participating in mastication and swallowing are intact and patients continue to be able to locate food particles on the lips, tongue, or gingiva. On the other hand, the sensory loss is permanent and durability of long-term relief is uncertain. Some modifications in the topography and degree of sensory deficit can be made post-tractotomy with medications. Levodopa will decrease the extent of the sensory deficit and thus potentially increase the amount of facial pain perceived while, conversely, methyldopa and the longer-acting L-tryptophan will increase the sensory deficit zone size and potentially decrease the pain experienced (Hodge & King 1976; King 1980).

The subnucleus caudalis is the rostral extension of the substantia gelatinosa, and there is overlap between the fibres of the trigeminal nerve and the upper cervical rootlets that may transmit painful sensations to higher centres over both trigeminothalamic and spinothalamic fibre systems. This is most marked at C2, since the sensory root at C1 may be small or absent and only a small group of fibres of the spinal tract of the trigeminal nerve enter C3. Addition of a partial cervical nucleotomy may be needed to destroy the pain fibres coming from the cervical roots. In patients with malignant pain in the distribution of V, VII, IX, or X, a cervical rhizotomy is also usually employed for more effective pain relief (King 1985; Plangger *et al.* 1987).

Nucleus caudalis dorsal root entry zone (DREZ) lesion

The original DREZ lesion described in the neurosurgical literature in 1976 (Nashold *et al.* 1976) was performed for brachial plexus avulsion and has since been expanded in concept to include deafferentation pain syndromes at all levels of the spinal cord and higher. Medical treatment and operations designed to interrupt the trigeminal nerve or root are rarely effective in deafferentation pain. The theoretical basis for performing DREZ lesions is the belief that central pain is localized to the secondary neurons. These are thought to be 'hyperirritable' and become destabilized after deafferentation, firing erratically and resulting in severe pain. The nucleus caudalis of the trigeminal nerve is the first relay station for central transmission of facial pain. The DREZ lesion is aimed at destroying Lissauer's tract and the five superficial Rexed layers of the dorsal horn, and differs from trigeminal tractotomy in that the lesions are placed in order to destroy the secondary neurons carrying nociceptive and thermal sensation (Nashold 1988).

Indications for DREZ lesions include post-herpetic neuralgia, anaesthesia dolorosa, malignancy, or intractable facial pain secondary to dental procedures, glaucoma, salivary stones, Caldwell–Luc procedures, facial trauma, or brainstem vascular lesions (Sampson & Nashold 1992). In general, DREZ lesions are thought to be most efficacious for deafferentation pain, and should probably be limited to patients failing the first-line procedures.

Results

Typically, DREZ lesions in the trigeminal nucleus caudalis result in hypaesthesia over the entire ipsilateral hemiface, including all three trigeminal divisions plus the cornea and variably the cheeks and anterior tongue. The nuclear afferents for VII, IX, X run along the dorsal aspect of the nucleus caudalis so that strategic inclusion of these can tailor therapy for pain from dental or oropharyngeal structures. Although these are used for a wide variety of dissimilar primary problems, certain generalizations may be made. Most patients seem to receive excellent immediate pain relief at the price of a nearly 100% chance of an undesired deficit of some sort (Ishijima *et al.* 1988; Spiegelmann *et al.* 1991; Sampson & Nashold 1992). At follow-up the pain-free percentage declines to 55% to 100% (Bernard *et al.* 1987, 1988; Ishijima *et al.* 1988; Sampson & Nashold 1992). In all of the reviewed studies, patients with post-herpetic neuralgia have the best results with 67% to 100% having satisfactory pain relief over the long term. Trigeminal neuralgia and atypical facial pain patients have more varied results with satisfactory pain relief in only approximately 50%. Patients with burning or sharp, lancinating pain have better outcomes than those with dull, aching pain. In addition, patients with painful symptoms lasting less than 4 years fare better than those with longer duration of symptoms. As with tractotomy, a better outcome can be expected if the preoperative symptoms were associated with minor or no sensory deficits. The number of trigeminal dermatomes operated upon has no bearing on the results as all ipsilateral divisions are covered by unilateral nucleus caudalis DREZotomy. Many patients continue to have satisfactory pain relief at follow-up 6 months to 4 years later. The DREZ lesion can be repeated for good effect if necessary.

Complications

As expected from the structures present in the vicinity of the operative target, many undesired lower cranial nerve and long tract lesions can be produced. Many patients will have transient ipsilateral dysmetria affecting arms more than legs due to involvement of the spinocerebellar tracts, which often improves somewhat and does not usually pose a serious functional problem. This can be reduced by 50% using the insulated tip nucleus caudalis DREZ electrode. Other reported complications include ataxia, ipsilateral Brown–Sequard syndrome, ipsilateral spinal accessory nerve palsy with torticollis, mild ipsilateral upper extremity monoparesis or ipsilateral hemiparesis, and ipsilateral hypaesthesia (Bernard *et al.* 1987; Spiegelmann *et al.* 1991; Sampson & Nashold 1992). Postoperative dysaesthesia has not thus far been reported, and mortality is very low and usually associated with other postoperative medical problems.

Discussion

Relatively few studies are available and those tend to be small clinical series combining patients with diverse primary diseases manifesting as 'facial pain'. The encouraging results seen with refractory post-herpetic craniofacial neuralgia support the theory that this entity may primarily involve the secondary afferent neurons in the nucleus caudalis, and represent an example of a 'central' pain phenomenon that is directly amenable to a procedure addressing the second order neurons. The nucleus caudalis is associated with the trigeminal, facial, glossopharyngeal, and vagal pathways. Therefore, DREZ lesions of the nucleus caudalis which involve all three divisions plus the nuclear efferents from VII, IX, X result in an extensive ipsilateral hemihypaesthesia to pinprick over the entire half of the face, oral and pharyngeal region. The most difficult technical feat is locating the rostral limit of destruction (Katusic *et al.* 1990). Failure to extend the lesion to or slightly above the obex may result in sparing of central facial sensation and persistent facial pain. One should take care not to injure the ascending spinocerebellar pathways, which are lateral and dorsal to the trigeminal pathways. Injury to this tract would result in ipsilateral ataxia, particularly of the upper extremity. The nucleus of XI, the crossed pyramidal tract, and dorsal columns are also in the immediate vicinity and attractive targets for a misguided probe. It has been suggested that this procedure be done awake to allow for patient input on pre-lesioning stimulation to avoid misplaced lesions and complications (Spiegelmann *et al.* 1991). DREZ has a significant learning curve and is best done at centres which frequently perform this procedure. In any case, it is prudent to consider a therapeutic trial of epidural narcotics before proceeding to tractotomy or DREZotomy (Anderson *et al.* 1991).

Novel regimens

Retrograde adriamycin sensory ganglionectomy

Peripheral intraneural administration of neurotoxins such as adriamycin results in rapid retrograde axoplasmic transport to the ganglion (Yamamoto *et al.* 1984), and it is thought that this could be useful for selectively inducing permanent lesions in target sensory ganglions. Preliminary studies have reported good short term results after treatment in patients with neuropathic pain who were treated with retrograde adriamycin transport (Kato *et al.* 1990). The indications and advantages over the other percutaneous procedures are not yet clear, but they merit further active investigation.

Chronic neurostimulation

Chronic electrical stimulation of the gasserian ganglion has been described for the treatment of severe deafferentation pain (Lazorthes *et al.* 1987). The electrodes are placed using the traditional approach of Hartel (1912) and connected to an external stimulator for a trial period. If the pain is effectively relieved, the electrodes are permanently implanted along with an impulse generator. Early studies report satisfactory pain relief in over 50% of patients with intractable facial pain, but also an 85% rate of technical or procedural complications. No patient had total relief (Lobato *et al.* 1990). Admittedly, these difficult patients are generally refractory to multiple therapeutic interventions, but in light of other highly effective procedures with better pain relief and fewer complications, the place for this modality in the treatment scheme for trigeminal neuralgia remains unclear. This procedure should not be a first or second line therapy for idiopathic trigeminal neuralgia, but it does bear further investigation by those centres actively researching it.

References

Adams, C. B. T. (1989). Microvascular compression: an alternative view and hypothesis. *J. Neurosurg.* **70**, 1–12.

Andersen, P., Cohen, J., Everts, E., Bedder, M. & Burchiel, K. (1991). Intrathecal narcotics for relief of pain from head and neck cancer. *Arch. Otolaryngol. Head Neck Surg.* **117**, 1277–80.

Bederson, J. & Wilson, C. B. (1989). Evaluation of microvascular decompression and partial sensory rhizotomy in 252 cases of trigeminal neuralgia. *J. Neurosurg.* **71**, 359–67.

Belber, C. & Rak, R. (1987). Balloon compression rhizolysis in the surgical management of trigeminal neuralgia. *Neurosurgery* **20**, 908–13.

Bergenheim, A., Hariz, M. & Laitinen, L. (1991). Selectivity of retrogasserian glycerol rhizotomy in the treatment of trigeminal neuralgia. *Stereotact. Funct. Neurosurg.* **56**, 159–65.

Bernard, E. Jr, Nashold, B. Jr, Caputi, F. & Moossy, J. (1987). Nucleus caudalis DREZ lesions for facial pain. *Br. J. Neurosurg.* **1**, 81–92.

Bernard, E. Jr, Nashold, B. Jr, & Caputi, F. (1988). Clinical review of nucleus caudalis dorsal root entry zone lesions for facial pain. *Appl. Neurophysiol.* **51**, 218–24.

Broggi, G., Franzini, A., Lasio, G., Giorgi, C. & Servello, D. (1990). Long-term results of percutaneous retrogasserian thermorhizotomy for 'Essential' trigeminal neuralgia. *Neurosurgery* **26**, 783–7.

Brown, J. & Preul, M. (1989). Percutaneous trigeminal ganglion compression for trigeminal neuralgia. *J. Neurosurg.* **70**, 900–4.

Burchiel, K., Steege, T., Howe, J. & Loeser, J. (1981). Comparison of percutaneous radiofrequency gangliolysis and microvascular decompression for the surgical management of tic douloureux. *Neurosurgery* **9**, 111–19.

Burchiel, K. (1988). Percutaneous retrogasserian glycerol rhizolysis in the management of trigeminal neuralgia. *J. Neurosurg.* **69**, 361–6.

Burchiel, K. J., Clarke, H., Haglund, M. & Loeser, J. (1988). Long-term efficacy of microvascular decompression in trigeminal neuralgia. *J. Neurosurg.* **69**, 35–8.

Burchiel, K. (1987*a*). Surgical treatment of trigeminal neuralgia: minor operative procedures. In *Medical and Surgical Management of Trigeminal Neuralgia*, ed. G. Fromm, pp. 71–99. Mount Kisco, New York: Futura.

Burchiel, K. (1987*b*). Surgical treatment of trigeminal neuralgia: major operative procedures. In *Medical and Surgical Management of Trigeminal Neuralgia*, ed. G. Fromm, pp. 71–99. Mount Kisco, New York: Futura.

Dandy, W. E. (1932). The treatment of trigeminal neuralgia by the cerebellar route. *Am. J. Surg.* **96**, 787–95.

Dandy, W. E. (1934). Concerning the cause of trigeminal neuralgia. *Am. J. Surg.* **24**, 447–55.

Gardner, W. J. & Miklos, M. V. (1959). Response of trigeminal neuralgia to 'decompression' of sensory root. Discussion of cause of trigeminal neuralgia. *JAMA* **170**, 1773–6.

De La Porte, C., Verlooy, J., Veeckman, G., Parizel, P., de Moor, J. & Selosse, P. (1990). Consequences and complications of glycerol injection in the cavum of Meckel. *Stereotact. Funct. Neurosurg.* **54, 55**, 73–5.

Fraoili, B., Esposito, V., Guidetti, B., Crucci, G. & Manfredi, M. (1984). Treatment of trigeminal neuralgia by thermocoagulation, glycerolization, and percutaneous compression of the gasserian ganglion and/or retrogasserial rootlets: long-term results and therapeutic protocol. *Neurosurgery* **24**, 239–45.

Fritz, W., Schafer, J. & Klein, H. (1988). Hearing loss after microvascular decompression for trigeminal neuralgia. *J. Neurosurg.* **69**, 367–70.

Fujimaki, T., Fukishima, T. & Miyazaki, S. (1990). Percutaneous retrogasserian glycerol injection in the management of trigeminal neuralgia. *J. Neurosurg.* **73**, 212–16.

Hakanson, S. (1978). Transoval trigeminal cisternography. *Surg. Neurol.* **10**, 137.

Hakanson, S. (1981). Trigeminal neuralgia treated by the injection of glycerol into the trigeminal cistern. *Neurosurgery* **9**, 638–46.

Hamlyn, P. & King, T. (1992). Neurovascular compression in trigeminal neuralgia. *J. Neurosurg.* **76**, 948–54.

Hardy, D. & Rhoton, A. Jr (1978). Microsurgical relationship of the superior cerebellar artery and the trigeminal nerve. *J. Neurosurg.* **49**, 669–78.

Hartel, F. (1912). Die Leitungsanasthesie und injections behandlung des ganglion gasseriund der trigeminusstame. *Arch. Klin. Chir.* **100**, 193–292.

Hodge, C. Jr & King, R. (1976). Medical modification of sensation. *J. Neurosurg.* **44**, 21–8.

Hosobuchi, Y. & Rutkin, B. (1971). Descending trigeminal tractotomy. Neurophysiological approach. *Arch. Neurol.* **25**, 115.

Hussein, M., Wilson, L. & Illingworth, R. (1982). Patterns of sensory loss following fractional posterior fossa Vth nerve section for trigeminal neuralgia. *J. Neurol. Neurosurg. Psychiatry* **45**, 786–90.

Ishijima, B. Shimoji, K., Shimuzu, H., Takahashi, H. & Suzuki, I. (1988). Lesions of spinal and trigeminal dorsal root entry zone for deafferentation pain. *Appl. Neurophysiol.* **51**, 175–87.

Jannetta, P. (1980). Neurovascular compression in cranial nerve and systemic disease. *Ann. Surg.* **192**, 518–25.

Jannetta, P. J. (1967). Arterial compression of the trigeminal nerve at the pons in patients with trigeminal neuralgia. *J. Neurosurg.* **26**, 159–62.

Kato, S., Otsuki, T., Yamamoto, T., Iwasaki, Y. & Yoshimoto, T. (1990). Retrograde adriamycin sensory ganglionectomy. *Stereotact. Funct. Neurosurg.* **54**, 86–9.

Katusic, S., Beard, C., Bergstrahl, E. & Kurland, L. (1990). Incidence and clinical feature of trigeminal neuralgia, Rochester Minnesota 1945–1984. *Ann. Neurol.* **27**, 89–95.

King, R. B. (1985). Medullary tractotomy for pain relief. In *Neurosurgery*, eds. R. H. Wilkins & S. S. Rengachary, pp. 2452–4. New York: McGraw Hill.

King, R. B. (1980). Pain and tryptophan. *J. Neurosurg.* **53**, 44–52.

Klun, B. (1992). Microvascular decompression and partial sensory rhizotomy in the treatment of trigeminal neuralgia. *Neurosurgery* **30**, 49–52.

Lazorthes, Y., Armengaud, J. P. & DaMotta, M. (1987). Chronic stimulation of the Gasserian ganglion for treatment of atypical facial neuralgia. *Pacing Clin. Electrophysiol.* **V10**, 257–65.

Lobato, R., Rivas, J., Sarabia, R. & Lamas, E. (1990). Percutaneous microcompression of the gasserian ganglion for trigeminal neuralgia. *J. Neurosurg.* **72**, 546–53.

Matsushima, T., Fukui, M., Sazuki, S. & Rhoton, A. Jr (1989). The microsurgical anatomy of the infratentorial lateral supracerebellar approach to the trigeminal nerve for tic douloureux. *Neurosurgery* **24**, 890–5.

Meglio, M., Cioni, B., Moles, A. & Visocchi, M. (1990). Microvascular decompression versus percutaneous procedures for typical trigeminal neuralgia. *Stereotact. Funct. Neurosurg.* **54**, **55**, 76–9.

Meglio, M., Cioni, B. & d'Annunzio, V. (1987). Percutaneous microcompression of the gasserian ganglion: Personal experience. *Acta Neurochir.* **39** (Suppl.), 142–3.

Meglio, M. & Cioni, B. (1989). Percutaneous procedures for trigeminal neuralgia: microcompression versus radiofrequency thermocoagulation. *Pain* **38**, 9–16.

Moraci, A., Buonaiuto, C., Punzo, A., Parlato, C. & Amalfi, R. (1992). *Neurochirurgica* **35**, 48–53.

Morley, T. P. (1985). Case against microvascular decompression in the treatment of trigeminal neuralgia. *Arch. Neurol.* **42**, 801–2.

Mullan, S. & Lichtor, T. (1990). A 10-year follow-up review of percutaneous microcompression of the trigeminal ganglion. *J. Neurosurg.* **72**, 49–54.

Mullan, S. & Lichtor, T. (1983). Percutaneous microcompression of the trigeminal ganglion for trigeminal neuralgia. *J. Neurosurg.* **59**, 1007–12.

Nashold, B. (1988). Neurosurgical technique of the dorsal root entry zone operation. *Appl. Neurophysiol.* **51**, 136–45.

Nashold, B. & Crue, B. (1982). Stereotaxic mesencephalotomy and trigeminal tractotomy. In *Neurological Surgery*, 2nd edn, ed. J. R. Youmans, p. 3702. Philadelphia; Saunders.

Nashold, B., Urban, B. & Zorub, D. (1976). Phantom pain relief by focal destruction of the substantia gelatinosa of Rolando. In *Advances in Pain Research and Therapy*, vol. 1, ed. J. Bonica, pp. 959–63. New York: Raven Press.

North, R., Kidd, D., Piantadosi, J. & Carson, B. (1990). Percutaneous retrogasserian glycerol rhizotomy. *J. Neurosurg.* **72**, 851–6.

Piatt, J. & Wilkins, R. (1984). Treatment of tic douloureux and hemifacial spasm by posterior fossa exploration: therapeutic implications of various neurovascular relationships. *Neurosurgery* **14**, 462–71.

Piquer, J., Joanes, V., Roldam, P., Barcia-Salario, J. & Masbout, G. (1987). Long-term results of percutaneous gasserian ganglion lesions. *Acta Neurochir.* **39**(Suppl.), 139–41.

Plangger, C., Fischer, J., Grunert, V. & Mohsenipour, I. (1987). Tractotomy and partial vertical nucleotomy: for treatment of special forms of trigeminal neuralgia and cancer pain of face and neck. *Acta Neurochirurg.* **39** (Suppl.), 147–50.

Pollack, I., Jannetta, P. & Bissonette, D. (1988). Bilateral trigeminal neuralgia: a 14-year experience with microvascular decompression. *J. Neurosurg.* **68**, 559–65.

Puca, A., Meglio, M., Cioni, B., Visocchi, M. & Lauretti, L. (1992). Intracerebral injury following thermocoagulation of the trigeminal ganglion. *Surg. Neurol.* **38**, 280–2.

Sampson, J. & Nashold, B. Jr (1992). Facial pain due to vascular lesions of the brain stem relieved by dorsal root entry zone lesions in the nucleus caudalis. *J. Neurosurg.* **77**, 473–5.

Sahni, K. S., Pieper, D., Anderson, R. & Baldwin, N. (1990). Relation of hypesthesia to the outcome of glycerol rhizolysis for trigeminal neuralgia. *J. Neurosurg.* **72**, 55–8.

Saini, S. S. (1987). Retrogasserian anhydrous glycerol injection thereapy in trigeminal neuralgia: observations in 552 patients. *J. Neurol. Neurosurg. Psychiatry* **50**, 1536–8.

Schvarcz, J. (1989). Craniofacial postherpetic neuralgia managed by stereotactic spinal trigeminal nucleotomy. *Acta Neurochirurg.* **46** (Suppl.), 62–4.

Shelden, C. H., Pudenz, R. H. & Freshwater, D. B. (1955). Compression rather than decompression for trigeminal neuralgia. *J. Neurosurg.* **12**, 123–6.

Schwartz, D. & Gennarelli, T. (1990). Delayed sensorineural hearing loss following uncomplicated neurovacular decompression of the trigeminal root entry zone. *Am. J. Otol.* **11**, 95–8.

Sindou, M., Fobe, J., Ciriano, D. & Fischer, C. (1992). Hearing prognosis and intraoperative guidance of brainstem auditory evoked potential in microvascular decompression. *Laryngoscope* **102**, 678–82.

Sjoqvist, O. (1938). Studies on pain conduction in the trigeminal nerve: a contribution to the surgical treatment of facial pain. *Acta Psychiatr. Neurol.* **17** (Suppl.), 1–139.

Spiegelmann, R., Friedmann, W., Ballinger, W. & Tedeschi, H. (1991). Anatomic examination of a case of open trigeminal nucleotomy for facial pain. *Stereotact. Funct. Neurosurg.* **56**, 166–78.

Sweet, W. H. & Wepsic, J. G. (1974). Controlled thermocoagulation of trigeminal ganglion and rootlets for differential destruction of pain fibres, part 1, trigeminal neuralgia. *J. Neurosurg.* **40**, 143.

Sweet, W. H. (1985). Trigeminal neuralgia: problems as to cause and consequent conclusions regarding treatment. In *Neurosurgery*, ed. R. H. Wilkins & S. S. Rengachary, pp. 366–72. New York: McGraw-Hill.

Szapiro, J. & Sindou, M. (1985). Prognostic factors in microvascular decompression for trigeminal neuralgia. *J. Neurosurg.* **17**, 920–9.

Tashiro, H., Kondo, A., Aoyama, I., Nin, K., Shimotake, K., Nishioka, T., Ikai, Y. & Takahashi, J. (1991). Trigeminal neuralgia caused by compression from arteries transfixing the nerve. *J. Neurosurg.* **75**, 783–6.

Tsubaki, S., Fukishima, T., Tamagawa, T., Miyazaki, S., Watanabe, K., Kuwana, N. & Shimuzu, T. (1989). Parapontine trigeminal cryptic angiomas presenting as trigeminal neuralgia. *J. Neurosurg.* **71**, 368–74.

Tytus, J. (1982). Treatment of trigeminal neuralgia through temporal craniotomy. In *Neurological Surgery*, 2nd edn, ed. J. Youmans, p. 3850. Philadelphia: Saunders.

Yamamoto, T., Iwasaki, Y. & Konno, H. (1984). Experimental sensory ganglionectomy by way of suicide axoplasmic transport. *J. Neurosurg.* **69**, 108–14.

Zhang, K., Zhao, Y., Shun, Z. & Li, P. (1990). Microvascular decompression by retromastoid approach for trigeminal neuralgia: experience in 200 patients. *Ann. Otol. Rhinol. Laryngol.* **99**, 129–30.

Zorman, G. & Wilson, C. (1984). Outcome following microsurgical decompression or partial sensory rhizotomy in 125 cases of trigeminal neuralgia. *Neurology* **34**, 1362–5.

28 Neurosurgical treatment for pain: spinal cord stimulation

ANDREW PARRENT

Introduction

The concept of electrically stimulating the spinal cord or peripheral nerve to treat chronic pain followed as a practical application of the gate control theory proposed by Melzack & Wall in 1965. They proposed that pain perception was determined by a balance of small-fibre and large-fibre input into a central 'gating' mechanism located in the dorsal horn of the spinal cord, and that chronic pain could be caused by conditions that skewed this balance toward small-fibre input (Melzack & Wall 1965).

In testing predictions of the gate control theory, Wall & Sweet stimulated their own infraorbital nerves with needle electrodes (Wall & Sweet 1967; Sweet & Wepsic 1968). This stimulation caused a non-painful buzzing in the distribution of the nerve as well as an elevation of the threshold for pinprick appreciation during stimulation and shortly after its discontinuation.

There was a succession of reports involving the use of peripheral nerve simulation, both transcutaneously (TENS) and directly for the treatment of chronic pain (Wall & Sweet 1967; Sweet & Wepsic 1968; Long 1974; Shealy 1973). Shealy *et al.* (1967*a,b*) suggested that stimulation of the dorsal columns of the spinal cord would affect a greater concentration of large-diameter fibres and might therefore inhibit pain more effectively. In 1967, they reported the first use of dorsal column stimulation for the treatment of chronic pain, and in 1970 they reported results in six patients with 'excellent' pain control in three and 'good' control in two patients.

Since the mechanisms by which dorsal column stimulation produces relief are not fully understood and the physiological basis of most chronic pain syndromes is not known, the use of dorsal column stimulation has evolved along empirical lines. Indications for spinal stimulation have changed as experience has been gained in this technique, and most publications stress the need for better patient selection.

Mechanisms of spinal cord stimulation

In spite of much experimental work, the mechanism by which dorsal column stimulation achieves chronic pain control is not known. Much of the experimental work involves acute nociceptive stimulation and many of the findings are at odds with the clinical experience with dorsal column stimulation.

In experimental animal models it has been shown that stimulation of the dorsal columns can block the activity of lamina V polymodal and nociceptive specific neurons in response to peripheral nociceptive input (Handwerker *et al.* 1975; Feldman 1975; Hilman & Wall 1969; Saade & Jabbur 1985), as well as nociceptive reflexes. In these studies, the effects do not outlast the duration of stimulation by more than a few seconds. Chronic pain patients treated with dorsal column stimulation frequently report latencies of many minutes before effective relief is obtained, and the post-stimulatory effect may last for minutes to hours. The threshold for the appreciation of acute pain is rarely elevated in these patients, in spite of suppression of chronic pain.

There has been much study of the pathways that may be affected by spinal cord stimulation and mechanisms by which they suppress pain. It has been proposed that spinal cord stimulation produces pain relief by causing a conduction block in spinothalamic tract fibres (Campbell 1981). Hoppenstein (1975) and Larson *et al.* (1975) demonstrated that by directly stimulating the ventral aspect of the spinal cord they could produce pain relief at thresholds 30–40 times lower than those required for relief from dorsal cord stimulation. It was noted that relief from ventral cord stimulation occurred in the absence of stimulation-induced paraesthesias and was associated with diminished appreciation of pinprick contralaterally below the level of stimulation. Larson *et al.* (1975) suggested that dorsal column stimulation produced its effect by producing a conduction block in the spinothalamic tract fibres. This does not account for the fact that dorsal column stimulation frequently produces persistent pain relief after cessation of stimulation, that there is rarely a change in the perception of acute pain and that sectioning of the dorsal columns below the level of stimulation in experimental animals abolishes its effectiveness even though the spinothalamic tract is intact (Foreman *et al.* 1976).

Dorsal column stimulation may act by antidromic activation of dorsal column collaterals causing inhibition of nociceptive neurons in the dorsal horn. Such inhibition has been observed in experimental animals (Handwerker *et al.* 1975; Hillman & Wall 1969) and the effect is abolished by sectioning the dorsal columns caudal to the site of the stimulating electrode (Foreman *et al.* 1976). However, this effect is very brief in duration and would not account for the prolonged pain relief reported by patients.

There is evidence that supraspinal mechanisms may be involved. Shetter & Atkinson (1977) demonstrated activation of neurons in the nucleus gigantocellularis during dorsal column stimulation, and proposed that this may result in the activation of pain inhibitory mechanisms. Saade & Jabbur (1985) showed that a rostral projection through the brainstem was responsible for the inhibition of nociceptive reflexes and dorsal horn nociceptive neurons seen with dorsal column stimulation in the cat and rat. Nyquist & Greenhoot (1975) added further support to possible supraspinal mechanisms when they showed that unilateral dorsal column stimulation suppressed centrum median nucleus responses to painful peripheral stimulation.

There is thus, evidence to support a 'gating' mechanism at a segmental, spinal or supraspinal level.

Patient selection

From literature review and personal experience, a number of statements can be made about the selection of patients for dorsal column stimulation.

Location of pain

In order to obtain pain relief from stimulation, paraesthesias must be produced to overlap the pain distribution. This is difficult to achieve with midline, deep or visceral pain, and is more difficult to achieve with bilateral than with unilateral extremity pain.

Aetiology of pain

Spinal cord stimulation seems to have a preferential effect on pain of neurogenic origin. This includes peripheral deafferentation (e.g. phantom limb pain) and the various causalgia-like pain syndromes associated with incomplete peripheral nerve injuries. Peripheral injuries associated with signs of sympathetic hyperfunction (so-called sympathetically maintained pain or reflex sympathetic dystrophy) also appear to respond. Pain secondary to injuries of the spinal cord and brain appears to respond less well than peripheral nerve injury. Certain injuries preclude the effective production of stimulation-induced paraesthesias in the pain distribution. For example, we have rarely been able to produce appropriate paraesthesias below the level of a complete spinal cord injury, and in some patients with high-level amputation. This implies that injuries which result in the loss of dorsal column fibres would preclude effective dorsal column stimulation. Pain associated with peripheral vascular disease is another entity that responds well to spinal stimulation.

Psychosocial factors

There is no doubt that psychological and social factors influence a patient's reaction to pain and response to treatment. Beyond ruling out overtly psychotic and manipulative patients and appropriately treating those with major affective disorders, there is no general consensus on the psychological factors that should be used to exclude patients from a trial of spinal stimulation. Psychological testing frequently demonstrates evidence of depression, anxiety and lack of sleep as part of the expected response to chronic pain. These findings have not been found to adversely affect the outcome of spinal cord stimulation.

Spinal stimulation trial

In the early years of spinal stimulation, electrodes were placed subdurally, endodurally (between the dural layers) or epidurally during an open procedure at which time a permanent stimulating system was also inserted. Reported success rates varied from 18% to 44%. Subsequently, attempts were made to carry out some form of trial stimulation in order to identify those patients who might derive benefit from spinal stimulation prior to implanting a permanent system. This was initially accomplished by inserting electrodes percutaneously into the subarachnoid space adjacent to the cord (Larson *et al.* 1975; Hoppenstein 1975; Erickson 1975; Long & Hagfors 1975) or into the substance of the posterior columns themselves (Hosobuchi *et al.* 1972) and carrying out brief (30–60 min) intraoperative stimulation. Overall it was felt that the effects of short-term stimulation administered in this manner were not predictive of longer-term success. In the mid to late 1970s better hardware was developed allowing the percutaneous insertion of an electrode into the epidural space. This could be externalized by a percutaneous extension and trial stimulation could then be carried out for days to weeks.

Currently, most centres carry out a trial of spinal stimulation before permanently implanting a stimulator. This can be done using a linear electrode inserted percutaneously into the epidural space under fluoroscopic control, or a paddle-type electrode inserted through a small laminotomy. The electrode should be positioned so as to produce paraesthesias that overlap the pain distribution. This is best accomplished by inserting the electrode under local anaesthesia so that the patient may provide intraoperative feedback about the localization of paraesthesias.

During the period of trial stimulation the patient is encouraged to be relatively active so that an accurate assessment of pain relief can be made. The criteria for considering the trial a 'success' are variable and largely subjective. It relies on the patient's report of stimulation-induced pain reduction and some means of quantifying the same, usually with a visual analogue pain scale. In those studies that specified their criteria for permanent implantation after a percutaneous trial, almost all required a minimum of 50% pain reduction (Meglio *et al.* 1989*b*; North *et al.* 1991*a*, 1993; Richardson *et al.* 1979; Sanchez-Ledesma *et al.* 1989; Waisbrod & Gerbershagen 1985).

Permanent stimulator implantation

There are two types of permanently implantable spinal stimulation systems. The first is a radio frequency (RF) coupled system. This requires the attachment of the spinal electrode to an RF receiver which is then implanted into a subcutaneous pocket created somewhere in the abdominal wall for thoracic cord stimulation or in the subclavicular area for cervical cord stimulation. In order to operate this system an external stimulator box generates the stimulation parameters which are then transmitted to the subcutaneous receiver through an antenna applied to the skin overlying the receiver. The second type is an implantable pulse generator. A pulse generator is attached to the spinal electrode and buried subcutaneously similar to the RF system. This device is self-powered and generates the stimulation signal without the need of an external system. The system can be turned off and on using an externally applied magnet, and can be programmed by an external device similar to that used to program a cardiac pacemaker. When the battery is depleted a new stimulator must be implanted.

Results of spinal stimulation

Results of spinal stimulation were compiled from 35 series and our own unpublished data (Tables 28.1, 28.2). Series were included only when a trial of percutaneous spinal stimulation was used for a number of days prior to permanent stimulator implantation and where results were presented according to pain aetiology.

An inherent difficulty in comparing results from different series is the different criteria by which successful stimulation is defined. In some reports, published trial stimulation was considered successful if patients reported greater than 50% pain reduction during the trial. Others required 'significant', 'satisfactory' or 'acceptable' pain relief. Similar difficulties are present when assessing the results after permanent stimulator implantation. A number of factors can be used, including: return to work status, analgesic use, patient satisfaction, continued stimulator use and pain relief as assessed by patient report or some type of pain scale. For each report we have used the author's judgement of success, and in reports that listed results by the percentage of pain relief we have considered more than 50% relief as success.

Results for spinal stimulation trials (Table 28.1) are presented separately from those following permanent implantation (Table 28.2). The former should give an indication of conditions that physiologically respond to spinal stimulation, while the latter should indicate the stability of that response over time.

The aggregate results for trial stimulation (Table 28.1) show that 70%–77% of candidates with peripheral vascular disease, peripheral nerve injury, stump pain and reflex sympathetic dystrophy have a beneficial effect from stimulation. The group of patients with post-amputation pain also showed a 70% response, but it is not clear from the original reports how many of these patients had phantom limb pain, stump pain or a combination of both. Only 48% of those with phantom limb pain showed a beneficial response to a trial of spinal cord stimulation. Patients with failed back syndrome, brachial plexus avulsion and plexus injuries showed a 62%–66% response rate.

Half or less of the patients with post-herpetic neuralgia, phantom limb pain and pain after spinal cord or brain lesions showed an initial response to spinal stimulation. The data also suggest that patients with pain due to traumatic spinal cord injury respond less well than those with other cord lesions (transverse myelitis, multiple sclerosis, tumour). We have found that in patients with complete sensory loss and pain below the level of a traumatic cord injury we have been unable to produce paraesthesias in the pain area. Cole *et al.* (1991) reported the same problem in three of four spinal cord-

Table 28.1. *Stimulator implantation after stimulation trial*

Reference	PHN	PVD	FBS	PN	RSD	Amp	Phant	Stump	BPA	Plexus	SCI	Cord	Brain
Barolat et al. (1987)					13/16								
Barolat et al. (1989)					15/18								
Broggi et al. (1987)		31/40			4/6								
Broseta et al. (1982)				3/3				5/5	1/1				
Broseta et al. (1986)		37/41								2/2			
Cole et al. (1991)	2/4										0/4		
De La Porte & Siegfried (1983)			38/94										
Demirel et al. (1984)			7/11			5/6				6/9	4/8	3/3	
Fiume (1983)		12/21											
Garcia-March et al. (1987)									6/6				
Hood & Siegfried (1984)									5/13	8/8			
Kumar et al. (1991)	0/1	4/5	57/66	4/5	2/3	0/2					1/2	10/11	
Meglio & Cioni (1982)	1/3												
Meglio et al. (1989b)		32/40	13/19										
Meglio et al. (1989a)	10/15			3/9									
North et al. (1993)			133/153										
Richardson et al. (1979)			8/9	3/3		2/3							1/1
Richardson et al. (1980)											5/7	1/3	
Robaina et al. (1988)		3/3			8/8								
Sanchez-Ledesma et al. (1989)	4/6			11/13	8/11		3/6	4/5	6/8				
Siegfried & Cetinlap (1981)					11/25					6/15	1/10		
Siegfried & Lazorthes (1982)			89/191										
Spiegelmann & Friedman (1992)	1/3		12/18	5/6					2/2			4/6	
Tallis et al. (1983)		5/10											
Tasker & Parrent (this series)	2/4	4/5	34/43	13/19			2/9	3/7	2/3	7/12		11/31	6/12
Urban & Nashold (1978)	1/2	2/3	3/10	1/1					0/1	0/1	2/2		
Vogel et al. (1986)	0/2		16/29				1/3	4/4				0/3	
Waisbrod & Gerbershagen (1985)			16/16										
Wester (1987)			10/11				5/5				3/3	4/7	
Winkelmuller (1981)	1/2	2/10	56/64		1/1	9/12					2/10	1/3	0/1
Totals	22/42 (52%)	134/180 (79%)	492/725 (68%)	43/59 (77%)	62/88 (70%)	16/23 (70%)	11/23 (48%)	16/21 (76%)	22/34 (65%)	29/47 (62%)	18/46 (39%)	34/67 (51%)	7/14 (50%)

PHN, post-herpetic neuralgia; PVD, peripheral vascular disease; FBS, failed back syndrome; PN, peripheral nerve injury; RSD, reflex sympathetic dystrophy; Amp, post-amputation pain (not specified); Phant, phantom limb pain; Stump, post-amputation stump pain; BPA, brachial plexus avulsion; Plexus, plexus injury; SCI, spinal cord injury (traumatic); Cord, pain from other cord lesions; Brain, pain after brain lesions.

Table 28.2. *Follow-up after stimulator implantation*

Reference	PHN	PVD	FBS	PN	RSD	Amp	Phant	Stump	BPA	Plexus	SCI	Cord	Brain
Barolat et al. (1987)					7/13								
Barolat et al. (1989)					11/15								
Broggi et al. (1987)		31/31			2/4			1/5	1/1	2/2			
Broseta et al. (1982)				3/3									
Broseta et al. (1986)		29/37											
De La Porte & Siegfried (1983)			18/38										
Demirel et al. (1984)	0/2		3/7			1/5				1/6	0/4	0/3	
Fiume (1983)		12/12											
Garcia-March et al. (1987)									3/6				
Hood & Siegfried (1984)									0/5	2/8			
Krainick et al. (1980)						14/61							
Kumar et al. (1991)		4/4	37/57	3/4	1/2						0/1	8/10	
Lazorthes & Verdie (1985)			29/57	4/10			0/3	2/3			0/4	3/6	
Long (1981)			18/24	1/1			1/1						
Meglio & Cioni (1982)	1/1		2/9									1/1	
Meglio et al. (1989b)		32/32									3/5		
Meglio et al. (1989a)	9/10			3/3									
North et al. (1991b)			26/50								2/5		
Ray et al. (1982)			27/50										
Richardson et al. (1979)			8/8	3/3		2/2							1/1
Richardson et al. (1980)											1/5	1/1	
Robaina et al. (1989)		3/3			7/8								
Sanchez-Ledesma et al. (1989)	3/4			11/11	8/8		1/3	3/4	3/6				
Siegfried & Cetinlap (1981)					4/9					3/4	0/1		
Siegfried (1991)	7/21	12/19	71/123	116/127		13/19					13/17	21/56	
Spiegelmann & Friedman (1991)	0/1	2/2							1/2			3/4	
Tallis et al. (1983)		5/5											
Tasker & Parrent (this series)	1/2	4/4	21/34	8/10			0/1	2/2	1/2	3/7		0/10	1/6
Urban & Nashold (1978)	0/1	0/2		1/1							1/2		
Vogel et al. (1986)			4/11				1/1	3/3					
Waisbrod & Gerbershagen (1985)			12/16								1/3		
Wester (1987)	1/1		6/8		1/1		2/5					0/4	
Totals	22/43 (51%)	134/151 (89%)	284/495 (57%)	153/173 (88%)	41/60 (68%)	30/87 (34%)	5/14 (36%)	11/17 (65%)	9/22 (41%)	11/27 (41%)	21/47 (45%)	37/95 (39%)	2/7 (29%)

PHN, post-herpetic neuralgia; PVD, peripheral vascular disease; FBS, failed back syndrome; PN, peripheral nerve injury; RSD, reflex sympathetic dystrophy; Amp, post-amputation pain (not specified); Phant, phantom limb pain; Stump, post-amputation stump pain; BPA, brachial plexus avulsion; Plexus, plexus injury; SCI, spinal cord injury (traumatic); Cord, pain from other cord lesions; Brain, pain after brain lesions.

injured patients. Richardson *et al.* (1980) noted the absence of paraesthesias in five patients with complete spinal cord injuries. However, he also noted that these patients experienced some degree of short-term relief from stimulation.

The results in Table 28.2 show that in patients with pain from peripheral vascular disease and peripheral nerve injury 89% and 88% respectively retained long-term benefit. In patients with post-herpetic neuralgia, failed back syndrome, stump pain and reflex sympathetic dystrophy 51%–68% maintained long-term benefit. It has been noted in a number of reports that in patients with failed back syndrome spinal stimulation tends to help the extremity component of the pain rather than the midline back pain. This may be due to the fact that it is difficult to produce paraesthesias in the midline low back region, or that the pathophysiology of the low back pain is different from the leg pain. North *et al.* (1991*a*) reported that paraesthesias overlapped the low back in 27% of his failed back patients. He also noted that the relief of low back pain was the same as the degree of relief of leg pain. Law (1992), using two lines of eight electrodes each, has reported more consistent production of low back paraesthesias and has noted equivalent relief in patients with predominantly low back pain and those with predominantly leg pain.

The remainder of diagnostic groups experienced more than a 50% decay in stimulator effectiveness in the long term. In patients with pain due to traumatic spinal cord injury and brain lesions long-term benefit was evident in only 23% and 29%, respectively. It appears that pain secondary to non-traumatic spinal cord damage responded better than traumatic cord injury with almost half the patients deriving long-term benefit.

Dorsal column stimulation failure

As noted in Table 28.2, a significant number of patients with initially beneficial effects from stimulation will ultimately lose that effectiveness. Some of these failures, particularly the early failures may be attributed to a placebo effect. North *et al.* (1993) reported that 22% of patients followed up after stimulator implantation reported that they had never experienced as much as 50% relief from their devices and one third of these claimed that they had never experienced any degree of relief even though they would have required more than 50% relief during trial stimulation to warrant implantation.

There is another group of patients who derive pain relief from stimulation but find that this relief diminishes over time in spite of appropriate overlap of stimulation-induced paraesthesias and their pain distribution (North *et al.* 1991*a*, 1993; Hosobuchi *et al.* 1981; Meyerson 1983; Lazorthes & Verdie 1985; Siegfried & Lazorthes 1982). In some patients the paraesthesias cease being pleasant or neutral and take on an unpleasant quality (Hosobuchi *et al.* 1981). Siegfried & Lazorthes (1982) reported an increasing failure rate over a 4-year period of time. Lazorthes & Verdie (1985) reported a progressive decrease in good and excellent results over their entire follow-up period without a tendency to stabilize. North *et al.* (1991*b*) noted that 45% of their patients reported an overall decrease in the degree of pain relief while 13% reported an increase over a mean follow-up period of 2.14 years. Kumar *et al.* (1991) reported diminishing pain relief in 34% of patients to the point of no longer deriving worthwhile benefit from stimulation. They found that this tended to occur in the first 4 years post-implant with the greatest decline in the first 2 years. They felt that those patients continuing to obtain worthwile relief at 4 years had an excellent long-term prognosis.

In our series of patients with the failed back syndrome, 21% reported a declining effect from stimulation 15 to 56 months after implanation, half of whom discontinued stimulator use as they no longer found it worthwhile. In contrast, 56% of patients reported stable beneficial effects over a mean follow-up period of 35 months (4–117 months).

The reason for the observed fall-off in stimulator effectiveness in some patients and not others is not known. It has been proposed that this may represent plasticity in the central nervous system (Meyerson 1983; Kumar *et al.* 1991) with a reorganization of the pain-transmitting or pain-inhibiting systems over time.

Complications and technical problems (Table 28.3)

When spinal electrodes were inserted intradurally or endodurally there were reports of neurological complications associated with their insertion (Krainick *et al.* 1980; Lazorthes & Verdie 1985; Meglio *et al.* 1989*b*; Sweet & Wepsic 1974), as well as delayed neurological problems related to proliferation of scar and granulation tissue around the electrode (Krainick *et al.* 1980; Pineda 1978). Whereas, we have found only a single report of dorsal column ataxia lasting 1 year following the insertion of an epidural electrode (Lazorthes & Verdie 1985).

Infection rates vary from 0 to 38% (Table 28.3) though usually less than 10%. Infection around any of the stimulator components necessitates their removal along with antibiotic treatment. Meningitis has rarely been reported (Lazorthes & Verdie 1985). Most centres use perioperative antibiotics during insertion of the stimulator, although not necessarily for the entire duration of the stimulation trial.

Pain and tenderness at the sites of hardware implantation have been reported in up to 20% of cases. Persistent pain requires revision of the subcutaneous pocket.

Technical problems with the stimulator hardware are unfortunately common, including lead migration, electrode fracture or failure and receiver failure (Table 28.3). The rate of electrode migration has varied from 2% to 77%. The type of electrode system appears to have some influence on the migration rate. North *et al.* (1993) found that migration rates in single channel systems sufficient to result in loss of appropriate paraesthesia distribution occurred in 22% over a 17-year period compared with a migration rate of less than 10% for multicontact electrodes. The use of multicontact electrodes allows one to compensate for minor changes in electrode position by changing electrode combinations thereby avoiding revision. Paddle-type electrodes were introduced to reduce the incidence of electrode migration, but there are no

Table 28.3. *Complications and technical problems with spinal cord stimulation*

Reference	Patients (n)	Lead extrusion (%)	Lead migration (%)	Infection (%)	Hardware pain (%)	Electrode fracture/failure (%)	Receiver failure (%)
Barolat et al. (1989)	18		6	0	22	17	
Broseta et al. (1986)	41		24				
De La Porte & Siegfried (1983)	38	24	55	26	11	5	5
Demirel et al. (1984)	33		33	0		9	
Koeze et al. (1987)	26		77	38		38	
Kumar et al. (1991)	94		27	9		12	2
Law & Kirkpatrick (1992)	241		5	2	8		
Lazorthes & Verdie (1985)	93	22	25	8		3	1
Meglio & Cioni (1982)	26		4	0			
Meglio et al. (1989b)	109		3	3			
North et al. (1991b)	62		2	11		13	
Racz et al. (1989)	26		69	8		23	12
Richardson et al. (1979)	36		14	3			
Sanchez-Ledesma et al. (1989)	36	3	3	0			
Simpson (1991)	60		27	5		7	12
Spiegelmann & Friedman (1991)	43		3	7		13	
Tasker & Parrent (this series)	102		48	7	9	19	
Wester (1987)	35		37	6	3		

reports indicating a lower migration rate compared with linear multicontact electrodes.

Summary

Spinal cord stimulation is a useful modality for the treatment of some chronic pain conditions. The best long-term results have been achieved in patients with pain from peripheral vascular disease and peripheral nerve injury. More than half the patients with post-herpetic neuralgia, failed back syndrome, reflex sympathetic dystrophy and post-amputation stump pain have derived long-term benefit following implantation. Notably poor results are seen in patients with phantom limb pain and pain associated with brain lesions and traumatic spinal cord injury.

With newer multicontact electrodes and multichannel stimulators many of the earlier technical problems have become rare. There still remains the unexplained problem of diminishing effectiveness of stimulation in some patients over time.

References

Barolat, G., Schwartzmann, R. & Woo, R. (1987). Epidural spinal cord stimulation in the management of reflex sympathetic dystrophy. *Appl. Neurophysiol.* **50**, 442–3.

Barolat, G., Schwartzmann, R. & Woo, R. (1989). Epidural spinal cord stimulation in the management of reflex sympathetic dystrophy. *Stereotact. Funct. Neurosurg.* **53**, 29–39.

Broggi, G., Servello, D., Franzini, A., Giorgi, C., Luccarelli, M., Ruberti, I., Cugnasca, M., Odero, A., Tealdi, D. & Denale, A. (1987). Spinal cord stimulation for treatment of peripheral vascular disease. *Appl. Neurophysiol.* **50**, 439–41.

Broseta, J., Barbera, J., de Vera, A., Barcia-Salorio, J. L., Garcia-March, G., Gonzalez-Darder, J., Robaina, F. & Joanes, V. (1986). Spinal cord stimulation in peripheral arterial disease. *J. Neurosurg.* **64**, 71–80.

Broseta, J., Roldan, P., Gonzalez-Darder, J., Bordes, V. & Barcia-Salorio, J. L. (1982). Chronic epidural spinal cord stimulation in the treatment of causalgic pain. *Appl. Neurophysiol.* **45**, 190–4.

Campbell, J. N. (1981). Examination of possible mechanisms by which stimulation of the spinal cord in man relieves pain. *Appl. Neurophysiol.* **44**, 181–6.

Cole, J. D., Illis, L. S. & Sedgwick, E. M. (1991). Intractable central pain in spinal cord injury is not relieved by spinal cord stimulation. *Paraplegia* **29**, 167–72.

De La Porte, C. & Siegfried, J. (1983). Lumbar spinal fibrosis (spinal arachnoiditis): its diagnosis and treatment by spinal cord stimulation. *Spine* **8**, 593–603.

Demirel, T., Braun, W. & Reimers, C. D. (1984). Results of spinal cord stimulation in patients suffering with chronic pain after a two-year observation period. *Neurochirurgia* **27**, 47–50.

Erickson, D. L. & Long, D. M. (1983). Ten-year follow-up of spinal cord stimulation. *Adv. Pain Res. Ther.* **5**, 583–9.

Feldman, R. A. (1975). Patterned responses of lamina V cells: cutaneous and dorsal funicular stimulation. *Physiol. Behav.* **15**, 79–84.

Fiume, D. (1983). Spinal cord stimulation in peripheral vascular disease. *Appl. Neurophysiol.* **46**, 290–4.

Foreman, R. D., Beall, J. A., Applebaum, A. E., Coulter, J. D. & Willis, W. D. (1976). Effects of dorsal column stimulation on primate spinothalamic tract neurons. *J. Neurophysiol.* **39**, 534–46.

Garcia-March, G., Sanchez-Ledesma, M. J., Diaz, P., Yague, L., Anaya, J., Goncalves, J. & Broseta, J. (1987). DREZ lesions versus spinal cord stimulation in the management of pain from brachial plexus avulsion. *Acta. Neurochir.* **39** (Suppl.), 155–8.

Handwerker, H. O., Iggo, A. & Zimmerman, M. (1975). Segmental and supraspinal actions on dorsal horn neurons responding to noxious and non-noxious stimuli. *Pain* **1**, 147–65.

Hillman, P. & Wall, P. D. (1969). Inhibitory and excitatory factors influencing the receptive fields of lamina 5 spinal cord cells. *Exp. Brain Res.* **9**, 284–306.

Hood, T. W. & Siegfried, J. (1984). Epidural vs. thalamic stimulation for the management of brachial plexus lesion pain. *Acta Neurochir.* **33** (Suppl.), 451–7.

Hoppenstein, T. (1975). Electrical stimulation of the ventral and dorsal columns of the spinal cord for the relief of chronic intractable pain, preliminary report. *Surg. Neurol.* **4**, 180–6.

Hosobuchi, Y., Adams, J. E. & Weinstein, P. R. (1972). Preliminary percutaneous dorsal column stimulation prior to permanent implantation. Technical note. *J. Neurosurg.* **37**, 242–5.

Hosobuchi, Y., Rutkin, B., Neilson, D. & Adams, J. E. (1981). Evoked potential study of dorsal column stimulator – a potential explanation for DCS failures. In *Indications for Spinal Cord Stimulation*, eds. Y. Hosobuchi & T. Corbin, pp. 97–107. Amsterdam: Excerpta Medica.

Koeze, T. H., de Williams, A. C. & Reiman, S. (1987). Spinal cord stimulation and the relief of chronic pain. *J. Neurol. Neurosurg. Psychiatry* **50**, 1424–9.

Krainick J. U., Thoden, U. & Riechert, T. (1980). Pain reduction in amputees by long-term spinal cord stimulation. *J. Neurosurg.* **52**, 346–50.

Kumar, K., Nath, R. & Wyant, G. M. (1991). Treatment of chronic pain by epidural spinal cord stimulation: a 10-year experience. *J. Neurosurg.* **75**, 402–7.

Larson, S. J., Sances, A., Cusick, J. F., Meyer, G. A. & Siontek, T. (1975). A comparison between anterior and posterior spinal implant systems. *Surg. Neurol.* **4**, 180–6.

Larson, S. J., Sances, A., Riegel, D. H., Meyer, G. A., Dallman, D. E. & Swionek, T. (1974). Neurophysiological effects of dorsal column stimulation in man and monkey. *J. Neurosurg.* **41**, 217–23.

Law, J. D. (1992). Clinical and technical results from spinal cord stimulation for chronic pain of diverse pathophysiologies. *Stereotact. Funct. Neurosurg.* **59**, 21–4.

Law, J. D. & Kirkpatrick, A. F. (1992). Update: spinal cord stimulation. *AJPM* **2**, 34–42.

Lazorthes, Y. & Verdie, J. C. (1985). Technical evolution and long-term results of chronic spinal cord stimulation. In *Neurostimulation: an Overview*, eds. Y. Lazorthes & A. Upton, pp. 67–86. New York: Futura.

Long, D. M. (1974). Cutaneous afferent stimulation for relief of chronic pain. *Clin. Neurosurg.* **21**, 257–68.

Long, D. (1981). Patient selection and results of spinal cord stimulation for chronic pain. In *Indications for Spinal Cord Stimulation*, eds. Y. Hosobuchi & T. Corbin, pp. 1–16. Amsterdam: Excerpta Medica.

Long, D. M. & Hagfors, N. (1975). Electrical stimulation of the nervous system: the current status of electrical stimulation of the nervous system for relief of pain. *Pain* **1**, 109–23.

Meglio, M. & Cioni, B. (1982). Personal experience with spinal cord stimulation in chronic pain management. *Appl. Neurophysiol.* **45**, 195–200.

Meglio, M., Cioni, B., Prezioso, A. & Talamonti, G. (1989a). Spinal cord stimulation in the treatment of postherpetic pain. *Acta Neurochir.* **46** (Suppl.), 65–6.

Meglio, M., Cioni, B. & Rossi, G. F. (1989b). Spinal cord stimulation in management of chronic pain – a 9-year experience. *J. Neurosurg.* **70**, 519–24.

Melzack, R. & Wall, P. D. (1965). Pain mechanisms: a new theory. *Science* **150**, 971–9.

Meyerson, B. A. (1983). Electrostimulation procedures: effects, presumed rationale, and possible mechanisms. *Adv. Pain Res. Ther.* **5**, 495–534.

North, R. B., Ewend, M. G., Lawton, M. Y., Kidd, D. H. & Piantadosi, S. (1991a). Failed back surgery syndrome: 5-year follow-up after spinal cord stimulator implantation. *Neurosurgery* **28**, 692–9.

North, R. B., Ewend, M. G., Lawton, M. T. & Piantadosi, S. (1991b). Spinal cord stimulation for chronic intractable pain: superiority of 'multi-channel' devices. *Pain* **44**, 119–30.

North, R. B., Kidd, D. H., Zahurak, M., James, C. S. & Long, D. M. (1993). Spinal cord stimulation for chronic, intractable pain: experience over two decades. *Neurosurgery* **32**, 384–95.

Nyquist, J. K. & Greenhoot, J. H. (1975). Responses evoked from the thalamic centrum medianum by painful input: suppression by dorsal funicular conditioning. *Exp. Neurol.* **39**, 215–22.

Pineda, A. (1978). Complications of dorsal column stimulation. *J. Neurosurg.* **48**, 64–8.

Racz, G. B., McCarron, R. F. & Talboys, P. (1989). Percutaneous dorsal column stimulation for chronic pain control. *Spine* **14**, 1–4.

Ray, C. D., Burton, C. V. & Lifson, A. (1982). Neurostimulation as used in a large clinical practice. *Appl. Neurophysiol.* **45**, 160–6.

Richardson, R. R., Meyer, P. R. & Cerullo, L. J. (1980). Neurostimulation in the modulation of intractable paraplegic and traumatic neuroma pains. *Pain* **8**, 75–84.

Richardson, R. R., Siqueira, E. B. & Cerullo, L. J. (1979). Spinal epidural neurostimulation for treatment of acute and chronic intractable pain: initial and long-term results. *Neurosurgery* **5**, 344–8.

Robaina, F. J., Dominguez, M., Diaz, M., Rodriguez, J. L. & de Vera, J. A. (1989). Spinal cord stimulation for relief of chronic pain in vasospastic disorders of the upper limbs. *Neurosurgery* **24**, 63–7.

Saade, N. E. & Jabbur, S. J. (1985). Dorsal column influence, through the brainstem, on spinal nociceptive input. In *Development, Organization, Processing in Somatosensory Pathways*, pp. 367–73. New York: Alan R. Liss.

Sanchez-Ledesma, M. J., Garcia-March, G., Diaz-Cascajo, P., Gomez-March, J. & Broseta, J. (1989). Spinal cord stimulation in deafferentation pain. *Stereotact. Funct. Neurosurg.* **53**, 40–5.

Shealy, C. N. (1973). Pain suppression through posterior column stimulation. In *Neural Organization and its Relevance to Prosthetics*, ed. W. S. Fields, pp. 251–60. New York: Intercontinental Medical Book Corp.

Shealy, C. N., Mortimer, J. T. & Reswick, J. B. (1967a). Electrical inhibition of pain by stimulation of the dorsal columns – preliminary clinical report. *Anesth. Analgesia* **46**, 489–91.

Shealy, C. N., Tashitz, N., Mortimer, J. T. & Becker, D. P. (1967b). Electrical inhibition of pain: experimental evaluation. *Anesth. Analgesia* **46**, 299–305.

Shetter, A. G. & Atkinson, J. R. (1977). Dorsal column stimulation: its effect on medial bulboreticular unit activity evoked by noxious stimuli. *Exp. Neurol.* **54**, 185–98.

Siegfried, J. (1991). Therapeutic neurostimulation – indications reconsidered. *Acta Neurochir.* **52** (Suppl.), 112–17.

Siegfried, J. & Cetinlap, E. (1981). Neurosurgical treatment of phantom limb pain: a survey of methods. In *Phantom and Stump Pain*, eds. J. Siegfried & M. Zimmerman, pp. 148–55. New York: Springer.

Siegfried, J. & Lazorthes, Y. (1982). Long-term follow-up of dorsal column stimulation for chronic pain syndrome after multiple lumbar operations. *Appl. Neurophysiol.* **45**, 201–4.

Simpson, B. A. (1991). Spinal cord stimulation in 60 cases of intractable pain. *J. Neurol. Neurosurg. Psychiatry* **54**, 196–9.

Spiegelmann, R. & Friedman, W. A. (1991). Spinal cord stimulation: a contemporary series. *Neurosurgery* **28**, 65–71.

Sweet, W. H. & Wepsic, J. G. (1968). Treatment of chronic pain by stimulation of fibres of primary afferent neuron. *Trans. Am Neurol. Assoc.* **93**, 103–5.

Sweet, W. H. & Wepsic, J. G. (1974). Stimulation of the posterior columns of the spinal cord for pain control – indications, technique and results. *Clin. Neurosurg.* **21**, 278–310.

Tallis, R. C., Illis, L. S., Sedgwick, E. M., Hardwidge, C. & Garfield, J. S. (1983). Spinal cord stimulation in peripheral vascular disease. *J. Neurol. Neurosurg. Psychiatry* **46**, 478–84.

Urban, B. J. & Nashold, B. S. (1978). Percutaneous epidural stimulation of the spinal cord for relief of pain. *J. Neurosurg.* **48**, 323–8.

Vogel, H. P., Heppner, B., Humbs, N., Schramm, J. & Wagner, C. (1986). Long-term effects of spinal cord stimulation in chronic pain syndromes. *J. Neurol.* **233**, 16–18.

Waisbrod, H. & Gerbershagen, H. U. (1985). Spinal cord stimulation in patients with a battered root syndrome. *Arch. Orthop. Trauma Surg.* **104**, 62–4.

Wall, P. D. & Sweet, W. H. (1967). Temporary abolition of pain in man. *Science* **155**, 108–9.

Wester, K. (1987). Dorsal column stimulation in pain treatment. *Acta. Neurol. Scand.* **75**, 151–5.

Winkelmuller, W. (1981). Experience with the control of low back pain by the dorsal column stimulation system and by the peridural electrode system. In *Indications for Spinal Cord Stimulation*, eds. Y. Hosobuchi & T. Corbin, pp. 34–41. Amsterdam: Excerpta Medica.

29 Stereotactic surgery for movement disorder

R.R. TASKER

Patients with movement disorders usually have disabling features not affected by surgery; for example, paraplegia in patients suffering from spasticity and ataxia in patients with cerebellar tremor. Relieving one aspect of the problem does not correct the patient's overall disability.

Similar problems affect assessment of surgery for movement disorders; a spastic paraplegic's life expectancy is not altered by successful baclofen infusion. One possible exception, the question as to whether 'successful' thalamotomy alters the course of Parkinson's disease will be discussed. The quantitative assessment of change in movement disorders is a major problem in clinical research. The plethora of protocols for assessing patients with Parkinson's disease for example, attests to difficulties with this process.

Hemifacial spasm, though regularly successfully treated by microvascular decompression is relatively infrequent in North America compared with the Far East, and therefore in the author's practice, so that it will not be discussed. This condition can also be treated with botulinum toxin injection, with favourable results, but direct comparison of medical and surgical therapy is lacking.

Surgery for movement disorders

Although a variety of surgical operations have been proposed for the treatment of movement disorders, those in common use today are all stereotactic except for microvascular decompression in hemifacial spasm, botulinus toxin injections and procedures for spasmodic torticollis. This author has no experience with these last modalities other than the use of multiple rhizotomies in spasmodic torticollis in which little recent information has accumulated. The bulk of published data in stereotactic surgery relates to Parkinson's disease, information concerning essential and cerebellar tremor and dystonia being so sparse as to make a survey of 'outcomes' difficult. Therefore this chapter will be devoted mainly to Parkinson's disease with brief comments on the other conditions.

When surgery for Parkinson's disease is considered, a number of options are available. Pallidotomy, the procedure of choice of the 1950s is being re-examined because of its apparent effect on bradykinesia which was not appreciated in the past (Laitinen *et al.* 1992). The operation is still under investigation and its true 'outcome' remains to be seen; however, it is promising.

Although instillation of a chronic brain stimulator in the thalamus has been used sporadically for a long time to treat tremor, as an alternative to thalamotomy, intensive use of this modality has only begun recently so that adequate outcome data are sparse (Siegfried & Rea 1988; Benabid *et al.* 1987). Transplantation of living cells into the brain is still an experimental operation.

Parkinson's disease

This chapter is not the venue to discuss the evolution of current practices in thalamotomy from Meyer's historic open surgery (Meyers 1940). Thalamotomy is an enigmatic procedure (Cooper & Bravo 1958*b*; Hassler & Reichert 1954). Developed as a supposed central extension of pallidotomy (Adams 1965), it proved more effective than the latter for the treatment of the tremor and rigidity of Parkinsonism and for most other dyskinesias. However, the preferred thalamic target turned out to be not the thalamic relay of the pallidum but some other more caudal structure, as yet undefined after nearly 40 years. The baffling fact of the procedure is that the same lesion, with minor variations, appears capable of abolishing or ameliorating a widely divergent group of disturbances of motor control: rest tremor of Parkinson's disease, essential tremor, tremor from damage to neocerebellar pathways, rigidity, chorea, athetosis, hemiballismus, secondary dystonia, dystonia musculorum deforman (DMD) and dopa dyskinesia. The only differences are that the tremor of Parkinson's disease and essential tremor are capable of complete and, if arrested for 3 months, permanent resolution (Tasker *et al.* 1983; Van Manen *et al.* 1984) while the other dyskinesias are less completely affected. The minimal lesion to relieve these two types of tremor may be smaller than that required to relieve other dyskinesias and the lesion for the relief of non-tremorous abnormalities such as rigidity and dopa dyskinesia may need to extend more rostrally than that for tremor (Hirai *et al.* 1983; Narabayashi 1988).

One of the problems with evaluating such surgery is a lack of understanding of how the thalamotomy lesion relieves so many different types of movement disorder. Even in the case of Parkinsonian tremor there is no consensus on just where the lesion should be and what it should destroy (Ohye & Narabayashi 1979; Lenz *et al.* 1987*b*; Ohye *et al.* 1989; Tasker *et al.* 1982*b*). Laitinen's review (Laitinen 1985) emphasizes the variability of location of lesion site used by different surgeons.

Particularly difficult to deal with from the point of view of outcome analysis is the fact that, except in essential tremor, thalamotomy is only partial treatment for the motor disorder in which it is used. Thalamotomy reduces but rarely eliminates the tremor of neocerebellar syndromes and has no effect on the accompanying ataxia. Thalamotomy is most effective for tremor and dyskinesia in distal limb joints but relatively ineffective for the relief of movements in proximal joints or in the neck or trunk. Many movement disorders are secondary to neurological disease; cerebellar tremor is most often caused by multiple sclerosis (MS). Craniocerebral injury (Bullard & Nashold 1984) and stroke (Jokura *et al.* 1990) can result in dystonia or tremor. Obviously the symptomatic treatment of the movement disorder in these situations has no effect on the underlying, usually disabling disease. Most dyskinesias progress with time: Parkinson's disease, DMD, tremor in MS, even secondary dystonia. The result of a thalamotomy can be assessed only at the moment in time that it is done. If disease progress is rapid, as in DMD and some cases of Parkinson's disease, any benefit from surgery may soon be 'eaten up' by such progress and it may be impossible to distinguish surgical complications from the effects of such progress (Tasker *et al.* 1988*a*). There is no evidence that thalamotomy arrests the progress of any movement disorder (Narabayashi 1988; Scott *et al.* 1970; Li *et al.* 1990). In the case of Parkinson's disease, rate of progress may vary enormously from that of the cases reported by Tetrud & Langston (1989) where deterioration occurred at the rate of 0.7 Hoehn and Yahr grades per year to that of postencephalitic or early (< 40 years) onset cases where little if any change can be detected over 20 years of follow-up (Li *et al.* 1990; Tasker *et al.* 1996). In fact the author has seen at least three unilateral young onset/postencephalitic cases with arrested hemi-Parkinsonism.

In addition to these features that confound the evaluation of results are the problems of outcome assessment. Is it realistic to evaluate activities of daily living as a measure of surgical outcome in a bradykinetic Parkinsonian operated on for tremor? How does one assess the patient with MS in whom the aim of surgery is to reduce ballistic ataxic tremor to the point the patient's arms no longer suffer abrasions or knock things on the floor even though they are still incapable of use? Finally, patients' capabilities and the degree of tremor, rigidity or other dyskinesias vary from one moment in time to the next, with the degree of cognitive activation and relative to drug intake. How can a baseline be established?

Indications

Thalamotomy is indicated in the treatment of Parkinsonian tremor that is disabling and which, as is usually the case, does not respond to medical therapy. It can be safely done into the eighth decade, avoiding patients with cognitive impairment, severe bradykinesia or medical problems such as bleeding diatheses.

Technique of thalamotomy

Thalamotomy is performed in a similar fashion to the stereotactic procedures described for pain (Tasker *et al.* 1982*a*). The location of the tactile relay nucleus of thalamus is identified first anatomically with reference to the patient's ACPC line determined by CT or MR imaging and a brain atlas. A probe is then introduced and its location corroborated physiologically with threshold electrical stimulation that produces paraesthesiae in appropriate body parts and/or microelectrode recording of the receptive fields of tactile neurons (Hardy *et al.* 1979; Lenz *et al.* 1988*b*; Hardy *et al.* 1981; Bertrand *et al.* 1967). The probe is then moved rostral to the anterior limit of the tactile nucleus into an area thought to lie in ventral intermediate nucleus (Vim) and, possibly, posterior ventral oral (Vop) nucleus where voluntary neurons firing in relation to contralateral voluntary movements (voluntary cells) (Hardy *et al.* 1980*b, c*; Jasper & Bertrand 1966; Lenz *et al.* 1988*a*, 1990; Raeva 1986; Tasker *et al.* 1987, 1988*b*; Ohye 1987; Ohye *et al.* 1982*a*, 1990), or kinaesthetic cells firing in response to passive movements are found along with other kinaesthetic cells that respond to deep pressure or squeezing of muscles and tendons. Many of these (and other unidentified) neurons fire in time with the patient's tremor or other dyskinesia (Lenz *et al.* 1985, 1988*a*, 1990*a*; Ohye *et al.* 1989).

Though the most exquisite information about probe localization is obtained with microelectrode recording, most surgeons proceed on the basis of stimulation alone. Stimulating kinaesthetic cells usually induces contralateral paraesthesiae in more or less the same body part as the RFs of the neurons; occasional sensations of movement are reported though no movement takes place. Stimulating voluntary cells causes a contralateral muscle contraction at the onset of a stimulus. But, more impressive, stimulation amongst tremor cells may suppress the tremor of Parkinson's disease, inhibit or more often drive other types of dyskinesias (Tasker *et al.* 1982*b*; Albe-Fessard *et al.* 1963; Reichert 1980; Lenz *et al.* 1985).

Strategies for choosing target sites vary with the surgeon and the physiological localization technique used. Some surgeons rely heavily on siting their lesion anatomically, 14–15 mm from midline, 2–3 mm above the ACPC line and about the junction of anterior two thirds and posterior one third (Laitinen 1966, 1985). But, in addition to anatomical criteria, it is preferable to utilize physiological data, especially choosing sites at which tremor cells occur and electrical stimulation at the lowest threshold most profoundly inhibits (or drives) the dyskinesia. A 4 to 5-mm diameter RF lesion is then made as in mesencephalic tractotomy.

The mechanism of thalamotomy for Parkinsonian tremor

The use of microelectrode data brings out the lack of consensus amongst different surgeons more clearly. Ohye and his group (Ohye 1985, 1987; Ohye & Narabayashi 1979; Ohye *et al.* 1982*a*, 1989, 1990) site their lesion on the basis of finding at least one or two kinaesthetic tremor cells along an electrode trajectory. When we have tried to use their criteria, we find up to 10–20 kinaesthetic tremor cells along a single electrode trajectory at any site along which stimulation may arrest tremor. We have found that making lesions at these sites may not ensure permanent tremor relief and may even result in postoperative ataxia (Jones & Tasker 1990). Lenz (Lenz *et al.* 1985, 1987*a,b*, 1988) has advocated making the lesion at the site at which firing of tremor cells has the tightest relationship to the pattern of the peripheral tremor. This occurs 2–3 mm above the ACPC line which happens to lie close to that advocated by others on anatomic grounds and by Albe Fessard and her associates (1963). Lenz's evidence suggests that the tremor cells in this area may be voluntary cells with receptive fields. We have attempted to further refine the choice of target site with diagnostic microinjections of lidocaine (Dostrovsky *et al.* 1993) and have found that there are many sites at which kinaesthetic tremor cells occur, stimulation induces tremor arrest, but where lidocaine injections (and presumably RF lesionmaking) have no effect on the tremor and sometimes lesions will stop tremor at sites where stimulation does not.

Further experimental evidence seems increasingly to support a cerebellar role for Parkinsonian, essential and of course, cerebellar tremor. The early work of Poirier and his colleagues (Poirier *et al.* 1969) suggested that one of the essential features of the ventromedial tegmental lesion that induced a Parkinson-like tremor in macaques was interruption of cerebellar pathways. We have shown that in rats cerebellar tremor from a variety of cerebellar lesions could be converted into a rest tremor after the injection of harmaline that increased muscle tone (Tasker & Sogabe *unpublished*). Recent studies with PET scanning suggest that essential tremor is associated with heightened regional cerebral blood flow (rCBF) in cerebellum bilaterally (Jenkins *et al.* 1993) and that thalamic stimulation that inhibits Parkinsonian tremor, but not ineffective stimulation, suppresses rCBF rostrally medially and bilaterally in cerebellum (Deiber *et al.* 1993). These observations tend to make us favour Lenz's (Lenz *et al.* 1987b) suggestion of an optimal target site amongst voluntary cells with receptive fields rather than kinaesthetic cells.

Outcome of thalamotomy for Parkinson's disease

Tables 29.1–29.3 review our own results (Tasker *et al.* 1983) in reduction of tremor and rigidity and on various motor functions, after unilateral thalamotomy in Parkinson's disease while Table 29.4 lists the complications.

In our experience thalamotomy is most effective for the relief of tremor, but also suppresses rigidity as our data show (Magaseki *et al.* 1986). Certain manual dextrous functions such as repetitive finger–thumb touching and rapid repetitive wrist rotation also improve, presumably because of elimination of tremor but other tasks such as finger–nose touching, rapid patting, writing, as well as speech, facial movements and locomotion show no significant improvement. Musculoskeletal pain is usually relieved opposite to the lesion, and when postencephalitic cases were still being treated, oculogyric crises were also relieved (Tasker 1967). After 3 months tremor abolition is virtually always permanent but there is a tendency for rigidity to recur and of course the disease worsens with time according to the worsening of the bradykinesia which most authors feel is not affected by thalamotomy. However, perusal of early results of thalamotomy (Cooper 1965) in the pre-L-dopa era suggests at least a transient improvement in bradykinesia similar to that seen after puncture of the basal ganglia for tissue transplantation (Van Manen *et al.* 1984; Tasker 1967). Perhaps the current use of L-dopa in virtually every patient masks such transient events; it will also be interesting to see what the final multicentre long-term evaluation of pallidotomy for bradykinesia will be.

Table 29.1. *Effect of unilateral thalamotomy on various functions in Parkinson's disease*

Function	Patients with function (%)					
	Preoperative		3 months postoperative		2 years postoperative	
	Normal	Near-normal	Normal	Near-normal	Normal	Near-normal
Finger–thumb touching	4	20	31	55	19	38
Finger–nose touching	11	40	27	63	19	67
Rapid patting	15	23	28	53	27	46
Rapid wrist rotation	6	13	30	49	.20	36
Handwriting	3	19	9	30	10	24
Speech	37	70	29	59	24	48
Locomotion	18	55	30	54	15	42
Facial movement	11	44	12	40	12	35

Table 29.2. *Unilateral thalamotomy for Parkinsonian rigidity*

Site	Patients with rigidity (%)					
	Preoperative		3 months postoperative		2 years postoperative	
	Absent	Absent or minimal	Absent	Absent or minimal	Absent	Absent or minimal
Manual digits	4	10	37	70	26	56
Wrist	3	7	30	41	22	30
Elbow, shoulder	8	27	37	56	37	67
Ankle, foot	31	45	41	51	22	37
Knee, hip	34	51	46	62	33	52

It has been suggested (Kelly & Gillingham 1980; Matsumoto *et al.* 1984; van Manen *et al.* 1984; Bosch 1986) that thalamotomy is less effective today than it was in the pre-dopa days (Gillingham 1964) because of the delaying effects of the almost inevitable current L-dopa therapy, but in our review of 55 Parkinsonian patients operated on bilaterally in a time-frame spanning the pre- and post-dopa eras, we found no significant difference in results (Li *et al.* 1990). Part of the problem is said to be related to the greater incidence of postoperative cognitive problems and to an increased incidence of permanent aggravation of ipsilateral tremor (44% upper, 25% lower extremity) in L-dopa-treated patients after thalamotomy (Van Manen *et al.* 1984).

One other feature of Parkinson's disease that thalamotomy benefits is L-dopa-induced dyskinesia on the side contralateral to the operation. We noted this early in the L-dopa era (Tasker 1970) and confirmed it again with our review of 55 patients operated upon bilaterally (Li *et al.* 1990). In the latter study, we examined the effect of the

Table 29.3. *Unilateral thalamotomy for Parkinson's disease*

Site	Patients with tremor (%)					
	Preoperative		3 months postoperative		2 years postoperative	
	Absent	Absent or minimal	Absent	Absent or minimal	Absent	Absent or minimal
Manual digits	15	28	72	82	82	89
Wrist	16	20	75	70	86	86
Elbow, shoulder	61	85	84	96	79	86
Ankle, foot	65	69	84	87	93	97
Knee, hip	80	93	93	97	82	97

Table 29.4. *Complications of unilateral thalamotomy for Parkinsonism*

Complication	Patients (%)
Mortality, significant permanent cognitive disorder	0
Intrathalamic haemorrhage	1.3
Persistent significant aggravation of dysarthria	1.3
Equinovarus deformity, transient arm ataxia	4.0
Equinovarus deformity, persistent arm ataxia	1.3
Subjective transient numbness	12.0
Persistent numbness	1.3
Transient hypotonia	6.0
Transient hand ataxia	4.0
Transient equinovarus deformity	1.3
Transient equinovarus deformity and transient hand ataxia	1.3
Transient dysphasia	1.3
Transient or mild aggravation of dysarthria	2.1
Transient confusion	12.0
Epileptic seizure	1.3
Scalp infection	2.1
Lightheadedness	1.3

procedure on the appearance of L-dopa dyskinesia during the patients' follow-up (as shown in Table 29.5): 18% of those with previous thalamotomy developed L-dopa dyskinesia, 63% of those without. The difference in incidence between the operated and unoperated patient sides is statistically significant.

Results in bilateral thalamotomy

It has been stated that if a patient is operated upon bilaterally (Krayenbühl *et al.* 1961, 1963), results on the first side are better than on the second (Walker 1982; Cooper 1969; van Manen *et al.* 1984). The author feels that this is more apparent than real since only the patients enjoying a successful first-side operation are likely to go on to second-side surgery. Thus first-side results are selected for success but not those of the second side.

Table 29.5. *Relationship between previous thalamotomy and occurrence of L-dopa dyskinesia: patient sides at risk*

	Previous thalamotomy	No thalamotomy
L-Dopa dyskinesia present	9(18%)	5 (63%)
L-Dopa dyskinesia absent	41	3

Table 29.6. *Effect of age of patient on complications of unilateral thalamotomy for Parkinson's disease (percentage of patients in age group)*

Age (years)	All transient and permanent complications	All major and minor permanent complications
< 50	24	5
50–60	54	20
> 60	62	43

In our 55 bilateral-operated patients there was no significant difference between sides if repeat operations were included and, of course, the chance of successful thalamotomy on both sides is the square of that on one side alone, i.e. if the success rate is 80% for one side, that for both is 64%.

Complications

The complications of thalamotomy fall into several groups:

(a) complications common to all surgery such as cardiovasculo-pulmonary problems which will not be further considered

(b) complications such as infection, haemorrhage, cognitive disorders, hemiparesis, dysphasia, hyperkinesis, epilepsy, numbness

(c) cerebellar complications including hypotonia, lateropulsion, manual ataxia, dysarthria, gait disturbance including equinovarus deformity of the foot.

Complications tend to be more frequent, the older the patient as shown in Table 29.6 (Tasker 1967).

Haemorrhagic complications are to some extent unavoidable but those associated with lesion-making have, in our hands, been least with radiofrequency as compared with leucotomy and cryoprobe lesions.

Cognitive disorders not obviously related to intracranial haemorrhage are commonest in older, disabled and already cognitively impaired patients. There is little advantage in operating on patients to relieve tremor unless they are cognitively and physically capable of exploiting that effect. Cognitive impairment has been shown to be present after thalamotomy by psychometric testing in patients in whom it is not clinically apparent (Riklan *et al.* 1960) but we abandoned routine psychometric testing in the 1970s after thalamotomy when we found no significant changes over dozens of thalamotomies (Tasker *et al.* 1983).

Significant infections are rarely reported and superficial scalp infections at stereotactic frame pin sites affect only 0.5%–1% of patients. It is often stated that thalamotomy enhances ipsilateral tremor (Walker 1982). Van Manen *et al.* (1984) found ipsilateral tremor increased in 44% of upper limbs and 25% of lower limbs but we were unable to identify it in our patients (Tasker *et al.* 1983). Dysphagia and pseudobulbar effects are rarely reported being problems only in severe, advanced cases. One author reported operation-induced Parkinsonian crisis in 8% of cases; we have seen it once or twice. Epilepsy is rare in Parkinsonian patients but more often seen in patients operated on for other dyskinesias.

Hyperkinesis, thought to be due to encroachment on and destruction of up to 20% of the subthalamic nucleus (Mundinger 1985; Mundinger & Kuhn 1982) has become rare in current experience, having been much more frequently seen in the early days of thalamotomy (Tasker 1967; Tasker *et al.* 1983; Modesti & Van Buren 1979; Laitinen 1966; Bravo *et al.* 1966). It appears to be a complication in patients with post-encephalitic rather than idiopathic disease, a type of Parkinson's disease much less often seen today (Bravo *et al.* 1966; Modesti & van Buren 1979).

Numbness is a common but usually insignificant complication probably reflecting encroachment of the lesion on the thalamic sensory relay nucleus. It rarely persists past a few months and thalamotomy is virtually never associated with neuropathic pain.

'Cerebellar' complications

There are several complications of thalamotomy that we believe are natural consequences of lesions placed in the part of the thalamus recognized as the target for thalamotomy which have been referred to as cerebellar complications. They appear reasonably attributable to interruption of the dentatothalamic and possibly spindle or kinaesthetic pathways. These are dysarthria, contralateral hypotonia, hand clumsiness and ataxia, and various gait disturbances including lateropulsion, and equinovarus deformity of the foot (Yasui *et al.* 1976, 1977; Yoshida *et al.* 1976–77; Zoll 1978; Mamo *et al.* 1965). These complications are of great concern since they result from properly located lesions, yet they are rarely addressed in the literature. They appear to be natural extensions of what many patients notice immediately postoperatively: a feeling of the limb not belonging and difficulty controlling it, leading to neglect. These effects usually disappear rapidly with concentrated use of the limbs which the patient 'had to learn to use all over again'. Why they persist in a few patients is uncertain; possibly lesion size or degree of interruption of a particular pathway play a part (Miyamoto *et al.* 1985). Zoll (1978) concluded that equinovarus deformity was the result of interfering with sensation and muscle tone in the face of pre-existing weakness.

Complications of bilateral thalamotomy

As in percutaneous cordotomy, the incidence of complications of bilateral thalamotomy are essentially the square of those of the unilateral procedure – except for dysarthria (Krayenbühl *et al.* 1961). Just as the patient can tolerate unilateral damage to the micturition pathway without great risk after cordotomy, unilateral thalamic lesions inflict a small incidence of speech disturbance. But bilateral thalamotomy carries a 30%–60% chance of increased dysarthria afterwards.

Effect on progress of Parkinson's disease

In patients with Parkinson's disease, one issue remains: does successful thalamotomy arrest the course of Parkinson's disease? Cooper originally thought that it did (Cooper & Bravo 1958*b*; Cooper 1965) but his study with Scott and Brody (Scott *et al.* 1970) suggested that any halting of progress was only apparent, based on the very slow progress seen in postencephalitic or youthful onset Parkinsonism, regardless of whether they underwent thalamotomy, an opinion shared by Narabayashi (1988). Matsumoto and his colleagues have reopened the question (Matsumoto *et al.* 1984; Matsumoto *et al.* 1976/77) reporting a series of 21 bilaterally operated Parkinsonians with impressive relief of tremor and rigidity of whom some seemed to enjoy lack of progress of the disease postoperatively; there was, of course, no control group.

Since we had operated bilaterally on 55 patients with Parkinson's disease up to that time (Li *et al.* 1990; Tasker *et al.* 1996) we undertook to review their courses with this issue in mind. It seemed that if thalamotomy were to influence the course of bilateral disease it would have to be performed on both sides of the brain since the effects of thalamotomy appear to be strictly contralateral. It seemed reasonable to suggest that if thalamotomy were to arrest the progress of the disease it should be a 'successful' thalamotomy that abolished tremor and rigidity, rather than 'unsuccessful', leaving residual tremor and/or significant rigidity. We developed criteria for adequate follow-up, 'successful' control of tremor and rigidity and arrest of progress of disease for our patients, some of whom had been followed for up to 30 years by the author after completion of bilateral thalamotomy using the same semiquantitative assessment protocol throughout.

We found that 13 of the 43 patients with adequate follow-up were 'stable' post-operatively, i.e. they did not progress over a significant follow-up using our criteria, six of the 13 with postencephalitic and/or youthful onset (before age 40) (PEY) disease and seven of the 42 with 'idiopathic' disease. The preponderance of stable PEY cases was striking suggesting as others had concluded, that PEY disease sometimes progressed so slowly that it could appear to be stable postoperatively. 'Stability' was not related to differences in elapsed time between onset and completion of surgery. We then studied 10 further PEY and 16 idiopathic cases undergoing only unilateral thalamotomy matched in date of surgery to the bilateral cases; 40% of the former and 6% (one patient) of the latter were postoperatively 'stable' thus strengthening our conviction that 'stability' merely reflected the slow progress of PEY disease.

Yet there were also 'stable' idiopathic cases. There was no difference in age of disease onset between 'stable' and 'unstable' idiopathic cases. To our amazement, when we related 'success' of surgery to postoperative 'stability', we found a statistically significant difference in the stability of PEY cases, unilaterally *or* bilaterally operated depending upon whether their surgery was 'successful' or not. For the bilaterally operated cases, four out of five with bilaterally 'successful', two out of five with unilaterally 'successful' surgery and none of three with bilaterally 'unsuccessful' surgery appeared not to progress postoperatively while, of the unilaterally operated cases, four out of six with unilaterally 'successful', none out of four with unilaterally 'unsuccessful' surgery became stable.

Results were similar with idiopathic disease: of bilaterally operated cases, six out of nine bilaterally 'successful', one out of nine unilaterally 'successful', none out of 12 bilaterally 'unsuccessful' became stable; of unilaterally operated cases, one out of nine unilaterally 'successful' and none out of seven unilaterally 'unsuccessful' failed to progress postoperatively.

When we recalculated the results of Matsumoto's group (Matsumoto *et al.* 1976/77, 1984) using the same criteria as in our study, only five of 22 of his bilaterally operated cases were 'stable', by our criteria, all but one (onset age 43) experiencing disease onset before 40, again reflecting slow progress of youthful onset disease. We could not evaluate 'success' using our criteria. Admittedly, interpretation of their data is difficult since several of their patients who were graded at the same or a better level at latest follow-up as that recorded at the time of completion of their second side surgery had shown poorer grades in the interim; we did not include them in the 'stable' group.

What does this mean other than the fact that PEY disease is relatively stable? It is difficult to believe that 'successful' thalamotomy affects the course of Parkinson's disease. I believe that these data simply show that there are patients, mostly, but not exclusively, with PEY disease, whose disease is characterized by little bradykinesia and slow progress in whom successful relief of tremor and rigidity eliminates the main features of their disease so that they appear stable after surgery; but the issue should be kept open.

Thalamotomy for essential and cerebellar tremor and dystonia

Parkinsonism is the chief indication for thalamotomy, relatively small numbers of procedures being done for other dyskinesias. In each case the technique is the same, except that in conditions other than essential tremor, the lesion probably must be made larger and to extend more rostrally (Mohadiger *et al.* 1990).

Essential tremor

This condition, whether familial or not, usually begins in youth and slowly progresses through life. It nearly always affects upper limbs, sometimes voice, rarely trunk or lower limbs. It is unaccompanied by deficit other than an action tremor and there is no known pathology. Investigations other than PET imaging studies which suggest overactivity of cerebellar pathways (Jenkins *et al.* 1993) reveal no abnormalities.

Indications

It is perhaps the best indication for thalamotomy or DBS (Cooper 1962). The tremor is usually distal so that it is readily relieved by thalamotomy and once that happens without complications the patient has no other deficit. Tremor relieved for 3 months never recurs, and the disease progresses very slowly on the other side. Milder cases may be controlled with propranolol; ethyl alcohol is even more effective but exposes patients to the risk of alcoholism. Otherwise medically intractable tremor that disables through loss of dextrous hand movements can only be treated surgically.

Cerebellar tremor

Cerebellar tremor arises as the result of craniocerebral injury, stroke, cerebellar degeneration, and most prominently, multiple sclerosis. The degree of disability is variable depending upon the extent of the lesion, ranging from a pure action tremor to a wild ballistic ataxic tremor as shown by Carpenter & Hanna (1962) in the macaque.

Indications

The role of thalamotomy in this disorder is limited since it has no effect on the ataxia and benefits only the tremor residing distally in the limb. In the case of MS especially, ataxia may be very severe and the worst tremor often affects the shoulder where, in our experience, thalamotomy is relatively ineffective. It is interesting that DBS in the dorsal part of Vim is effective in proximal tremor, ventral stimulation in distal cerebellar tremor (Goldman & Kelly 1992*a,b*). Furthermore, tremor is often only one small part of the problem. The patient with MS also faces cognitive dysfunction, spastic paresis, sensory loss, and visual impairment. Reported series often mix patients with tremor of differing causes, usually do not specify tremor sites, nor identify other features that thalamotomy cannot correct.

Results and complications

Because of the widespread neurological lesions present in MS patients, who constitute the commonest group undergoing thalamotomy for cerebellar tremor, postoperative cognitive dysfunction and dysphagia are more likely than in Parkinson's disease and essential tremor. And there is the risk of precipitating an acute MS event, a complication which we seem to have prevented with prophylactic steroid therapy.

Dystonia

Indications

The phasic or tonic activity of dystonia musculorum deformans (DMD) or secondary dystonia that occurs distally in limbs can also be ameliorated by thalamotomy but not, in this author's experience, proximal limb, nuchal or truncal dystonia (Tasker *et al.*

1988*a*). In both DMD and secondary dystonia, if the disease is progressing rapidly at the time of surgery, this progress may soon cancel out any benefit from surgery or even cause new motor deficits so soon postoperatively that they may be mistaken for complications.

One caution stems from the fact that patients with DMD have normal brains, no abnormalities being demonstrable by investigation and no neurological deficits being present outside their dystonia. As a result they have a narrow thalamus and third ventricle so that the internal capsule lies closer to midline than in the usual Parkinsonian patient (Hawrylyshyn *et al.* 1976/77). Unless microelectrode recording is done, capable of distinguishing fibres from neurons, a typical thalamotomy lesion 14–15 mm from midline, as in Parkinson's disease based on radiology or stimulation studies, may damage the internal capsule and produce hemiparesis.

Finally, as in two of our patients with bilateral secondary dystonia, particularly as seen after cerebral palsy, widespread neurological damage may be present so that an additional thalamic lesion may inflict cognitive disturbances, pseudobulbar effects and dysphagia. These neurologically precarious patients have little neurological reserve with which to cope with any postoperative problems such as hypotonia and related gait disturbance.

Results and complications

Tables 29.7 and 29.8 list our results and complications with thalamotomy for DMD and secondary dystonia (Tasker *et al.* 1988*a*).

It is apparent that the operation benefits chiefly limb phasic or tonic dystonia both in DMD and secondary dystonia. Benefit in other categories is so infrequent as to be negligible (Cooper 1976*a*, 1976*b*; Andrew *et al.* 1983).

Of the complications, those related to worsening of pseudobulbar deficit (death, tracheotomy, dysphagia, dysarthria) are of note. They tend to occur in disabled bilaterally neurologically involved patients even if operated on unilaterally (Gros *et al.* 1976).

As with Parkinson's disease bilateral thalamotomy carries a significant risk of permanent speech deterioration.

Finally, particularly in patients with DMD, it is difficult to decide if deterioration in speech and gait postoperatively is the result of often rapid disease progress or of the surgery.

We made an attempt to determine 'risk factors' for dystonia patients undergoing thalamotomy. Since thalamotomy improves only limb dystonia, progress of the disease can obscure any benefits derived from surgery. The more widespread the disease, the more disabled the patient so that we analysed the effect of numbers of limbs involved. We also checked to see whether fixed tonic deformities responded less well than phasic dystonia (Table 29.9). Patient groups with less than 25% and with over 50% overall postoperative benefit showed little difference in numbers of limbs affected, nor in presence of tonic features. Bad results apparently correlated with trunk and neck

Table 29.7. *Complications of thalamotomy for dystonia (percentage of 49 patients)*

Complication	DMD ($n=20$)	Secondary dystonia ($n=29$)
Death (aggravation of pseudobulbar effects)	0	3.4
Permanent tracheotomy	0	3.4
Persistent mild/moderate hemiparesis	10	0
Transient dysphagia	5	6.9
Persistent significant worsening of dysarthria	20[a]	6.9[a]
Persistent mild worsening of dysarthria	30[a]	6.9[b]
Transient mild worsening of dysarthria	20	6.9
Persistent gait disturbance	20	6.9
Transient gait disturbance	0	20.7
Transient hand ataxia	15	3.4
Transient dysphasia	0	3.4
Transient numbness	20	17.2
Superficial wound infection	5	6.9
Epileptic seizure	5	3.4

DMD, dystonia musculorum deformous
[a] Thirty-five percent of this 50% with permanent speech impairment had undergone bilateral thalamotomy.
[b] This 13.8% with persistent speech impairment constituted four (80%) of the five patients undergoing bilateral thalamotomy.

Table 29.8. *Effect of thalamotomy on features of dystonia musculorum deformans (DMD)*

Feature	Percentage of 20 patients significantly improved
Speech	2
Facial movement	22
Neck movement	29
Trunk movement	28
Locomotion	13
Dexterity	38
Upper limb movements	
Phasic	53
Tonic	57
Lower limb movements	
Phasic	39
Tonic	69

involvement and good results with sparing of trunk and neck (Table 29.10). Surprisingly, rate of disease progress had little relevance to results.

Conclusion

In summary, we have reviewed published data for several neurosurgical procedures for the relief of intractable pain and for thalamotomy for movement disorders. In each case salient issues have been raised that might be expected to lead to difficulties with

Table 29.9. *Effect of thalamotomy on features of secondary dystonia*

Feature	Percentage of 29 patients significantly improved
Speech	12
Facial movements	35
Neck movements	19
Trunk movements	31
Locomotion	12
Dexterity	17
Upper limb movements	
Phasic	52
Tonic	50
Lower limb movements	
Phasic	53
Tonic	41

Table 29.10. *Possible 'risk' factors in thalamotomy for dystonia musculorum deformans (DMD) and secondary dystonia*

Degree of improvement	Number of limbs affected		Involvement of trunk, neck		Disease progress at time of surgery		Tonic dystonia present	
	1–2	3–4	Yes	No	Yes	No	Yes	No
< 25%	33%	67%	89%	11%	33%	67%	22%	78%
> 50%	40%	60%	30%	70%	10%	90%	20%	80%

outcome analysis. The solution, the establishment of a more reliable set of criteria for outcome reporting, remains elusive.

References

Adams, J. E. & Rutkin, B. B. (1965). Lesions of the centrum medianum in the treatment of movement disorders. *Confin. Neurol.* **26**, 231–6.

Albe-Fessard, D., Guiot, G. & Hardy, J. (1963). Electrophysiological localization and identification of subcortical structures in man by recording spontaneous and evoked activities. *EEG Clin. Neurophysiol.* **15**, 1052–3.

Andrew, J., Fowler, C. J. & Harrison, M. J. G. (1983). Stereotaxic thalamotomy in 55 cases of dystonia. *Brain* **106**, 981–1000.

Benabid, A. L., Pollak, P., Louveau, A., Henry, B. & de Rougemont, J. (1987). Combined (thalamotomy and stimulation) surgery of the VIM thalamic nucleus for bilateral Parkinson disease. *Appl. Neurophysiol.* **50**, 344–6.

Bertrand, C., Jasper, H. & Wong, A. (1967). Microelectrode study of the human thalamus: functional organization in the ventrobasal complex. *Confin. Neurol.* **29**, 81–6.

Bosch, D. A. (1986). *Stereotactic Techniques in Clinical Neurosurgery.* Vienna: Springer-Verlag.

Bravo, G., Parera, C., Sequeira, G. (1966). Neurological side-effects in a series of operations on the basal ganglia. *J. Neurosurg.* **24**, 640–7.

Bullard, D. E. & Nashold, B. S. Jr (1984). Stereotaxic thalamotomy for treatment of post-traumatic movement disorders. *J. Neurosurg.* **61**, 316–21.

Caparros-Lefebvre, D., Blond, S., Vermersh, P., Pécheux, N., Guieu, J. D. & Petit, H. (1993). Chronic thalamic stimulation improves tremor and levodopa induced dyskinesias in Parkinson's disease. *J. Neurol. Neurosurg. Psychiatry* **56**, 268–73.

Carpenter, M. B., Hanna, G. R. (1962). Effects of thalamic lesions upon cerebellar dyskinesia in the Rhesus monkey. *J. Comp. Neurol.* **119**, 127–47.

Cooper, I. S. (1962). Heredofamilial tremor; abolition by chemothalamectomy. *Arch. Neurol.* **7**, 129–31.

Cooper, I. S. (1965). Surgical treatment of Parkinsonism. *Ann. Rev. Med.* **16**, 309–30.

Cooper, I. S. (1969). *Involuntary Movement Disorders*, pp. 160–292. New York: Hoeber.

Cooper, I. S. (1976a). 20-year follow-up study of the neurosurgical treatment of dystonia musculorum deformans. In *Dystonia*, eds. R. Eldridge & S. Fahn, pp. 423–52. *Advances in Neurology* **14**. New York: Raven Press.

Cooper, I. S. (1976b). Dystonia: surgical approaches to treatment and physiological implications. In *The Basal Ganglia*, ed. M. D. Yahr, pp. 364–83. New York: Raven Press.

Cooper, I. S. & Bravo, G. J. (1958). Implications of a five-year study of 700 basal ganglia operations. *Neurology* **8**, 701–7.

Deiber, M. P., Pollak, P., Passingham, R., Landais, P., Gervason, C., Cinotti, L., Frislon, K., Frackowiak, R., Mauguière, F. & Benabid, A. L. (1993). Thalamic stimulation and suppression of parkinsonian tremor. Evidence of a cerebellar deactivation using positron emmision tomography. *Brain* **116**, 267–79.

Dostrovsky, J. O., Sher, G. D., Davis, K. D., Parrent, A., Hutchison, W. D. & Tasker, R. R. (1993). Microinjection of lidocaine into human thalamus: a useful tool in stereotactic surgery. *Stereotact. Funct. Neurosurg.* **60**, 168–74.

Gillingham, F. J. (1964). Bilateral stereotaxic lesions in the management of Parkinsonism and the dyskinesias. *BMJ* **II**, 656–9.

Goldman, M. S. & Kelly, P. J. (1992a). Symptomatic and functional outcome of stereotactic ventralis lateralis thalamotomy for intention tremor. *J. Neurosurg.* **77**, 223–9.

Goldman, M. S. & Kelly, P. J. (1992b). Stereotactic thalamotomy for medically intractable essential tremor. *Stereotact. Funct. Neurosurg.* **58**, 22–5.

Gros, C., Frerebeau, P. H., Perez-Dominguez, E., Bagin, M. & Privat, J. M. (1976). Long-term results of stereotaxic surgery for infantile dystonia and dyskinesia. *Neurochirurgia* **19**, 171–8.

Guiot, G., Derome, P. & Trijo, J. C. (1967). Le tremblement d'attitude: indication la meilleure de la chirurgie stéréotaxique. *Press. Med.* **75**, 2513–18.

Hardy, T. L., Bertrand, G. & Thompson, C. J. (1979). Thalamic recordings during stereotactic surgery. II. Location of quick-adapting touch-evoked (novelty) cellular responses. *Appl. Neurophysiol.* **42**, 198–202.

Hardy, T. L., Bertrand, G. & Thompson, C. J. (1980a). Passive position and organization of the thalamic cellular activity during diencephalic recording. II. Joint- and muscle-evoked activity. *Appl. Neurophysiol.* **43**, 28–36.

Hardy, T. L., Bertrand, G. & Thompson, C. J. (1980b). Topography of bilateral movement-evoked thalamic cellular activity found during diencephalic recording. *Appl. Neurophysiol.* **43**, 67–74.

Hardy, T. L., Bertrand, G. & Thompson, C. J. (1981). Touch-evoked thalamic cellular activity. The variable position of the anterior border of somesthetic SI thalamus and somatotopography. *Appl. Neurophysiol.* **44**, 302–13.

Hassler, R. & Riechert, T. (1954). Indikationen und Lokalizationsmethode der gezielten. Hirnoperationen Nervenarzt **25**, 441–7.

Hawrylyshyn, P. A., Tasker, R. R. & Organ, L. W. (1976–77). Third-ventricular width and the thalamocapsular border. *Appl. Neurophysiol.* **39**, 34–42.

Hirai, T., Miyazaki, M., Nakajima, H., Shibazaki, T. & Ohye, C. (1983). The correlation between tremor characteristics and the predicted volume of effective lesions in stereotaxic nucleus ventralis intermedius thalamotomy. *Brain* **106**, 1001–18.

Jasper, H. H. & Bertrand, G. (1966). Thalamic units involved in somatic sensation and voluntary and involuntary movement in man. In *The Thalamus*, eds. D. P. Purpura & M. D. Yabr, pp. 365–90. New York: Columbia University Press.

Jenkins, I. H., Bain, P. G., Colebatch, J. G., Thompson, P. D., Findley, L. J., Frackowiak, R. S. J., Marsden, C. D. & Brooks, D. J. (1993). A positron emission tomography study of essential tremor: evidence for overactivity of cerebellar connections. *Ann. Neurol.* **34**, 82–90.

Jokura, H., Otsuki, T., Niizuma, H., Nakasalo, N., Takahashi, H., Yoshimoto, T. & Saso, S. (1990). Long-term results of Vim thalamotomy for postapoplectic tremor. *Stereotact. Funct. Neurosurg.* **54–55**, 216.

Jones, M. W. & Tasker R. R. (1990). The relationship of documented destruction of specific cell types to complications and effectiveness in thalamotomy for tremor in Parkinson's disease. *Stereotact. Funct. Neurosurg.* **54–55**, 207–11.

Kandel, E. I. (1982). Treatment of hemihyperkinesias by stereotactic operations on basal ganglia. *Appl. Neurophysiol.* **45**, 225.

Kelly, P. J. & Gillingham, F. J. (1980). The long-term results of stereotaxic surgery and L-dopa therapy in patients with Parkinson's disease. A 10-year follow-up study. *J. Neurosurg.* **53**, 332–7.

Kelly, P. J., Ahlskog, J. E., Goerss, S. J., Daube, J. R., Duffy, J. R. & Kall, B. A. (1987). Computer-assisted stereotactic ventralis lateralis thalamotomy with microelectrode recording control in patients with Parkinson's disease. *Mayo Clin. Proc.* **62**, 655–64.

Krayenbühl, H., Wyss, O. A. M. & Yasargil, M. G. (1961). Bilateral thalamotomy and pallidotomy as treatment for bilateral Parkinsonism. *J. Neurosurg.* **18**, 429–44.

Krayenbühl, H., Siegfried, J. & Yasargil, M. G. (1963). Résultats tards des opérations stéréotaxiques dans le traitement de la maladie de Parkinson. *Rev. Neurol.* **108**, 485–94.

Laitinen, L. V. (1965). Stereotactic treatment of hereditary tremor. *Acta Neurol. Scand.* **41**, 74–9.

Laitinen, L. V. (1966). Thalamic targets in the stereotaxic treatment of Parkinson's disease. *J. Neurosurg.* **24**, 82–5.

Laitinen, L. V. (1985). Brain targets in surgery for Parkinson's disease. *J. Neurosurg.* **62**, 349–51.

Laitinen, L. V. (1988). Mesencephalotomy and thalamotomy for chronic pain. In *Modern Stereotactic Neurosurgery*, ed. L. D. Lunsford, pp. 269–77. Boston: Martinus Nijhoff.

Laitinen, L. V., Bergenheim, A. T. & Hariz, M. I. (1992). Leksell's posteroventral pallidotomy in the treatment of Parkinson's disease. *J. Neurosurg.* **76**, 53–61.

Lenz, F. A., Tasker, R. R., Kwan, H. C., Schnider, S., Kwong, R. & Murphy, J. T. (1985). Cross-correlation analyses of thalamic neurons and EMG activity in Parkinsonian tremor. *Appl. Neurophysiol.* **48**, 305–8.

Lenz, F. A., Schnider, S., Tasker, R. R., Kwong, R., Kwan, H., Dostrovsky, J. O. & Murphy, J. T. (1987*a*). The role of feedback in the tremor frequency activity of tremor cells in the ventral nuclear group of human thalamus. *Acta. Neurochir.* **39** (Suppl.), 54–6.

Lenz, F. A., Tasker, R. R., Kwan, H. C., Schnider, S., Kwong, R., Dostrovsky, J. O. & Murphy, J. T.

(1987*b*). Selection of the optimal lesion site for the relief of Parkinsonian tremor on the basis of spectral analysis of neuronal firing patterns. *Appl. Neurophysiol.* **50**, 338–43.

Lenz, F. A., Tasker, R. R., Kwan, H. C., Schnider, S., Kwong, R., Murayama, M., Dostrovsky, J. O. & Murphy, J. T. (1988*a*). Single unit analysis of the human ventral thalamic nuclear group; correlation of thalamic 'tremor cells' with the 3–6 Hz component of Parkinsonian tremor. *J. Neurosci.* **8**, 754–64.

Lenz, F. A., Dostrovsky, J. O., Tasker, R. R., Yamashiro, K., Kwan, H. C. & Murphy, J. T. (1988*b*). Single-unit analyses in the human ventral thalamic nuclear group: somatosensory responses. *J. Neurophysiol.* **59**, 299–316.

Lenz, F. A., Dostrovsky, J. O., Tasker, R. R., Yamashiro, K., Kwan, H. C. & Murphy, J. T. (1990*b*). Single-unit analysis of the human ventral thalamic nuclear group: somatosensory responses. *J. Neurophysiol.* **59**, 299–316.

Lenz, F. A., Kwan, H. C., Dostrovsky, J. O., Tasker, R. R., Murphy, J. T. & Lenz, Y. E. (1990*a*). Single unit analysis of the human ventral thalamic nuclear group. Activity correlated with movement. *Brain* **113**, 1795–821.

Lenz, F. A., Martin, R., Kwan, H. C., Tasker, R. R. & Dostrovsky, J. O. (1990*b*). Thalamic single-unit activity occurring in patients with hemidystonia. *Stereotact. Funct. Neurosurg.* **54–55**, 159–62.

Li, J. C. S., De Carvalho, G. & Tasker, R. R. (1990). Does VIM thalamotomy affect the course of Parkinson's disease? *Stereotact. Funct. Neurosurg.* **54–55**, 192.

Mamo, H., Dondey, M., Cophignon, J., Pidloux, P., Fontelle, P. & Houdait, R. (1965). Latéropulsion transitoire au décours des coagulation sousthalamiques et thalamiques chez des parkinsoniens. *Rev. Neurol.* **112**, 509–20.

Matsumoto, K., Asano, T., Baba, T., Miyamoto, T. & Ohmoto, T. (1976–77). Long-term follow-up results of bilateral thalamotomy for Parkinsonism. *Appl. Neurophysiol.* **39**, 257–60.

Matsumoto, K., Shichijo, F. & Fukami, T. (1984). Long-term follow-up review of cases of Parkinson's disease after unilateral or bilateral thalamotomy. *J. Neurosurg.* **60**, 1033–44.

Meyers, R. (1940). A surgical procedure for the alleviation of postencephalitic tremor with notes on the physiology of the premotor fibres. *Arch. Neurol. Psychiatry* **44**, 455–9.

Miyamoto, T., Bekku, H., Moriyama, T. & Suchida, S. (1985). Present role of stereotactic thalamotomy for Parkinsonism. Retrospective analysis of operative results and thalamic lesion in computed tomograms. *Appl. Neurophysiol.* **48**, 294–304.

Modesti, L. M. & Van Buren, J. M. (1979). Hemiballismus complicating stereotactic thalamotomy. *Appl. Neurophysiol.* **42**, 267–83.

Mohadiger, M., Goerkett, H., Milios, E., Etou, A. & Mundinger, F. (1990). Long-term results of stereotaxy in the treatment of essential tremor. *Stereotact. Funct. Neurosurg.* **54–55**, 125–9.

Mundinger, F. I. (1985). Postoperative and long-term results of 1561 stereotactic operations in Parkinsonism. *Appl. Neurophysiol.* **48**, 293.

Mundinger, F. & Kühn, I. (1982). Postoperative and long-term results after stereotactic operations for action myoclonia in cases of encephalomyelitis disseminata. *Appl. Neurophysiol.* **45**, 299–305.

Nagaseki, Y., Shibazaki, T., Hirai, T., Kawashuma, Y., Hirato, Y., Wada, H., Miyazaki, M. & Ohye, C. (1986). Long-term follow-up results of selective VIM-thalamotomy. *J. Neurosurg.* **65**, 296–302.

Narabayashi, H. (1988). Lessons from stereotaxic surgery using microelectrode techniques in understanding Parkinsonism. *Mt Sinai J. Med.* **55**, 50–57.

Ohye, C. (1985). Neurons of the thalamic ventralis intermedius nucleus: their special reference to tremor. *Adv. Neurol. Sci.* **29**, 224–31.

Ohye, C. (1987). Stereotactic surgery in movement disorders: choice of patient, localization of lesion with microelectrodes, and long-term results. In *Neurosurgery. Stereotactic Surgery, State of the Art Reviews*, 2(1) May, ed. R. R. Tasker, pp. 193–208. Hanley and Belfus.

Ohye, C. H. & Narabayashi, H. (1979). Physiological study of presumed ventralis intermedius neurons in the human thalamus. *J. Neurosurg.* **50**, 290–7.

Ohye, C., Hirai, T., Miyazaki, M., Shitazaki, T. & Nakahima, H. (1982a). Vim thalamotomy for the treatment of various kinds of tremor. *Appl. Neurophysiol.* **45**, 275–80.

Ohye, C., Miyazaki, M., Hirai, T. *et al.* (1982b). Primary writing tremor treated by stereotactic selective thalamotomy. *J. Neurol. Neurosurg. Psychiatry* **45**, 988–97.

Ohye, C., Shibazaki, T., Hirai, T., Wada, H., Hirato, M. & Kawashura, Y. (1989). Further physiological observations in the ventralis intermedius neurons in the human thalamus. *J. Neurophysiol.* **61**, 488–500.

Ohye, C., Shibazaki, T., Hirato, M., Kawashima, Y. & Matsumura, M. (1990). Strategy of selective Vim thalamotomy guided by microrecording. *Stereotact. Funct. Neurosurg.* **54–55**, 186–91.

Poirier, L. J., Bouvier, G., Bedard, P., Boucher, R., Larochelle, L., Olivier, A. *et al.* (1969). Essai sur les circuits neuronaux impliqués dans le tremblement postural et l'hypokinésie. *Rev. Neurol.* **120**, 15–40.

Raeva, S. N. (1986). Localization in human thalamus of units triggered during 'verbal commands', voluntary movements and tremor. *EEG Clin. Neurophysiol.* **63**, 160–73.

Riechert, T. (1962). Long-term follow-up of results of stereotactic treatment of extrapyramidal disorders. *Confin. Neurol.* **22**, 356–63.

Riechert, T. (1980). *Stereotactic Brain Operations: Methods, Clinical Aspects, Indications.* Bern: Hoeber.

Riklan, M., Diller, L., Weimer, H. & Cooper, I. S. (1960). Psychological studies on effects of chemosurgery of the basal ganglia in Parkinsonism. I. Intellectual functioning. *Arch. Gen. Psychiatry* **2**, 22–31.

Schnider, S. M., Kwong, R. H., Lenz, F. A., Kwan, H. L. (1989). Detection of feedback in the central nervous system using system identification technique. *Biol. Cybernet.* **60**, 203–12.

Scott, R. M., Brody, J. A. & Cooper, I. S. (1970). The effect of thalamotomy on the progress of unilateral Parkinson's disease. *J. Neurosurg.* **32**, 286–8.

Siegfried, J. (1988). La place actuelle de la neurochirurgie stéréotaxique dans le traitement des movements involuntaires. *Ther. Umschau/Rev. Ther.* **45**, 50–5.

Siegfried, J. & Rea, G. L. (1988). Deep brain stimulation for the treatment of motor disorders. In *Modern Stereotactic Neurosurgery*, ed. L. D. Lunsdorf, pp. 409–12. Boston: Martinus Nijhoff.

Spiegel, E. A., Wycis, H. T., Szekely, E. G. *et al.* (1962). Campotomy. *Trans. Am. Neurol. Assoc.* **87**, 240.

Stellar, S. & Cooper, I. S. (1968). Mortality and morbidity in cryothalamectomy for Parkinson's disease. A statistical study of 2868 consecutive operations. *J. Neurosurg.* **28**, 459–67.

Tasker, R. R. (1963). Preliminary report on stereotactic surgery. *Bull. Acad. Toronto.*

Tasker, R. R. (1967). Surgical aspects. Symposium on extrapyramidal disease. *Appl. Therapeutic.* **9**, 454–62.

Tasker, R. R. (1970). Significance and etiology of induced abnormal movements: physiological implications. In *L-dopa and Parkinsonism*, eds. A. Barbeau & F. H. McDowell, pp. 159–63. Philadelphia: Davis.

Tasker, R. R. (1990). Thalamotomy. In *Stereotactic Neurosurgery. Neurosurgery Clinics of North America*, vol. 1, ed. W. A. Friedman, pp. 841–64. Philadelphia: Saunders.

Tasker, R. R. (1994a). Movement disorders. In *Brain Surgery: Complication Avoidance and Management*, ed. M. Apuzzo, pp. 1509–24.

Tasker, R. R., Organ, L. W., Hawrylyshyn, P. A. (1982a). *The Thalamus and Midbrain of Man. A Physiological Atlas Using Electrical Stimulation.* Springfield: Thomas.

Tasker, R. R., Organ, L. W. & Hawrylyshyn, P. (1982b). Investigation of the surgical target for alleviation of involuntary movement disorders. *Appl. Neurophysiol.* **45**, 261–74.

Tasker, R. R., Siqueira, J., Hawrylyshyn, P. A. & Organ, L. W. (1983). What happened to VIM thalamotomy for Parkinson's disease? *Appl. Neurophysiol.* **46**, 68.

Tasker, R. R., Lenz, F. A., Dostrovsky, J. O. *et al.* (1987). The physiological basis of VIM thalamotomy for involuntary movement disorders. In *Clinical Aspects of Sensory Motor Integration*, eds. A. Struppler & A. Weindl, p. 265. Berlin: Springer-Verlag.

Tasker, R. R., Doorly, T. & Yamashiro, K. (1988a). Thalamotomy in generalized dystonia. In *Advances in Neurology 50, Dystonia 2*, eds. S. Fahn *et al.*, pp. 615–631. New York: Raven Press.

Tasker, R. R., Yamashiro, K., Lenz, F. & Dostrovsky, J. O. (1988b). Thalamotomy for Parkinson's Disease. In *Modern Stereotactic Neurosurgery*, ed. L. D. Lunsford, pp. 297–314. Boston: Martinus Nijhoff.

Tasker, R. R., DeCarvalho, G. C., Li, C. S. & Kestle, J. R. W. (1996). Does thalamotomy alter the course of Parkinson's disease? In *Advances in Neurology*, Vol. 69, eds. L. Battistin, G. Scarlato, T. Caraceni & S. Ruggieri, pp. 563–83. Philadelphia: Lippincott-Raven.

Tetrud, J. W. & Langston, J. W. (1989). The effect of deprenyl (selegitine) on the natural history of Parkinson's disease. *Science* **245**, 519–22.

Van Manen, J., Speelman, J. D. & Tans, R. J. J. (1984). Indications for surgical treatment of Parkinson's disease after levodopa therapy. *Clin. Neurol. Neurosurg.* **86**, 207–12.

Walker, A. E. (1982). Stereotaxic surgery for tremor. In *Stereotaxy of the Human Brain. Anatomical, Physiological and Clinical Applications*, eds. G. Schaltenbrand & A. E. Walker, pp. 515–21. Stuttgart: Thieme.

Wester, K., Haughlie-Hanssen, E. (1990). Stereotaxic thalamotomy: experiences from the levodopa era. *J. Neurol. Neurosurg. Psychiatry* **53**, 427–30.

Yasui, N., Narabayashi, H., Kondo, T. & Ohye, C. (1976–77). Slight cerebellar signs in stereotactic thalamotomy and subthalamotomy for Parkinsonism. *Appl. Neurophysiol.* **39**, 315.

Yoshida, M., Okuda, K., Watanabe, M. & Kuramoto, S. (1976–77). Analysis of tremulous movement after thalamotomy correlated to intrathalamic therapeutic lesions. *Appl. Neurophysiol.* **39**, 311.

Zoll, J. G. (1978). Inversion or pronation of the foot following thalamotomy for Parkinson's disease. *Appl. Neurophysiol.* **41**, 232–6.

30 Neuropsychology: recovery after brain lesions

IAN H. ROBERTSON

This chapter will attempt to answer three questions: (1) what are the neuropsychological processes which may be involved in recovery of function following brain damage? (2) What are some of the courses of recovery following various types of brain damage? (3) Is there any evidence that neuropsychological rehabilitation can accelerate recovery?

What are the neuropsychological processes which may be involved in recovery of function following brain damage?

The cerebral cortex may show a greater degree of plasticity than has hitherto been recognized. Merzenich *et al.* (1984), for example, found that somatosensory fields in owl monkey altered in such a way as to apparently 'use up' space 'vacated' by amputated fingers. Similarly, if the postcentral gyrus was damaged, they found a redistribution of receptive fields for other fingers so that they all 'had a share', albeit with less acuity because of having fewer representational neurons per finger. Jenkins *et al.* (1990) also demonstrated reorganization of the somatosensory fields after damage to somatosensory cortex in monkeys. Parts of the field which never before responded to specific fingers began to do so after the responsible areas were ablated. Also, simple, tactile training extensively altered the cortical maps. Many other studies have come to similar conclusions (e.g. Pons *et al.* 1991), but it is outwith the scope of the present chapter to review this literature in detail.

Animal studies also suggest that such plasticity can be influenced by post-damage experience (Gentile *et al.* 1978; Slavin *et al.* 1988), a finding with clearly important implications for human neurorehabilitation. Furthermore, Mayer *et al.* (1992) showed that rats given striatal neural transplants only benefited from the transplants when they were given the opportunity for learning. These studies suggest that the behavioural loss apparent after damage to the brain may not reflect simple and irrevocable loss of underlying neural functioning – experience and perhaps training may modify not only the behavioural deficit, but also the underlying neural representation.

LeVere & LeVere (1982) provided animal evidence to suggest that behavioural deficits after brain injury may arise from failure to use the injured neural system and that a behavioural deficit may be caused not by a neural deficit, but because the compensatory strategy is interfering with residual capacities in the damaged system. Such a formulation rests on two assumptions, argued LeVere & LeVere, namely that: first, individuals, both normal and brain injured, are optimizers, i.e. they make best use of existing sensory, motor and cognitive resources. After a lesion, there will be some loss in some of these, and so they will readjust to make up for this. Second, compensation may work in certain situations, but will fail when specific behaviour which is crucially dependent on the undamaged but underutilized neural system is required.

LeVere & LeVere argued that one cannot assume that neurological losses yield commensurate behavioural losses, and the importance of environmental, learning and motivational variables in moderating the behavioural manifestations of brain damage are becoming increasingly recognized. While setting aside the possibility of learning affecting underlying neural structure as well as vice versa, there are a number of possible neuropsychological mechanisms which are important in determining the degree of neuropsychological recovery following brain damage. These are inhibition, compensation, motivation and functional adaptation, each of which will be discussed in turn.

Inhibition

Sprague (1966) demonstrated that hemianopia in cats could be ameliorated by destroying the superior colliculus on the side opposite to initial visual input, thereby freeing the lesioned hemisphere from the collicular inhibition of the intact hemisphere and allowing ipsilesional circuits to operate.

Parallel findings in the human literature are now also available. Butter & Kirsch (1992) showed that unilateral neglect in patients suffering from right hemisphere strokes could be temporarily reduced if the ipsilesional eye was patched. Butter based his research on an argument made by Rafal (Posner & Rafal 1987), namely that, given that eye–colliculus connections are completely crossed, patching the right eye should cut off sensory input to the left (contralesional) superior colliculus. The effect of this would be to reduce inhibition of the right hemisphere superior colliculus and thereby increase the attentional functioning of the right hemisphere via improved right collicular activation.

Robertson and North (1992, 1993) showed that unilateral left neglect following right hemisphere stroke could be improved if patients were required to make minimal movements with left limbs in left hemispace. When they made identical movements with *both* hands, however, this effect disappeared (Robertson & North 1994), and the authors argued that this was because the activation of the intact hemisphere overshadowed or extinguished the activation of the damaged hemisphere, the implication being that bilateral limb use may prevent underutilized potential from being realized in the damaged hemisphere.

In summary, therefore, some neuropsychological recovery may take place, or fail to take place, because of inhibitory processes from intact to impaired circuits in the brain. This has considerable implications for the rehabilitative aspects of neuropsychological recovery.

Compensation

Brain-lesioned animals can show suboptimal performance because of compensation strategies learned early post-lesion which outlive their usefulness later in the course of recovery and which end up being obstacles to efficient performance because of a lack of use of underutilized but nevertheless functioning circuits (e.g. LeVere & LeVere 1982). Clear evidence for this type of phenomenon is absent in humans, though Beauvois (1982) showed that in a case of optic aphasia, tactile recognition could be improved by taping closed the lips of the patient to prevent implicit verbalization. She proposed that an intact tactile object recognition system was inhibited by the patient's attempts to use an impaired verbal system as a compensatory aid.

A clinical example of maladaptive compensation is apparent in the following case seen by the author. The patient had complete left homonymous hemianopia, with no sparing of the macula. He had some perceptual problems, for instance, depth perception difficulties, and subjectively reported problems in missing the left side of written items such as price labels in shops, 'losing' the ball while watching soccer on television and risking serious injury when crossing the road by failing to notice cars coming from both right and left.

The subject was given a computerized visual search task, where he was found to make more omissions of targets on the left than on the right, while at the same time being much *slower* to detect targets on the right side. It transpired that this slowness on the right arose because of an over-conscientiously applied leftward scanning strategy with which he had learned to try to compensate for the left-sided errors which he knew he made. This strategy involved a painstaking item-by-item search of the left side, leading to long delays before he reached the right, and this technique was partially the cause of him narrowly escaping being mown down by cars coming from the right as well as from the left!

The recommended solution was to modify his compensation strategy, so as to quickly scan to the right at the beginning of a search, return to the systematic left search, return to the right and to do this a few times so as to make sure that the relatively intact ability to scan right was not underused. Implementation of this strategy with the computer search led to a marked speeding up of right search times, without any change in left errors or search time. There was also a 30% drop in rated effort of carrying out the search.

Functional adaptation

Sometimes a particular modular circuit underlying a given neuropsychological function is to all intents and purposes non-functioning, and there has to occur a reorganization of intact circuits such as to produce a comparable behavioural outcome based on a different arrangement of underlying neuropsychological systems. According to Luria (1963) this is the major mechanism underlying recovery of function following brain injury.

A study by Goodale *et al.* (1990) provides an example of such functional adaptation. They studied a group of nine subjects who had suffered unilateral right hemisphere lesions a mean of 21 weeks after the onset of the lesion. Many of these patients had previously shown signs of unilateral neglect, but by the time they were tested by the authors, there was no clinically significant neglect.

The experiment consisted of two tasks, one involving reaching out and touching one of a number of lighted targets presented on a vertical screen in front of the subjects, and the other consisted of requiring the subjects to bisect the distance between two specified targets on the screen. The brain-damaged patients showed no difference from the controls on their accuracy of touching the targets, while they did show a significant tendency to bisect to the right of the true mid-point of the distance between adjacent targets, suggesting the existence of an enduring subclinical manifestation of left unilateral neglect which was not revealed by standard clinical testing.

More interestingly, however, were the trajectories of the hand as it reached into the targets. In both the target and bisection conditions, kinematic video analysis of the reaching movements was made. This revealed that the patients made a wide right arc into the final target, a pattern which was not apparent in the controls; Figure 30.1 shows the movements of patient D55 of the Goodale *et al.* series during bisection. These results suggest that even after the apparent recovery of neglect, underlying distortions in spatial or attentional mechanisms still exist (for instance, the deficit may have been attributable to a persisting 'hypokinesia', namely a difficulty in making movements in the contralesional direction). It may be the case that the patients had learned to compensate for their neglect by compensatory visual control. When the patients first sent their arms out on ballistic trajectories, it appears that they did so on the basis of a distorted body-referenced spatial system.

The rightward trajectory may then have been corrected by a compensatory visual feedback system which the subjects had spontaneously learned to use to correct the spatial errors of which they may have been unaware. Alternatively, they may not have been aware of the deficits, and these compensatory visual responses may have been elicited by some kind of conditioning process along the lines of those which have been hypothesized in hemianopics spontaneously learning to compensate for their visual field deficits (e.g. Williams & Gassell, 1962; Meienberg *et al.* 1980).

If it is true that underlying deficits still persist which are obscured by compensatory mechanisms, then it should be possible to cause the basic deficit to re-emerge by presenting a task which is attentionally demanding or requires a high degree of spatial thought. An example of the former may be the results for a case reported in Robertson & Frasca (1992) described above, where left–right differences in response latency only emerged during an attentionally demanding secondary task performance. An example

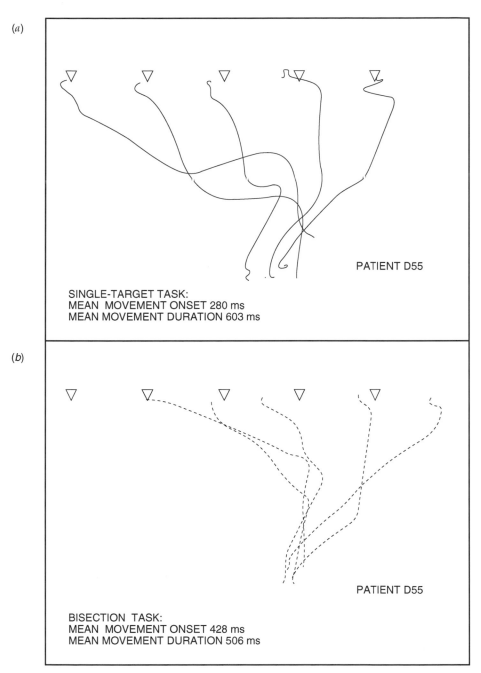

(a)

SINGLE-TARGET TASK:
MEAN MOVEMENT ONSET 280 ms
MEAN MOVEMENT DURATION 603 ms

PATIENT D55

(b)

BISECTION TASK:
MEAN MOVEMENT ONSET 428 ms
MEAN MOVEMENT DURATION 506 ms

PATIENT D55

Fig. 30.1a,b. Representative trajectories (in the X-Y plane) of reaches made by patient D55 using the right hand (ipsilateral to the damaged hemisphere). Notice that, when reaching into the left or right hemispace, the movements made showed a pronounced rightward heading, vis-à-vis the correct endpoint. These initial rightward errors were largely corrected for in the target task (solid lines in **a**), but not in the bisection task (broken lines in **b**). (Reprinted with permission from the Canadian Journal of Psychology, vol. 44, 1990.)

of the latter may be the poor performance of Goodale *et al.*'s subjects on the bisection task compared with the target pointing task. Functional adaptation takes place in all neuropsychological functions following brain injury, including memory, attention, perception, motor control and thinking. The above example will suffice for the purpose of this review in illustrating the principle.

Motivation and emotion

A study by Parsons and Stewart (1966) is important in illustrating the role of motivation in neuropsychological function. They compared 20 brain-injured people and 20 neurotics on perceptual-motor performance over three testing sessions. They compared two interviewing styles during testing: one disinterested/factual, and the other supportive. While the neurotic group showed no significant interview-type effect on test performance over the three trials, the brain-damaged group whose testers were supportive showed a significantly greater test-retest practice effect than those interviewed in a distinterested manner.

Suffering a brain injury has corrosive effects on morale and self-esteem, both because of the loss of abilities which arise, but also because of the loss of important work, family, social or sexual roles. Depression is known to depress cognitive functions and hence it is apparent that in some cases, secondary emotional and motivational factors play a part in determining a particular neuropsychological performance. Hence some but not all types of neuropsychological rehabilitation may have positive effects through affecting morale, mood and self-confidence more than through any specific training of cognitive functions.

Some aspects of the course of recovery following neuropsychological impairment

Any insult to the brain will produce both local and diffuse effects. The location of any specific site will influence the type of the deficits shown, and different types of deficits have different courses of remission, as a study by Hier *et al.* (1983) showed. In the following selective review, the example of unilateral neglect will predominate in illustrating some of the principles underlying recovery of neuropsychological function.

Hier *et al.* found that recovery of a variety of neuropsychological deficits in a series of 41 patients suffering right hemisphere stroke seemed to depend on whether or not the functions were subserved by complex processes with widely distributed anatomical substrata. For instance, recovery was rapid for left neglect, prosopagnosia, anosognosia, while it was slowest for hemianopia, hemiparesis, motor impersistence and extinction. Recovery rates were intermediate for constructional dyspraxia and dressing dyspraxia. A plateau for arm weakness was reached at 16 weeks post-stroke, for instance, with less than a 50% probability of recovery. For hemianopia it was 32 weeks, with a less than 70% chance of recovery. In the case of unilateral spatial neglect by drawing, on the other hand, by 12 weeks more than 70% of patients had recovered, while anosognosia had all but disappeared by 17 weeks post-stroke. These findings seem to support Luria's contention that recovery depends largely on reorganization of complex neuropsychological systems. Where the underlying process is more modular and specific – e.g. in the case of hemianopia or primary motor loss – there is less possibility that such reorganization can occur.

The frontal lobes are thought to be the basis of the brain's executive functions, concerned with sequencing and monitoring ongoing activity, including learning. One would therefore predict that damage to frontal structures should predict poor outcome following brain injury. Hier *et al.* (1983) did indeed find this to be the case, in a series of 41 right brain damaged patients, though Ogden *et al.* (1994) did not find that any particular location of subarachnoid haemhorrage was predictive of good or poor recovery.

In their study, Ogden *et al.* followed up 89 patients 10 weeks and 12 months post-subarachnoid haemorrhage (SAH). No significant predictors of outcome in terms of lesion location, clinical grade and vasospasm were found. A high proportion had mild to moderate psychosocial impairments at 10 weeks, and while there was recovery over the next 8 months, 86% of subjects still suffered from excessive fatigue and 55% from hypersensitivity to noise at the 12 months assessment. Of the subjects employed at the time of SAH, 59% were either unemployed or working reduced hours at 12 months follow-up.

Motor impersistence, a measure of ability to sustain a simple act such as protruding the tongue for a specified period without taking it in, has been shown to be a significant predictor of outcome following stroke, indeed this measure together with a verbal memory test were the strongest predictor of discharge outcome in 134 stroke patients (Novack *et al.* 1987). This is probably a measure of alertness or vigilance, which recent research suggest may be a function located partly in the right frontal lobe (Wilkins *et al.* 1987; Pardo *et al.* 1991), and which also predicts recovery of motor function following right hemisphere stroke (Robertson *et al.* 1999).

Among stroke patients, the presence of unilateral neglect has consistently been found to be a predictor of poor outcome in activities of daily living (ADL). (Denes *et al.* 1982; Wade *et al.* 1983; Henley *et al.* 1985; Fullerton *et al.* 1986; Kinsella & Ford 1980; Smith *et al.* 1983). Indeed the Denes *et al.* study found that the presence of neglect a mean of 53 days post-stroke was the *only* significant predictor of activities of daily living (ADL) functioning: severity of lesion, dysphasia, intellectual capacity all failed to show a significant relationship with ADL. A further Italian study (Gialanella & Mattioli, 1992) suggests, however, that the presence of anosognosia for the neglect may be a crucial variable in explaining why neglect is a poor prognostic factor. Only those neglect subjects who had anosognosia showed poorer prognosis for motor and functional recovery, while those with unilateral neglect in the absence of anosognosia had no worse outcome than other types of neuropsychological disorder.

A number of studies of head injury have shown that pre-accident intelligence and educational level is predictive of much better post-accident outcome (Cullum & Bigler 1986; Brooks & McKinley 1987), and Grafman (1986) found that among Vietnam veterans with brain injuries caused mainly by missile wounds, pre-accident intelligence was the single best predictor of good outcome. The duration of posttraumatic amnesia and of duration and depth of coma are also important predictors of eventual outcome following closed head injury, with the prevailing problems being those of memory, attention, information processing speed, interpersonal and personality changes, irritability and fatigue. Most people suffering a severe closed head injury (posttraumatic amnesia of greater than 24 hours) will be left with permanent problems in some or all of these areas (see Brooks 1989, for a review).

Teuber (1975) studied the effects of traumatic lesions from the Korean war on a large sample of soldiers, comparing tests given 1 week post-injury with those given 20 years post-injury. Roughly 40% showed some recovery of motor deficits, 30% from somatosensory deficits, 40% from visual deficits, and only 20% showed some recovery from their initial dysphasia. Kertesz (1979) asserts, however, that aphasia following closed head injury shows rapid and often complete recovery in contrast to aphasia following stroke, and this difference compared with the Teuber paper is probably because of the penetrating nature of the wounds in many of Teuber's series. Kertesz finds that most recovery in aphasia takes place in the first 3 months, with further, but less recovery taking place in the next 6 months, and with recovery being rare after a further 3 months post-injury.

Memory is another important predictor of outcome following neurological damage. Wilson (1991) found that 5–10 years after rehabilitation, 60% of a group of 43 people with severe memory disorders showed no improvement in their memory function, and that only one third had shown any improvement. The causes of the memory disorders were mainly closed head injury and stroke, though the sample included encephalitis, Korsakoff syndrome and hypoxic patients. The Rivermead Behavioural Memory Test (RBMT) administered at follow-up discriminated almost perfectly between those people who were living independently (defined as in paid employment or full-time education or living alone) and those who were not. This was not true for other memory tests; furthermore, the RBMT scores 5–10 years previously, at the end of rehabilitation, were significantly related to independence status at follow-up.

Is there any evidence that neuropsychological rehabilitation can accelerate recovery of neuropsychological deficits?

A recent well-conducted meta-analytic review of stroke rehabilitation studies which evaluated treatments of motor, cognitive, language and visuoperceptual functions concluded that rehabilitation may improve functional performance in some patients (Ottenbacher & Jannell 1993). A meta-analysis was carried out of 36 trials of stroke rehabilitation aimed at language, visuoperceptual, motor, functional daily activity and general cognitive processes. In truly randomized designs, the effect size did not vary significantly according to whether or not there was blind outcome assessment, whereas in both quasi-experimental and pre-experimental designs, significantly bigger effect sizes were obtained when there was no blind assessment than when the assessment was blind. The analysis concluded that the average patient receiving a program of focused stroke rehabilitation performed better than approximately 65% of patients in comparison groups.

Benedict (1989) reviewed the literature on cognitive rehabilitation programmes for closed head injury, with the main areas that have been covered being attention problems, self-regulation difficulties and memory problems. He concludes that there may be some evidence for improvement in self-regulation and attention skills, though the research has been methodologically limited in the main, and this is not a firm conclusion. He further concludes that the effectiveness of memory rehabilitation has not been consistently demonstrated, though two studies published since his review have yielded more promising results as far as memory rehabilitation is concerned (Ruff *et al.* 1989; Berg *et al.* 1991). The effectiveness of computer-aided cognitive rehabilitation for a variety of neuropsychological disorders has also not been clearly established (Robertson 1990), though computer training aimed at teaching specific skills in amnesia has been shown to be effective (e.g. Glisky 1992).

McGlynn (1990) reviewed the literature on behavioural approaches to neuropsychological rehabilitation, and concluded that 'there is considerable evidence suggesting that behavioural techniques can be successfully applied to a variety of problems following neurological impairment'. These problems included inappropriate social behaviour, attention and motivation, lack of awareness of deficits, memory, language and speech and motor disturbance.

If neuropsychological rehabilitation is to fulfill its promise, then practical treatments will have to be more closely tied to theories of underlying neuropsychological systems impaired by the brain damage. One example of such an attempt is as follows. Joanette & Brouchon (1984) described a 64-year-old woman who suffered a right brain cerebrovascular accident (CVA) and who tended to point to stimuli on her left as if she had seen them on her right. Interestingly, an interaction appeared between the side of space upon which the stimulus appeared and the arm which was used. Only when the right arm was used in response to a left-sided stimulus did the allaesthesia appear. When the other arm was used in response to the same stimulus on the same side, there was no allaesthetic response; performance was reasonably accurate. A subsequent series of cases (Joanette *et al.* 1986) found that it was not only allesthetic problems which revealed such an interaction. In a standard stimulus identification procedure, neglect was less severe when the limb contralateral to the lesion was used to point to the target stimuli than when the limb ipsilateral to the lesion was used.

These findings are in line with the theoretical position of Rizzolatti & Camarda (1987), who propose that spatial attention is based upon a series of circuits largely independent from one another which program motor plans in a spatial framework. Spatial attention is not seen as a supraordinate function controlling whole-brain activity, but as a property intrinsically linked to premotor activity and distributed among a range of centres.

The potentially therapeutic effects of left arm activation were experimentally examined by Robertson & North (1992, 1993). Left hand finger movement was compared with an instruction to visually anchor perception on the left arm during letter cancellation. Only the finger movements significantly reduced neglect. Another comparison was between 'out of sight' finger movements of the left hand in left and right hemispace respectively. Only left hemispace 'blind' finger movements significantly reduced neglect compared with the standard condition. Third, blind left finger movements in left hemispace were compared with passive visual cueing (reading a changing number) and again it was found that only the finger movements reduced neglect. Finally, right finger movements in left hemispace were compared with left finger movements in left hemispace: only the latter reduced neglect. This suggests that the potent effect of moving the hemiplegic side is not simply that of cueing attention to the neglected side, but rather the fact of making movements by the left limb in left hemispace. Robertson & North interpreted the results by reference to the work of Rizzolatti and his colleagues (Rizzolatti & Berti 1990). Rizzolatti and his colleagues suggest that multiple and dissociable spatial frames of reference exist in both humans and animals, and these may be selectively impaired. Rizzolatti has demonstrated in monkeys that space is coded in dissociable ways by different brain centres, and that damage to one centre may result in unilateral neglect for one spatial system but not another. For instance, frontal eye field neurons use visual information to control purposeful eye movements, while inferior area 6 neurons use somatosensory and peripersonal visual information to organize purposeful somatic movements. Lesions in these different areas produce correspondingly different types of spatial deficit. A recent case study demonstrates related dissociations between neglect for peripersonal and locomotor space in humans (Halligan & Marshall 1990).

Rizzolatti proposes the existence of multiple representations of space by these different spatial systems, interacting together to produce a coherent spatial reference system against which purposeful motor movements are calibrated and organized. It is the parallel activity of these different perceptuomotor neural maps which produces the representation of space, and, conversely, it is their breakdown which creates distorted representations. Applying this theory to the data reported by Robertson & North (1992, 1993), the subject may have been suffering neglect with respect to *at least* two independent but nevertheless integrated spatial systems – a 'personal' space related in some way to some somatosensory representation of his body, and a peripersonal or 'reaching' space within which he manifested such deficits as neglecting the left in letter cancellation.

By inducing the subject to make voluntary movements with the left hand in left hemispace, it is possible that the left half of the somatosensory spatial sector was in some way activated or enhanced. Because of the integration of the somatosensory and peripersonal spatial sectors, this in turn produced enhanced activation of the impaired half of peripersonal space. Such is the interpretation which would follow from Riz-zolatti's work. But why did not left hand movements in right hemispace similarly activate the left side of peripersonal space? After all, though left hemispace may not have been activated, the left side of the body was activated. One possibility is that reciprocal activation of more than one corresponding spatial sector of the closely linked neuronal maps in the brain must be activated to overcome the deficit in representing the left side of space. In other words, cueing/recruitment of the hemis-patial system was inadequate on its own. So also for the hemi-corporeal ('personal') system. Only when both were activated simultaneously did some improvement of spatial perception of the left arise, possibly by reciprocal activation across the related neuronal systems (Robertson & Frasca 1992).

This experimental and theoretical analysis led to a series of treatment evaluations (Robertson *et al.* 1992), whose aim was to induce minimal movements of left limbs by using a 'neglect alert device', which emitted random sounds which the patient had to prevent or terminate by pressing a switch with some movement of a left limb. The results of this training were positive and daily ratings of mobility difficulties arising from the neglect showed improvements in line with the onset of treatment. These ratings improved as the training commenced, and patients also showed improvements on standardized tests.

This series of experiments constitutes just one example of the attempt to forge theories of neuropsychological recovery leading to effective rehabilitation which hope-fully in the future will lead to improvements in the neuropsychological outcome following brain damage of various types.

Conclusion

Returning to the three questions posed at the beginning of this chapter, provisional answers to these can be summarized thus:

What are the neuropsychological processes which may be involved in recovery of function following brain damage? A number of discrete neuropsychological processes underlying recovery of function, and these include (a) overcoming dysfunctional com-pensatory mechanisms, (b) overcoming inhibition by functionally linked intact brain regions, (c) compensatory mechanisms and functional adaptation, and (d) moti-vational and emotional changes.

What are some of the courses of recovery following various types of brain damage? There are very variable courses of recovery following neuropsychological damage, and these depend on a number of factors including the complexity and redundancy of neuropsychological processes underlying a particular function, as well as on the degree to which executive and attentional functions are intact in the damaged brain.

Is there any evidence that neuropsychological rehabilitation can accelerate recovery? The evidence in favour of this proposition is scant but promising.

Acknowledgments
I would like to thank Dr Barbara Wilson and Dr Tony Ward for their helpful comments on an earlier draft of this chapter.

References

Beauvois, M. F. (1982). Optic aphasia: a process of interaction between vision and language. *Phil. Trans. R. Soc. Lond.* **B298**, 35–47.

Benedict, R. H. B. (1989). The effectiveness of cognitive rehabilitation remediation strategies for victims of traumatic head injury: a review of the literature. *Clin. Psychol. Rev.* **9**, 605–26.

Berg, I. J., Koning-Haanstra, M. & Deelman, B. G. (1991). Long-term effects of memory rehabilitation: a controlled study. *Neuropsychol. Rehabil.* **1**, 97–112.

Brooks, D. N. (1989). Cognitive deficits. In *Rehabilitation of the Adult and Child with Traumatic Brain Injury*, 2nd edn, eds. M. Rosenthal, M. R. Bond, E. R. Griffith & J. D. Miller, Philadelphia: Davis.

Brooks, D. N. & McKinlay, W. (1987). Return to work within the first seven years of severe head injury. *Brain Inj.* **1**, 5–15.

Butter, C. M., & Kirsch, N. (1992). Combined and separate effects of eye patching and visual stimulation on unilateral neglect following stroke. *Arch. Phys. Med. Rehabil.* **73**, 1133–39.

Cullum, M. & Bigler, E. D. (1986). Late effects of haematoma on brain morphology and memory in closed head injury. *Int. J. Neurosci.* **28**, 279–86.

Denes, F. G., Semenza, C., Stoppa, E. & Lis, A. (1982). Unilateral spatial neglect and recovery from hemiplegia: A follow-up study. *Brain* **105**, 543–52.

Fullerton, J., McSherry, C., & Stout, M. (1986). Albert's test: A neglected test of perceptual neglect. *Lancet*, 430–32.

Gentile, A. M. Green, S., Neiburgs, A., Schmelzer, W. & Stein, D. G. (1978). Disruption and recovery of locomotor and manipulatory behaviour following cortical lesions in rats. *Behav. Biol.* **22**, 417–55.

Gialanella, B. & Mattioli, F. (1992). Anosognosia and extrapersonal neglect as predictors of functional recovery following right hemisphere stroke. *Neuropsychol. Rehabil.* **2**, 169–78.

Glisky, E. L. (1992). Acquisition and transfer of declarative and procedural knowledge by memory-impaired patients: a computer data-entry task. *Neuropsychologia* **30**, 899–910.

Goodale, M. A., Milner, A. D., Jakobson, L. S. & Carey, D. P. (1990). Kinematic analysis of limb movements in neuropsychological research: subtle deficits and recovery of function. *Can. J. Psychol.* **44**, 180–95.

Grafman, J. (1986). The relationship of brain tissue loss volume and lesion location to cognitive deficit. *J. Neurosci.* **6**, 301.

Halligan, P. W. & Marshall, J. C. (1990). Left neglect for near but not far space in man. *Nature* **350**, 498–500.

Henley, S., Pettit, P., Todd-Pokropek, L., & Tupper, J. (1985). What goes home? Predictive factors in stroke recovery. *J. Neurol. Neurosurg. Psychiatry*, **48**, 1–6.

Hier, D. B., Mondlock, J. & Caplan, L. R. (1983). Recovery of behavioural abnormalities after right hemisphere stroke. *Neurology* **33**, 345–50.

Jenkins, W. M., Merzenich, M. M. & Reconzone, G. (1990). Neocortical representational dynamics in adult primates: implications for neuropsychology. *Neuropsychologia* **28**, 573–84.

Joanette, Y. & Brouchon, M. (1984). Visual allesthesia in manual pointing: some evidence for a sensori-motor cerebral organization. *Brain Cognit.* 3, 152–65.

Joanette, Y., Brouchon, M., Gauthier, L. & Samson, M. (1986). Pointing with left versus right hand in left visual field neglect. *Neuropsychologia* 24, 391–6.

Kertesz, A. (1979). *Aphasia and Associated Disorders.* New York: Grune and Stratton.

Kinsella, S. & Ford, B. (1980). Acute recovery patterns in stroke patients. *Med. J. Australia* 2, 660–6.

LeVere, N. D. & LeVere, T. E. (1982). Recovery of function after brain damage: support for the compensation theory of the behavioural deficit. *Physiol. Psychol.* 10, 165–74.

Luria, A. R. (1963). *Restoration of Function after Brain Injury.* Oxford: Pergamon Press.

McGlynn, S. M. (1990). Behavioural approaches to neuropsychological rehabilitation. *Psychol. Bull.* 108, 420–1.

Mayer, E., Brown, V. J., Dunnett, S. B. & Robbins, T. W. (1992). Striatal graft-associated recovery of a lesion-induced performance deficit in the rat requires learning to use the transplant. *Eur. J. Neurosci.* 4, 119–26.

Meienberg, O., Zangmeister, W., Rosenberg, M., Hoyt, W. & Stark, L. (1980). Saccadic eye movement strategies in patients with homonymous hemianopia. *Ann. Neurol.* 9, 537–44.

Merzenich, M. M., Nelson, R. J., Stryker, M. P., Cynader, M. S., Schoppmann, A. & Zook, J. M. (1984). Somatosensory cortical map changes following digit amputation in adult monkeys. *J. Comp. Neurol.* 224, 591–605.

Novack, T. A., Haban, G., Graham, K. & Satterfield, W. T. (1987). Prediction of stroke rehabilitation outcome from psychologic screening. *Arch. Phys. Med. Rehabil.* 68, 729–34.

Ogden, J. A., Mee, E. W. & Henning, M. (1994). A prospective study of psychosocial adaptation following subarachnoid haemorrhage. *Neuropsychol. Rehabil.* 4, 7–30.

Ottenbacher, K. J. & Jannell, M. S. (1993). The results of clinical trials in stroke rehabilitation research. *Arch. Neurol.* 50, 37–44.

Pardo, J. V., Fox, P. T. & Raichle, M. E. (1991). Localization of a human system for sustained attention by positron emission tomography. *Nature* 349, 61–4.

Parsons, O. & Stewart, K. (1966). Effects of supportive versus disinterested interviews on perceptual-motor performance in brain-damaged and neurotic patients. *J. Consult. Psychol.* 30, 260–6.

Pons, R. P., Garraghty, P. E., Ommaya, A. K., Kaas, J. H., Taub, E. & Mishkin, M. (1991). Massive cortical reorganisation after sensory deafferentation in adult macaques. *Science* 252, 1857–60.

Posner, M. I. & Rafal, R. D. (1987). Cognitive theories of attention and the rehabilitation of attentional deficits. In *Neuropsychological Rehabilitation*, ed. M. J. Meier, A. L. Benton & L. Diller. Edinburgh: Churchill Livingstone.

Rizzolatti, G. & Berti, A. (1990). Neglect as neural representation deficit. *Rev. Neurol.* 146, 626–34.

Rizzolatti, G. & Camarda, R. (1987). Neural circuits for spatial attention and unilateral neglect. In *Neurological and Neuropsychological Aspects of Neglect*, ed. M. Jeanerod. Amsterdam: North-Holland.

Robertson, I. (1990). Anomalies in the lateralisation omissions in unilateral left neglect: implications for an attentional theory of neglect. *Neuropsychologia* 27, 157–65.

Robertson, I. & Frasca, R. (1992). Attentional load and visual neglect. *Int. J. Neurosci.* 62, 45–56.

Robertson, I. & North, N. (1992). Spatio-motor cueing in unilateral neglect: the role of hemispace, hand and motor activation. *Neuropsychologia* 30, 553–63.

Robertson, I. H. & North, N. (1993). Active and passive stimulation of left limbs: influence on visual and sensory neglect. *Neuropsychologia* 31, 293–300.

Robertson, I. H. & North, N. T. (1994). One hand is better than two: motor extinction of left hand advantage in unilateral neglect. *Neuropsychologia* **32**, 1–11.

Robertson, I. H., Halligan, P. W., Bergego, C., Homberg, V., Pizzamiglio, L., Weber, E. & Wilson, B. A. (1994). Right neglect following right brain damage? *Cortex* **30**, 199–214.

Robertson, I., North, N. & Geggie, C. (1992). Spatio-motor cueing in unilateral neglect: three single case studies of its therapeutic effectiveness. *J. Neurol. Neurosurg. Psychiatry* **55**, 799–805.

Robertson, I. H., Ridgeway, V., Greenfield, E. & Parr, A. (1997). Motor recovery after stroke depends on intact sustained attention: a two-year follow-up study. *Neuropsychology* **11**, 290–5.

Ruff, R. M., Baser, C. A., Johnston, J., Marshall, L. F., Klauber, S. K., Klauber, M. R. & Minteer, M. (1989). Neuropsychological rehabilitation: an experimental study with head-injured patients. *J. Head Trauma Rehabil.* **4**, 20–36.

Slavin, M.D., Held, J. M., Basso, D. M., Lesensky, S., Curran, E., Gentile, A. M. & Stein, D. G. (1988). Fetal brain tissue transplants and recovery of locomotion following damage to the sensorimotor cortex in rats. In *Transplantation into the Mammalian CNS*, eds. D. M. Gash & J. R. Sladek. New York: Elsevier.

Smith, D. L., Akhtar, A. J. & Garraway, W. M. (1983). Proprioception and spatial neglect after stroke. *Age Ageing* **12**, 63–9.

Sprague, J. M. (1966). Interaction of cortex and superior colliculus in mediation of visually guided behaviour in the cat. *Science* **153**, 1544–7.

Teuber, H. L. (1975). Recovery of function after brain injury in man. In *Outcome of Severe Damage to the Nervous System*. Ciba Foundation Symposium 34. Amsterdam: Elsevier.

Wade, D., Skilbeck, C. & Langton Hewer, R. (1983). Predicting Barthel ADL score at 6 months after acute stroke. *Arch. Phys. Med. Rehab.* **64**, 24–28.

Wilkins, A. J., Shallice, T. & McCarthy, R. (1987). Frontal lesions and sustained attention. *Neuropsychologia* **25**, 359–65.

Williams, D. & Gassell, M. (1962). Visual function in patients with homonymous hemianopia, part 1, the visual fields. *Brain* **85**, 175–250.

Wilson, B. A. (1991). Long-term prognosis of patients with severe memory disorders. *Neuropsychol. Rehabil.* **1**, 117–34.

31 Rehabilitation outcomes in neurological and neurosurgical disease

DERICK T. WADE

Introduction

Rehabilitation is integral to all neurological and neurosurgical management because almost every patient has some alteration in behaviour, function or life style as part of their illness and rehabilitation is concerned with these aspects of illness. Thus almost every clinician is necessarily involved in some rehabilitation, particularly as many patients with neurological or neurosurgical disease are unfortunately left with life-long neurological loss. Specialist rehabilitation might help many of these patients to gain maximum benefit from their surgery or medicine but specialist services are often not available, in the UK at least. Therefore it becomes the responsibility of the initial clinician to be actively involved in the rehabilitation of many of their patients. This is often quite appropriate because it maintains continuity of care and expertise, and it may be essential in the absence of specialized services.

Thus this chapter is aimed primarily at the neurologist and neurosurgeon, not the rehabilitation specialist. The purpose of this chapter is to help clinicians judge the effectiveness of rehabilitation both in research literature and in local practice. It will first explain what the aims of rehabilitation are, because often these are not discussed or recognized. An understanding of the aims is essential if the outcomes from rehabilitation are to be measured. Then the chapter will discuss the processes involved because in practice rehabilitation is often monitored (audited) through measures of process. Third, the chapter discusses some of the processes, and reviews the evidence relevant to intervention where that exists. However, it must be recognized that the quantity and quality of rehabilitation research is limited.

Two major theses are put forward. First, rehabilitation is integral to the successful management of all disabling diseases throughout their course, and cannot be seen in isolation. Furthermore the factors which influence rehabilitation outcome extend well beyond matters under the control of Health Services (whatever Health Care system is in place). Second, although there is little doubt that the process of rehabilitation does work, we do not know which specific interventions are effective. In this chapter most of the evidence put forward relates to stroke, for two reasons: most good specific rehabili-

Table 31.1. *A model of disabling illness*

Level affected	Name given to abnormal state	Comment
Organ or organ system	Pathology	The abnormality is usually in the structure or function of cells. Synonyms include *disease* and *diagnosis*
Organism (whole body)	Impairment	Synonymous with *symptoms and signs*. Independent of environment. Reflects integrated function of body/person
Behaviour: interaction of person with environment	Disability	The 'functional consequences'. Meaningful behaviours altered. Relates to environment. *Manifest as dependence*
Social position: roles fulfilled	Handicap	The social and societal consequences. Relates to *meaning* attributed to observed behaviours

tation research has involved stroke: and the author knows most in that field! However, the principles are likely to be generally applicable.

A model of illness

Rehabilitation needs to work within a model or framework, and it is essential that the framework is agreed and understood before discussing the process. A model of illness derived from the World Health Organization's (WHO) International Classification of Impairments, Disabilities and Handicap (ICIDH) (WHO 1980; Badeley 1993) will be discussed.

Any *illness* (the personal experience of disease) can, using concepts derived from General Systems Theory (Checkland 1981) be considered to have four hierarchical, interconnected levels. At each level emergent properties may arise and abnormalities may occur (Table 31.1). It is important to notice that the names given to each level apply not to the level (system) itself but to the disordered state at that level associated with illness. There are no words specifically referring to normality or the absence of changes associated with illness. Also it is vital to notice that *disability* refers to observed interaction between the patient and the environment (in its widest sense) and that it is manifest and usually measured as dependence, either upon people or upon 'special' equipment. In this model patients with insulin-dependent diabetes may be considered 'disabled' in that they depend upon syringes and injections of insulin which are not part of 'normal' life.

Within this model of illness, rehabilitation is best considered as being synonymous with 'the management of disability'. The overall *aims of rehabilitation* can be defined as:

1. Maximizing the patient's social role functioning (i.e. minimizing handicap)
2. Minimizing the distress felt by the patients (i.e. control of somatic and emotional pain)
3. Minimizing the distress of and stress on carers (the family).

Table 31.2. *Objectives of rehabilitation*

1 To maximize the patient's behavioural repertoire
    Independence in personal activities of daily living
    Independence in domestic and community activities
    The range of independent leisure activities available
    The range of productive (work) skills available
    The normality of social interaction skills, including basic communication

2 To optimize the physical and personal environment for role fulfillment
    Identifying accommodation
    Arranging aids and equipment
    Identifying and supplying personal care needs

3 To help adaptation by patient and family
    Giving information and advice
    Giving emotional support

4 To minimize physical stress of patient and family
    Identifying and supplying personal care needs
    Identifying causes of somatic distress and treating them

It is worth stressing that the *aim of rehabilitation* is not to maximize independence in daily activities (a commonly held assumption). This is often a major *objective*, important in achieving the aims but it should not be the final aim. The usual objectives of rehabilitation are shown in Table 31.2.

The *process of rehabilitation* is a reiterative, educational, problem-solving process which focuses on disability. Like any problem-solving process, it comprises the following stages:

1. *Assessment*: the identification of problems, their causes and prognostic (treatment-determining) factors; the identification of any strengths the patient may have; the collection of other relevant information concerning the environment, including the family; and the determination of the wishes and aspirations of all interested parties
2. *Goal-planning*: the setting of long-term aims, medium-term objectives and short-term targets, in conjunction with the patient and all involved parties
3. *Intervention*, which has two components: *care*, that which is needed simply to maintain the status quo (life and safety); and *treatment*, any action intended to affect the process of change
4. *Reassessment*: evaluation of the intervention, making rehabilitation reiterative, and further goal setting.

It must be stressed that rehabilitation is not synonymous with 'therapy'. Therapy is a term which applies (I think) to 'hands-on' (i.e. person-to-person) treatment, usually practising some skill such as sitting, walking or dressing but extending to counselling and social skill retraining. Instead rehabilitation is a process which may involve many professions and many agencies, and certainly extends to include organizing or supplying suitable housing (for example).

This model of illness and rehabilitation has been put forward in more detail elsewhere (Wade 1990, 1992), and does lead to several insights which can be useful. However, here it will hopefully be accepted as a basis for discussion because this model and definition of rehabilitation leads to some important conclusions relevant to this chapter.

Measuring rehabilitation effectiveness

The model described above will now be used to discuss some aspects of measuring the effectiveness of rehabilitation. Unfortunately the discussion may sound like a series of excuses for poor proof of effectiveness, but it is intended to illustrate some difficulties.

Effectiveness is often, and now increasingly sought through audit which can concentrate upon one or more of three factors (Hopkins 1990): structure (the resources available); process (the organization and use of the resources); and outcome (the final effect) which in audit is not usually tested scientifically against any alternative structure or process. Audit of rehabilitation is not easy to undertake (Wade, 1994).

In terms of structure, rehabilitation is sometimes judged by the number of therapists available, the presence of specific professions (e.g. orthotists), the presence of certain facilities (e.g. hydrotherapy), etc. There is no evidence to link effectiveness of a rehabilitation service with specific quantitative aspects of structure, although (as will be seen later) the organizational structure probably is important. A service may be limited by the absence of some features, but can obtain the input from elsewhere. Therefore aspects of the rehabilitation structure itself do not equate with outcome measured as quality or quantity.

In terms of process, rehabilitation could be judged by the time patients spend 'in therapy'. However rehabilitation is not synonymous with therapy or treatment. Instead it is an approach to problems, a process which happens to include 'therapy' but also includes prescription of drugs, provision of aids and equipment and counselling among other interventions. The essence of the process is the ability to identify, analyse and resolve the problems. This is difficult to measure, but it is worth stressing that fewer experienced (expert) staff are likely to be more effective than a mass of inexpert staff, a point often overlooked by purchasers of health services (and politicians). Much stroke research demonstrates that better outcomes are often associated with less time spent in direct therapy (e.g. Kalra *et al.* 1993; Wade 1993).

Next, rehabilitation might be judged more globally by costing resources used. While this is fair, it needs careful interpretation because disability, the focus of rehabilitation, is manifest and measured primarily in terms of dependence either upon other people or/and upon special features of the environment. The level of dependence in turn determines the amount of care needed. And it is the care needs of patients which dominate resource use by 'disabled people'. Therefore, if rehabilitation is to be subjected to any analysis of cost-effectiveness it is important to remove the cost of care which would have to be met regardless of whether or not 'rehabilitation' is used. Indeed one benefit of rehabilitation should be a reduction in care costs although these might only show up later after rehabilitation.

Measurement of outcome itself is best, but if the aims of rehabilitation given above are accepted then many factors complicate the measurement and evaluation of outcome. There are no agreed measures of handicap; most so-called measures of handicap are focused primarily on disability (Wade 1992). Furthermore, handicap necessarily relates to the circumstances of the individual patient, and there are no normal values for social role attainment. One possible approach is to measure satisfaction with life which may relate to handicap (Vitanen *et al.* 1988; Fugi-Meyer *et al.* 1991). Assessing distress in the patient or relatives is more straightforward using one of many measures such as the General Health Questionnaire (Goldberg & Hillier 1979).

However, rehabilitation, the management of neurological disability, must involve all agencies and not simply health services. The outcome is inevitably affected by factors well outside the control of health services such as the general level of service provision for the disabled, the attitudes of people, employment prospects, availability of suitable housing. Therefore in practice it is very difficult to measure the outcome of rehabilitation, and it is especially difficult because the long-term 'steady-state' might not be reached for many months or years after the rehabilitation input. Furthermore, interpretation of any findings is difficult (except in the context of a randomized controlled trial). There are no 'normal' values for such outcomes as handicap or stress. Many factors such as disease severity, coexisting diseases, patient and family expectations and resources, and cultural and social factors all may affect the outcome.

Thus one must be more pragmatic and instead of judging rehabilitation against its aims, one must judge its effectiveness against the various objectives outlined in Table 31.2. In other words, one may assess outcome at the level of disability accepting that it is a surrogate measure of effectiveness. Assessment could cover a range of activities from the most basic, such as personal Activities of Daily Living (ADL) or gait speed to the more complex such as ability to work or independence in domestic ADL. This approach assumes that role fulfilment is related to independence in various activities which is probably true to a limited extent. In addition one could measure patient adaptation, both satisfaction with their situation and also their experience of pain and emotional distress. These outcomes should be measured at least 3 months and preferably 12 months after intervention has ceased to ensure that outcomes are sustained.

In conclusion it is obviously important to start assessing the effectiveness of rehabilitation by measuring some outcomes, provided the difficulties in interpreting data are recognized. Some suggested crude outcome measures are given in Table 31.3; the single questions are not validated in any way and are purely suggestions.

Determinants of outcome

The pathological diagnosis is a crucial determinant of rehabilitation outcome. Knowledge of diagnosis is vital both to the daily practice of rehabilitation and to the interpre-

Table 31.3. *Outcome after rehabilitation*

Domain	Suggested measures (single question alternative in brackets underneath)
Personal activities of daily living (ADL)	Barthel ADL index (Collin *et al.* 1988) (Do you bath or shower yourself without help?)
Mobility	Rivermead Mobility Index (Collen *et al.* 1991) (Do you walk outdoors more than 15 minutes independently?)
Extended ADL	Nottingham extended ADL index (Nouri & Lincoln 1987) Frenchay Activities Index (Schuling *et al.* 1993) (Have you returned to your previous employment/level of domestic activities?)
Patient emotion	General Health Questionnaire (Goldberg & Hillier 1979) Hospital Anxiety and Depression scale (Zigmond & Snaith 1983) (Are you more depressed or worried?)
Carer stress	General Health Questionnaire (Are you coping with the patient?)
Living situation	Accommodation (compared with before) (Are you living in the same place?)
Overall	Life Satisfaction Questionnaire (Fugi-Meyer *et al.* 1991) (Have you recovered fully?)

tation of any outcome data. Management aims can only be set and plans can only be made in the context of the known or expected future which is primarily determined by the underlying disease. For example, rehabilitation of a 40-year-old man who has minimal disability 3 weeks after a stroke will be quite different from that of a similar man with a known glioma, or motor neuron disease or even with Parkinson's Disease.

Knowledge of the disease is obviously also important when interpreting outcome data. For example a failure to return to work after lumbar discectomy would be unusual but it would be common after a stroke. Of course it must be acknowledged that the pathology does not determine the precise prognosis, but it does determine the prognostic field and also can allow one to identify specific prognostic variables to use when interpreting outcome data.

Age is often assumed to be an important determinant of outcome, but age itself is not very important in determining responsiveness to therapy. It does have an important influence, but only through the many important determinant factors which are associated with age (Wade & Hewer 1986). Many elderly people have concomitant disease which may limit both the speed and extent of recovery. Elderly patients and their families may have lower expectations. Their social role functioning may have been very limited beforehand. Many elderly people have reduced cognitive skills, making learning (which is integral to rehabilitation) slow. However, (old) age itself should not be used to determine access to rehabilitation. Instead the patient's specific state should always be considered. One has to be aware of the factors associated with the patient's age (whatever the age) and seek them out. It is the cognitive impairment, social isolation, heart failure, etc. suffered by that patient which is important, not their age.

The importance of other demographic factors is certain but unquantified. Gender determines, to an extent, the available roles and likely activities undertaken; for example, few men undertake ironing of clothes. Personal finances may determine the resources available to overcome or ameliorate some impairments and disabilities; richer people can afford adapted cars or houses. Housing and social support have a major influence even on simple things like length of stay in hospital (Epstein *et al.* 1988, 1990).

More specific determinants are known for some specific diseases. The presence of urinary incontinence shortly after stroke predicts a worse outcome both in terms of mortality and morbidity (Wade & Hewer 1985). Patients with multiple sclerosis presenting with sensory impairments have a lower likelihood of becoming wheelchair-dependent. Prognosis after head injury is broadly determined by the duration of posttraumatic amnesia. However, in all diseases where prognosis has been studied the predictions are unreliable for individual patients and certainly cannot be used (rationally or fairly) to decide on treatment. They may be useful for studying case-mix.

Therefore, when interpreting data on disability outcome after rehabilitation it is important to take account of the many factors known to influence outcome. The outcome can only be interpreted satisfactorily in the knowledge of the underlying diagnosis; specific measures of disease severity (or prognosis) where known; associated diseases and impairments; and many social factors including the availability of personal resources. All determine outcome.

'Does rehabilitation work?': evidence on effectiveness

Table 31.4 shows a range of studies on rehabilitation which used a controlled design, usually randomized, and a few others. It must be emphasized that many of the studies were very small (under 50 subjects) and therefore could not have drawn any firm conclusions; the reader is strongly recommended to read the original papers. Table 31.4 does not include any of the single-case studies, some of which do provide convincing evidence for specific interventions. Lastly Table 31.4 does not claim to be comprehensive, and both major and minor studies might have been omitted. Nonetheless it does show that many randomized studies have been carried out demonstrating that such studies are possible. Most have been focused on stroke because it is most common and attracts more funds. The available evidence will now be reviewed selectively.

The evidence that rehabilitation works is strongest at the two ends of the spectrum: for individual patients, and for large heterogeneous groups of patients. It is weakest when focusing on specific components of the process. Most studies have taken reduction in dependence to be the measure of success, and none have investigated the effect upon handicap or distress.

A recently published single-case study illustrates that rehabilitation does work for individual patients (Jantra *et al.* 1992), but shows the problem in trying to answer this question. The patient was seen 7 years after a cerebellar stroke, still house-bound by ataxia. Over a 7-week period of assessment with various interventions being tried on an

Table 31.4. *Rehabilitation effectiveness; evidence*

Author(s)	Topic	Method	Conclusion
Reviews and meta-analyses			
Langhorne *et al.* 1993	Stroke rehabilitation	FMA	Organized services improve outcome at less cost
Ottenbacher & Jannell 1993	Stroke rehabilitation	MA	Rehabilitation is associated with better outcome
Wade 1993	Stroke rehabilitation	Review	Organized services improve outcome at less cost
Organization studies			
Stevens *et al.* 1984	Stroke: general hospital v. separate unit rehabilitation	RCT	Separate stroke unit did not affect outcome.
Garraway *et al.* 1980	Stroke: medical ward v. stroke unit rehabilitation	RCT	Stroke unit achieved same outcome for less
Wade *et al.* 1985	Stroke: extra services at home	CT	Extra service did not affect outcome or use of hospital
Indredavik *et al.* 1991	Stroke: general hospital RCT v. stroke unit rehabilitation	RCT	Outcome better in unit: uniform organized system is cost-effective
Kalra *et al.* 1993	Stroke: medical ward v. stroke ward rehabilitation	RCT	Stroke ward more cost-effective
Studies on approach			
Feldman *et al.* 1962	Stroke: 'Medical' v. 'special' rehabilitation	RCT	Patients did as well on disability-orientated medical ward after stroke
Wood-Dauphinee *et al.* 1984	Stroke: team approach on general hospital wards	RCT	Team approach more effective (but study analysis too complex)
Jongbloed *et al.* 1989	Stroke: functional or sensorimotor integrative approach	RCT	Functional approach after stroke as effective as sensorimotor integrative approach
Neistadt (1992)	Head injury: task-specific training	RCT	Task-specific training more effective. Supports functional approach
Young & Forster 1992, 1993	Stroke: domiciliary or day hospital therapy after discharge	RCT	Physiotherapy at home was more effective and cheaper.
Sunderland *et al.* 1992, 1994	Stroke: arm function & acute enhanced therapy after stroke	RCT	Enhanced therapy after stroke increases early recovery of arm function; not sustained
Specific aspects			
Stern *et al.* 1970	Stroke: PNF	RCT	PNF approach did not alter outcome
Taylor *et al.* 1971	Stroke (left hemiplegia): perceptual training	RCT	Additional perceptual training did not help
Inaba & Piorkowski 1972	Post-stroke shoulder pain: ultrasound & exercises	RCT	Ultrasound and range of movement exercises no better than placebo
Inaba *et al.* 1973	Stroke hemiparesis: strength training	RCT	Improving power speeded functional recovery
Meikle *et al.* 1979	Stroke aphasia: speech therapy or volunteers	RCT	No difference found
Weinberg *et al.* 1979	Stroke, right brain damage: scanning training	RCT	Minimal difference in severe neglect
Carter *et al.* 1980	Elderly with cognitive failure: skill remediation	RCT	Specific skills changed, function did not

Table 31.4 (*cont.*)

Author(s)	Topic	Method	Conclusion
Smith *et al.* 1981	Stroke: intensity of therapy after hospital discharge	RCT	More intense therapy after discharge reduced decline
Weinberg *et al.* 1982	Stroke, right brain damage: visual scanning training	RCT	Minor effect only
David *et al.* 1982	Stroke aphasia: speech therapy or volunteers?	RCT	Special therapy as effective as volunteers. Assessment helped recovery
Lincoln *et al.* 1982	Stroke aphasia: operant training	RBD	Operant training no more effective than standard therapy
Logigian *et al.* 1983	Stroke hemiparesis: facilitation approach	RCT	Facilitation (Bobath or PNF) no more effective than functional approach
Carter *et al.* 1983	Stroke: cognitive skill training	RCT	Trained skills improved, but no generalization
Lincoln & Pickersgill 1984	Stroke aphasia: PIOT	RCD	PIOT no more effective
Lincoln *et al.* 1984	Stroke aphasia: speech therapy service delivered	RCT	Service delivered did not affect outcome
Lincoln *et al.* 1985	Stroke neglect: perceptual training	RCT	No significant differences. Small groups
Sivenius *et al.* 1985	Stroke: intensity of acute therapy	RCT	More intense therapy might speed recovery
Wertz *et al.* 1986	Stroke aphasia: speech therapy v. volunteers v. nil	RCT	Any therapy helped; no treatment group worse
Hartmann & Landau 1987	Stroke aphasia: speech therapy or counselling	RCT	No difference: linguistic exercises may not help
Evans *et al.* 1988	Stroke: counselling and/or education	RCT	Counselling & education leads to better adjustment
Jobst 1989	Ataxia (any cause): biofeedback training	RCT?	Training on balance platform more effective than physical training
Brindley *et al.* 1989	Stroke aphasia: intense therapy	SCSD	Intense therapy late after stroke helps some patients
Towle *et al.* 1989	Stroke: social work intervention after discharge	RCT	Social work input did not affect outcome
Robertson *et al.* 1990	Neglect: computerized training	RCT	No effect detected
Ruff & Nieman 1990	Head injury: cognitive remediation	RCT	After 8 weeks, no difference from day treatment
Jongbloed & Morgan 1991	Stroke: occupational therapy & leisure	RCT	No benefit found
Mackenzie 1991	Stroke aphasia: intense therapy	SCSD	Intense therapy leads to definite long-lasting improvement
Friedland & McColl 1992	Stroke: social support intervention	RCT	No effect detected
Wade *et al.* 1992	Stroke immobility: physiotherapy late after stroke	RCT	Physiotherapy given at home late after stroke reduces decline in mobility; not sustained
Yekutiel & Guttman 1993	Stroke: sensory retraining	CT	Impairment reduced: disability not assessed
Faghri *et al.* 1994	Stroke shoulder subluxation: functional electrical stimulation (FES)	RCT	FES 6 hours daily reduced shoulder subluxation after stroke. Clinical benefit unclear

CT, controlled trial; FES, functional electrical stimulation; FMA, formal meta-analysis; MA, meta-analysis (other); PNF, proprioceptive neuromuscular facilitation; PIOT, programmed instruction and operant training; RCT, randomized controlled trial; RBD, randomized block design; RCD, randomized cross-over design; SCSD, single-case study design.

empirical basis, a method of walking was developed which gave the patient great freedom, reducing the need for care. The final technique used is not the subject of any randomized controlled trial and might suit few other individuals but clearly benefited this patient (and society).

Second, an uncontrolled study many years ago investigated the effect of rehabilitation on 33 patients, and the results suggested that the process of rehabilitation was able to increase independence (Lehmann *et al.* 1975). Thirty-three patients admitted more than 6 months after their stroke (i.e. after any 'spontaneous' recovery was complete) were studied. At discharge and at subsequent follow-up there were increases in independence in continence, transfers, walking and dressing. Furthermore there was a significant cost-benefit advantage from rehabilitation, as admission to the rehabilitation unit enabled some patients to move from state-supported institutional care to unsupported community care. A more recent study of similar design came to the same conclusion (Dam *et al.* 1993).

At the other end of the spectrum, several more-or-less formal overview analyses of stroke rehabilitation have been conducted (Langhorne *et al.* 1993; Ottenbacher & Jannell 1993; Wade 1993). All concluded that well-organized rehabilitation services (which all included physical therapy) lead to a better outcome (faster recovery of independence and/or a greater level of independence) at less cost and often with less indirect input. Furthermore, a formal meta-analysis has shown that mortality after stroke is also reduced by 18%, making organized rehabilitation the only intervention known to reduce the stroke fatality rate (Langhorne *et al.* 1993).

It is important to note that the studies reviewed have all involved therapists from all professions; that all the staff were experienced and interested; and that no single therapeutic approach was common to the studies. Therefore it is unlikely that a particular method of treatment is needed. The important components appear to be organizational: the patients should have easy access to a wide range of experts in a coordinated service. Therefore one can conclude that being seen by a specialist team of rehabilitation experts does increase independence more than occurs 'naturally', and that this may occur through solving the individual problems of each patient in individual ways.

Specific components

It is much more difficult to determine which components of the service are effective and (more importantly) which are totally ineffective or even counterproductive. Nonetheless relevant evidence for each part will be reviewed, but larger texts should be consulted for more detail (e.g. Greenwood *et al.* 1993).

First, simply being involved with a rehabilitation service and being assessed might itself improve outcome. The only evidence was revealed incidentally in a randomized trial of speech therapy; the process of assessment of aphasia appeared to improve communication (David *et al.* 1982). Further research into all aspects of assessment is urgently required.

Goal planning has also not been subject to much investigation, and indeed the process of goal planning in rehabilitation has only recently been explored (McGrath & Davis 1992). One study investigated the effect of introducing discharge planning on length of stay in hospital and found no benefit (Cable & Mayers, 1983) which is ironic given the increased emphasis on case management being introduced in the UK at least. Again research into all aspects of goal planning and case management is urgently needed.

There is minimal research into the most cost-effective way of delivering care. Issues which need consideration include the location of the patient (home, hospital, nursing home, etc.), the utility of, and indications for, different pieces of equipment (hoists, pressure-relieving matresses, gastrostomy tubes, etc.), the skill-mix of staff needed (qualified or unqualified nurses, relatives, etc.).

Further considerations of great practical importance relate to the funding of care, and at present clinical considerations are often overruled by budgetary considerations. For example, in the UK one is supposed to distinguish between 'social' and 'medical' care (an impossible distinction) as well as deciding who is reponsible for funding what piece of equipment and deciding who is 'allowed' to undertake what aspects of care. Studies into the most efficient ways of allocating resources and responsibilities are urgently needed.

Next, in the management of any illness, treatment interventions may be directed at any level. Pathology-based treatment (surgical or pharmacological) has been discussed in the rest of this book, although in many diseases there is at present little scope for reducing cerebral damage.

Impairment

Interventions may be directed at impairment. Examples of impairment-level interventions include anti-spastic agents, analgesia for pain, foot-drop splints, tendon transfers, drugs to control urinary urgency, etc. Good evidence on the effectiveness of and indications for most of these interventions is limited or non-existent.

Spasticity is one common impairment for which there are many interventions available: botulinum toxin injection, drugs (e.g. baclofen), local destructive nerve injections, tenotomies, ice, splints, 'correct' handling, etc. There is little doubt that drugs such as baclofen reduce the hypersensitivity of the stretch reflex (McLellan 1977) but there is no good evidence that the routine use of anti-spastic agents after stroke improves outcome (Katrak et al. 1992).

Botulinum toxin certainly reduces muscle strength, and tenotomies and nerve destruction certainly reduce muscle tightness but none of this necessarily supports the use of these interventions 'for spasticity'. Therefore the use of anti-spastic agents in selected patients may be effective in reducing dependence or distress, or in easing care, but specific evidence on who should be treated and how is absent. At present one should not treat the impairment of spasticity but should focus on resolving the secondary problem which might be pain, difficulty in cleaning a hand, poor balance when walking, spasms, or frustration because of dependence. Often spasticity itself is not the major cause or 'real' problem but if it is then one or more of these treatments can be tried on an empirical basis.

Disability

The range of interventions aimed at disability is vast and includes, for example, providing and teaching to use a wheelchair, teaching to dress one-handed, teaching relatives how to transfer, providing stair-rails and social skills retraining. The evidence relating to most specific actions is sparse.

It is probable that some interventions such as giving a wheelchair to someone who cannot walk are so obvious that research is considered unnecessary. The provision of a wheelchair after stroke is an example which nonetheless highlights some interesting issues. Some therapists believe that a wheelchair should be provided late, only when all else fails (because a wheelchair reduces motivation to walk). Others give wheelchairs early (because it increases freedom and self-esteem). This policy division could be investigated. Moreover, it highlights the issue of considering the aim of rehabilitation. Providing a wheelchair will not improve walking, but it might increase mobility, reduce distress and increase role fulfilment. Depending upon the outcome measure used it might be deleterious or very useful.

Even when simply considering therapists and therapy, there are in fact many interventions undertaken by therapists which are not considered (by some) to be part of therapy: giving advice, teaching carers how to care, referring on to other agencies, liaising with others, etc. Furthermore therapists are necessarily involved in assessment; they will undertake their own goal planning and should be involved in team goal-planning which is crucial to successful rehabilitation; they may need to give care (e.g. if someone needs the toilet while at speech therapy); they will give treatment; and they will reassess. All of these processes occur throughout any involvement, and 'therapy' cannot be seen in isolation. Confirming this, the evidence from rehabilitation centres shows that 'hands-on therapy' constitutes a small proportion of treatment and, equally important, there is good evidence that patients spend little time in direct contact with therapists. One study in a relatively well-staffed stroke unit in Bristol found that patients spent about 3%–4% of waking time in therapy (Tinson 1989) and the commonest activity for many patients was and remained looking into space vacantly. Despite this low direct input most patients improved.

The use of speech therapists seems to arouse most controversy. Their functions include assessment of all aspects of communication and, in conjunction with others, assessment of swallowing, giving advice, identifying and teaching the use of communication aids, and trying to maximize communication. The evidence that the therapy given by generic speech therapy services available in the UK has any effect on language function is weak (Lincoln *et al.* 1984). This may be because the amount is too little, and there is evidence that a high input can improve communication in a few selected patients. There is evidence that assessment does lead to improved communication (David *et al.* 1982), though this has not been proven in randomized controlled trials.

Physical therapy covers both physiotherapy and occupational therapy. There is evidence that intervention of a physiotherapist late after stroke can reduce the decline in mobility seen (Wade *et al.* 1992). Other research has shown that active intervention in the early stages can improve recovery of arm function in some patients (Sunderland *et al.* 1992), although the difference is small and not sustained. 'Disability-centred' interventions can be directed not only at the patient but also at the environment. This ranges from the obvious, such as providing a wheelchair or walking stick to the provision of very specific and/or complex adaptations including new or adapted housing, communication aids and special cars. Further, one may need to provide a specific social environment (e.g. sheltered housing, group homes) either to support the patient or to give opportunities for social interaction. After head injury, for example, a few patients are most appropriately placed in an institution which provides a structured day and social contacts.

Orthoses are pieces of equipment which minimize impairment in some way. In neurological rehabilitation the best examples are ankle-foot orthoses (AFOs, foot-drop splints), calipers and various arm orthoses. There is little research into effectiveness, but AFOs have been assessed after stroke and in cerebral palsy and shown to improve mobility (Lehman *et al.* 1987). Most research is into the technology of orthoses.

Lastly, one important issue in rehabilitation is that of generalization. This term covers several specific issues. First, improvements seen in one setting may not necessarily translate to other settings; in fact they rarely do. In principle treatment in the home setting is likely to be most effective, and recent research suggests that treatment given at home is more cost-effective (Young & Forster 1993). Second, improvements in one skill (impairment) do not necessarily lead to reduced dependence; in other words treatments successful at reducing impairment may not necessarily have any effect whatsoever on behaviour (disability). Third, the results of one study may not generally apply to other settings.

Handicap

Interventions aimed at the level of handicap are generally in the power of politicians, because they involve such matters as providing income support, supported employment, day centres, good public transport and sympathetic public attitudes. Many of these interventions are undertaken by non-therapists (as usually considered).

Conclusions

If it is accepted that rehabilitation is a problem-solving process, then its success must be judged by how well the problems are resolved. Each patient's problem profile is unique. The limited evidence available suggests that rehabilitation given in a well-organized way by experienced staff is successful at resolving problems to reduce dependence. Its success at reducing handicap is unknown. However, if rehabilitation is simply equated with the specific interventions given, then there is much less evidence to support any particular treatment.

References

Badley, E. M. (1993). An introduction to the concepts and classifications of the international classification of impairments, disabilities and handicaps. *Disabil. Rehabil.* **15**, 161–78.

Cable, P. R. & Mayers, S. P. (1983). Discharge planning effect on length of hospital stay. *Arch. Phys. Med. Rehabil.* **64**, 57–60.

Carter, L., Caruso, J., Languirand, M. & Berard, M. (1980). Cognitive skill remediation in stroke and non-stroke elderly. *Clin. Neuropsychol.* **2**, 109–13.

Carter, L., Howard, B. & O'Neill, W. (1983). Effectiveness of cognitive skill retraining in acute stroke patients. *Am. J. Occup. Ther.* **37**, 320–6.

Checkland, P. (1981). *Systems Thinking, Systems Practice.* Chichester: Wiley.

Collen, F. M., Wade, D. T., Robb, G. F. & Bradshaw, C. M. (1991). The Rivermead Mobility Index: a further development of the Rivermead Motor Assessment. *Int. Disabil. Stud.* **13**, 5–54.

Collin, C., Wade, D. T., Davis, S. & Horne, V. (1988). The Barthel ADL index: a reliability study. *Int. Disabil. Stud.* **10**, 61–3.

Dam, M., Tonin, P., Casson, S., Ermani, M., Pizzolato, G., Iaia, V. & Battistin, L. (1993). The effects of long-term rehabilitation therapy on poststroke hemiplegic patients. *Stroke* **24**, 1186–91.

David, R., Enderby, P. & Bainton, D. (1982). Treatment of acquired aphasia: speech therapists and volunteers compared. *J. Neurol. Neurosurg. Psychiatry* **45**, 957–61.

Epstein, A. M. *et al.* (1988). The association of patients' socioeconomic characteristics with the length of hospital stay and hospital charges within disagnosis-related groups. *N. Engl. J. Med.* **318**, 1579–85.

Epstein, A. M., Stern, R. S. & Weissman, J. S. (1990). Do the poor cost more? A multihospital study of patients' socioeconomic status and use of hospital resources. *N. Engl. J. Med.* **322**, 1122–8.

Evans, R. L., Matlock, A.-L., Bishop, D. S., Strahan, S. & Pederson, C. (1988). Family intervention after stroke: does counselling or education help? *Stroke* **19**, 1243–9.

Feldman, D. J., Lee, P. R., Unterecker, J., Lloyd, K., Rusk, A. & Toole, A. (1962). A comparison of functionally orientated medical care and formal rehabilitation in the management of patients with hemiplegia due to cerebrovascular disease. *J. Chron. Dis.* **15**, 297–310.

Friedland, J. F. & McColl, M. A. (1992). Social support intervention after stroke: results of a randomised trial. *Arch. Phys. Med. Rehabil.* **73**, 573–81.

Fugl-Meyer, A. R., Branholm, I. & Fugl-Meyer, K. S. (1991). Happiness and domain-specific life satisfaction in adult Northern Swedes. *Clin. Rehabil.* **5**, 25–33.

Garraway, W. M., Akhtar, A. J., Hockey, L. & Prescott, R. J. (1980). Management of acute stroke in the elderly: follow-up of a controlled trial. *BMJ* **281**, 827–9.

Goldberg, D. P. & Hillier, V. F. (1979). A scaled version of the General Health Questionnaire. *Psychol. Med.* **9**, 139–45.

Greenwood, R., Barnes, M. P., McMillan, T. M. & Ward, C. D. (eds.) (1993). *Neurological Rehabilitation.* Edinburgh: Churchill Livingstone.

Hartman, J. & Landau, W. M. (1987). Comparison of formal language therapy with supportive counselling for aphasia due to vascular accident. *Arch. Neurol.* **44**, 646–9.

Hopkins, A. (1990). *Measuring the Quality of Medical Care*. London: Royal College of Physicians.

Inaba, M. K. & Piorkowski, M. (1972). Ultrasound in treatment of painful shoulders in patients with hemiplegia. *Phys. Ther.* **52**, 737–41.

Inaba, M. K., Edberg, E., Montgomery, J. & Gillis, K. (1973). Effectiveness of functional training, active exercise and resistive exercise for patients with hemiplegia. *Phys. Ther.* **53**, 28–35.

Indredavik, B., Bakke, F., Solberg, R., Rosketh, R., Haahein, L. L. & Holme, I. (1991). Benefit of a stroke unit: a randomised controlled trial. *Stroke* **22**, 1026–31.

Jantra, P., Monga, T. K., Press, J. M. & Gervais, B. J. (1992). Management of apraxic gait in a stroke patient. *Arch. Phys. Med. Rehabil.* **73**, 95–7.

Jongbloed, L. & Morgan, D. (1991). An investigation of involvement in leisure activities after a stroke. *Am. J. Occup. Ther.* **45**, 420–7.

Kalra, L., Dale, P. & Crome, P. (1993). Improving stroke rehabilitation. A controlled study. *Stroke* **24**, 1462–7.

Katrak, P. H., Cole, A. M. D., Poulos, C. J. & McCauley, J. C. K. (1992). Objective assessment of spasticity, strength and function with early exhibition of dantrolene sodium after cerebrovascular accident: a randomised double-blind study. *Arch. Phys. Med. Rehabil.* **73**, 4–9.

Langhorne, P., Williams, B. O., Gilchrist, W. & Howie, K. (1993). Do stroke units save lives? *Lancet* **342**, 395–8.

Lehmann, J. F., DeLateur, B. J., Fowler, R. S. *et al.* (1975). Stroke: does rehabilitation affect outcome? *Arch. Phys. Med. Rehabil.* **56**, 375–82.

Lehmann, J. F., Condon, S. M., Price, R. & DeLateur, B. J. (1987). Gait abnormalities in hemiplegia: their correction by angle-foot orthoses. *Arch. Phys. Med. Rehabil.* **68**, 763–71.

Lincoln, N. B. & Pickersgill, M. J. (1984). The effectiveness of programmed instruction with operant training in the language rehabilitation of severely aphasic patients. *Behav. Psychother.* **12**, 237–48.

Lincoln, N. B., Pickersgill, M. J., Hankey, A. I. & Hilton, C. R. (1982). An evaluation of operant training and speech therapy in the language rehabilitation of moderate aphasics. *Behav. Psychother.* **10**, 162–78.

Lincoln, N. B., McGuirk, E., Mulley, G. P., Lendrem, W., Jones, A. C. & Mitchell, J. R. A. (1984). Effectiveness of speech therapy for aphasic stroke patients: a randomised controlled trial. *Lancet* **1**, 1197–200.

Lincoln, N. B., Whiting, S. E., Cockburn, J. & Bhavnani, G. (1985). An evaluation of perceptual retraining. *Int. Rehabil. Med.* **7**, 99–101.

Logigian, M. K., Samuels, M. A. & Falconer, J. (1983). Clinical exercise trial for stroke patients. *Arch. Phys. Med. Rehabil.* **67**, 88–91.

McGrath, J. R. & Davis, A. M. (1992). Rehabilitation: where are we going and how do we get there? *Clin. Rehabil.* **6**, 225–35.

Mackenzie, C. (1991). An aphasia group efficacy study. *Br. J. Disord. Commun.* **26**, 275–91.

McLellan, D. L. (1977). Co-contraction and stretch reflexes in spasticity during treatment with baclofen. *J. Neurol. Neurosurg. Psychiatry* **40**, 30–8.

Neistadt, M. E. (1992). Occupational therapy treatments for constructional deficits. *Am. J. Occup. Ther.* **46**, 141–8.

Nouri, F. M. & Lincoln, N. B. (1987). An extended activities of daily living scale for stroke patients. *Clin. Rehabil.* **1**, 301–5.

Ottenbacher, K. J. & Jannell, S. (1993). The results of clinical trials in stroke rehabilitation research. *Arch. Neurol.* **50**, 37–44.

Robertson, I., Gray, J., Pentland, B. & Waite, L. (1990). A randomised controlled trial of computer-based cognitive rehabilitation for unilateral left visual neglect. *Arch. Phys. Med. Rehabil.* **71**, 663–8.

Ruff, R. M. & Niemann, H. (1990). Cognitive rehabilitation versus day treatment in head-injured adults: is there an impact on emotional and psychosocial adjustment? *Brain Inj.* **4**, 339–47.

Schuling, J., de Haan, R., Limburg, M. & Groenier, K. H. (1993). The Frenchay Activities Index. Assessment of functional status in stroke patients. *Stroke* **24**, 1173–7.

Sivenius, J., Pyorala, K., Heinonen, O. P., Salonen, J. T. & Riekkinen, P. (1985). The significance of intensity of rehabilitation of stroke – a controlled trial. *Stroke* **16**, 928–31.

Smith, D. S., Goldenberg, E., Ashburn, A., Kinsella, G., Sheikh, K., Brennan, P. J., Meade, T. W., Zutshi, D. W., Perry, J. D. & Reeback, J. S. (1981). Remedial therapy after stroke: a randomised controlled trial. *BMJ* **282**, 517–20.

Stern, P. H., McDowell, F., Miller, J. M. & Robinson, M. (1970). Effects of facilitation exercise techniques in stroke rehabilitation. *Arch. Phys. Med. Rehabil.* **51**, 526–31.

Stevens, R. S., Ambler, N. R. & Warren, M. D. (1984). A randomised controlled trial of a stroke rehabilitation ward. *Age Ageing* **13**, 65–75.

Sunderland, A., Tinson, D. J., Bradley, E. L., Fletcher, D., Langton-Hewer, R. & Wade, D. T. (1992). Enhanced physical therapy improves recovery of arm function after stroke: a randomised controlled trial. *J. Neurol. Neurosurg. Psychiatry* **55**, 530–5.

Sunderland, A., Tinson, D. J., Bradley, E. L., Fletcher, D., Langton-Hewer, R. & Wade, D. T. (1994). Enhanced physical therapy improves recovery of arm function after stroke: follow-up to a randomised controlled trial. *J. Neurol. Neurosurg. Psychiatry* **57**.

Tinson, D. J. (1989). How do stroke patients spend their day: an observational study of the treatment regime offered to patients in hospital with movement disorders following stroke. *Int. Disabil. Stud.* **11**, 45–9.

Towle, D., Lincoln, N. B. & Mayfield, L. M. (1989). Service provision and functional independence in depressed stroke patients and the effect of social work intervention on these. *J. Neurol. Neurosurg. Psychiatry* **52**, 519–22.

Viitanen, M., Fugl-Meyer, K. S., Bernspang, B. & Fugl-Meyer, A. R. (1988). Life satisfaction in long-term survivors after stroke. *Scand. J. Rehabil. Med.* **20**, 17–24.

Wade, D. T. (1990). Neurological rehabilitation. In *Recent Advances in Clinical Neurology* **6**, ed. C. Kennard, pp. 133–56. Edinburgh: Churchill Livingstone.

Wade, D. T. (1992). *Measurement in Neurological Rehabilitation.* Oxford: Oxford University Press.

Wade, D. T. (1993). Is stroke rehabilitation worthwhile? *Curr. Opin. Neurol. Neurosurg.* **6**, 78–82.

Wade, D. T. (1994). Audit in neurological rehabilitation. In *Neurological Rehabilitation*, ed. L. S. Ellis. Oxford: Blackwell Scientific.

Wade, D. T. & Hewer, R. L. (1985). Outlook after an acute stroke: urinary incontinence and loss of consciousness compared in 532 patients. *Q. J. Med.* **221**, 601–8.

Wade, D. T. & Hewer, R. L. (1986). Stroke: associations with age, sex, and side of weakness. *Arch. Phys. Med. Rehabil.* **67**, 540–5.

Wade, D. T., Langton-Hewer, R., Skilbeck, C. E., Bainton, D. & Burns-Cox, C. (1985). Controlled trial of home care service for acute stroke patients. *Lancet* **1**, 323–6.

Wade, D. T., Collen, F. M., Robb, G. F. & Warlow, C. P. (1992). Physiotherapy intervention after stroke and mobility. *BMJ* **304**, 609–13.

Weinberg, M., Diller, L., Gordon, W. *et al.* (1979). Training sensory awareness and spatial organisation in people with right brain damage. *Arch. Phys. Med. Rehabil.* **60**, 491–6.

Weinberg, M., Piasetsky, E., Diller, L. & Gordon, W. (1982). Treating perceptual organisation deficits in non-neglecting RBD stroke patients. *J. Clin. Neuropsychol.* **4**, 59–75.

Wood-Dauphinee, S., Shapiro, S., Bass, E., Fletcher, C., Georges, P., Hensby, V. & Mendelsohn, B. (1984). A randomised trial of team care following stroke. *Stroke* **15**, 864–72.

World Health Organization (1980). International Classification of Impairments, Disabilities and Handicaps. Geneva: WHO.

Yekutiel, M. & Guttman, E. (1993). A controlled trial of the retraining of the sensory function of the hand in stroke patients. *J. Neurol. Neurosurg. Psychiatry* **56**, 241–4.

Young, J. B. & Forster, A. (1992). The Bradford community stroke trial: results at six months. *BMJ* **304**, 1085–9.

Young, J. B. & Forster, A. (1993). Day hospital and home physiotherapy for stroke patients: a comparative cost-effectiveness study. *J. R. Coll. Phys.* **27**, 252–7.

Zigmond, A. & Snaith, P. (1983). The Hospital Anxiety and Depression Scale. *Acta Psychiatr. Scand.* **67**, 361–70.

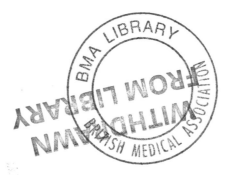